SKELETAL TRAUMA IN CHILDREN

VOLUME THREE

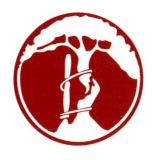

SKELETAL TRAUMA IN CHILDREN

VOLUME THREE

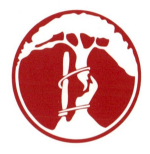

Neil E. Green, M.D.
Professor and Vice Chairman
Department of Orthopaedic Surgery
Head of Pediatric Orthopaedics
Vanderbilt University School of Medicine
Nashville, Tennessee

Marc F. Swiontkowski, M.D.
Professor and Vice Chairman
University of Washington
Department of Orthopaedics
Chief of Orthopaedic Traumatology
Harborview Medical Center
University of Washington
Seattle, Washington

W.B. SAUNDERS COMPANY
A Division of Harcourt Brace & Company
Philadelphia • London • Toronto • Montreal • Sydney • Tokyo

W.B. SAUNDERS COMPANY
A Division of Harcourt Brace & Company

The Curtis Center
Independence Square West
Philadelphia, Pennsylvania 19106

Library of Congress Cataloging-in-Publication Data

Skeletal trauma in children / [edited by] Neil E. Green, Marc F. Swiontkowski.
    p. cm.
ISBN 0-7216-5129-1
    1. Fractures in children.   2. Dislocation in children.
[DNLM: 1. Dislocations—in infancy & childhood.   2. Fractures—in infancy & childhood.   WE 175 S6273]
RD101.S55   1993
617.1′5′083—dc20
DNLM/DLC   92-11622

SKELETAL TRAUMA IN CHILDREN   ISBN 0-7216-5129-1

Copyright © 1994 by W.B. Saunders Company

All rights reserved. No part of this publication may be reproduced or transmitted in any form or by any means, electronic or mechanical, including photocopy, recording, or any information storage and retrieval system, without permission in writing from the publisher.

Printed in the United States of America

Last digit is the print number: 9   8   7   6   5   4   3   2   1

We dedicate this book to our teachers and our families for their patience, support, sacrifices, and education throughout our academic life.

    Lesley Nield Green

        Bruce Arthur Green

        Lisa Beth Green

    Beth Ellen Swiontkowski

        Timothy Ian Swiontkowski

        Jeffrey Neal Swiontkowski

        Ellen Rose Swiontkowski

Contributors

Peter F. Armstrong, M.D., F.R.C.S.C., F.A.C.S., F.A.A.P.
Professor of Orthopedic Surgery, University of Utah; Chief of Staff, Shriners Hospitals for Crippled Children, Salt Lake City, Utah
Pediatric Fractures of the Forearm, Wrist, and Hand

Fred Behrens, M.D.
Department of Orthopaedics, University of Medicine and Dentistry of New Jersey, New Jersey Medical School, Newark, New Jersey
Fractures of the Tibia and Fibula

S. Terry Canale, M.D.
Professor, Campbell Clinic–University of Tennessee Department of Orthopaedic Surgery; Chief of Pediatric Orthopaedics, LeBonheur Children's Medical Center; Active Staff, Baptist Memorial Hospital; Consulting Staff, Regional Medical Center, Memphis, Tennessee
Physeal Injuries

Howard M. Clarke, M.D., Ph.D., F.R.C.S.C., F.A.C.S., F.A.A.P.
Assistant Professor of Surgery, Division of Plastic Surgery, University of Toronto; Active Staff Surgeon, The Hospital for Sick Children, Toronto, Ontario
Pediatric Fractures of the Forearm, Wrist, and Hand

Alvin H. Crawford, M.D., F.A.C.S.
Professor of Pediatrics and Orthopaedic Surgery, University of Cincinnati College of Medicine; Director of Orthopaedic Surgery, Children's Hospital Medical Center, Cincinnati, Ohio
Fractures and Dislocations of the Foot and Ankle

Neil E. Green, M.D.
Professor and Vice Chairman, Department of Orthopaedic Surgery; Head of Pediatric Orthopaedics, Vanderbilt University School of Medicine, Nashville, Tennessee
Fractures and Dislocations Above the Elbow; Child Abuse

Robert N. Hensinger, M.D.
Professor, Department of Surgery, University of Michigan Medical School; Chief, Pediatric Orthopaedics, Mott Children's Hospital, Ann Arbor, Michigan
Complications of Fractures in Children

Eric T. Jones, M.D., Ph.D.
Clinical Professor of Orthopedic Surgery, West Virginia University Health Science Center; West Virginia University Hospitals, Monongalia General Hospital, Mountain View Rehabilitation Hospital, Morgantown, West Virginia
Skeletal Growth and Development as Related to Trauma

V. Elaine Joughin, M.D., F.R.C.S.C.
Clinical Professor of Surgery, Division of Orthopaedic Surgery, University of Calgary; Alberta Children's Hospital, Calgary, Alberta
Pediatric Fractures of the Forearm, Wrist, and Hand

William W. Robertson, Jr., M.D.
Professor of Orthopaedic Surgery, Professor of Pediatrics, George Washington University School of Medicine; Chairman, Department of Pediatric Orthopaedic Surgery, Children's National Medical Center, Washington, D.C.
Pathologic Fractures and Tumors

M. L. Chip Routt, Jr., M.D.
Assistant Professor of Orthopedic Surgery, University of Washington; Harborview Medical Center, Seattle, Washington
Fractures of the Femoral Shaft

J. Andy Sullivan, M.D.
Professor and Chair, Department of Orthopedic Surgery and Rehabilitation, University of Oklahoma College of Medicine; Children's Hospital of Oklahoma, Oklahoma Medical Center, Oklahoma University Health Sciences Center, Oklahoma City, Oklahoma
Fractures of the Spine in Children

Marc F. Swiontkowski, M.D.
Professor and Vice Chairman, University of Washington Department of Orthopaedics; Chief of Orthopaedic Traumatology, Harborview Medical Center, Seattle, Washington
Fractures and Dislocations About the Hip and Pelvis

George H. Thompson, M.D.
Professor of Orthopaedic Surgery and Pediatrics, Case Western Reserve University; Director, Pediatric Orthopaedics, Rainbow Babies and Children's Hospital, Cleveland, Ohio
The Multiply Injured Child; Fractures of the Tibia and Fibula

Vernon Tolo, M.D.
John C. Wilson, Jr., Professor of Orthopaedics, University of Southern California School of Medicine; Head, Division of Orthopaedics, Children's Hospital, Los Angeles, California
Fractures and Dislocations Around the Knee

Lawrence X. Webb, M.D., F.A.C.S.
Associate Professer of Surgical Sciences, Department of Orthopaedics, and Chief of Orthopaedic Traumatology, Wake Forest University Medical Center, Winston-Salem, North Carolina
Fractures and Dislocations About the Shoulder

John H. Wilber, M.D.
Assistant Professor of Orthopaedic Surgery, Case Western Reserve University; Director of Orthopaedic Trauma, University Hospital of Cleveland, Cleveland, Ohio
The Multiply Injured Child

Foreword

For many years the gravity of and potential for lifelong complications from skeletal trauma in children were not fully appreciated. Children's fractures were, for the most part, treated in the same way as their adult counterparts, or it was assumed that all fractures in children would heal with simple conservative treatment. Only a few "fractures of necessity" were considered for operative treatment. With a better understanding of the structure and function of the physes and the effects of trauma on these growth mechanisms, a tremendous body of literature concerning skeletal trauma in children has been developed. Numerous procedures and devices have been proposed for treating various injuries, with equally varied results.

It is because of this proliferation of information and innovation that concise, well-founded guidelines for treatment are especially important. To sort through the myriad possibilities for treatment of skeletal trauma in a child and to choose the best method for that patient requires a thorough understanding of the special anatomy and physiology of children as well as a clear comprehension of the results and complications that can be expected from each method. This text presents a foundation of basic information about skeletal growth and physeal function that allows a clear progression through the discussions of treatment of specific skeletal injuries.

Appropriate treatment of skeletal trauma in children is especially important because its effects will last a lifetime. The recommendations of the 17 authors of this text are based on knowledge gained over many years of treating skeletal trauma in children. Their experience will prove helpful to any physician involved in the care of children, from pediatricians to general orthopaedists to pediatric orthopaedic specialists. The goal of the editors, Drs. Green and Swiontkowski, who have over 50 years of combined experience, and authors of this text is to help physicians choose the methods of treatment of skeletal trauma in children that will obtain the best possible results and will perhaps prevent complications or sequelae that might affect a child for the rest of his or her life.

S. TERRY CANALE, M.D.

Preface

Orthopaedic surgery is becoming highly subspecialized, with increasing numbers of graduating residents seeking subspecialty training in the form of postresidency fellowships. In spite of this trend toward a focused practice within orthopaedic surgery, most orthopaedic surgeons continue to care for the traumatized patient. This volume is therefore designed with the practitioner in mind. Our goal was to produce a practical yet comprehensive text that covered the field of pediatric musculoskeletal trauma. The design of the chapters allows the reader to quickly find the pertinent information about a specific injury without the distraction of too much historical perspective. Extensive bibliographies have been provided so that in-depth research may be undertaken if desired. We have sought to provide the reader with up-to-date concepts concerning the treatment of fractures in children. The chapter authors have been selected because of their expertise in specific areas of pediatric orthopaedic trauma. Half of the contributors are orthopaedic trauma surgeons with an interest in pediatric orthopaedic trauma, and the other half are pediatric orthopaedic surgeons who are involved in the care of musculoskeletal trauma in the pediatric patient.

Some forms of treatment may still be controversial, and alternative means of therapy are described. Nevertheless, treatment that today is considered on the cutting edge may well become the standard tomorrow. Until recently, operative treatment of children's fractures was rarely considered appropriate except in the case of open fractures. We have come to realize, however, that some fractures in children may be best managed operatively. We have reflected this trend in the writing of this text.

This text has been written to accompany the first two adult volumes entitled *Skeletal Trauma*. *Skleletal Trauma in Children*, however, is able to stand alone because it deals entirely with pediatric orthopaedic trauma.

NEIL E. GREEN, M.D.
MARC F. SWIONTKOWSKI, M.D.

Acknowledgments

Although many individuals played an important role in the development, writing, and editing of this text, we would like to thank some in particular. The staff of the W. B. Saunders Company worked with us throughout the entire process. The artist Philip Ashley expertly illustrated this text.

Dr. Neil E. Green would like to personally thank many of the people who helped throughout the production of the book. Joan Lorber was instrumental in communicating with the publisher and the authors and in coordinating the final revisions of the chapters. Holly Quick and Pat Post provided expertise in collating data and in typing and editing the final manuscripts, and Debbie Chessor's photography reproduced beautifully. Dr. Green would very much like to express how much his father, Dr. H. Howard Green, meant to him and how much he influenced the direction of his academic career. As a practicing orthopaedic surgeon, he showed enormous compassion for his patients, intellect, and medical ability that he passed on to three sons.

Dr. Marc F. Swiontkowski realizes that the material presented in this text has been edited based on the extensive experience that the orthopaedic group at Harborview Medical Center in Seattle, Washington, has collectively gathered. He especially wants to recognize his teachers, Drs. F. N. Elliott, J. P. Harvey, Jr., and S. T. Hansen, Jr., whose examples at critical points in his career have had a deep and lasting effect. In particular, he would like to acknowledge the contributions made by Stephen K. Benirschke, M.D., Sigvard T. Hansen, Jr., M. Bradford Henley, M.D., and Keith A. Mayo, M.D., as well as the other full-time faculty, fellows, and national and international visitors. Harborview is a truly amazing place; no one can help but continually learn from the collective excellence there. Without the competence and attention to detail of Rebecca Lessard, this volume would have never been completed.

Contents

1
Skeletal Growth and Development as
Related to Trauma 1
Eric Jones, M.D., Ph.D.

2
Physeal Injuries 15
S. Terry Canale, M.D.

3
Pathologic Fractures and Tumors 57
William W. Robertson, Jr., M.D.

4
The Multiply Injured Child 65
John H. Wilber, M.D.
George H. Thompson, M.D.

5
Complications of Fractures in Children 99
Robert N. Hensinger, M.D.

6
Pediatric Fractures of the Forearm, Wrist,
and Hand 127
Peter F. Armstrong, M.D., F.R.C.S.C., F.A.C.S.
V. Elaine Joughin, M.D., F.R.C.S.C.
Howard M. Clarke, M.D., Ph.D., F.R.C.S.C.

7
Fractures and Dislocations About the
Elbow 213
Neil E. Green, M.D.

8
Fractures and Dislocations About the
Shoulder 257
Lawrence X. Webb, M.D.

9
Fractures of the Spine in Children 283
J. Andy Sullivan, M.D.

10
Fractures and Dislocations About the Hip
and Pelvis 307
Marc F. Swiontkowski, M.D.

11
Fractures of the Femoral Shaft 345
M. L. Chip Routt, Jr., M.D.

12
Fractures and Dislocations Around the
Knee 369
Vernon Tolo, M.D.

13
Fractures of the Tibia and Fibula 397
George H. Thompson, M.D.
Fred Behrens, M.D.

14
Fractures and Dislocations of the Foot and Ankle 449
Alvin H. Crawford, M.D., F.A.C.S.

15
Child Abuse 517
Neil E. Green, M.D.

Index 533

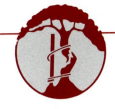

Eric Jones, M.D.

1

Skeletal Growth and Development as Related to Trauma

The effect of growth on trauma to the musculoskeletal system may be positive or negative. Adult bone is dynamic; it is constantly involved in bone turnover and remodeling in response to aging and changes in stress on the skeleton. Bone in children undergoes a very rapid, steady state of change. The pediatric skeleton not only remodels in response to alterations in stress but also grows in length and width in addition to changing shape, alignment, and rotation as it matures. An understanding of these changing forces and their effect on skeletal trauma in children is important in determining treatment of injured bones and joints.

Factors affecting the growth of bone and particularly the physis are variable and incompletely understood. The physis responds to various growth-inducing hormones, for instance, thyroxin, estrogen, and testosterone.[3] Diurnal variation in growth of bone has been shown to reflect the levels of the different hormones.[3] Mechanical factors also have control over growth rates. This is particularly evident in femoral overgrowth, in which disruption of the periosteal sleeve and increasing vascularity to the bone by fracture will increase longitudinal growth.[3,12] It has been postulated that mechanical factors, such as tension within the surrounding periosteum, may have some control over growth rate.[12,15]

The principles of fracture treatment are the same for all ages, anatomic alignment being the primary concern. The fracture should not be malaligned or malrotated. Although some angulation is acceptable when treating fractures in children, it is best to keep the amount of angulation as small as possible by routine fracture treatment methods, whatever the patient's age. The small amount of angulation associated with torus or "buckle" fractures in children can virtually always be accepted. Marked bowing, which can be seen in greenstick fractures in the forearm, should usually be corrected by completing the fracture and restoring alignment.[10]

Bone healing in children is usually very rapid, primarily because of the thickened, extremely osteogenic periosteum. The age of the patient directly affects the rate of healing of any fracture. The younger the child, the more rapidly the fracture heals. At birth, femoral shaft fractures heal in 3 or 4 weeks. As the child ages, the healing rate approaches that of an adult. An adolescent sustaining a femoral shaft fracture heals in 12 to 16 weeks (Fig. 1–1).

Injuries to the growth plate heal more rapidly than do shaft fractures. Physeal injuries, in almost all parts of the body, heal in approximately 3 weeks.[16] The age-related rate of healing is due to the osteogenic activity of the periosteum. The periosteum thins as the child grows older, thereby lessening osteogenic activity.

Treatment of trauma to the pediatric skeleton is generally routine. Dislocations and ligamentous injuries, however, are very uncommon in children compared with adults. Ligamentous injuries may occur in older children, in whom the epiphysis and the metaphysis are more securely attached. Most injuries, however, are simple fracture patterns caused by low-velocity trauma, such as falls. In most cases, closed reduction followed by a short time in a cast will restore normal function to a pediatric extremity. However, a number of pitfalls can make treatment of pediatric fractures very difficult and

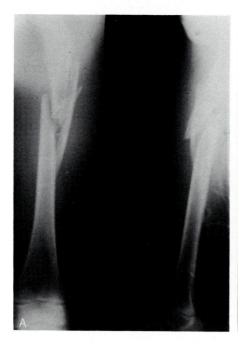
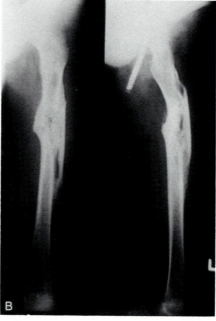

Figure 1–1

Radiograph of a comminuted subtrochanteric fracture of the femur in an 11-year-old boy (A). Ten weeks following fracture the bone is healed (B). In an adult this fracture would be difficult to treat nonoperatively and would require 3 to 6 months to heal.

demanding—this is particularly true of fractures to the growth plate.

History and Diagnosis

In infants, a history is usually not available, and the child will not always cooperate with either the physical examination or the treatment. Radiographs of an infant can be very difficult to obtain and interpret (Fig. 1–2), especially of bones in the elbow and hip region, which may require comparison views. An anteroposterior view as well as a lateral view to include joints above and below the injured area constitutes a minimal radiographic evaluation. Often in an infant, two views of the side opposite the injury are necessary. An arthrogram or other special radiographic studies may also be required to identify the exact injury.

Fractures through the growth plate in children can be difficult to interpret if the fracture is not displaced. A thorough physical examination can usually identify this type of injury, which occurs most commonly at the distal radius or distal fibula. Palpation at the tip of the lateral malleolus can usually identify a ligament injury; swelling and tenderness at the growth plate region can identify a fracture undetected by radiographs. Often, a small metaphyseal fragment on the radiograph suggests physeal injury.

The dependence of healing capacity on age is very significant. Every age group has its typical injury.

Most infants and newborns (up to age 2 years) sustain their fractures by having someone else injure them. Above age 2 years the child is walking and running and beginning to pursue various activities. Children most commonly fracture the forearm and usually the distal radius.[11, 14] Clavicular fractures are common in infancy and the preschool age group. The incidence of clavicular fractures decreases with increasing age. Forearm fractures, while very common in young children, show a progressive increase into the teenage years.

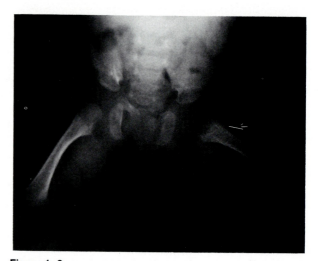

Figure 1–2

Anteroposterior radiograph of the pelvis of a 1-month-old infant who sustained an intertrochanteric fracture (arrow) of the left hip. Initially, the child was diagnosed as having a septic hip.

Most injuries occur when the child is playing with relatively simple toys. The more severe injuries are caused by automobiles, lawnmowers, all-terrain vehicles, and the like. As a child approaches the midteens, injuries are very much like those of an adult. The age at which the growth plates close varies greatly and depends on hereditary factors and hormonal variations. Skeletal age is an important factor in the consideration of injuries in children. The closer the child is to the end of growth the less prominent is the role of the growth plate in the treatment of the injury.

The effect of growth on fracture healing usually aids the orthopaedist in fracture treatment. A certain amount of angulation and deformity will remodel with growth. This amount is dependent on the age of the child, location of the injury in the bone, degree of deformity, and whether or not the deformity is in the plane of motion of the adjacent joint.[2] Increased blood flow to the injured area can result in accelerated growth of the injured bone (as well as surrounding bones), which can lead to overgrowth (usually associated with the femur or humerus). Growth, however, can produce deformity if the growth plate is injured or if trauma has altered muscle forces on an extremity, as it does in a head-injured child.

Finally, child abuse must be considered in all children's injuries and should always be suspected when treating this age group for fracture.[8] Care must be taken to ensure that the child is checked for abuse on initial assessment and for possible subsequent injuries during follow-up. Parents or guardians of children who are not brought back for follow-up appointments for fractures should be contacted and asked to schedule a return visit.

Formation of Bone

Embryonic bone forms through either membranous or enchondral ossification. In the former, mesenchymal cells proliferate to form membranes primarily in the region in which flat bones will be fabricated.[15] Primary bone is formed within an ossification center, which is then invaded by blood vessels. Ossification continues in the membrane, and a sheet of bone covered by mesenchymal cells is formed. Surface cells become the periosteum. Primary bone is remodeled and transformed into cancellous bone, to which the periosteum adds a compact cortical bone cover. This type of growth continues and is most important in formation of bones such as the scapula, skull, and, in part, the clavicle and pelvis.

MEMBRANOUS BONE FORMATION

All bones are involved in membranous bone formation. As enchondral ossification lengthens bones, the diaphyseal portion of the bone enlarges by proliferation of the bone beneath the periosteum. This constantly enlarges the diaphyseal cortex of the bone via membranous bone growth. This type of bone formation is apparent in injury to bone in which periosteal bone forms around hematoma from fracture as well as around subperiosteal infection (Fig. 1-3).

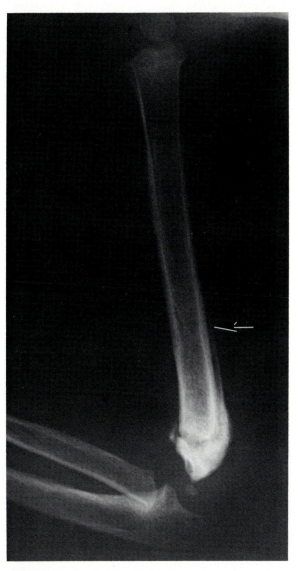

Figure 1-3

Radiograph of a healing supracondylar fracture illustrating the periosteum stripped (arrow) to nearly the midshaft of the humerus. The bridging periosteal bone stabilizes this fracture in about 3 weeks.

ENCHONDRAL OSSIFICATION

Enchondral ossification is bony replacement of a cartilage model and is the mode of formation of long bones. Early in gestation, mesenchymal cells aggregate to form models of the future long bones. A cartilage model is formed, and the peripheral cells organize into a perichondrium.[12, 15] The cartilage cells enlarge and degenerate, and the matrix surrounding them calcifies. The enveloping perichondrium of the region converts to a periosteum and deposits a layer of compact bone peripherally, through membranous ossification.

As these events occur, a vascular bud enters the ossification center, bringing with it new mesenchymal cells that will modulate into osteoblasts, chondroclasts, and osteoclasts. These cells align themselves on the calcified cartilage and deposit bone. Primary cancellous bone is thus formed. The center of ossification, located in the diaphysis, extends toward both metaphyseal regions. The terminal ends of the cartilage model continue to grow in length by cartilage cell proliferation.

Long bone growth continues in this manner until after birth, when secondary ossification centers develop (epiphyses). The mass of cartilage found between the epiphyseal and diaphyseal bone in later postnatal development thins to become the epiphyseal plate, which continues as the principal contributor to growth (in length) of long bones until maturation is reached. The girth of the long bone is provided by the cambium layer of the periosteum.[12] Successive surfaces of compact bone are added to the exterior while remodeling by resorption of the interior (endosteal) surface takes place.

Once the physis is established between the epiphysis and metaphysis, the periosteal ring becomes relatively firmly attached at the level of the zone of hypertrophied cells. This periphyseal periosteal collar is referred to as the fibrous ring of Lacroix.[12] The zone of Ranvier, the cellular segment responsible for growth in diameter of the physis,[12] is located in the same area. The periosteum is firmly attached at this level. Even when the periosteum is torn over the diaphysis, it usually remains attached at the physis.

Injury to bones results in an acceleration of both enchondral and membranous bone formation. This occurs particularly in the area of injury, but normal growth in surrounding bones likewise may be increased by the greater blood flow to an injured extremity.[6]

Fracture healing in children involves membranous as well as enchondral ossification. The major process is the formation of membranous bone by the periosteum around the hematoma that forms at the site of fracture. Blood clot accumulates within the bone at the fracture site and beneath the periosteum. Blood may also spill extraperiosteally if the periosteum has been injured. In children the periosteum strips readily away from the underlying bone, allowing blood to spread along a larger area, raise the periosteum, and stimulate new bone formation beneath the periosteum that has been elevated.

When bone is injured, bone dies for a few millimeters on either side of the fracture. The more diaphyseal the fracture, the thicker the cortex, the lower the blood supply, and the longer the time required for the inflammatory response to occur to initiate healing. In the area of the metaphysis, where the blood supply is greater, this process happens faster. If an injury occurs through the growth plate, only one side of the fracture suffers any ill effects because the growth plate does not require a blood supply and is not involved in necrosis. Hence, fractures through the epiphyseal plate heal very readily. Fractures through the metaphysis heal more rapidly than those through the diaphysis. Because a child has more vascular bone, healing is more rapid than in an adult with a diaphyseal injury.

Injuries to the pediatric skeleton may involve the bone as well as a variable amount of soft tissue. The blood supply to the bone is a very important part of fracture healing, and significant soft tissue injury will delay healing. The normal process of fracture healing in any part of the bone follows a set chronological order. Any of these phases may be disrupted or delayed by excessive adjacent soft tissue injury.

The initial phase of bone healing is the inflammatory phase, followed by the reparative phase, and then the remodeling phase. Cartilage does not heal in the same phases as bone. When the physis is injured, it does not heal by formation of callus. There is an inflammatory and a reparative phase in cartilage healing but not a remodeling phase.[3, 12]

Following a fracture, the inflammatory phase is initiated almost immediately. There is bleeding from the injured bone, and if the periosteum is torn, there is bleeding into the soft tissues adjacent to the periosteum. Hematoma accumulates within the medullary canal at the fracture site as well as in the surrounding periosteum. One of the primary differences between pediatric and adult bone is the very thick periosteum in children. The periosteum around the fracture site contains hematoma and is stripped from the bone as bleeding occurs. This is a primary factor in the amount of new bone formed around a fracture. The area of bone necrosis on either side of the fracture surface must be replaced by viable bone through the process of bone resorption and deposition. This process leads to an initial radiographic appearance of sclerosis at the fracture because of new bone being formed on the existing necrotic bone. The area around the necrotic bone elicits an inflammatory response. Because pediatric bone is more vascular than adult bone, the inflammatory (hyperemic) response is more rapid and significant. Fever as high as 40°C may be seen immediately following major long bone fractures. This hyperemic inflammatory reaction is also responsible for growth stimulation, which may result in overgrowth of the bone. Because of this response, the early stage of fracture healing is much faster in a child than in an adult.[3, 12, 14, 16]

The initial cellular repair process with organization of hematoma and fibrovascular tissue growth is of much greater importance in adult than in pediatric bone. Periosteal callus bridges this area long before the underlying hematoma forms a cartilage anlage that goes on to ossify.

Once cellular organization from the hematoma has passed through the inflammatory process, there is initial repair of the bone in the area of fracture. In children, the periosteum is the primary producer of new bone through membranous ossification. This process supplements considerably the (organizing hematoma) enchondral bone formation. In most children, by 10 days to 2 weeks after fracture a rubber-like bone forms around the fracture, making it very difficult to manipulate. The fracture site is still tender, however, and not yet ready for mobilization of the adjacent joints.

As part of the reparative phase, cartilage formed as the hematoma organizes is eventually replaced by bone through the process of enchondral bone formation, much as enchondral bone is formed in utero.

The remodeling phase of fracture healing may go on for some time, particularly in more displaced fractures. Remodeling is accelerated by motion of the adjacent joints and use of the extremity. The stresses and strains of regular use of the bone directly promote remodeling of the fractured bone into a bone that closely resembles the original structure. Because the mechanisms involved in fracture healing are the same as those in the growth process, particularly in the remodeling phase, bone heals much more rapidly in children than in adults.

The hematoma, which forms in the inner portion of the bone, is invaded by inflammatory cells and subsequently by collagen. Enchondral bone may be formed deep in a fracture while the membranous (periosteal) bone will be rapidly and abundantly bridging the fracture peripherally.

The major reason for the increased speed of healing of children's fractures is the periosteum, which contributes the largest part of new bone formation around a fracture. Children have significantly greater osteoblastic activity in this area because bone is already being formed beneath the periosteum as part of normal growth. This already active process is readily accelerated.

In radiographs of bones that have been fractured several months previously, transverse lines may be seen in the metaphyseal region. These lines are usually referred to as Harris growth arrest lines[7] or transverse lines of Park.[13] These transversely oriented trabeculae occur in bones that normally are rapidly growing (e.g., femur, tibia) and in those in which the trabeculae are usually predominantly longitudinally oriented (Fig. 1–4). When a growth

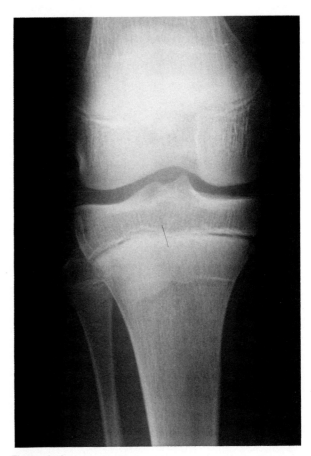

Figure 1–4

Arrest lines parallel to the physis in the metaphyseal area of the distal femur and proximal tibia and fibula 6 months following a femoral shaft fracture in a 12-year-old child. The temporary depression of growth at the time of injury results in more horizontal trabeculae being laid down, increasing the density of bones at that level.

deceleration occurs, as happens immediately following fracture to an extremity, the bone is, in effect, standing still and making transversely oriented trabeculae, formations that increase local bone density and are evident radiographically after further growth. Arrest lines should parallel the physeal contour. If they do not, it may indicate an area of physeal damage or an osseous bridge.[13]

Usually, these transverse trabeculae are transmitted symmetrically throughout the skeleton, as the growth slowdown is systemic. The physes that grow more rapidly (e.g., distal femur, proximal tibia) have arrest lines farthest from the physis. In the metaphyseal areas of bones, where the slowest growth occurs, the transverse trabeculae may be difficult to see radiographically or may not form at all.

Physes that do not grow rapidly under normal circumstances form primarily transversely oriented trabeculae, so the arrest lines are not often seen in these slower growing bones. Transversely oriented Harris lines may result from any type of stress on bone that causes a temporary slowdown in the formation of the longitudinally oriented bone. This includes systematic illness, fever, and starvation.[13]

Anatomy of Pediatric Bones

As the skeleton of a child grows it develops from a relatively elastic and rubbery type of biomechanical material to the more rigid structure of an adult. Because of the amount of radiolucent cartilage material in pediatric bone, comparison films are often necessary to determine whether a radiograph is abnormal. The type of injury also may be different in children; for example, ligamentous injuries and dislocations are rarely seen. Valgus stress injuries around the knee frequently lead to ligamentous and intraarticular ligamentous and meniscal injuries in adults. In children, in contrast, usually the distal femoral physis or proximal tibial physis will be disrupted depending on the age of the child, relative force velocity, and relative stress to the knee. Ligament injuries in the skeletally immature are uncommon but do occur. The distal femoral or proximal tibial growth plate would usually be the first to fail with a three-point stress across the knee (Fig. 1–5).

Pediatric bony injuries are more often treated by closed reduction than by open reduction because of the short time to union and the ease of obtaining and maintaining an anatomic reduction.

REMODELING

The remodeling ability of bone in children may make reduction accuracy somewhat less important than in an adult. Remodeling may occur readily in the plane of a joint (Fig. 1–6). However, it occurs far less readily, if at all, for rotational deformity and angular deformity not in the plane of the joint.[2, 15]

Angulation in the midportion of long bones is usually not acceptable and will not remodel very well. In children under the age of 8 to 10 years, angulation near the joint is more acceptable. If the angulation is less than 30 degrees and is within the plane of the joint, remodeling toward normal alignment can be expected.[12] Side-to-side (bayonet) apposition of bone is very acceptable as long as alignment is accurate (Fig. 1–7). This position will lead to prompt strong union with solid periosteal bone bridging.

The younger the child the greater the amount of remodeling that can be expected. The capacity for remodeling should not be cause to treat injuries less than completely. Age of the child, distance from the end of the bone, and amount of angulation are

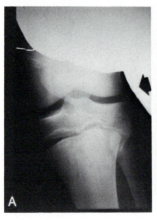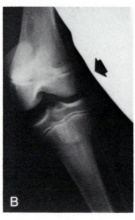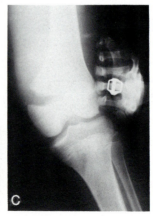

Figure 1–5

Stress films illustrating injury to the proximal tibial physis (A), the medial collateral ligament (B), and the distal femoral physis (C) in skeletally immature children.

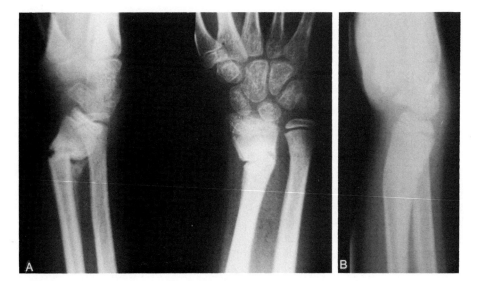

Figure 1-6

Radiograph of the distal radius in an 11-year-old girl at the time of cast removal 6 weeks after injury *(A)*. Lateral radiograph taken 3 months later showing considerable remodeling of the fracture in the plane of the joint *(B)*.

the primary considerations. Remodeling will not occur in displaced intraarticular fractures. In children, remodeling is relied on in the treatment of injuries of the proximal humerus and distal radius. Although operative treatment would be required for best initial radiographic alignment, remodeling will usually result in excellent restoration of the anatomy.

Delayed union and nonunion very rarely, if ever, occur in children. In a series of over 2000 fractures in children, there was not a single case of nonunion.[1] Probably the only exception to this would be in the case of open injuries in older children that become infected. Refracture is uncommon, although in malaligned forearm fractures refracture may occur following mobilization. Myositis ossificans and stiffness

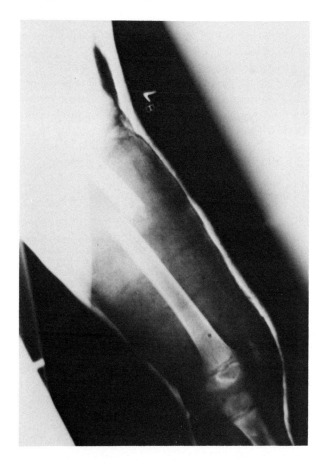

Figure 1-7

Radiograph of a femoral shaft fracture in a 12-year-old boy in a cast. The fracture was placed in about 1 cm of overlap (bayonet apposition) to allow for expected overgrowth of the extremity following fracture.

in joints secondary to fractures are exceedingly rare except in head-injured children.

Anatomic Differences

The most obvious anatomic difference in the pediatric skeleton is the presence of growth plates and the thick periosteum. Growth plate injuries and epiphyseal injuries can lead to growth disturbance that may be significant. Often injury to the growth plate and epiphysis parallels the adult intraarticular injury. Just as adult intraarticular injuries require anatomic reduction, so do pediatric articular injuries. As noted earlier, periosteum in children is much thicker, more active, less readily torn, and more easily stripped from the bone than in adults. The periosteum helps both in reduction and in maintenance of reduction and contributes immensely to rapid fracture healing.

The periosteum in children is much less frequently disrupted around the entire circumference of the bone and exhibits a much greater osteogenic potential than in adults. The intact periosteum helps reduce the amount of displacement and is, in general, the primary reason for more stable fractures in children. Callus forms much more quickly in children, and bones heal faster because of the osteogenic periosteum and the greater vascularity of growing bone.

Occasionally plain x-rays are not sufficient to demonstrate the anatomy of a pediatric joint injury, and it may be necessary to obtain an arthrogram to adequately visualize the fracture of a child, particularly around the elbow or in the newborn hip. Each part of the developing bone has its own characteristic injuries, growth, and remodeling patterns.

EPIPHYSIS

At birth most epiphyses are completely cartilaginous structures. The length of time for formation of the secondary ossification center within the epiphysis varies, with the distal femur being formed first.[2] A global type of growth plate is present in the epiphysis. When the epiphysis is completely cartilaginous, the physis is almost completely protected from injury. Once bone is formed within the epiphysis, it is more likely to be broken. When the epiphysis is very nearly all bone, it is subject to injury much like the remainder of the bone.

PHYSIS

The growth plate remains cartilaginous throughout development. As the child grows older, the physis becomes thinner and it is easier to disrupt the growth plate by injury. In infants and newborns, there are fewer mamillary processes that stabilize the epiphysis on the metaphysis. However, with further growth, particularly in the distal femoral region, very prominent mamillary processes help the physis secure the epiphysis to the metaphysis. The proximal femoral physis changes considerably and forms into what are essentially two separate physeal areas, the capital femoral epiphysis and, below it, the trochanteric apophysis.

METAPHYSIS

The metaphysis is the trumpet-shaped end of long bones. It has a thinner cortical area and increased trabecular bone and is wider than the corresponding diaphyseal part of the bone. Porosity in the metaphyseal area is greater than in the diaphyseal area, and the periosteum is more firmly attached in the metaphyseal area as it gets closer to the physis.

Most bone remodeling occurs in the metaphyseal region of bone following fracture. Periosteal bone forms in the area joining the diaphysis to the epiphysis. This area progressively transforms back into trumpet-shaped metaphyseal cortex with longitudinal growth.

DIAPHYSIS

The diaphysis is the principal portion of the long bone. It is extremely vascular in the newborn. With further growth it becomes less vascular and the cortical bone thickens. The diaphysis grows by periosteum-mediated membranous bone formation.

Biomechanical Differences

Pediatric bone is less dense and more porous and is penetrated by more vascular channels than is adult bone.[9, 15] It has a comparatively lower modulus of elasticity, lower bending strength, and lower mineral content.[4] Immature bone has greater porosity on cross section, and immature cortical bone has a greater number of osteon systems traversing the cortex when compared with mature bone. The periosteum is very strong and can serve as a hinge for reduction and maintenance of fracture reduction. The increased porosity of pediatric bone helps prevent propagation of fracture lines. It is very uncommon to see comminuted fractures in children. Load-deformation curves of fractures comparing pediatric and adult bone show a long plastic phase in children.[4] The porosity and rough mechanical fracture surface prolong the time and energy absorption before bone is broken. Adult bone almost always fails in tension, whereas bone in children can fail either in tension or in compression.

When bones are bent, stress on the tension side is about the same as on the compression side. Because bone has a lower yield stress in tension than in compression, bone yields first on the tensile side. As the bending continues, a crack travels across the bone from the tension side toward the compression side.

Depending on the amount of energy to be absorbed, the large pores in growing bone may stop the propagation of the fracture line, which may leave a portion of the cortex intact on the compression side and result in a greenstick fracture.[10] If there is enough plastic deformity in the remaining cortex, it may be necessary to complete the fracture as part of treatment. Completing the fracture is usually done by reversing the deformity so the remaining cortex is placed on the tension side.

Bone is said to be elastic if it returns to its original shape after load is removed. If bone does not return to its original shape and residual deformity remains after the load is released, bone has undergone plastic deformation. This results from failure in compression on one side of the bone and failure in tension on the opposite side. Incomplete failure in tension in which the fracture line does not propagate through bone results in plastic deformity of bone (Fig. 1–8).

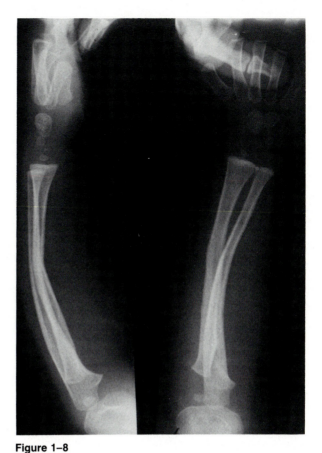

Figure 1–8

Plastic deformation in the radius and ulna of a 2-year-old following a fall. The bones are plastically deformed at midshaft, with volar compression and dorsal tension failure but without fracture propagation.

Classification of Children's Fractures

Pediatric fractures can be classified into five types: (1) plastic deformation, (2) buckle fracture (near the metaphysis), (3) greenstick fracture, (4) complete fracture, and (5) epiphyseal fracture.

PLASTIC DEFORMATION

Plastic deformation of bone, rare in adults, is essentially unique to children. It is most commonly seen in the ulna and, occasionally, the fibula. If bending of bone occurs to such a degree that there is microscopic failure in compression on the concavity of the bone and tension on the convexity, but a fracture on the tension side does not propagate, then permanent deformation of the bone ensues when the force is removed. If there is no hematoma, there may be no periosteal elevation and no significant callus formation, but the bone may be permanently deformed in a plastic fashion. If the deformity occurs in a child less than 4 years old or if the deformation is less than 20 degrees, the angulation will usually correct with growth.[10]

BUCKLE FRACTURES

Buckle fracture, also an injury primarily of childhood, is a compression failure of bone that usually occurs at the junction of the metaphysis and diaphysis. In the metaphysis, where porosity is greatest, bone in compression may be buckled by the denser bone of the diaphysis (Fig. 1–9). This injury is similar to the diaphyseal greenstick fracture. Failure on the tension side propagates the fracture, and failure on the compression side buckles the more cortical diaphyseal bone into the more membranous metaphyseal bone. This injury is commonly referred to as a torus fracture because of its similarity to the raised band around the base of a classical Greek column.

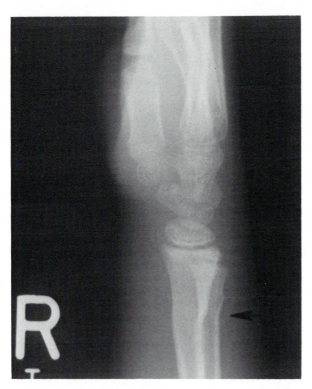

Figure 1–9

Torus fractures usually occur at the junction (arrow) of the metaphyseal and diaphyseal bone. The more porous metaphyseal bone fails in compression.

GREENSTICK FRACTURES

Greenstick fractures occur when a bone is bent and there is failure on the tension side of the bone. The bone begins to fracture, but the fracture line does not propagate entirely through the bone. Failure on the compression side of the bone allows plastic deformity to occur. In an adult, without porous bone and compression side deformity, the fracture line virtually always propagates through the bone. Because compressive bone undergoes plastic deformation, it does not recoil to an anatomic position and must be completely broken to restore normal alignment.

Complete Fractures

Fractures that propagate completely through a bone may be described in several ways, as follows.

SPIRAL FRACTURES

Spiral fractures are usually created by a rotational force on the bone. They are low-velocity injuries commonly associated with child abuse. An intact periosteal hinge enables the orthopaedic surgeon to reduce the fracture by reversing the rotational injury.

OBLIQUE FRACTURES

Oblique fractures occur diagonally across diaphyseal bone, usually at about 30 degrees to the axis of the bone.[16] Analogous to complete fractures in an adult, these injuries usually cause significant disruption to the periosteum. Because the fractures are unstable and may be difficult to hold in anatomic reduction, alignment is important. Fracture reduction is attempted by immobilizing the extremity while applying traction.

TRANSVERSE FRACTURES

Transverse fractures through pediatric bone usually occur from three-point bending and are readily reduced by utilizing the periosteum on the concave side of the fracture force. Periosteum on the side opposite the apex of the force is torn. The three-point bending type of immobilization usually maintains this diaphyseal fracture in a reduced position (Fig. 1–10).

Butterfly fragments are not common in pediatric injuries but result from a mechanism similar to that causing a transverse fracture, with the butterfly fragment remaining on the side of the apical force of the three-point bend. This injury occurs in the

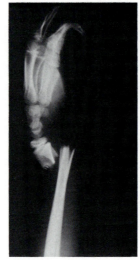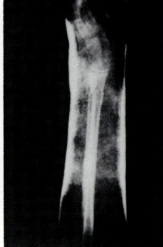

Figure 1–10

Lateral radiograph of a dorsally displaced distal radius and ulna fracture, which is easily reduced by utilizing the intact dorsal periosteum to aid in locking the distal fragments in place.

highly cortical area of the diaphysis—usually in the midshaft of the femur, tibia, or ulna (Fig. 1–11).

EPIPHYSEAL FRACTURES

Injuries to the epiphysis of a bone usually involve the growth plate. Problems after injury to the growth plate are not common, but anytime the physis is injured, the potential for deformity exists. The distal radial physis is the most frequently injured physis.[11] Usually the growth plate repairs well and rapidly, and most physeal injuries are healed in 3 to 6 weeks. Damage to the plate can occur by crushing, vascular compromise to the physis, or bone growth bridging from the metaphysis to the bony portion of the epiphysis. The damage can result in progressive angular deformity, limb length discrepancy, or joint incongruity.

Injury to the physis has been studied by many researchers over the years.[3, 5, 14, 17] Their studies show a change in the stability of the epiphysis on the metaphysis that depends on age. The physis and epiphyses are very firmly connected externally by periosteum and connected internally by the mamillary processes. The physis is a hard rubbery material more susceptible to injury by rotation than by angulation or traction.

Injuries involving the growth plate usually occur at the junction of the cartilage cells that are calcifying with those that are uncalcified.[17] With epiphyseal injury the growth plate is usually attached to the epiphyseal side of the fracture, and anatomic reduction of the joint surface usually results in anatomic reduction of the growth plate. In distal femoral epiphyseal injuries, the germinal part of the plate is often "scraped off" the epiphyseal portion of the fracture either in fracture or in fracture reduction. These injuries are likely to result in growth plate damage.

Epiphyseal injuries are usually classified by the Salter and Harris classification system,[17] a scheme based on the radiographic appearance of the fracture (Fig. 1–12). Injury may occur to the epiphysis and growth plate or to the perichondrial ring. In a type I fracture, the epiphysis separates completely from the metaphysis without any radiographically evident fracture through bone.

The plane of cleavage in a type I fracture is usually through the zone of hypertrophic and degenerating cartilage cell columns. The remaining growth plate remains attached to the epiphysis. The fracture plane does not always propagate directly through the hypertrophic zone but may at some places undulate into the germinal zone of the physis or into segments of the metaphysis. Changes in contour are caused by the mamillary processes extending into the metaphysis. The distal femoral growth plate is shaped such that often fragments of metaphysis are broken off when the growth plate is injured.

In type I injuries the periosteum usually remains attached to the growth plate, preventing significant displacement of the epiphysis. If there is very little periosteal disruption, slight widening of the physis may be the only radiographic sign of an injury through the physis (Fig. 1–13). Although type I injuries are usually not associated with vascular change, a complete separation of the capital femoral epiphysis can result in avascular necrosis and growth arrest of the proximal femur. The larger the ossifi-

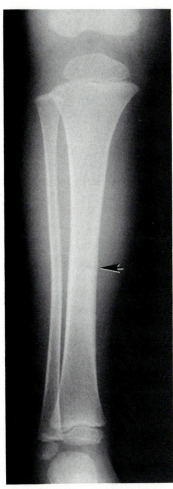

Figure 1–11

Radiograph of a tibia of a 2-year-old with incomplete fracture of the tibia *(arrow)* and plastic deformity of the fibula. The lateral apex three-point stress to the tibia resulted in a tension-generated fracture whose propagation was halted before it reached the lateral cortex. The injury lacked sufficient energy to generate a butterfly fragment on the lateral side.

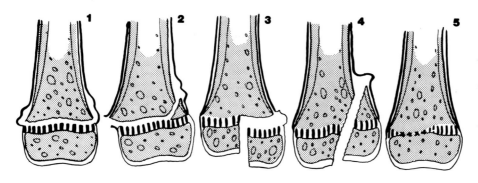

Figure 1–12

Illustration of Salter and Harris classification of epiphyseal injuries (see text). (From Salter RB, Harris WR: Injuries involving the epiphyseal plate. J Bone Joint Surg 45A:587, 1963.)

cation center, the greater the tendency of the injury to produce a metaphyseal fragment on the compression side of the injury.

In a type II fracture, the injury passes through the growth plate and out through a portion of the metaphysis. The periosteum is usually damaged on the tension side, but the fracture leaves the periosteum intact in the region of the metaphyseal fragment.

As in a type I injury the line of fracture separation occurs along the hypertrophic and calcified zones of the physis. However, propagation along this junction is more variable with a type II injury. As the fracture line courses toward the compression side of the injury the fracture line propagates through the metaphyseal area. The periosteal attachment along

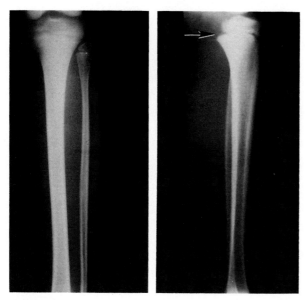

Figure 1–13

Anteroposterior and lateral radiograph of the tibia of a 10-year-old child who had proximal tibial pain and swelling. This proximal tibial epiphyseal injury *(arrow)* was missed in the emergency room. Salter I injuries are often subtle and require close correlation between the physical examination and the radiograph.

the metaphyseal fragment can be utilized to aid reduction of the injury.

Growth disruption secondary to type I and type II injuries is very infrequent, although it can occur, particularly if the circulation to the epiphysis is disrupted. Anatomic reduction is generally not required with type I and type II injuries. These injuries are adjacent to the joint, and the entire growth plate is intact. Remodeling will usually occur rapidly if the bone is angulated.

A type III fracture is intraarticular and passes through the epiphysis until it reaches the growth plate. Then the fracture line courses through the growth plate to the periosteal surface. The same layer of the growth plate is usually involved in the physeal portion of the fracture as in type I and type II injuries. This fracture usually occurs when the growth plate is beginning to undergo closure. Problems relative to growth arrest may not be major. This is particularly true of distal fibula injuries but may not be true of injuries around the elbow. With anatomic reduction of the articular surface, the physis is usually anatomically reduced as well. In that situation, growth arrest is generally not a problem, even in the skeletally immature.

A type IV injury is also intraarticular and involves the epiphysis as well as the metaphysis. The fracture line crosses through the growth plate. The injury is similar to a type III fracture in that the articular surface must be anatomically reduced. A vertical split of all zones of the physis occurs, and the physis must be anatomically reduced to restore the architecture of the growth plate and minimize the risk of osseous bridge formation.

Considerable debate exists concerning type V injuries. The original type V injury as described by Salter was a crush injury to the growth plate.[17] A type V fracture may be difficult to recognize on the initial radiographs because it may appear to be a type I. These injuries are very uncommon, but any injury that shows clinical swelling and tenderness around the growth plate and is associated with considerable axial load should be suspected to be a Type V.

The Salter-Harris classification is useful as a rapid way to describe an epiphyseal injury based on radiographic interpretation. A more complex and inclusive classification scheme was proposed by Ogden.[14] It includes nine types of fractures that are further divided into subtypes A through D, and so forth. Since its introduction, however, the Ogden classification has not been used to any extent because of its complexity.

Other injuries to the epiphysis are avulsion injuries of the tibial spines and injuries to the muscle attachments to the pelvis. Osteochondral fractures from the articular surface of the femur, patella, and talus are among other epiphyseal injuries that do not involve the growth plate.

Summary

Injury to the growing skeleton is common both as an isolated event and in the multiply injured child. Skeletal injuries heal rapidly and should be treated as early as possible because they begin to mend as soon as the injury has occurred. Growth usually aids the orthopaedist who is caring for a traumatized extremity. Growth speeds fracture healing because the repair processes are ongoing and no time is lost in calling up the repair troops. The thick osteogenic periosteum aids in reduction of the fracture and rapidly provides a bridge over the broken bone.

Porous growing bone affords fracture patterns that are biomechanically different from those of adult bone but that are, in general, easier to treat. Nearly all fractures in children can be treated in a cast without worry about stiff joints or the need for physical therapy to mobilize injured joints.

Although growing bone is well equipped to deal with trauma, some injuries may damage the growth mechanisms so severely that they cannot recover. Others have that potential if the orthopaedist is not wary and ready to act rapidly to restore normal growth as well as function.

REFERENCES

1. Beckman, F.; Sulivan, J. Some observations of fractures of long bones in children. Am J Surg 51:722–741, 1941.
2. Blount, W. Fractures in Children. Baltimore, Williams & Wilkins, 1955.
3. Brighton, C. T. The growth plate and its dysfunctions. AAOS Instr Course Lect 36:3–25, 1987.
4. Currey, J. D.; Butler, G. The mechanical properties of bone tissue in children. J Bone Joint Surg 57-A:810–814, 1975.
5. Dale, G. G.; Harris, W. R. Prognosis of epiphysial separation: An experimental study. J Bone Joint Surg 40-B:116–122, 1958.
6. Edvardson, P.; Syversen, S. M. Overgrowth of the femur after fractures of the shaft in childhood. J Bone Joint Surg 58-B:339–346, 1976.
7. Harris, H. A. The growth of long bones in childhood. Arch Intern Med 38:785–793, 1926.
8. King, J.; Diefendorf, D.; Apthorp, J. Analysis of 429 fractures in 189 battered children. J Pediatr Orthop 51:722–741, 1941.
9. Light, T. R.; Ogden, D. A.; Ogden, J. A. The anatomy of metaphyseal torus fractures. Clin Orthop 188:103–111, 1984.
10. Mabrey, J. D.; Fitch, R. D. Plastic deformation in pediatric fractures: Mechanism and treatment. J Pediatr Orthop 9:310–314, 1989.
11. Neer, C. S., II; Horwitz, B. Z. Fractures of the epiphyseal plate. Clin Orthop Rel Res 41:24–32, 1965.
12. Ogden, J. A. Anatomy and physiology of skeletal development. In: Ogden, J. A., ed. Skeletal Injury in the Child. Philadelphia, Lea & Febiger, 1982, pp. 16–40.
13. Ogden, J. A. Growth slowdown and arrest lines. J Pediatr Orthop 4:409–415, 1984.
14. Ogden, J. A. Injury to growth mechanisms of the immature skeleton. Skeletal Radiol 6:237–253, 1963.
15. Ogden, J. A. The uniqueness of growing bones. In: Rockwood, C. A., Jr., Wilkins, K. E.; King, R. E., eds. Fractures in Children, Vol. 3. Philadelphia, J. B. Lippincott, 1984, pp. 1–86.
16. Rang, M. Injuries of the epiphysis, growth plate and perichondrial ring. In: Rang, M., ed. Children's Fractures. Philadelphia, J. B. Lippincott, 1983, pp. 10–25.
17. Salter, R. B.; Harris, W. R. Injuries involving the epiphyseal plate. J Bone Joint Surg 45-A:587–622, 1963.

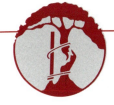

S. Terry Canale, M.D.

2

Physeal Injuries

The physes appear to be the weakest area in children's bone and also are the structures that must be preserved if normal growth is to occur. Because there are no noninvasive methods for assessing the histologic level of injury to the physeal potential for renewal and longitudinal growth, it is mandatory to treat all physes as gently as possible and to delay prognosis after injury until the time for growth disturbance has passed. Just as all children are different, so do injuries to different physes respond differently. To provide the best care, each physeal injury must be approached as a distinct entity, keeping in mind the patient's age, the location of the injury, the type of injury, the growth potential of the affected area, the degree of displacement, and the time from injury to treatment. It also should be remembered that the management of complications of physeal injuries is difficult and complex.

Pathology

RELEVANT ANATOMY

The physis is the primary center for growth of the skeleton. Initially, primary physes are relatively discoid areas of rapidly maturing cartilage, but with increasing biomechanical stresses, especially shear stresses, the physes develop changes in contour, or undulations. Planar physes contribute primarily to longitudinal growth, and spherical physes contribute almost exclusively to circumferential expansion of the bone. The physes also differ in morphology according to their location in the skeleton. The rapidly growing distal femoral physis, for example, has elongated cell columns in contrast to the shortened cell column formation in the slowly growing phalangeal physis.

Cartilage cells grow continually on the side of the physis facing the epiphysis of a long bone, while on the metaphyseal side cartilage continually breaks down and is replaced by bone. When the skeleton has achieved its adult size, the physes are resorbed and replaced by bone that joins the epiphysis permanently to the metaphysis. In males, most fusions are complete at about age 20 years; in females, growth in length of the bones ceases about 2 years earlier. The annual rate of bone renewal during the first 2 years of life is 50%, compared with 5% in adults.

The physis may be divided into zones according to function (Fig. 2–1). The zone of growth is concerned with both longitudinal and circumferential growth of the bone. The zone of matrix formation undergoes several biochemical changes necessary for eventual ossification. In the zone of cartilage transformation, tissue is mineralized to create bone matrix (the primary spongiosa), and the original bone surrounding the cartilaginous septum is gradually removed and replaced by a more mature secondary spongiosa that no longer contains remnants of the cartilaginous precursor. Ranvier described a circumferential notch containing cells, fibers, and a bony lamina that is located at the periphery of the physis and is an area of active peripheral cellular addition to the physis contributing to latitudinal growth (appositional growth). The periosteal sleeve is firmly attached to each end of a bone at the zone of Ranvier and the perichondrium of the epiphysis; it appears to be an anatomic restraint to rapid, uncontrolled longitudinal growth.

Physes have been described as either pressure (compressive) or traction (tensile) responsive; the

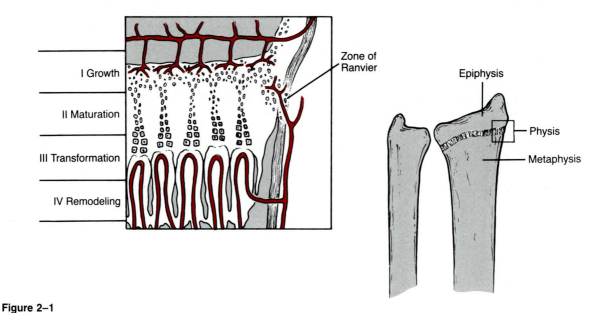

Figure 2–1
Zones of the physis according to function. I—Growth; II—maturation; III—transformation; IV—remodeling. (Redrawn from Ogden, J. A. Skeletal Injury in the Child, ed 2. Philadelphia, Lea & Febiger, 1990.)

latter have been referred to as apophyses. Recent studies have demonstrated significant histologic differences in the two types of physes in the tibial tuberosity, and similar structural changes are believed to exist in other apophyses.

The metaphysis is the area of most rapid change in bone structure. As the physis is replaced by primary spongiosa this bone is apposed to the surfaces of the longitudinal matrix between the cell columns, where it is rapidly remodeled and replaced by more mature bone. The metaphysis represents the transition zone from the wider physis to the narrow diaphysis.

The blood supply of the physis is from three sources: epiphyseal circulation, metaphyseal circulation, and perichondrial circulation. Epiphyseal circulation varies with the location and growth of the secondary ossification center. Vessels enter and disperse throughout the chondroepiphysis within cartilage canals. These canals course throughout the epiphysis, except for the avascular articular cartilage region, and branch out into the germinal cell regions of the physis. The vessels may occasionally communicate with the metaphyseal circulation. Each canal contains a central artery, veins, and a complex capillary network surrounding the central vessels. As ossification progresses, these vessels are incorporated into the osseous vasculature; one or two vessels usually develop as the predominant blood supply.

INCIDENCE

Mann and Rajmaira reported that of 2650 long bone fractures in children, approximately 30% involved the physes.[121] Neer and Horowitz reported 2500 consecutive physeal injuries, almost half of which (43.8%) occurred in the distal radius.[136] The next most frequently injured physis was that of the distal humerus (13%), followed by the physes of the distal fibula, distal tibia, distal ulna, proximal humerus, distal femur, proximal tibia, and proximal fibula. Chadwick and Bentley, in a report of 103 physeal injuries, found 27% of fractures in the distal tibia and 25% in the distal radius.[46] Several other studies have shown that in all long bones the distal physes are injured more often than the proximal physes. Physeal injuries occur more frequently in boys than in girls, probably because the physes remain open longer in boys and are exposed to more trauma through athletic activities. Most physeal fractures occur in boys between the ages of 12 and 15 years, and in girls between the ages of 9 and 12 years.

Although athletics play an important role in physeal injuries, Collins reviewed 2137 athletic injuries and found only 58 physeal injuries, most of which were acute Osgood-Schlatter lesions.[52] Some specific physeal injuries are associated with specific sports, such as "Little League elbow" and "gymnast's wrist." Yong-Hing and colleagues[207] and Albanese and co-workers[3] described stress injuries of the distal radius and ulna in competitive adolescent gymnasts.

They found radiologic evidence of premature closure of the physis with later shortening of the radius. Repetitive compressive loading of the distal radial physis was believed to cause this injury. The increasing number of children participating in organized athletic activities will undoubtedly cause an increase in the number of physeal injuries. Apple and McDonald reported that chronic, repetitive, cyclic loading in the lower extremity produced no harmful effect on the physes and that young runners experienced no more injuries than did adult runners.[5] Micheli also found no deleterious effects from weight training in immature athletes.[128] Turz and Crost, however, reported that 12% of the children in their study who required hospitalization for a sports injury experienced angulation or shortening of a limb or limited joint motion.[193]

MECHANISM OF INJURY

The strengh of the physis is related to its morphology and to the intercellular matrix. In the first two zones of the physis, the cartilage matrix is abundant and the physis is strong. In the third zone, the enlarged chondrocytes decrease the capacity to withstand shearing, bending, and tension stresses. This appears to be the weakest part of the physis. Harris demonstrated in the proximal tibial epiphysis that when the epiphysis separated from the metaphysis, the plane of cleavage passed consistently through this third zone.[82] The fourth zone is reinforced by calcification but is still weaker than the first and second zones. Fractures generally involve the third and fourth zones. Trabecular formation in the metaphysis also contributes to the strength of the physis, but the metaphysis is susceptible to compression or torus forces. As long as the epiphysis is cartilaginous, it serves as a sort of shock absorber, transmitting forces directly into the metaphysis that result in torus fractures. As the epiphysis ossifies, this shock-absorbing ability lessens and forces are transmitted more directly into the physis, where shearing may occur through the third and fourth zones.

The dense periosteal attachments around the periphery of the physis also appear to increase the resistance to shear and tensile forces, especially as they blend into the epiphyseal perichondrium and joint capsule–ligament complex. The periosteum is attached relatively loosely to the metaphysis; the diaphyseal periosteum is even more loosely attached and does not appear to offer any mechanical protection for the diaphysis. Bright and Elmore showed that the load-to-failure value of epiphyseal cartilage with intact periosteum is almost twice that of epiphyseal cartilage with the periosteum removed.[25] As a checkrein on the epiphysis once the physis has failed, the periosteum may prevent marked displacement if its fibers are not ruptured. This function may explain why epiphyseal injury often occurs without roentgenographic evidence of significant displacement.

The mechanism of injury to the physeal structures depends to some extent on the age of the child. Bright and associates showed experimentally that the tensile strength of the physis increases with age.[26] Chung and associates found that the perichondrial complex provides significant strength to the physis in childhood but less so in adolescence.[49a] In infancy and early childhood, when the physis is relatively thick, shearing or avulsion forces are most commonly involved. In older children and adolescents, physeal fracture-separation is most often caused by a combination of shearing and angulatory forces. Near the end of skeletal growth, when part of the physis has closed, intraarticular shearing forces, with or without angulatory forces, may cause intraarticular fracture. Momentary, transient dislocation or near-dislocation of a joint, caused by an avulsion or shearing force, also may cause an intraarticular fracture. A severe abduction or adduction angulatory force applied to a joint that normally only flexes or extends exerts a severe compression force on the physis.

The role of compression in physeal injuries is still controversial. Brashear in 1959 proposed that compression was a component in all physeal injuries,[21] and Ogden recognized this in his modified classification:[144] Peterson and Burkhart questioned the existence of a "pure" compression injury unassociated with fracture of the physis.[162] When a compression force is applied, fracturing occurs first in the metaphyseal region; continued compressive forces may force the metaphyseal bone up into the physis, damaging all its layers. Peterson and Burkhart also have challenged the idea of a Salter-Harris V (pure compression) injury.[162]

Keret and co-workers, however, described asymmetric premature closure of the proximal tibial physis in a patient with fractures of the contralateral tibia and ankle; the physeal injury was not diagnosed at the time of injury.[100] Hresko and Kasser reported seven physeal arrests about the knee in patients who had nonphyseal injuries of the lower extremities.[91] Their patients were between the ages of 10 and 12 years, and all physeal arrests involved the posterolateral part of the distal femur or the anterior part of the proximal tibia. No patient had evidence of iatrogenic trauma to the physis, such as that caused by pin placement or other surgical procedure. Recognition of the physeal injury was delayed for an average of 1 year and 10 months until a gross angular deformity appeared. These reports seem to support the concept of a Salter-Harris type V injury caused by compression alone. Adolescents with fractures of the lower extremities, even if they do not appear to involve the physes, should be evaluated and followed closely to detect any physeal injury about the knee that may become evident only with growth.

In addition to trauma, the growth mechanisms may be damaged by surgical procedures, such as the penetration of pins or screws; by irradiation; by disease, such as infection or neoplasm; or by congenital conditions, such as metabolic or hematologic disorders.

CONSEQUENCES OF INJURY

The most obvious and catastrophic consequence of physeal injury is disruption of longitudinal growth of the bone. Complete growth arrest may result in significant limb length inequality with functional impairment. Partial growth arrest may result in angular deformity or progressive shortening. Nonunion (as after fractures of the lateral humeral condyle [Fig. 2–2]), malunion, and avascular necrosis (as after injury to the capital femoral epiphysis), also may occur. Infrequently, arteriovenous malformation may cause accelerated growth.

Several reports have demonstrated that the prognosis for future growth is dependent on the location of the lesion in the physis. If the fracture is limited to the layer of hypertrophic cells, healing is usually uneventful. However, Salter and Harris showed that if the fracture reaches the layer of germinal cells or crosses the entire physis, growth disturbance is more likely (Fig. 2–3). Shapiro and colleagues reported that growth disturbance after injury depends on the presence of vascular communication between the epiphyseal and metaphyseal osseous compartments, which may lead to formation of bony bridges between the two.[181] Gomes and co-workers, in an experimental study in rats, correlated growth disturbance with the Salter-Harris type of fracture.[71] They found that after types I and II fractures, there was transitory growth arrest and an increased thickening of the zone of hypertrophic cells but that a nearly normal physis was seen within 25 days. After type III injuries, an angular deformity occurred that increased with time. After type IV injuries, a step-off developed on the articular surface and became more severe with time. According to these investigators, no compressive force was applied to produce the bony bridges; this suggests that these alterations are secondary and may be triggered by the presence of the osseous callus itself, which fills the gap and maintains the interruption of the growth cartilage, thus establishing a bony bridge between the epiphyseal and metaphyseal bone.[71] Circulation plays an important role in the genesis of these deformities because the bony bridge is preceded by early anastomosis between the epiphyseal and metaphyseal vessels through the gap in the growth cartilage. These findings support the impression of other investigators that permanent damage to the physis and the consequent bone deformity in these two types of injuries (Salter-Harris types III and IV) are caused by the establishment of early anastomotic connections between the epiphyseal and metaphyseal vessels.

Complete Growth Arrest

Complete cessation of growth after physeal injury is infrequent, and its significance depends on the age of the patient. In an adolescent near the end of skeletal growth, there may be no functional sequelae; however, in younger children a substantial limb length discrepancy may develop.

Partial Growth Arrest

Partial growth arrest produces angular and longitudinal growth abnormalities. The arrest occurs when a bridge of bone forms across the physis from the metaphysis to the epiphysis, tethering growth. Growth of the remaining physis causes angular deformity. The size and location of the bony bar determine the clinical deformity. For example, laterally situated bony bars about the knee produce genu valgus deformities, while anterior bars produce genu recurvatum. If the bar is in the center of the physis, growth of the periphery may cause "cupping," "tenting," or "dip deformity" of the metaphysis and relative shortening of the bone with little angular deformity.

Bright classifies partial growth arrests as peripheral, central, and combined and reported that 60% of partial growth arrests in his series of 225 patients were caused by peripheral lesions.[22] Partial arrests occur almost twice as often in boys as in girls. The physes of the distal femur, distal and proximal tibia, and distal radius are most frequently affected.

All bony bars result from damage to the physeal cells, most commonly from fracture. They also may occur after other kinds of physeal damage such as

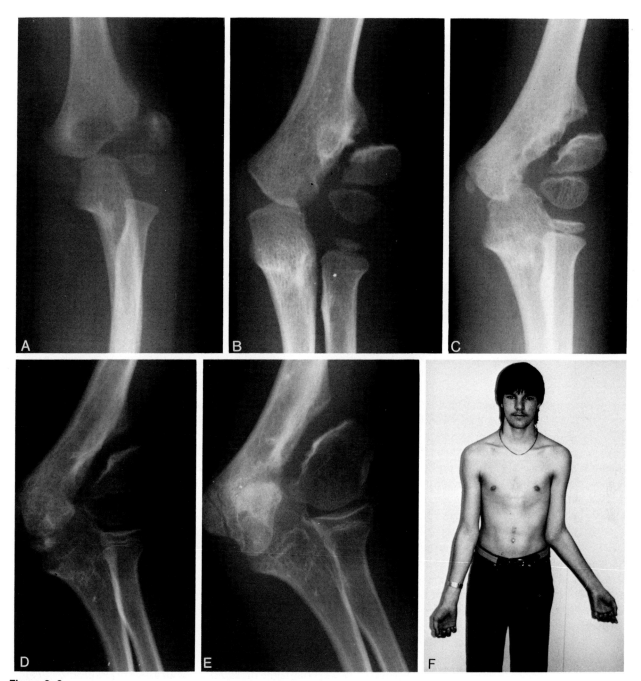

Figure 2–2

A, Fracture of lateral humeral condyle in a 5-year-old child, treated with observation only. *B,* One year after fracture, there is established nonunion. *C,* Three years after fracture, the capitellum and condyle appear to be migrating proximally. *D,* Five years after fracture, established cubitus valgus in addition to nonunion. *E,* Ten years after fracture, severe cubitus valgus deformity; the patient suffered mild ulnar nerve symptoms. *F,* Eleven years after fracture, the patient has unsightly cubitus valgus deformity. (From Canale, S. T.; Beaty, J. H., eds. Operative Pediatric Orthopaedics. St. Louis, Mosby-Yearbook, 1991.)

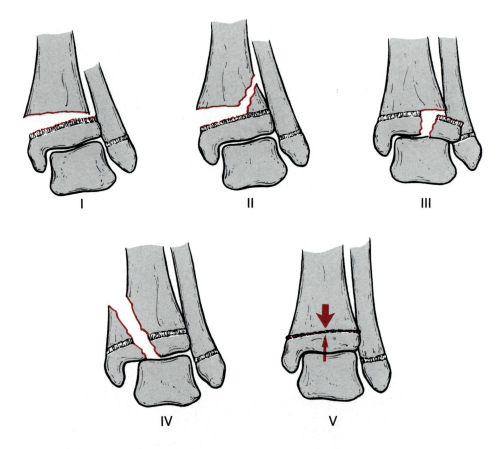

Figure 2-3

Salter-Harris classification of physeal injury. I—Pure separation through physis; II—metaphyseal spike; III—separation through physis and vertically through epiphysis; IV—fracture through metaphysis, through physis, and vertically through epiphysis; V—pure compression injury.

infection, tumors, irradiation, thermal burns, and the insertion of metal across the physis. Neural and vascular abnormalities also have been shown to alter physeal growth, and some bony bars have been found in which no cause was apparent. Of all the causes of bony bars, perhaps the only preventable one is iatrogenic damage from metal pins or screws placed across the physis. A small, smooth pin placed perpendicularly across the center of the physis for a short time (2 to 3 weeks) rarely causes growth arrest; however, a threaded wire placed obliquely across a physis and left in place for a few weeks usually results in a bony bar.

COMMONLY ASSOCIATED INJURIES

The injuries most commonly associated with physeal fractures are those to the neurovascular and ligamentous structures near the physis. Avulsion of the physis caused by ligamentous injury occurs most often at the tibial spine, at the ulnar styloid, and in the phalanges. Neurovascular injuries are most common with supracondylar humeral and proximal tibial fractures. Dislocation of the joint or an ipsilateral shaft fracture is seen most frequently with medial epicondylar fractures, about half of which are associated with partial or complete elbow dislocation; however, ipsilateral fractures of the shafts of other long bones often are seen with the physeal injury.

Combinations of physeal injury and ligamentous disruption are most common about the knee. Bertin and Goble reported that of 29 patients with epiphyseal separations, 14 had associated ligamentous instability at follow-up.[14] Avulsion of the tibial spine is often associated with injury to the cruciate ligaments. Posterior displacement of a fracture fragment may cause impingement, occlusion, intraluminal damage, or transection of the popliteal artery (Fig. 2-4).

CLASSIFICATION

The first classification scheme for physeal fractures was proposed by Foucher in 1863.[66] In 1898, Poland advanced his four-part classification,[163] and Aitken in 1965 divided these fractures into three types (Fig. 2-5).[2] The Salter-Harris classification, presented in 1963, has been the most widely used.[175] It is based

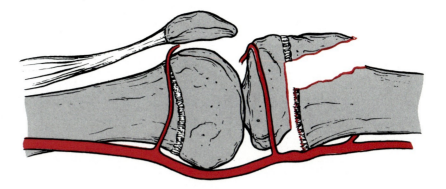

Figure 2–4

Displacement of fracture fragment may cause impingement, occlusion, intraluminal damage, or transection of the popliteal artery after posterior displacement of the tibia in Salter-Harris type I physeal injury.

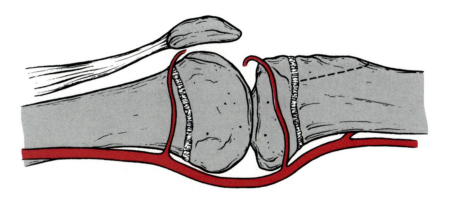

on the mechanism of injury, the relationship of the fracture line to various cellular layers of the physis, and the prognosis concerning subsequent growth disturbance.

This roentgenographic classification includes five types of fractures: type 1—complete separation of the epiphysis and physis from the metaphysis, with fracture through the zone of hypertrophic cells (Fig. 2–6); type 2—similar to type 1, except that a metaphyseal fragment is present on the compression side of the fracture (Thurston-Holland sign) (Fig. 2–7); type 3—physeal separation with fracture through the epiphysis into the joint (Fig. 2–8); type IV—fracture through the metaphysis, physis, and epiphysis and into the joint (Fig. 2–9); and type V—compression or crushing injury to the physis.

Rang added a type VI to the Salter-Harris classification[165]: avulsion injury to the peripheral portion of the physis, after which bony bridge formation may result in considerable angular deformity because of its peripheral location (Fig. 2–10). Weber added intraarticular and extraarticular designations to the Salter-Harris classification.[197]

Ogden included injuries to other growth mechanisms, such as the metaphysis, diaphysis, periosteum, zone of Ranvier, and perichondrium, in his extensive nine-part classification scheme, which follows (see Fig. 2–5).[144]

Type 1. The epiphysis and some of the contiguous physis separate from metaphysis with osseous fragments (type 1A); the fracture line undulates through a zone of hypertrophic cartilage cells; and there is little or no displacement of the epiphyseal fragment. Type 1B fractures occur in children with systemic disorders affecting the ossification of the metaphysis. Type 1C fractures have an associated injury to the germinal portion of the physis.

Type 2. This is the most common physeal injury. The line of fracture passes through hypertrophic and provisionally calcified zones; propagation across the physeal-metaphyseal junction is variable; a small, triangular metaphyseal fragment (Thurston-Holland sign) is diagnostic and displacement is variable. Type 2B involves further propagation of fracture forces on the tensile side to create a free metaphyseal fragment. Type 2C includes a thin layer of metaphysis along with, or instead of, the triangular fragment, traversing most of the metaphysis. Type 2D

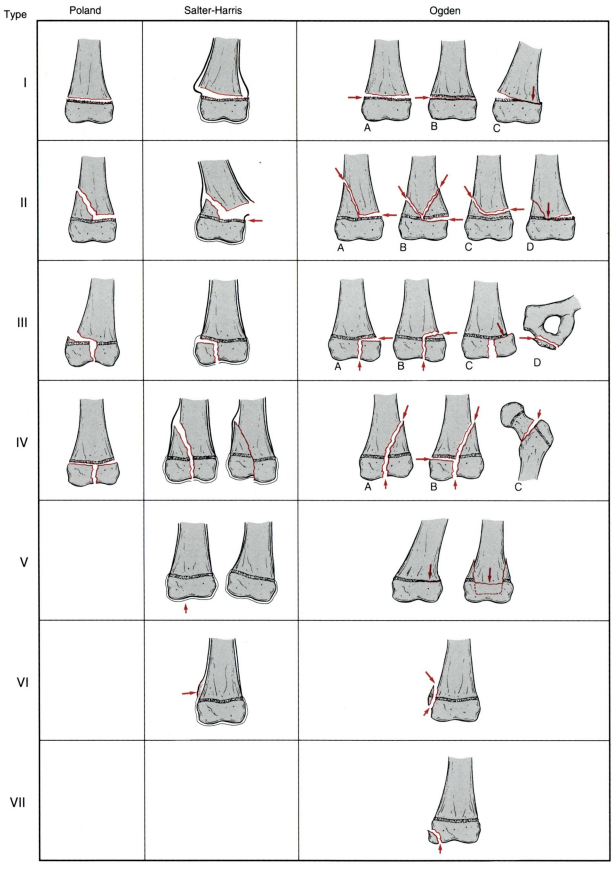

Figure 2–5

See legend on opposite page

Figure 2–6

Salter-Harris type I injury with physeal separation through zone of hypertrophic cells.

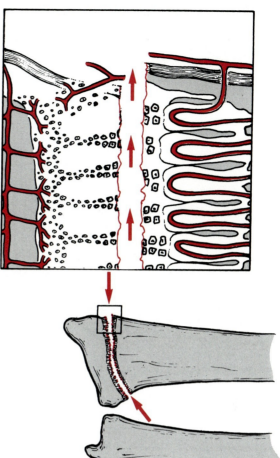

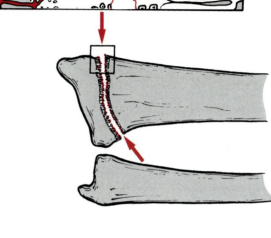

Figure 2–7

Salter-Harris type II injury is similar to type I but has metaphyseal spike.

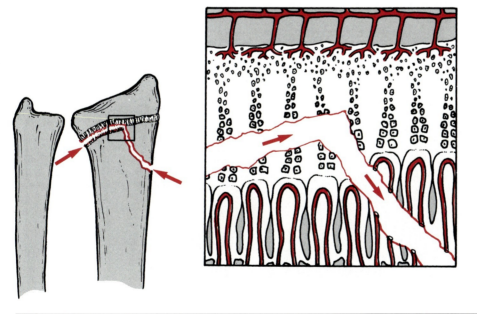

Figure 2–5

Classification of physeal injuries by Poland, Salter and Harris, Weber, and Ogden. All four systems are similar but from left to right are increasingly complex. The Salter-Harris classification is a refinement of Poland's system; the Weber classification adds extraarticular and intraarticular designations; Ogden's classification, which is all-inclusive, adds more subclasses. (From Canale, S. T. Fractures in children. In: Crenshaw, A. H., ed. Campbell's Operative Orthopaedics, ed 7. St. Louis, C. V. Mosby, 1987.)

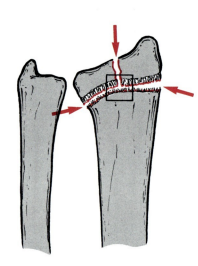
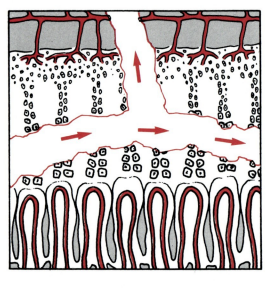

Figure 2–8
Salter-Harris type III injury with physeal separation and extension across epiphysis into joint.

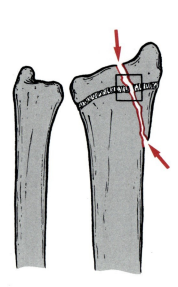
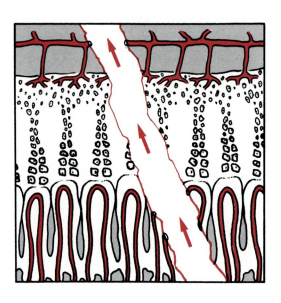

Figure 2–9
Salter-Harris type IV injury with metaphyseal spike; the physis and epiphysis are both involved.

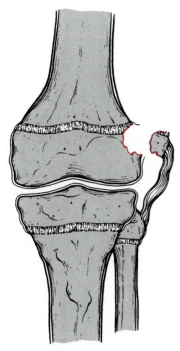

Figure 2–10

Example of type VI fracture, as described by Rang: avulsion of attachment of fibular collateral ligament at the physis, which can cause peripheral growth arrest and severe angular deformity. (Redrawn from Weber, B. G.; Brunner, C.; Freuler, F. Treatment of Fractures in Children and Adolescents. New York, Springer-Verlag, 1980.)

includes compression of the metaphysis into the physis.

Type 3. This lesion is an intraarticular fracture involving the epiphysis, with the plane of fracture occurring from the articular surface through the epiphysis, epiphyseal ossification center, and physis. In type 3A, the fracture line extends along the hypertrophic zone of the physis toward the periphery. In type 3B, transverse fracture propagation is through the primary spongiosa, leaving a thin layer of metaphyseal bone with the epiphyseal fragment. Type 3C includes injuries to epiphyses that have developed major contour changes, such as the ischial tuberosity, in which epiphyseal fracture propagation may not involve a joint (Fig. 2–11).

Type 4. The fracture line involves the articular surface, extends through the epiphysis, across the full thickness of the physis, and through a segment of the metaphysis (type 4A), causing a complete longitudinal split of all zones of the physis. In type 4B, further propagation of the fracture through the remaining portion of the physis creates an additional free fragment. In type 4C, the epiphyseal fracture propagates through radiolucent cartilage. Type 4D fracture results in multiple metaphyseal-physeal-epiphyseal fragments.

Type 5. A compression force is transmitted through segments of the epiphysis and physis, disrupting germinal regions of the chondrocytes and adjacent hypertrophic regions and damaging the vascular supply; this pattern is difficult, if not impossible, to appreciate on plain roentgenograms. Type 5 injuries include those caused by electrical shock, irradiation, and frostbite.

Type 6. This fracture involves the peripheral region of the physis, especially the zone of Ranvier, and may result from a glancing type of trauma primarily involving avulsion of overlying skin or subcutaneous tissue, such as might occur from a bicycle or lawnmower accident, deep extension of infection, or severe burn. Rang described this fracture as occurring in sports injuries secondary to avulsion of the ligamentous attachments adjacent to the physis.[165]

Type 7. These fractures are completely intra-epiphyseal, with propagation from the articular surface through the epiphyseal cartilage and into the secondary ossification center. Type 7A involves propagation of the fracture through both the epiphyseal and articular cartilage and the bone of the secondary ossification center (Fig. 2–12). Type 7B involves propagation of the fracture primarily through the cartilaginous portions, with involvement of some of the preossifying regions.

Type 8. These injuries affect metaphyseal growth and remodeling mechanisms and cause transient vascular compromise.

Type 9. This type comprises selective injuries to the diaphyseal growth mechanism of appositional, membranous bone formation from the periosteum. These injuries may be associated with severe fragmentation of portions of the diaphysis.

Several authors have devised classification schemes for specific anatomic locations: distal tibial injuries—Chadwick and Bentley[45]; tibial tuberosity fractures—Watson-Jones[196]; proximal humeral fractures—Neer and Horowitz[136]; lateral condylar fractures—Milch[132]; medial condylar fractures—Kilfoyle[101]; distal humeral epiphyseal separations—DeLee and co-workers[58]; olecranon epiphyseal fractures—Grantham and Kiernan[73] and Wilkins[200]; radial neck fractures—Vostal,[195] Newman,[138] O'Brien,[140] Jeffrey,[97] and Wilkins[200]; Monteggia fractures—Bado,[7] Wiley and Galey,[199] and Letts and co-workers[115]; thumb metacarpal fractures—O'Brien[139]; and phalangeal physeal fractures—Wood[204] and O'Brien.[139] More recently, Scu-

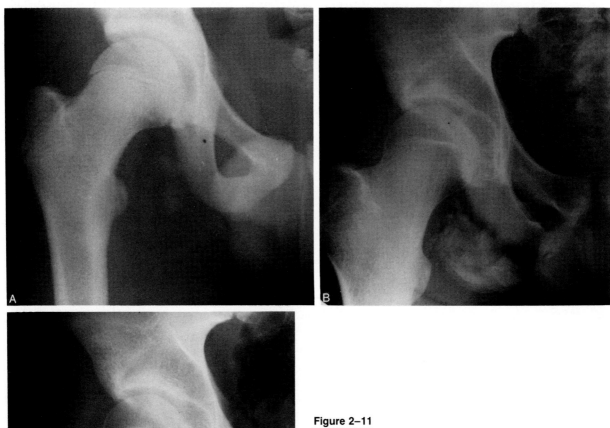

Figure 2-11

Ischial tuberosity fracture. *A,* Large avulsion of ischial tuberosity in a 13-year-old female. *B,* Six months after injury, large area of ossification. *C,* Three years after injury, ununited ischial tuberosity.

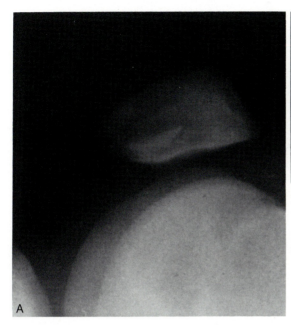
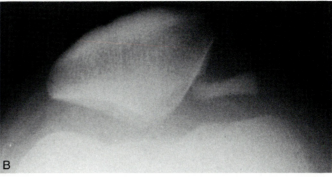

Figure 2–12

A–B, Osteochondral fracture of the patella in a child (Ogden type 7A).

deri and Bronson described a classification of triradiate cartilage fractures (Fig. 2–13).[178] These specific classification schemes are discussed in the chapters that deal with specific injuries.

For most physeal injuries, the Salter-Harris classification is adequate and is most easily applied. More complicated injuries may benefit by more specific classification according to one of the more detailed systems.

Diagnosis

HISTORY AND PHYSICAL EXAMINATION

Most patients with physeal injury relate a specific traumatic incident. Pain and localized tenderness are the most common symptoms. Swelling and effusion are variable signs, depending on the severity and anatomic location of the injury. Children, however, are not good historians, and physeal injuries can present in a variety of ways. In addition to specific trauma, the physes may be damaged by infection (Brodie's abscess), pathologic processes (tumor, pathologic fracture, chondromalacia, bone cyst), metabolic disease, congenital abnormalities such as neurofibromatosis or syphilis, endocrine disorders, or child abuse (Fig. 2–14).

RADIOGRAPHIC EVALUATION

Because of the chondro-osseous nature and the irregular contours of the physes, some acute physeal injuries are not clearly seen on plain roentgenograms. Slight widening of the physis may be the only sign of minimal displacement of an epiphyseal fragment. The small metaphyseal fragment (Thurston-Holland sign) may be difficult to appreciate. Two views taken at 90 degree planes to each other may help delineate the fracture, and comparison films of the opposite extremity are invaluable to determine if physeal injury has occurred. Oblique views may be helpful in injuries of the forearm or lower leg. Varus and valgus stress views are useful for injuries about the knee and elbow to demonstrate gapping between the epiphysis and metaphysis. Identical views of the contralateral extremity can help establish whether occult separation of the physis (Salter-Harris type I injury) has occurred.

SPECIAL STUDIES

Tomograms may be necessary in acute injuries to delineate fragmentation and orientation of fragments. The tomogram cuts should be made at 0.5 cm intervals rather than the standard 1 cm. Computed tomographic (CT) scanning, especially with sagittal and coronal reconstruction, may be necessary to determine the exact nature of severely comminuted epiphyseal and metaphyseal fractures that are not clearly seen on plain radiographic views. Nuclear bone scanning may not be especially helpful in physeal fractures because the physes are normally relatively active on nuclear scans of children; increased uptake may occur at several physes in an

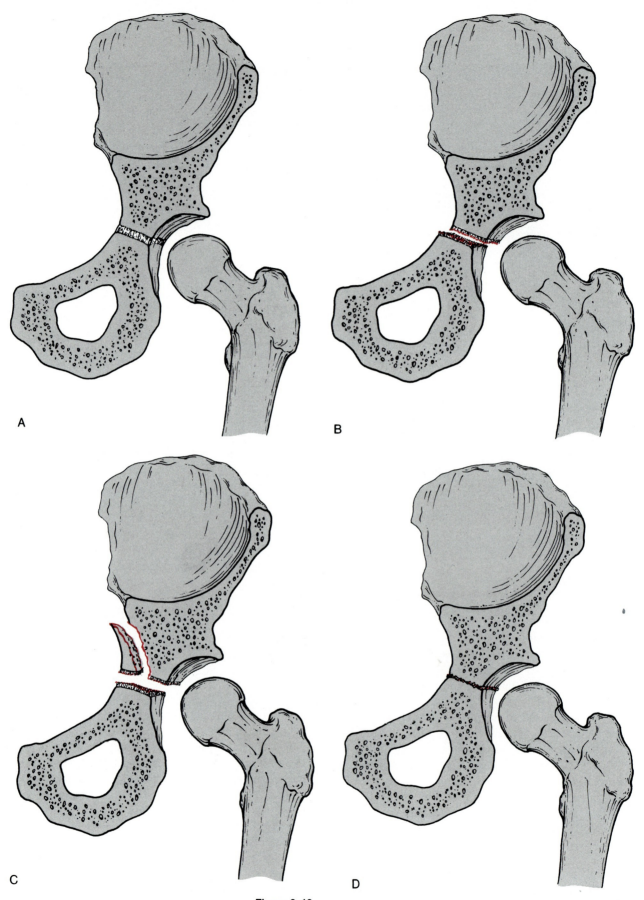

Figure 2-13

See legend on opposite page

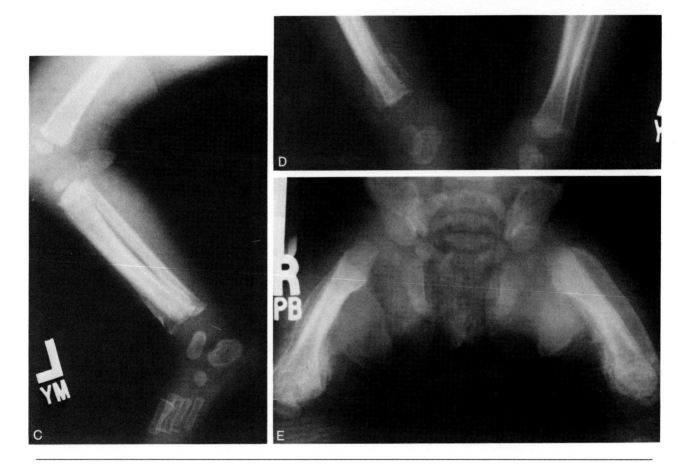

Figure 2–14

Physeal fractures caused by child abuse in an infant. *A,* Bilateral transepiphyseal hip fractures. *B,* Distal and proximal femoral physeal fractures. *C–D,* Distal tibial physeal fractures. *E,* Six months after injuries, with proliferative callus formation in femur.

Figure 2–13

Classification by Scuderi and Bronson of triradiate cartilage fractures. *A,* Normal; *B,* Salter I fracture; *C,* Salter II fracture; *D,* Salter V fracture. (From Scuderi, G.; Bronson, M. J. Triradiate cartilage injury; report of two cases and review of the literature. Clin Orthop 217:179, 1987.)

extremity secondary to trauma, infection, or neoplasm. Magnetic resonance imaging (MRI) has not proved reliable for evaluation of physeal injuries, except in the evaluation of avascular necrosis after separation of the capital femoral epiphysis. Ultrasound has been reported to document soft tissue injury without fracture; Boker and Burbach described the use of ultrasound for diagnosis of separation of the proximal humeral epiphysis in newborns.[18] Arthrography may be necessary to confirm suspected physeal injuries, especially in the hip and elbow. An arteriogram may be indicated if vascular injury is suspected.

DIFFERENTIAL DIAGNOSIS

Physeal fractures may be simulated by variations in normal growth patterns (Fig. 2–15), infection, congenital conditions, metabolic disorders, or neoplasms.

Management

The treatment of physeal injuries is based on the severity of the injury, its anatomic location, and the age of the patient. Many concepts of remodeling after angulation of a fracture have been described. Ryöppy and Karaharju listed several factors contributing to the remodeling process in a long bone, including asymmetric epiphyseal growth, changes in the process of resorption, and opposition in the metaphysis.[173] Longitudinal growth generally is accepted as a major modality of remodeling, as is the stimulation of growth by a diaphyseal fracture. Abraham demonstrated that after osteotomy the radius and tibia of an immature monkey remodeled 5 degrees each year until maturity and that the periosteum and growth plate contribute equally to the correction.[1] Valgus, varus, and flexion deformities corrected to the same degree. Epiphysiodesis of the adjacent physes did not prevent correction of the shaft of the bone. Remodeling of the osteotomy site was characterized radiographically by bone deposition on the concave side with no significant resorption on the convex side. Pauwels demonstrated that the physis responds eccentrically to change and pressure and that it will, through selective growth in different regions, attempt to remodel itself perpendicular to the major traction forces moving across the physis.[158] This characteristic may explain the gradual correction of some deformities, in accordance with the Heuter-Volkmann principle.

An injury that may cause disabling sequelae in a young child may result in little or no impairment in an adolescent nearing the end of skeletal growth. If a child has several years of growth remaining before closure of the physes, and if the epiphyses are still capable of growth, most deformities in the plane of motion of the joint will remodel.

Different physes have different growth potentials. Pritchett used teleroentgenograms of the upper extremities of 244 healthy, well-nourished children, taken at 6-month intervals from the age of 7 years until skeletal maturity, to determine the growth remaining at both physes of the humerus, radius, and ulna.[164] He determined that in this time span the humerus grows approximately 1.2 cm each year in girls and 1.3 cm in boys; the ulna grows approximately 1 cm each year in girls and 1.1 cm in boys; and the radius grows approximately 0.9 cm each year in girls and 1.0 cm in boys. These data allow accurate predictions of growth and growth discrepancy in the upper extremity and help determine more precisely the appropriate time for equalization procedures.

The greatest discrepancy between the physes of the same bone probably exists in the humerus. In this bone, the distal physis provides only 20% of the longitudinal growth and is therefore less capable of correcting angular deformity except in the sagittal plane. Conversely, the proximal physis provides 80% of the growth of the diaphysis and often can completely remodel the entire proximal humerus within a year. In the femur, the reverse is true. The distal physis contributes 70% of the growth of the femur, while the capital femoral physis contributes only 30% of the entire length of the femur. For this

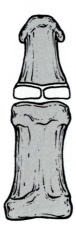

Figure 2–15

Fissuring of epiphysis of proximal phalanx of the great toe is not a fracture. (Redrawn from Lyritis, G. Developmental disorders of the proximal epiphysis of the hallux. Skeletal Radiol 10:250, 1983.)

reason, proximal femoral physeal arrest in the older child rarely causes significant leg length inequality and only minimal coxa vara deformity. Injury to the distal femoral physis may cause significant limb shortening and angulation. In the tibia, the proximal physis contributes considerably more growth than the distal physis; conversely, the distal radial physis contributes more growth than the proximal physis.

Most children's fractures heal twice as fast as adults' fractures, and most purely epiphyseal separations heal in half the time of a long bone fracture in a child. Thus, whereas an adult tibial fracture may require 12 to 18 weeks for healing, the same fracture in a child may require only 6 to 9 weeks, and a purely epiphyseal separation only 3 to 5 weeks. Supracondylar femoral fractures in adults may require 20 weeks for healing, whereas in children 8 to 10 weeks are sufficient. Only 5 to 6 weeks of immobilization usually are required for Salter-Harris type I or II fractures of the distal femoral physis.

The time between injury and initial treatment is also an important factor. For closed reductions, the injury ideally should be only several hours old. When the injury is several days old, the decision must be made as to whether the deformity is sufficient to warrant an initial reduction or, if the original reduction has been lost, whether a second closed reduction is indicated. The age of the patient, the severity of the deformity, and the plane of the deformity should all be considered. The younger the patient, the more correction that can be anticipated, especially if the angulation is in the plane of flexion or extension.

Establishing the time of the last oral intake of the child also is important in deciding whether general anesthesia is feasible. Serious complications from aspiration have been reported when a child with a full stomach is anesthetized for reduction of a closed fracture, which may have been unnecessary. Although regional anesthesia, such as axillary blocks or Bier blocks, is difficult in children, it may be supplemented with a "pediatric cocktail." Often, for simple epiphyseal separations, no anesthesia is preferable to multiple anesthetic injections into the fracture site. In any case, a gentle reduction is mandatory. Traction rather than forceful manipulation should be used to avoid physeal damage. Multiple attempts at closed reduction should be avoided. If, under local or regional anesthesia, the fracture cannot be reduced with one or two gentle attempts, closed reduction with general anesthesia should be considered. If significant deformity persists after closed reduction, especially of Salter-Harris types III and IV injuries, open reduction and internal fixation may be indicated.

If open reduction and internal fixation are indicated, the periosteum around the epiphysis may be resected for better exposure and more accurate reduction; however, the fragment should not be completely denuded of soft tissue attachments, through which it receives its blood supply. If the periosteum is elevated near the epiphysis, Bright recommends carefully resecting for about 1 cm on either side of the physis to prevent bony bridge formation between the epiphysis and metaphysis.

Treatment of specific physeal injuries is described in later chapters; general guidelines are given here based on the Salter-Harris classification of physeal fractures.

Type I (separation of the epiphysis from the metaphysis) injuries usually can be treated with closed reduction and casting because the periosteal sleeve generally is intact. At sites where the periosteum is thin (such as the femur or radius), internal fixaton may be required after open or closed reduction. Occasionally, closed reduction cannot be obtained because of interposed periosteum (medial malleolus) or muscle or tendon (deltoid or biceps in the proximal humerus).

Type II (fracture-separation of the epiphysis, fracture of metaphysis) fractures usually can be reduced closed by using the intact hinge of periosteum.

Types III and IV (intraarticular fracture involving the physis, epiphysis, and metaphysis) fractures require anatomic reduction, usually involving open reduction and internal fixation with smooth pins that avoid the physis.

Type V (compression) fractures rarely are diagnosed acutely, and treatment is delayed until the development of a bony bridge across the physis is apparent.

Some important points to remember in the treatment of physeal injuries include the following:

1. Often displacement is minimal or absent; however, if there is any doubt, the extremity should be splinted and the injury reexamined at 1 or 2 weeks for periosteal reaction indicating a Salter-Harris type I physeal injury.

2. When attempting closed reduction through manipulation and traction, great care must be taken to obtain a gentle reduction with the musculature as relaxed as possible to avoid "grating" the physis on metaphyseal or epiphyseal fragments. To avoid physeal damage, the reduction should be 75% traction and 25% manipulation.

3. Restoration of the congruency of both the

32   2 / Physeal Injuries

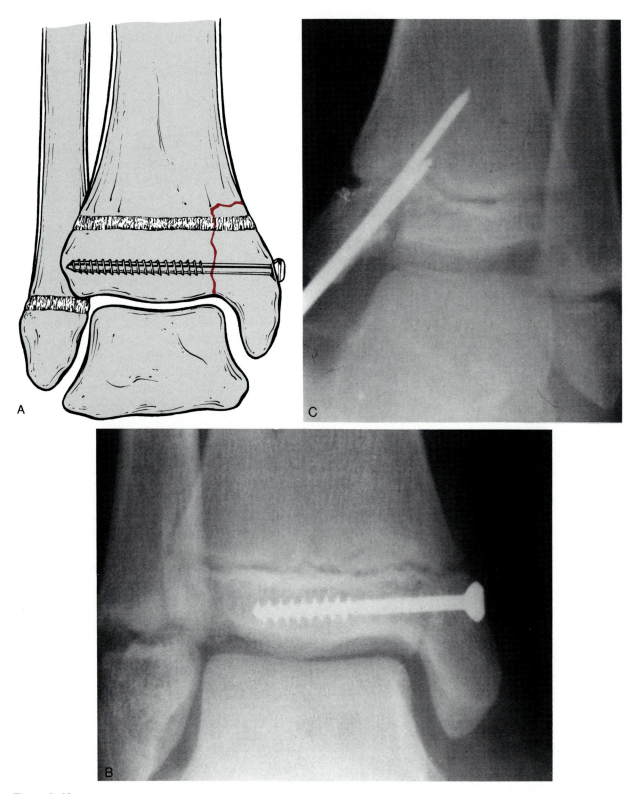

Figure 2–16

A, Cancellous screw should be placed in the epiphysis only, parallel to the physis. B, Roentgenogram showing screw in place. C, Smooth pins may cross the physis, as in this Salter-Harris type III fracture, even though parallel transverse pins are preferred when possible.

articular surface and the physis is essential if it has been disrupted, especially in young children. After a Salter-Harris type I or II injury without intraarticular disruption and in the plane of motion of the joint, a considerable amount of remodeling can be expected; a less than satisfactory reduction can and should be accepted in preference to repeated attempts at reduction that may damage the germinal cells of the physis. No definite degree of angulation can be called acceptable in children's fractures. In general, greater angular deformity can be tolerated in the upper extremity than in the lower; more valgus deformity can be tolerated than varus deformity; and more flexion deformity can be tolerated than extension deformity. In the lower extremity, more deformity can be tolerated proximally than distally (the same varus angle in the hip can be better compensated than in the knee and is least compensated in the ankle). Spontaneous correction of angular deformities is greatest when the angulation is in the plane of motion of a nearby hinged joint; for example, in fractures just proximal to the knee, elbow, or wrist, angulation with its apex toward the flexor aspect of the joint usually results in surprisingly little deformity. Function usually returns to normal unless the fracture occurs near the end of growth. Angulation in any other direction probably will persist to some extent. Rotational deformities are permanent.

4. The undulating contours of the physes must be borne in mind. Before open reduction and internal fixation are undertaken, the surgical approaches to and anatomy of the physes should be known. Birch and colleagues have published an excellent description of major physes and the most appropriate approach to each.[15]

5. Internal fixation should be adequate—but not more than necessary—and should be easily removable.

6. Smooth rather than threaded pins should be used, and the physis should be avoided if possible (Fig. 2–16A); pins should parallel the physis in the epiphysis and metaphysis. Smooth oblique pins should be inserted across the physis only if satisfactory internal fixation cannot be achieved with transverse fixation (Fig. 2–16B). Bostman and co-workers reported the experimental use of biodegradable pins (cylindrical rods made of polylactide-glycolide

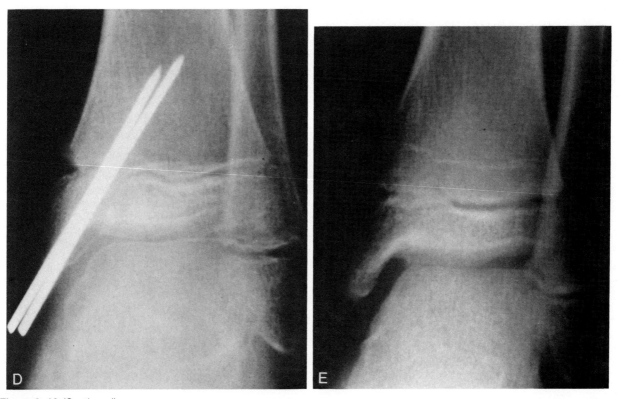

Figure 2–16 *(Continued)*

D, At the time of union and pin removal. *E,* At 2 years, symmetric growth (note parallel "injury line" proximally) and no bony bridge formation. (*B–E* from Canale, S. T.; Beaty, J. H., eds. Operative Pediatric Orthopaedics. St. Louis, Mosby-Yearbook, 1991.)

copolymer) for transepiphyseal fracture fixation, thus avoiding the need for removal of implants.[19] They reported the use of this device in three supracondylar fractures of the elbow and three fractures of the physes of the first metatarsal, distal tibia, and medial humeral epicondyle. Preliminary results at 1 year show no evidence of growth impairment or failure of fixation. The authors believe that because the cross-sectional area of the pin is only 1.8 mm, which falls within the experimentally observed safe limit of 3% of the physis, this device will not damage the physis; conclusive evidence requires larger numbers of patients and longer follow-up, however.

7. Neurovascular status must be carefully evaluated before treatment, after treatment, and during convalescence. Unfortunately, uncertainty about the neurovascular status of an extremity before treatment and resultant neurovascular compromise after treatment are common and can cause medicolegal problems.

8. Parents should be warned of the possibility of complications such as bony bridge formation, angular deformity, and avascular necrosis.

9. Long-term follow-up is essential to determine if complications will occur. All physeal separations, regardless of type, should be checked within the first week after reduction to ensure that reduction has not been lost or to allow a second reduction, if necessary, before healing has occurred. After 7 to 14 days, Salter-Harris types I and II fractures generally can be expected to heal without loss of reduction. Salter-Harris types III and IV fractures treated with closed reduction should be carefully examined every 5 to 7 days for the first 3 weeks to be sure

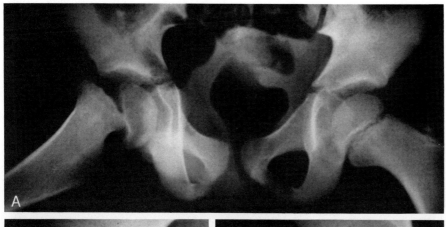
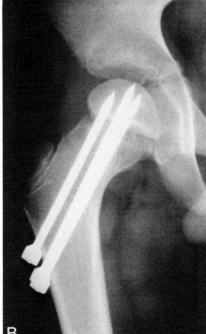
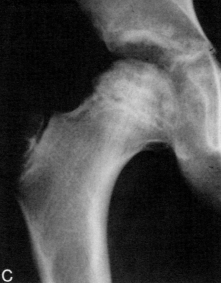

Figure 2–17

A, Type I transepiphyseal fracture in a 6-year-old child. *B*, After closed reduction and fixation with smooth pins. *C*, One year after fracture, pins have been removed and avascular necrosis has developed.

that fracture fragments are not displaced. If adequate radiographs cannot be made through the plaster cast, the cast should be removed. Depending on the type and location of the fracture, long-term follow-up is essential. Parents should be informed of the possibility of growth arrest and angulation deformity, and the importance of returning for follow-up examination at 6 to 12 months should be emphasized. At long-term follow-up, Harris growth lines should be examined to make sure that they are parallel to the physis (see further on).

Characteristics of Some Commonly Injured Physes

Proximal Femur. In epiphyseal separations of the hip joint, with or without displacement of the fragment from the acetabulum, avascular necrosis will occur in a large percentage of patients regardless of treatment (Fig. 2–17). In older children (10 years and above) closed reduction and pinning can be performed; premature physeal closure causes little limb length discrepancy.

Distal Femur. Salter-Harris types III and IV fractures of the distal femoral physis often cause significant shortening and angular deformity. Type II lesions, which usually are benign lesions in other physes, are especially prone to complications such as premature physeal closure. The portion of the physis attached to the metaphyseal fragment does not fuse prematurely or form bony bridges, whereas the unattached portion may.

Proximal Tibia. Unrecognized Salter-Harris type III fractures cause premature physeal closure with resulting varus or valgus deformity. Anterior closure results in hyperextension deformity. Salter-Harris type I or II fractures with posterior displacement may cause catastrophic vascular compromise of the popliteal vessels. Chow and co-workers reported 16 patients with avulsion fractures of the proximal tubercle, two thirds of which were Salter-Harris types I and II injuries and were treated conservatively; type III fractures involving the knee joint were internally fixed.[48] Final results were good in all patients, except for minor complications such as a prominent, uncomfortable tibial tubercle (Fig. 2–18).

Distal Tibia. Salter-Harris types III and IV fractures almost always occur at the medial plafond. Fixation should be obtained with transverse pins through the epiphysis or metaphyseal spike; oblique pins may cause premature physeal closure and bony bridge formation. After reviewing Salter-Harris type IV fractures of the distal tibial physis, with emphasis on those involving the medial malleolus, Cass and Peterson recommended open reduction and internal fixation because of severe complications of displaced fractures.[42] Fixation should be with smooth Kirschner wires or screws that do not cross the physis but traverse only the metaphysis and epiph-

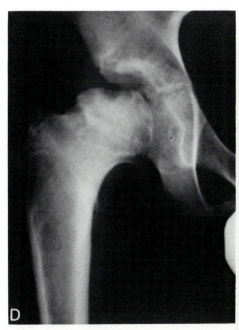
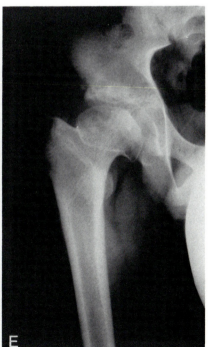

Figure 2–17 (Continued)

D, During course of abduction treatment. E, Four years after treatment for avascular necrosis, the femoral neck is short because of premature physeal closure; however, the head is reasonably well shaped and the result is acceptable. (From Canale, S. T.; Beaty, J. H., eds. Operative Pediatric Orthopaedics. St. Louis, Mosby-Yearbook, 1991.)

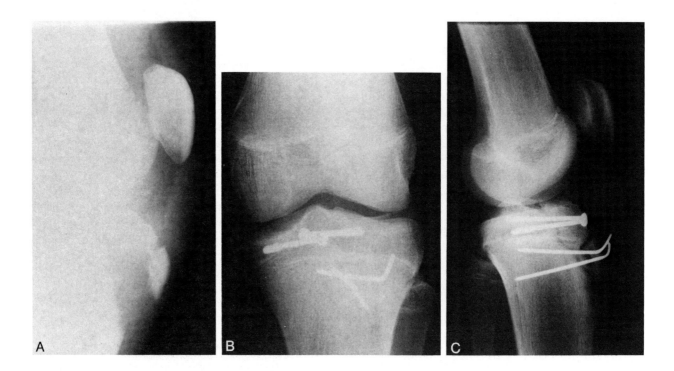

Figure 2-18

A, Severe Salter-Harris type III or IV fracture of proximal tibial physis. *B-C,* After open reduction and internal fixation.

ysis (Fig. 2-19). Types I and II fractures usually can be treated closed. However, if a large fragment of periosteum is caught in the fracture site, preventing adequate reduction and resulting in an unacceptable varus or valgus deformity, open reduction and internal fixation may be necessary (Fig. 2-20).

Proximal Humerus. Fractures at this location most commonly are Salter-Harris type II injuries, occur in younger children, and will remodel satisfactorily (Fig. 2-21A). Baxter and Wiley reviewed 57 fractures of the proximal humeral physis and found that, regardless of treatment, the maximum shortening of the humerus was 2 cm and residual varus angulation was insignificant.[12] They believe that manipulation of displaced fresh fractures does not improve humeral growth or function and that open reduction generally is not indicated. Open or percutaneous pin fixation is rarely necessary except when soft tissue (such as the deltoid, biceps tendon, or periosteum) is interposed in the fracture site (Fig. 2-21B).

Distal Humerus. Fracture-separation of the entire

Figure 2-19

A, Salter-Harris type IV fracture of distal tibial physis. *B,* After open reduction and internal fixation with cancellous screws.

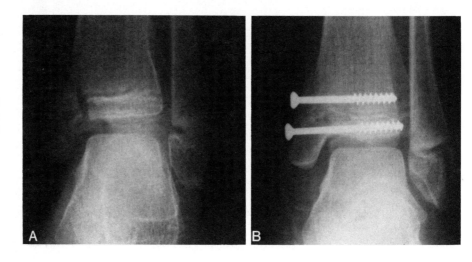

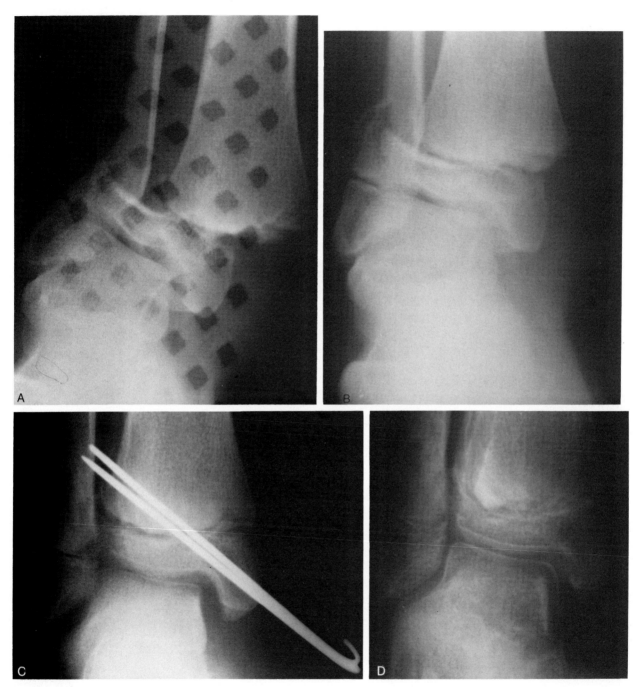

Figure 2-20

A, Salter-Harris type I fracture of distal tibial physis in an older child. B, After closed reduction, residual angulation is 17 degrees. C, Following open reduction and internal fixation with smooth pins; flap of periosteum was found caught in fracture. D, At early follow-up there was no evidence of bony bridge. (From Canale, S. T.; Beaty, J. H., eds. Operative Pediatric Orthopaedics. St. Louis, Mosby-Yearbook, 1991.)

38 2 / Physeal Injuries

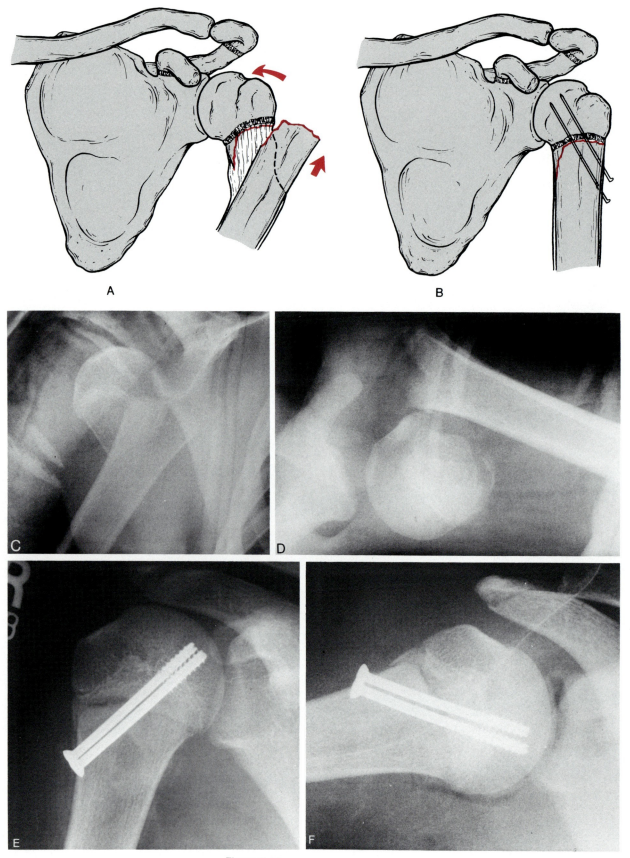

Figure 2–21

See legend on opposite page

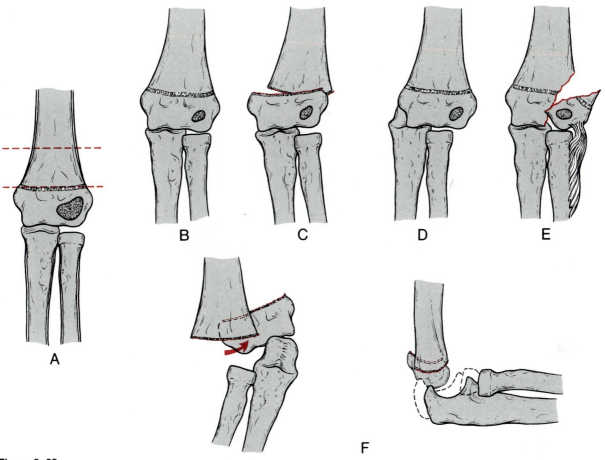

Figure 2–22

Elbow injuries that may be confused clinically. *A,* Horizontal lines indicate area proximally where supracondylar fracture occurs, and distally where epiphyseal fracture-separation occurs in wide part of the distal humerus in young children. *B,* Normal elbow before three centers of ossification appear. *C,* Separation of entire distal humeral epiphysis. *D,* Dislocation of elbow. *E,* Fracture of lateral condyle. *F,* Fracture-separation of entire distal humeral epiphysis displaced posteromedially; note radial head and proximal ulna displacing as a unit in relation to the distal humerus. (*A–E* redrawn from Mizuno, K.; Hirohata, K.; Kashiwagi, D. Fracture-separation of the distal humeral epiphysis in young children. J Bone Joint Surg 61A:570, 1979. *F* redrawn from Barrett, W. P.; Almquist, E. A.; Staheli, L. T. Fracture separation of the distal humeral physis in the newborn. J Pediatr Orthop 4:618, 1984.)

distal humerus should not be confused with elbow dislocation or fracture of the lateral condyle (Fig. 2–22). Lateral condylar fractures almost always require open reduction and internal fixation (Fig. 2–23). Rutherford reported 39 lateral humeral condylar fractures treated with open reduction and internal fixation.[172] He found that physeal arrest was rare despite malreduction and that the fishtail deformity commonly associated with malreduction did not necessarily predict avascular necrosis.

Medial epicondylar fractures are relatively uncommon. Fracture fragments may be caught in the joint after elbow dislocation but generally can be reduced with closed maneuvers (Fig. 2–24). Salter-Harris types I and II fractures of the radial neck usually can be treated closed with manual reduction

Figure 2–21

A, Remodeling potential of proximal humeral epiphyseal fracture because of periosteal sleeve. *B,* Closed reduction and percutaneous pinning of proximal humeral epiphyseal separation: Two wires cross physis. *C–D,* Anteroposterior and lateral views of displaced proximal humeral fracture in unacceptable position. *E–F,* After limited open reduction and internal fixation. (*A* redrawn from Ogden, J. A. Skeletal Injury in the Child. Philadelphia, Lea & Febiger, 1982. *B* redrawn from Magerl, F. Fractures of the proximal humerus. In: Weber, B. G.; Brunner, C.; Freuler, F., eds. Treatment of Fractures in Children and Adolescents. Berlin, Springer-Verlag, 1980.)

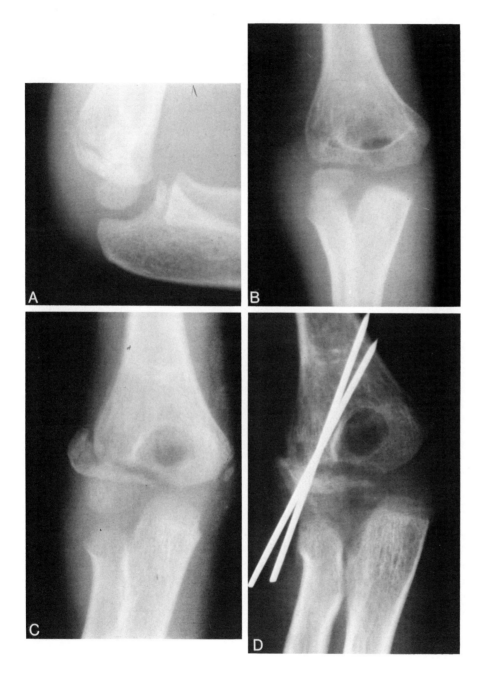

Figure 2–23

A–B, Undisplaced lateral condylar fracture was treated in long arm cast. *C,* "Jones view" at 3 weeks shows displacement.

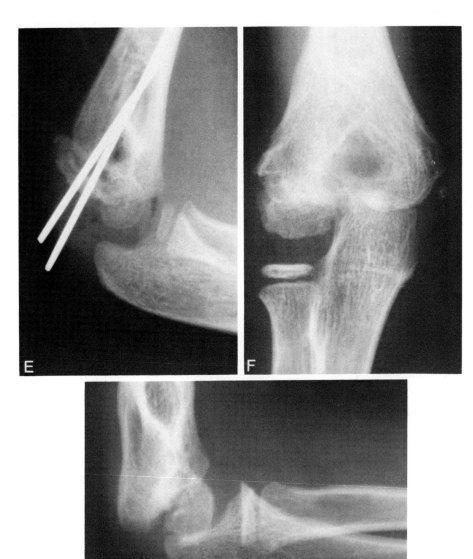

Figure 2–23 *Continued*

D–E, Following open reduction and fixation with smooth wires. *F–G,* At 6 months, wires have been removed and union is complete. (From Canale, S. T.; Beaty, J. H., eds. Operative Pediatric Orthopaedics. St. Louis, Mosby-Yearbook, 1991.)

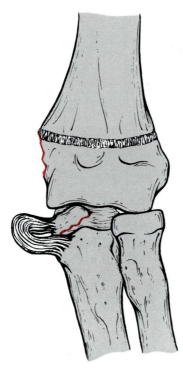

Figure 2–24

Medial epicondylar fracture fragment may be entrapped in joint after reduction of elbow dislocation.

or manipulation with a percutaneous pin to achieve an acceptable position of less than 45 degrees of angulation. Papavasiliou and associates reported 15 medial epicondylar fractures; displaced fractures were treated with open reduction and Kirschner wire fixation, and undisplaced fractures were immobilized in plaster.[155] Both methods produced good results. If open reduction and internal fixation are indicated, adequate fixation should be used to maintain the reduction. Normal secondary ossification centers of the olecranon should not be confused with physeal fractures (Fig. 2–25). Significant olecranon physeal fractures should be treated as in adults. Closed treatment by lengthy immobilization with the arm in extension to allow apposition and healing may permanently impair flexion of the elbow.

Distal Radius. Most Salter-Harris types I and II fractures in this area can be reduced by closed manipulation; the periosteal hinge that is usually present allows easy closed reduction. Rarely, a periosteal flap may prevent reduction, and open reduction and internal fixation may be necessary. Conversely, both-bone fractures of the distal forearm may be completely displaced and difficult to "hook on" with closed methods.

Complications

GROWTH ACCELERATION

Fracture of the physis with displacement of the epiphysis rarely may result in accelerated growth of the affected bone. Because of the rapid healing of the physis, increased vascular response to injury usually is briefer than after other fractures, and increased growth rarely is significant. Growth acceleration after physeal injury may be associated with the use of implants or fixation devices that may stimulate longitudinal growth. For the rare limb length discrepancy caused by accelerated growth that requires treatment, epiphysiodesis may be performed in young patients, or a shortening procedure may be done in skeletally mature patients.

GROWTH ARREST

Complete cessation of growth after physeal injury is uncommon. If it occurs near the end of skeletal growth, it causes no significant impairment. In younger patients, however, complete physeal arrest may lead to a substantial limb length discrepancy. The younger the child, the greater the problem. In adolescents, epiphysiodesis of the contralateral physis may be indicated if this can be done without producing disproportionate extremities. If more than 6 cm of correction is required, epiphysiodesis probably is not indicated. If epiphysiodesis is not feasible, a lengthening procedure may be considered. Ilizarov[95] and De Bastiani and co-workers[56] have described a technique of limb lengthening by slow distraction using a dynamic axial fixator (cal-

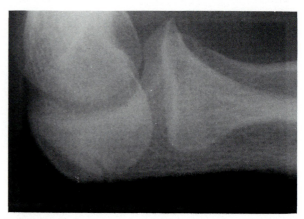

Figure 2–25

Delayed fusion of secondary ossification center may be confused with olecranon fracture. (From Canale, S. T.; Beaty, J. H., eds. Operative Pediatric Orthopaedics. St. Louis, Mosby-Yearbook, 1991.)

lotasis). Callus is formed in response to proximal submetaphyseal corticotomy when distraction is begun 2 weeks later. Once the desired length is obtained, the fixator is worn without distraction until callus formation is evident on radiographs. De Bastiani and associates reported mean lengthening of 22% in 100 bony segments in 50 patients with limb length inequality and in 23 with achondroplasia.[56]

These investigators also reported lengthening by chondrodiastasis or controlled symmetric distraction of the physis with the dynamic axial fixator.[57] Fjeld and Steen, however, noted growth retardation after experimental lengthening by physeal distraction.[65] In 7 of their 22 animal models, the physes of the lengthened bones appeared to close earlier than those of the controls, and growth retardation ranging from 40% to 70% occurred in all animals. They concluded that physeal distraction is a valid method of limb lengthening but appears to have a consistently harmful effect on the physis and should be used only in patients near skeletal maturity. Transplantation of a physis on a vascular pedicle has been reported, but this is not a well-established option.

Premature partial arrest of growth of a physis produces angular and longitudinal abnormalities of the involved bone and is much more common than complete growth arrest. The partial arrest occurs when a bridge of bone forms across the physis from the metaphysis to the epiphysis. This bar tethers growth in one area, and as the remaining physis grows, angular deformity occurs. The size and location of the bar determine the clinical deformity.

Any injury to the physeal cells may cause formation of a bony bar. The most common cause is fracture, although infection, tumors, irradiation, thermal burns, and metal implants across the physis also may result in bony bar formation. Some authors have suggested factors such as neural and vascular abnormalities, reduced vascular supply from any cause, and metabolic abnormalities. The most common sites of bony bars are the proximal tibial and distal femoral physes, which account for 60% and 70% of the growth of their respective bones.

Clinical signs of bony bar formation usually are angular deformity and shortening of the involved extremity. Growth disturbance lines (Harris lines), associated with episodes of illness or injury in children and adolescents, appear in the long bones after shaft fractures. Fractures of the femur, tibia, or fibula cause growth disturbance lines at all the fast-growing physes in both the fractured and the contralateral extremities.[72] O'Brien and colleagues related the appearance of these lines to the condition of the physis.[141] Hynes and O'Brien described Harris lines after injury to the distal tibial physis and related their appearance to the prognosis of these injuries.[94] Closure of the periphery of the physis or partial arrest after trauma results in a tilt deformity of the extremity; analysis of the character and displacement of Harris lines aids in the diagnosis of physeal arrest. The sclerotic line first appears 6 to 12 weeks after fracture. If the line extends across the width of the metaphysis parallel to the physis in both planes, growth of the entire physis is likely (Fig. 2–26). Focal defects in the line may indicate areas of growth impairment. If the line remains parallel to the physis, angular deformity is unlikely. An oblique line, not parallel to the physis, is an early warning that growth arrest, especially at the periphery, may occur. If the entire physis is involved, comparison of the location of the Harris lines in the injured extremity with those in the contralateral extremity and adjacent physis is also helpful.

In addition to routine radiographs, scanograms should be obtained to document lengths of the extremities. Bone age must be determined to assess the potential for remaining growth. Huurman and colleagues reported a simple, rapid, and accurate method for measuring limb length discrepancies with computed tomography (CT).[93] With their technique, the patient receives less radiation; some of the computation errors are eliminated; the cost is comparable to that of scanograms; and joint contractures do not prohibit accurate measurements. Polytomograms are helpful to determine the configuration and area involved by the bony bar and to delineate the configuration and area of the remaining normal physis.

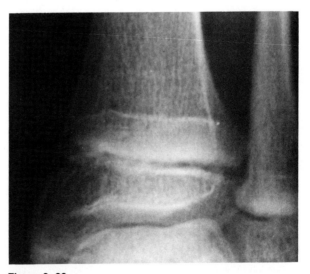

Figure 2–26

Growth disturbance line parallel to physis indicates no partial or total growth arrest.

Carlson and Wenger described a method for producing a schematic cross-sectional map on graph paper from data obtained from biplane polytomography (Fig. 2–27).[40] They report that this map helps identify the lesions that should be treated surgically and aids in planning the surgical approach and resection. They advise that the best results are obtained when 2 years of longitudinal growth remain and the physeal bar involves less than half the physis. Broughton and co-workers reported the results of epiphyseolysis (bony bar resection) in 13 children with partial growth arrest, eight of whom were followed to skeletal maturity and the other five for at least 4 years.[27] They found epiphyseolysis most effective for small bars and those affecting only the central area of the physis. Ogden has noted that if more than 40% to 50% of the area of the physis is involved with a bony bridge, an acceptable result is unlikely.[145] Surgery must be done meticulously and requires familiarity with physeal anatomy in general and the specific anatomy of the bony bridge to be treated.

Treatment of bony bars depends on the age of the patient, the specific physis, and the area of the physis involved. In adolescents with little remaining growth, observation may be the best treatment. In younger patients with significant growth remaining, surgical options include (1) arrest of the remaining growth of the injured physis, which should be considered in older children with mild angular deformity and expected minor limb length discrepancy; (2) arrest of the remaining physis and of the physis of the adjacent bone; (3) arrest of the remaining growth of the injured physis, the physis of the adjacent bone, and the corresponding physes of the contralateral bones; (4) combinations of physeal arrests with opening or closing wedge osteotomies to correct angular deformity; (5) opening or closing wedge osteotomy without physeal arrests, which may require several osteotomies because of recurrence of the deformity; (6) lengthening or shortening of the involved bone (shortening should be considered only for the femur); (7) resection of the bony bar and insertion of interposition material; (8) resection of the bony bar and osteotomy for correction of angular deformity; and (9) various combinations of these techniques.

Bright has classified partial growth arrest into three types, according to location and treatment: type I—peripheral; type II—central; and type III—combined.[22] Type I lesions can be approached through a peripheral incision; the periosteum is elevated and the bony bridge resected through a small window (Fig. 2–28). Type II lesions require a

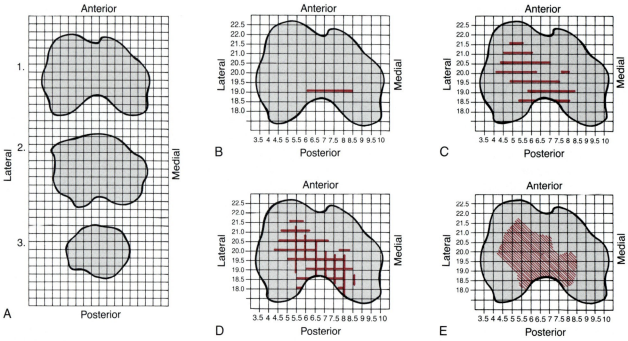

Figure 2–27

Carlson and Wenger method of mapping physeal bars. *A*, Outlines: 1, Distal femoral physis; 2, proximal tibial physis; 3, distal tibial physis. *B*, Anteroposterior projection level indicated by thick straight line. *C*, All anteroposterior levels plotted from tomograms. *D*, Lateral projection levels plotted. *E*, Final cross-sectional map of physeal bar. (Redrawn from Carlson, W. O.; Wenger, D. R. A mapping method to prepare for surgical excision of a partial physeal arrest. J Pediatr Orthop 4:232, 1984.)

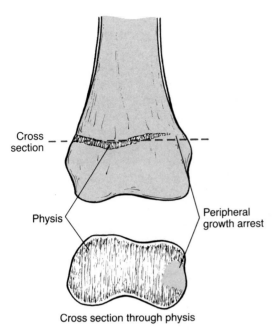

Figure 2–28

Type I peripheral growth arrest may cause rapid angular deformity. (Redrawn from Bright, R. W. Physeal injuries. In: Rockwood, C. A., Jr.; Wilkins, K. E.; King, R. E., eds. Fractures in Children. Philadelphia, J. B. Lippincott, 1984.)

more extensive and difficult approach. The skin incision is the same, but the periosteal flap is kept entirely on the metaphyseal side of the physis. A metaphyseal window is made close to the bony bridge, through which it is removed with a curette and dental burr (Fig. 2–29). Type III lesions cause extensive angular deformities and require removal of the bony bridge and osteotomy for correction (Fig. 2–30). According to Bright, varus or valgus angulation of 15 degrees or less does not require corrective osteotomy in young children if adequate bony bridge resection is accomplished. Both Bright[22] and Langenskiold[107] recommend osteotomy for angulation only if it is more than 25 to 30 degrees for deformities in the plane of motion of the adjacent joint (Fig. 2–31). Bright reports that angular deformities correct within a year of restoration of longitudinal growth and more quickly if the deformity is in the plane of joint motion.[22]

Resection with interposition material to prevent bony bar formation was evaluated experimentally by Peterson.[160] Among those interposition materials tested were gold leaf, rubber film, Gelfoam, bone wax, methylmethacrylate, muscle, fat, and cartilage. Results of his study and those of other authors, including Langenskiold and Bright, are varied, but evidence suggests that formation of the bony bar can be prevented or inhibited by the use of fat or other interposition materials; conversely, when no interposition material is used, bar formation recurs consistently. Peterson reported the successful use of methylmethacrylate with barium (Cranioplast) as an interposition material in 68 patients.[160] Olin and associates developed a procedure for transplanting free autogenous iliac crest physeal grafts into defects in the lateral aspect of the distal femoral physes of rabbits.[153] The transplant was composed of a fibrocartilaginous layer, cartilage similar to the physeal cartilage, and a physis. Their results showed that such a transplant can prevent bony bridge formation, growth arrest, or development of a valgus deformity when placed in the lateral femoral condyle after excision of a focal bony bridge.

Langenskiold and co-workers reported that osseous cavities of skeletally immature pigs filled with autogenous fat elongated with growth and, as the cavity elongated, the fat expanded to fill the defect.[109, 110] Histologic analysis demonstrated living adipose tissue, which has been shown to have an inhibitory effect on osteogenesis. Langenskiold also prefers fat for interposition, believing that the chemical and physical properties of fat contribute more than simple interposition to prevent recurrence of the bony bridge.[107, 108] Ogden has reported the use

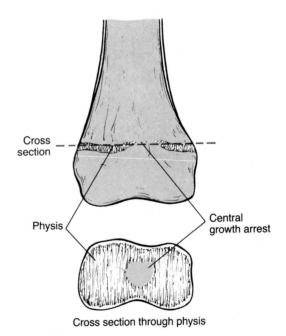

Figure 2–29

Type II central growth arrest with physeal tenting into metaphysis; entire perichondrial ring is open and intact to provide longitudinal growth. (Redrawn from Bright, R. W. Physeal injuries. In: Rockwood, C. A., Jr.; Wilkins, K. E.; King, R. E., eds. Fractures in Children, Philadelphia, J. B. Lippincott, 1984.)

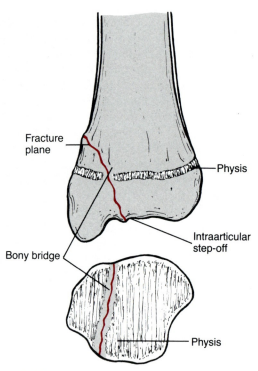

Figure 2–30

Type III combined growth arrest usually follows Salter-Harris type III or IV fracture that was incompletely reduced. (Redrawn from Bright, R. W. Physeal injuries. In: Rockwood, C. A., Jr.; Wilkins, K. E.; King, R. E., eds. Fractures in Children. Philadelphia, J. B. Lippincott, 1984.)

of fat interposition in open reduction and internal fixation of acute Salter-Harris type IV fractures.[144] He recommends, in addition to fat interposition, removal of the metaphyseal side of the small type IV fracture fragment (Thurston-Holland sign), especially at the malleoli, to convert the fracture to a type III and help prevent bony bridge formation. Enough fat usually can be taken at the edge of the operative site, but when the bridge resection is large, fat may be taken from the gluteal area.

Physeal transfer may someday offer a method of replacing the damaged physis. Lalanandham and associates monitored the viability and metabolism of cartilage transplanted to the physeal regions of rabbits.[106] In addition to measuring growth, they performed histochemical and autoradiographic studies. Their results indicated that avascular cartilage transplants could remain viable, could synthesize proteoglycan, and were associated with growth, although less than normal growth. Nettelblad and co-workers, in 1984, showed that free microvascular physeal transfers were superior to nonmicrovascular transfers in rabbits.[137] They found that a vascularized physeal graft could be transplanted from its normal site to the contralateral site with maintenance of normal growth capacity. However, they believe that clinical applications are minimal until further investigations determine how the transplanted physis reacts when transferred to a heterotopic anatomic site with altered stresses. More recently, Bowen and colleagues developed a method for transferring the metaphysis and epiphysis of the distal ulna in dogs and microsurgically revascularizing them from the pedicle of the anterior interosseous vessels.[20] When both circulations were revascularized, the grafts retained their structural integrity and growth continued at rates only slightly lower than normal (mean of 85%). If either or both circulations were not revascularized, growth rates were lower and skeletal collapse of the ischemic bone was frequent. These

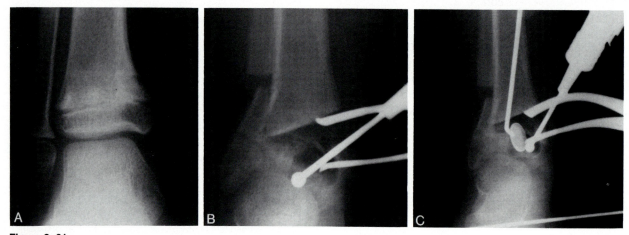

Figure 2–31

A, Bony bridge in distal tibial epiphysis causing varus deformity. B–C, Bridge was resected through osteotomy site with the aid of a laminar spreader; a dental mirror and bur assure removal of all of bridge.

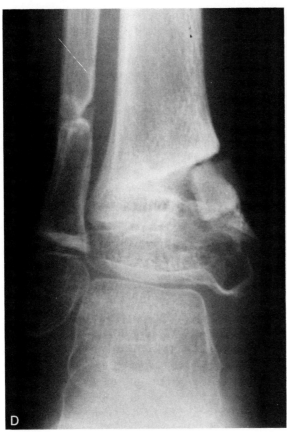
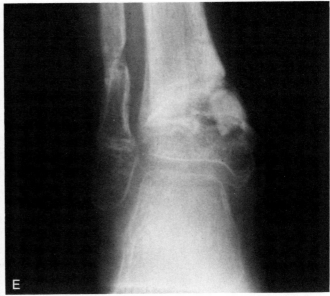

Figure 2–31 (Continued) D–E, At early follow-up.

investigators also developed a method of skeletal fixation but found long-term clinical results unsatisfactory because of fracture of the graft after a mean of 8.2 weeks.

Whatever surgical technique is chosen, a knowledge of the underlying physeal anatomy and the relationship of overlying structures to the physis is essential. Birch and colleagues examined by anatomic dissection the most commonly affected physes—those of the distal radius, distal femur, proximal tibia, and distal tibia and fibula—and described their surgical anatomy.[15] Their observations and recommendations are summarized below.

Distal Radial Physis. The physis of the distal radius is completely extracapsular and is easily exposed by any direct approach on its volar, dorsal, or radial aspect; it is obscured by the ulna medially. The volar metaphysis is cloaked by the pronator quadratus and is best exposed through the volar approach of Henry, but with the radial artery retracted radially rather than ulnarly.

Distal Femoral Physis. The synovial reflection of the suprapatellar pouch obscures portions of the anterior, medial, and lateral aspects of the distal femur and must be bluntly dissected anteriorly. The capsular attachment extends to the level of the physis anteriorly and posteriorly. The insertion of the adductor magnus tendon medially and the intermuscular septum laterally serve as landmarks to the level of the physis. This physis is best exposed through a posteromedial approach as described by Trickey[191] and a direct posterior exposure, mobilizing and protecting the neurovascular bundle.

Proximal Tibial Physis. The physis of the proximal tibia is completely extracapsular. The medial aspect of the physis is covered by the medial collateral ligament and tendons of the pes anserinus; in direct exposure these can be mobilized and retracted without difficulty. The anterolateral and anteromedial aspects of the metaphysis are easily accessible, but care must be taken to avoid injury to the apophysis of the tibial tubercle. The posterior aspects of the physis and the metaphysis are obscured in the midline by the popliteus muscle, and this posterolateral region is the least surgically accessible. The posteromedial aspect of the metaphysis can be approached through a modification of the Banks and Laufman exposure of the posteromedial tibia.[9] After developing the interval between the semitendinosus and the medial aspect of the gastrocnemius, the popliteus muscle is mobilized and reflected distally and laterally.

Distal Tibial and Fibular Physes. The distal tibial physis is entirely extracapsular. The anterior and posterior tibiofibular ligaments insert across the anterolateral and posterolateral aspects of the physis of the distal fibula. Direct exposure is difficult only on the lateral aspect of the tibia, where the physis is obscured by the overlying fibula.

APOPHYSEAL INJURIES

An apophysis is defined as a bony prominence onto which muscles or tendons are attached. In children, the apophysis is connected to the bone through a histologically recognizable physis. The shape and size of an apophysis are influenced by the forces placed on it by its muscle or tendon attachments. Because of the forces affecting them, these structures are called traction apophyses. Some apophyses have only a single muscle or tendon attachment, while others are attached to whole muscle groups.

Initially, the apophyses appear as cartilaginous prominences at the ends of or along the sides of bones; later they develop centers of ossification similar to other physes. The ossification centers then either fuse with an associated epiphysis, such as the tibial tubercle fusing with the proximal tibial epiphysis, or remain as isolated centers of ossification. Eventually the physeal plate between the ossification center and the shaft of the bone disappears as bony fusion is accomplished. Because the attachments to the apophysis are very strong, excessive forces usually cause avulsion or fracture through the apophysis rather than pulling the tendon from its insertion.

Most commonly, problems with the apophyses are inflammation or partial avulsion caused by repetitive microtrauma (traction apophysitis). This condition is common in the knee (Osgood-Schlatter disease and Sinding-Larsen-Johansson syndrome), heel (Sever's disease), medial epicondyle of the humerus (Little League elbow), ischial tuberosity, and spine.

Osgood-Schlatter disease is a traction apophysitis of the tibial tubercle, commonly occurring in boys 13 to 14 years of age and in girls 10 to 11 years of age. Inflammation and new bone formation at the tendon insertion are characteristic. Differential diagnoses include patellar peritendinitis, Sinding-Larsen-Johansson syndrome, avulsion fracture of the tibial tuberosity, tumor, and infection. The diagnosis of Osgood-Schlatter disease is based on clinical signs and symptoms, such as pain, heat, tenderness, and usually local swelling and prominence in the area of the tibial tuberosity. Pain typically occurs when the knee is extended against resistance. The most important radiographic sign is soft tissue swelling anterior to the tibial tuberosity. The condition usually resolves within 1 to 2 years, but in about 10% of patients the formation of a discrete ossicle and bursa causes pain and tenderness.

Reduction of stress on the apophysis is the objective of management. This usually can be obtained with some restriction of activity and the use of knee pads for sports in which direct knee contact occurs. If pain is severe, the extremity may be immobilized in a commercial knee immobilizer for 6 weeks. In chronic conditions, the ossicle may become so painful as to require excision. Avulsion fracture of the proximal tibial apophysis is relatively uncommon but does occur. Zimbler and Merkow described a genu recurvatum deformity caused by Osgood-Schlatter disease[211]; this was originally described in 1952 by Stirling as a complication of Osgood-Schlatter disease.[189] It rarely requires treatment.

Sinding-Larsen-Johansson syndrome is a traction apophysitis of the distal pole of the patella and is the juvenile equivalent of "jumper's knee" seen in mature patients. It also occurs in patients with cerebral palsy who walk in a crouched position. According to Medlar and Lyne, the condition occurs most commonly in males between the ages of 10 and 13 years, is usually unilateral, and requires 3 to 12 months for resolution.[124] Inflammation is localized to the tendon attachment of the distal patellar pole and is followed by calcification in distinct radiographic stages. Treatment is the same as for Osgood-Schlatter disease.

Sever's disease (calcaneal apophysitis) is a frequent overuse syndrome in growing children. It is most often seen in those who are in a growth spurt and are involved in vigorous physical activity. The calcaneal apophysis appears in boys at an average age of 7.9 years and in girls at an average age of 5.6 years. It is initially an area of irregular ossification of lesser density than the surrounding bone and is located in the lower portion of the posterior surface of the calcaneus. The most frequent differential diagnosis is retrocalcaneal bursitis. In calcaneal apophysitis, the heel is tender when the apophysis is compressed on its medial and lateral sides, and dorsiflexion of the ankle is limited. In retrocalcaneal bursitis, the point of maximal tenderness is immediately anterior to the Achilles tendon at the superior border of the calcaneus when compression is applied from the medial and lateral sides. Radiographic findings in Sever's disease are controversial. Some believe the appearance of the calcaneal apophysis is changed in symptomatic patients, whereas others believe that radiographs reflect normal variations due to skeletal age, weight, activity, and flexibility. In patients with unilateral heel pain, radiographs may help rule out other pathologies, such as tumor, infection, or fracture. Treatment consists of activity restriction and the use of heel cups and Plastizole inserts. Immobilization in a short leg cast for 4 to 6 weeks may be indicated for patients with acute symptoms.

Iliac apophysitis was reported in 18 adolescent runners by Clancy and Foltz in 1976.[50] They postulated that the mechanism of injury was an inflammatory reaction of the unfused iliac apophysis caused either by repetitive muscular contraction or by subclinical stress fractures of the apophysis. All their patients were able to return to running after 4 to 6 weeks of rest. Lombardo and co-workers re-

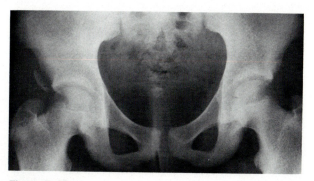

Figure 2–33

Avulsion of anteroinferior iliac spine in soccer player caused by resisted flexion of hip.

ported a bilateral radiographic abnormality, "discontinuity" of the anterior part of the iliac apophysis, in 9 of 13 adolescent athletes with a diagnosis of "hip-pointer" injuries.[117] They believe this discontinuity to be an anatomic anomaly, vulnerable to injury by either repetitive or acute trauma. The discontinuity disappeared at skeletal maturity in all nine patients; eight of the nine improved with a regimen of reduced activities, with total resolution of symptoms in 1 to 8 months. One cross-country runner continued to have symptoms for 4 years.

Avulsion of the pelvic apophysis is usually caused by sudden contraction of the hamstrings, adductor magnus, iliopsoas, and hip flexors in athletes participating in sports such as sprinting, long jumping, or hurdling, in which there is a high contraction rate or forceful hamstring stretch (Fig. 2–32). These avulsions have been classified as apophysiolysis (undisplaced), acute avulsion fractures, and old ununited avulsions (Fig. 2–33). Pain in the groin and buttock is the most common symptom. With separation of the ischial apophysis, the gap is palpable and should be sought after any suspected hamstring injury. Radiographs will confirm the diagnosis (see Fig. 2–11). Conservative management generally is sufficient if displacement is minimal; wide separation of the fracture fragments may require surgical intervention if symptoms persist. Wooton and associates reported chronic disability in three athletes with nonunions of avulsions of the ischial tuberosity; all resumed their sport after open reduction and internal fixation of the fracture.[206] These workers also successfully treated one acute fracture with wide displacement by open reduction and internal fixation and recommend this for acute fractures with more than 2 cm of displacement.

Vertebral apophysitis, or "atypical Scheuermann's disease," is frequently associated with repetitive

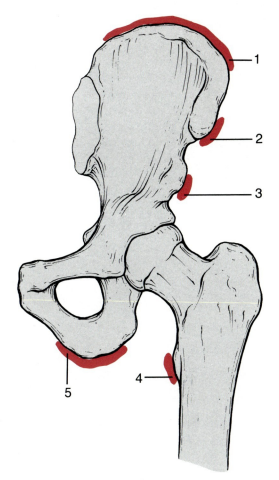

Figure 2–32

Sites of pelvic avulsion fractures reported by Fernbach and Wilkinson. 1, Iliac crest; 2, anterosuperior iliac spine; 3, anteroinferior iliac spine; 4, lesser trochanter; 5, ischium/ischial apophysis. (Redrawn from Fernbach, S. K.; Wilkinson, R. J. Avulsion injuries of the pelvis and proximal femur. AJR 137:581, 1981.)

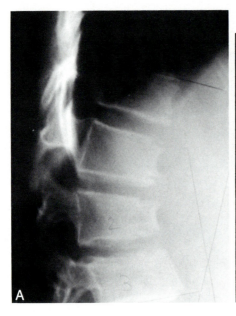
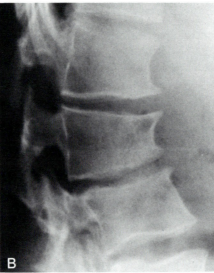

Figure 2–34

A, Roentgenogram of 12-year-old gymnast with nagging back pain shows thoracolumbar Scheuermann's disease. *B,* At age 19 years, she is pain free, but roentgenogram shows permanent wedging.

sports activity and may represent repetitive microtrauma compression fractures, most commonly in the thoracolumbar spine (Fig. 2–34). Acute injuries of the vertebral ring apophyses and intervertebral disks also have been reported in adolescent athletes, especially those involved in "jumping" sports, such as gymnastics, and in weightlifting. The ring apophysis is separated from the vertebral body by a cartilaginous layer and may be displaced by trauma. Although radiographs may be normal initially, injury to the vertebral ring apophysis may be followed by prolapse of disk material, reduction of disk height, and disk degeneration; thus, long-term follow-up of athletes with back symptoms is essential.

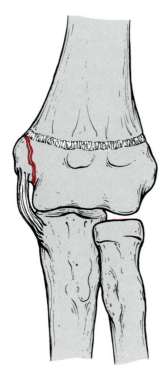

Figure 2–35

Medial epicondylar apophysitis.

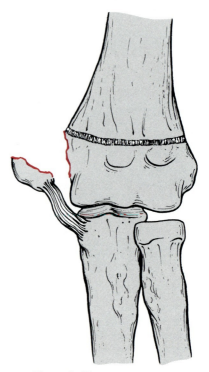

Figure 2–36

Medial epicondylar avulsion.

Olecranon apophysitis may be caused by abnormal stresses of the triceps attachment on the olecranon apophysis. Kovach and co-workers[103] and Micheli and associates[131] have reported persistence of the separated olecranon secondary ossification center into adulthood.

Medial epicondylar apophysitis occurs most frequently in children and adolescents involved in throwing sports, especially baseball, but has been reported in other sports, including gymnastics, wrestling, and weightlifting (Fig. 2–35). Repetitive microtrauma is caused by tension stresses across the medial epicondyle and collateral ligaments. With excessive throwing actions, the medial epicondyle may become prominent and painful. Active adolescent baseball pitchers frequently have accelerated growth and widening of the medial epicondylar apophysis; fragmentation of the apophysis is occasionally noted. Pain generally resolves with rest; usually there are no significant sequelae.

Avulsion of the medial epicondyle may result from a valgus injury to the elbow or occasionally from forceful pull of the forearm flexor muscles. These avulsions usually are minimally displaced and can be treated with 2 to 3 weeks of immobilization (Fig. 2–36). If valgus instability is suspected, stress radiographs should be obtained. Surgical treatment may be required for instability, entrapment of the fragment within the joint, or ulnar nerve dysfunction.

REFERENCES

1. Abraham, E. Remodeling potential of long bones following angular osteotomies. J Pediatr Orthop 9:37, 1989.
2. Aitken, A. P. Fractures of the epiphyses. Clin Orthop 41:19, 1965.
3. Albanese, S. A.; Palmer, A. K.; Kerr, D. R.; et al. Wrist pain and distal growth plate closure of the radius in gymnasts. J Pediatr Orthop 9:23, 1989.
4. Alford, B. A.; Oshman, D. G.; Sussman, M. D. Radiographic appearances following surgical correction of the partially fused epiphyseal plate. Skeletal Radiol 15:146, 1986.
5. Apple, D. F., Jr.; McDonald, A. Long-distance running and the immature skeleton. Orthopedics 3:929, 1981.
6. Backx, F. J. G.; Erich, W. B. M.; Kemper, A. B. A.; Verbeck, A. L. M. Sports injuries in school-aged children: an epidemiologic study. Am J Sports Med 17:234, 1989.
7. Bado, J. L. The Monteggia lesion. Clin Orthop 50:71, 1967.
8. Balthazar, D. A.; Pappas, A. M. Acquired valgus deformity of the tibia in children. J Pediatr Orthop 4:538, 1984.
9. Banks, S. W.; Laufman, H. An Atlas of Surgical Exposures of the Extremities. Philadelphia, W. B. Saunders, 1953.
10. Barnett, L. S. Little League shoulder syndrome proximal humeral epiphysiolysis in adolescent baseball pitchers. J Bone Joint Surg 67-A:495, 1985.
11. Baxter, M. P.; Wiley, J. J. Fractures of the proximal humeral epiphysis: their influence on humeral growth. J Bone Joint Surg 68-B:570, 1986.
12. Baxter, M. P.; Wiley, J. J. Fractures of the tibial spine in children: an evaluation of knee stability. J Bone Joint Surg 70-B:228, 1988.
13. Beck, C. L.; Burke, S. W.; Roberts, J. M.; et al. Physeal bridge resection in infantile Blount disease. J Pediatr Orthop 7:161, 1987.
14. Bertin, K. C.; Goble, E. M. Ligament injuries associated with physeal fractures about the knee. Clin Orthop 177:188, 1983.
15. Birch, J. G.; Herring, J. A.; Wenger, D. R. Surgical anatomy of selected physes. J Pediatr Orthop 4:224, 1984.
16. Blair, V.; Walker, S.; Sheridan, J.; et al. Epiphysiodesis: a problem of timing. J Pediatr Orthop 2:281, 1982.
17. Blair, W.; Hansen, C. Traumatic closure of triradiate cartilage. J Bone Joint Surg 61-A:144, 1979.
18. Boker, F. H. L.; Burbach, T. Ultrasonic diagnosis of separation of the proximal humeral epiphysis in the newborn. J Bone Joint Surg 72-A:187, 1990.
19. Bostman, O.; Makela, E. A.; Tormala, P.; Rokkanen, P. Transphyseal fracture fixation using biodegradable pins. J Bone Joint Surg 71-B:706, 1989.
20. Bowen, C. V. A.; Ethridge, G. P.; O'Brien, B. McC., et al. Experimental microvascular growth plate transfers. Part 2—investigation of feasibility. J Bone Joint Surg 70-B:311, 1988.
21. Brashear, H. R., Jr. Epiphyseal fractures: a microscopic study of the healing process in rats. J Bone Joint Surg 41-A:1055, 1959.
22. Bright, R. W. Partial growth arrest: identification, classification, and results of treatment. Abstract. Orthop Trans 6:65, 1982.
23. Bright, R. W. Surgical correction of partial growth plate closure: laboratory and clinical experience. Orthop Rev 8:149, 1978.
24. Bright, R. W. Operative correction of partial epiphyseal plate closure by osseous-bridge resection and silicone-rubber implant: an experimental study in dogs. J Bone Joint Surg 56-A:655, 1974.
25. Bright, R. W.; Elmore, S. M. Physical properties of epiphyseal plate cartilage. Surg Forum 19:463, 1968.
26. Bright, R. W.; Burstein, A. H.; Elmore, S. M. Epiphyseal-plate cartilage: a biomechanical and histological analysis of failure modes. J Bone Joint Surg 56-A:688, 1974.
27. Broughton, N. S.; Dickens, D. R. V.; Cole, W. G.; Menelaus, M. B. Epiphyseolysis for partial growth plate arrest: results after four years or at maturity. J Bone Joint Surg 71-B:13, 1989.
28. Bucholz, R. W.; Ezaki, M.; Ogden, J. A. Injury to the acetabular triradiate physeal cartilage. J Bone Joint Surg 64-A:600, 1982.
29. Bueche, M. J.; Phillips, W. A.; Gordon, J.; et al. Effect of interposition material on mechanical behaviour in partial physeal resection: a canine model. J Pediatr Orthop 10:459, 1990.
30. Burkus, R.; Ogden, J. Development of the distal femoral epiphysis: a microscopic, morphological investigation of the zone of Ranvier. J Pediatr Orthop 4:661, 1984.
31. Busch, M. T. Sports medicine in children and adolescents. In: Morrissy, R. T., ed. Lovell and Winter's Pediatric Orthopaedics, ed 3. Philadelphia, J. B. Lippincott, 1990.
32. Caffey, J. Traumatic cupping of the metaphyses of growing bones. AJR 108:451, 1970.

33. Cahill, B. R. Stress fracture of the proximal tibial epiphysis: a case report. Am J Sports Med 6:180, 1976.
34. Campbell, J.; Almond, H. G. A. Fracture-separation of the proximal humeral epiphysis. J Bone Joint Surg 59-A:262, 1977.
35. Canadell, J.; de Pablos, J. Breaking bony bridges by physeal distraction: a new approach. Int Orthop 9:223, 1985.
36. Canale, S. T. Fractures and dislocations. In: Canale, S. T.; Beaty, J. H., eds. Operative Pediatric Orthopaedics. St. Louis, C. V. Mosby, 1990.
37. Canale, S. T. Special techniques. In: Canale, S. T.; Beaty, J. H., eds. Operative Pediatric Orthopaedics. St. Louis, C. V. Mosby, 1990.
38. Canale, S. T. Sports medicine. In: Canale, S. T.; Beaty, J. H., eds. Operative Pediatric Orthopaedics. St. Louis, C. V. Mosby, 1990.
39. Canale, S. T.; Russell, T.; Holcomb, R. Percutaneous epiphysiodesis: experimental study and preliminary clinical results. J Pediatr Orthop 6:150, 1986.
40. Carlson, W. O.; Wenger, D. R. A mapping method to prepare for surgical excision of a partial physeal arrest. J Pediatr Orthop 4:232, 1984.
41. Carter, S. R.; Aldridge, M. J. Stress injury of the distal radial growth plate. J Bone Joint Surg 70-B:834, 1988.
42. Cass, J. R.; Peterson, H. A. Salter-Harris type IV injuries of the distal tibial epiphyseal growth plate, with emphasis on those involving the medial malleolus. J Bone Joint Surg 65-A:1059, 1983.
43. Cassebaum, W. H.; Patterson, A. H. Fractures of the distal femoral epiphysis. Clin Orthop 41:79, 1965.
44. Caudle, R. J.; Crawford, A. H. Avulsion fracture of the lateral acetabular margin: a case report. J Bone Joint Surg 70-A:1568, 1988.
45. Chadwick, C. J. Spontaneous resolution of varus deformity of the ankle following adduction injury of the distal tibial epiphysis. J Bone Joint Surg 64-A:774, 1982.
46. Chadwick, C. J.; Bentley, G. The classification and prognosis of epiphyseal injuries. Injury 18:157, 1987.
47. Chamay, A.; Tschantz, P. Mechanical influences in bone remodeling: experimental research on Wolff's law. J Biomech 5:173, 1972.
48. Chow, S. P.; Lam, J. J.; Leong, J. C. Y. Fracture of the tibial tubercle in the adolescent. J Bone Joint Surg 72-B:231, 1990.
49. Christie, M. J.; Dvonch, V. M. Tibial tuberosity avulsion fracture in adolescents. J Pediatr Orthop 1:391, 1981.
49a. Chung, S. M. K.; Batterman, S. C.; Brighton, C. T. Shear strength of the human femoral capital epiphyseal plate. J. Bone Joint Surg. 58-A:94, 1976.
50. Clancy, W. G., Jr.; Foltz, A. S. Iliac apophysitis and stress fractures in adolescent runners. Am J Sports Med 4:214, 1976.
51. Clement, D. A.; Colton, C. L. Overgrowth of the femur after femoral fractures in childhood. J Bone Joint Surg 68-B:534, 1986.
52. Collins, H. R. Epiphyseal injuries in athletes. Cleve Clin Q 42:285, 1975.
53. Cooperman, D. R.; Spiegel, P. G.; Laros, G. S. Tibial fractures involving the ankle in children: the so-called triplane epiphyseal fracture. J Bone Joint Surg 60-A:1040, 1978.
54. Cowell, H. R.; Hunziker, E. B.; Rosenberg, L. The role of hypertrophic chondrocytes in enchondral ossification and the development of secondary centers of ossification. Editorial. J Bone Joint Surg 69-A:159, 1987.
55. Czitrom, A. A.; Salter, R. B.; Willis, R. B. Fractures involving the distal femoral epiphyseal plate of the femur. Int Orthop 4:269, 1981.
56. De Bastiani, G.; Aldegheri, R.; Renzi-Brivio, L.; Trivella, G. Limb lengthening by callus distraction (callotasis). J Pediatr Orthop 7:129, 1987.
57. De Bastiani, G.; Aldegheri, R.; Renzi-Brivio, L.; Trivella, G. Chondrodiastasis-controlled symmetrical distraction of the epiphyseal plate. Limb lengthening in children. J Bone Joint Surg 68-B:550, 1986.
58. DeLee, J. C.; Wilkins, K. E.; Rogers, L. F.; Rockwood, C. A. Fracture-separation of the distal humeral epiphysis. J Bone Joint Surg 62-A:46, 1980.
59. Dias, L. S.; Giegerich, C. R. Fractures of the distal tibial epiphysis in adolescence. J Bone Joint Surg 65-A:438, 1983.
60. Eady, J. L.; Cardenas, C. D.; Sopa, D. Avulsion of the femoral attachment of the anterior cruciate ligament in a seven-year-old child. J Bone Joint Surg 64-A:1376, 1982.
61. Ehrlich, M. G.; Strain, R. E., Jr. Epiphyseal injuries about the knee. Orthop Clin North Am 10:91, 1979.
62. Ertl, J. P.; Barrack, R. L.; Alexander, A. H.; Van Buecken, K. Triplane fracture of the distal tibial epiphysis: long-term follow-up. J Bone Joint Surg 70-A:967, 1988.
63. Eyre-Brook, A. L. The periosteum: its function reassessed. Clin Orthop 189:300, 1984.
64. Fernbach, S. K.; Wilkinson, R. J. Avulsion injuries of the pelvis and proximal femur. AJR 137:581, 1981.
65. Fjeld, T. O.; Steen, H. Growth retardation after experimental limb lengthening by epiphyseal distraction. J Pediatr Orthop 10:463, 1990.
66. Foucher, M. De la divulsion des epiphyses. Congr Med France (Paris) 1:63, 1863.
67. Fries, J. Growth following epiphsyeal arrest: a simple method of calculation. Clin Orthop 114:316, 1976.
68. Gepstein, R.; Weiss, R. E.; Hallel, T. Acetabular dysplasia and hip dislocation after selective premature fusion of the triradiate cartilage: an experimental study in rabbits. J Bone Joint Surg 66-B:334, 1984.
69. Gill, J. G.; Chakrabarti, J. H.; Becker, S. J. Fracture of the proximal tibial epiphysis. Injury 14:324, 1983.
70. Godshall, R. W.; Hansen, C. A. Incomplete avulsion of a portion of the iliac apophysis. J Bone Joint Surg 55-A:1301, 1973.
71. Gomes, L. S.; Volpon, J. B.; Gonclaves, R. P. Traumatic separation of epiphyses: an experimental study in rats. Clin Orthop 236:286, 1988.
72. Garn, S. M.; Silverman, F. N.; Hertzog, K. P.; Rohmann, C. G. Lines and bands of increased density: their implication to growth and development. Med Radiogr Photogr 44:58, 1968.
73. Grantham, S. A.; Kiernan, H. A. Displaced olecranon fractures in children. J Trauma 15:197, 1975.
74. Greco, F.; de Palma, L.; Specchia, N.; Mannarini, M. Growth-plate cartilage metabolic response to mechanical stress. J Pediatr Orthop 9:520, 1989.
75. Green, N. E. Tibia valga caused by asymmetrical overgrowth following a nondisplaced fracture of the proximal tibial metaphysis. J Pediatr Orthop 3:235, 1983.
76. Greene, T. L.; Hensinger, R. N.; Hunter, L. Y. Back pain and vertebral changes simulating Scheuermann's disease. J Pediatr Orthop 5:1, 1985.
77. Greiff, J.; Bergman, F. Growth disturbance following fractures of the tibia in children. Acta Orthop Scand 51:315, 1980.
78. Grogan, D. P.; Love, S. M.; Ogden, J. A.; et al. Chondro-

osseous growth abnormalities after meningococcemia: a clinical and histopathological study. J Bone Joint Surg 71-A:920, 1989.
79. Gugenheim, J. J.; Stanley, R. F.; Woods, G. W.; Tullos, H. S. Little League survey: the Houston study. Am J Sports Med 4:189, 1976.
80. Hall, B. K. The embyronic development of bone. Am Sci 76:174, 1988.
81. Hand, W. L.; Hand, C. R.; Dunn, A. W. Avulsion fractures of the tibial tubercle. J Bone Joint Surg 53-A:1579, 1971.
82. Harris, H. The vascular supply of bone, with special reference to the epiphyseal cartilage. J Anat 64:3, 1929.
83. Harvey, J. S. Overuse syndromes in young athletes. Pediatr Clin North Am 29:1369, 1982.
84. Havranek, P. Injuries of the distal clavicular physis in children. J Pediatr Orthop 9:213, 1989.
85. Heeg, M.; Visser, J. D.; Oostvogel, H. J. M. Injuries of the acetabular triradiate cartilage and sacroiliac joint. J Bone Joint Surg 70-B:34, 1988.
86. Heikel, H. V. A. Has epiphyseodesis in one end of a long bone a growth-stimulating effect on the other end? An experimental study. Acta Orthop Scand 31:18, 1961.
87. Herring, J. A.; Birch, J. Instructional case: whither the bar. J Pediatr Orthop 7:722, 1987.
88. Herring, J. A.; Moseley, C. Posttraumatic valgus deformity of the tibia. J Pediatr Orthop 4:654, 1984.
89. Hines, R. F.; Herndon, W. A.; Evans, J. P. Operative treatment of medial epicondyle fractures in children. Clin Orthop 223:170, 1987.
90. Howard, F. M.; Piha, R. J. Fractures of the apophysis in adolescent athletes. JAMA 192:150, 1965.
91. Hresko, M. T.; Kasser, J. S. Physeal arrest about the knee associated with non-physeal fractures in the lower extremity. J Bone Joint Surg 71-A:698, 1989.
92. Hunziker, E. B.; Schenk, R. K.; Cruz-Orive, L-M. Quantitation of chondrocyte performance in growth-plate cartilage during longitudinal bone growth. J Bone Joint Surg 69-A:162, 1987.
93. Huurman, W. W.; Jacobsen, F. S.; Anderson, J. C.; Chu, W-K. Limb-length discrepancy measured with computerized axial tomographic equipment. J Bone Joint Surg 69-A:699, 1987.
94. Hynes, D.; O'Brien, T. Growth disturbance lines after injury of the distal tibial physis: their significance in prognosis. J Bone Joint Surg 70-B:231, 1988.
95. Ilizarov, G. A. The tension-stress effect on the genesis and growth of tissues. Part I. The influence of stability of fixation and soft-tissue preservation. Clin Orthop 238:249, 1989.
96. Jackson, D. W.; Cozen, L. Genu valgum as a complication of proximal tibial metaphyseal fractures in children. J Bone Joint Surg 53-A:1571, 1971.
97. Jeffrey, C. C. Fracture of the head of the radius in children. J Bone Joint Surg 32-B:314, 1950.
98. Jordon, S. E.; Alonso, J. E.; Cook, F. F. The etiology of valgus angulation after metaphyseal fractures of the tibia in children. J Pediatr Orthop 7:450, 1987.
99. Kärrholm, J.; Hansson, L. I.; Slevik, G. Roentgen stereophotogrammetric analysis of growth pattern after supination-adduction ankle injuries in children. J Pediatr Orthop 2:271, 1982.
100. Keret, D.; Mendez, A. A.; Harcke, H. T.; MacEwen, G. D. Type V physeal injury: a case report. J Pediatr Orthop 10:545, 1990.
101. Kilfoyle, R. M. Fracture of the medial condyle and epicondyle of the elbow in children. Clin Orthop 41:43, 1965.
102. Kling, T. F., Jr.; Bright, R. W.; Hensinger, R. N. Distal tibial physeal fractures in children that may require open reduction. J Bone Joint Surg 66-A:647, 1984.
103. Kovach, J., II; Baker, B. E.; Mosher, J. F. Fracture separation of the olecranon ossification center in adults. Am J Sports Med 13:105, 1985.
104. Kujala, U. M.; Kvist, M.; Heinonen, O. Osgood-Schlatter's disease in adolescent athletes: retrospective study of incidence and duration. Am J Sports Med 13:236, 1985.
105. Labelle, H.; Bunnell, W. P.; Duhaime, M.; Poitras, B. Cubitus varus deformity following supracondylar fractures of the humerus in children. J Pediatr Orthop 2:539, 1982.
106. Lalanandham, T.; Ehrlich, M. G.; Zaleske, D. J.; et al. Viability and metabolism of cartilage transplanted to physeal regions. J Pediatr Orthop 10:450, 1990.
107. Langenskiold, A. Surgical treatment of partial closure of the growth plate. J Pediatr Orthop 1:3, 1981.
108. Langenskiold, A. The possibilities of eliminating premature partial closure of an epiphyseal plate caused by trauma or disease. Acta Orthop Scand 38:267, 1967.
109. Langenskiold, A.; Osterman, K.; Valle, M. Growth of fat grafts after operation for partial bone growth arrest: demonstration by computed tomography scanning. J Pediatr Orthop 7:389, 1987.
110. Langenskiold, A.; Videman, T.; Nevalainen, T. The fate of fat transplants in operations for partial closure of the growth plate: clinical examples and an experimental study. J Bone Joint Surg 68-B:234, 1986.
111. Larson, R. L.; Singer, K. M.; Bergstrom, R.; Thomas, S. Little League survey: the Eugene study. Am J Sports Med 4:201, 1976.
112. Lawson, J. P.; Ogden, J. A.; Bucholz, R. W.; Hughes, S. A. Physeal injuries of the cervical spine. J Pediatr Orthop 7:428, 1987.
113. Lennox, D. W.; Goldner, R. D.; Sussman, M. D. Cartilage as an interposition material to prevent transphyseal bone bridge formation: an experimental model. J Pediatr Orthop 3:207, 1983.
114. Lesko, P. D.; Georgis, T.; Slabaugh, P. Case report. Irreducible Salter-Harris type II fracture of the distal radial epiphysis. J Pediatr Orthop 7:719, 1987.
115. Letts, M.; Locht, R.; Wiens, J. Monteggia fracture-dislocations in children. J Bone Joint Surg 67-B:724, 1985.
116. Letts, R. M. The hidden adolescent ankle fracture. J Pediatr Orthop 2:161, 1982.
117. Lombardo, S. J.; Ratting, A. C.; Kerlan, R. K. Radiographic abnormalities of the iliac apophysis in adolescent athletes. J Bone Joint Surg 65-A:444, 1983.
118. Lorenzi, G.; Rossi, P.; Quaglia, F.; et al. Growth disturbances following fractures of the femur and tibia in children. Ital J Orthop Traumatol 11:133, 1985.
119. Lowrey, J. J. Dislocated lumbar vertebral epiphysis in adolescent children: report of three cases. J Neurosurg 38:232, 1973.
120. Makela, E. A.; Vainionpaa, S.; Vihtonen, K.; et al. The effect of trauma to the lower femoral epiphyseal plate: an experimental study in rabbits. J Bone Joint Surg 70-B:187, 1988.
121. Mann, D. C.; Rajmaira, S. Distribution of physeal and non-physeal fractures of long bones in children aged 0 to 16 years. J Pediatr Orthop 10:713, 1990.
122. Marcus, R. E.; Mills, M. F.; Thompson, G. H. Multiple injury in children. J Bone Joint Surg 65-A:1290, 1983.
123. McGuigan, J. A.; O'Reilly, M. J. G.; Nixon, J. R. Popliteal

artery thrombosis resulting from disruption of the upper tibial epiphysis. Injury 16:49, 1984.
124. Medlar, R. C.; Lyne, E. D. Sinding-Larsen-Johansson disease. J Bone Joint Surg 60-A:1113, 1978.
125. Metzmaker, J. N.; Pappas, A. M. Avulsion fractures of the pelvis. Am J Sports Med 13:349, 1985.
126. Meyers, M. H. Isolated avulsion of the tibial attachment of the posterior cruciate ligament of the knee. J Bone Joint Surg 57-A:669, 1975.
127. Micheli, L. J. The traction apophysitises. Clin Sports Med 6:389, 1986.
128. Micheli, L. J. Overuse injuries in children's sport: the growth factor. Orthop Clin North Am 14:337, 1983.
129. Micheli, L. J. Low-back pain in the adolescent: differential diagnosis. Am J Sports Med 7:361, 1979.
130. Micheli, L. J.; Ireland, M. L. Prevention and management of calcaneal apophysitis in children: an overuse syndrome. J Pediatr Orthop 7:34, 1987.
131. Micheli, L. T.; Santori, R.; Stanitski, C. L. Epiphyseal fracture of the elbow in children. Am Fam Physician 22:107, 1980.
132. Milch, H. Fractures and fracture-dislocations of humeral condyles. J Trauma 4:592, 1964.
133. Mital, M. A.; Matza, R. A.; Cohen, J. The so-called unresolved Osgood-Schlatter lesion. J Bone Joint Surg 62-A:732, 1980.
134. Mizuta, T.; Benson, W. M.; Foster, B. K.; et al. Statistical analysis of the incidence of physeal injuries. J Pediatr Orthop 7:518, 1987.
135. Morrissy, R. T.; Wilkins, K. E. Deformity following distal humeral fracture in childhood. J Bone Joint Surg 66-A:557, 1984.
136. Neer, C. S.; Horowitz, B. Fractures of the proximal humeral epiphyseal plate. Clin Orthop 41:24, 1965.
137. Nettelblad, H.; Randolph, M. A.; Weiland, A. J. Free microvascular epiphyseal-plate transplantation. J Bone Joint Surg 66-A:1421, 1984.
138. Newman, J. H. Displaced radial neck fractures in children. Injury 9:114, 1977.
139. O'Brien, E. T. Fractures of the hand and wrist region. In: Rockwood, C. A., Jr.; Wilkins, K. E.; King, R. E., eds. Fractures in Children. Philadelphia, J. B. Lippincott, 1984.
140. O'Brien, P. I. Injuries involving the radial epiphysis. Clin Orthop 41:51, 1965.
141. O'Brien, T.; Millis, M. B.; Griffin, P. P. The early identification and classification of growth disturbances of the proximal end of the femur. J Bone Joint Surg 68-A:970, 1986.
142. O'Driscoll, S. W.; Keeley, F. W.; Salter, R. B. Durability of regenerated articular cartilage produced by free autogenous periosteal grafts in major full-thickness defects in joint surfaces under the influence of continuous passive motion: a follow-up report at one year. J Bone Joint Surg 70-A:595, 1988.
143. Ogden, J. A. Development and maturation of the neuromusculoskeletal system. In: Morrissy, R. T., ed. Lovell and Winter's Pediatric Orthopaedics, 3rd ed. Philadelphia, J. B. Lippincott, 1990.
144. Ogden, J. A. Skeletal Injury in the Child, 2nd ed. Philadelphia, Lea & Febiger, 1990.
145. Ogden, J. A. Current concepts review: the evaluation and treatment of partial physeal arrest. J Bone Joint Surg 69-A:1297, 1987.
146. Ogden, J. A. The uniqueness of growing bones. In: Rockwood, C. A.; Wilkins, K. E.; King, R. E., eds. Fractures in Children. Philadelphia, J. B. Lippincott, 1984.
147. Ogden, J. A. Growth slowdown and arrest lines. J Pediatr Orthop 4:409, 1984.
148. Ogden, J. A. Skeletal growth mechanism injury patterns. J Pediatr Orthop 2:371, 1982.
149. Ogden, J. A. Changing patterns of proximal femoral vascularity. J Bone Joint Surg 56-A:941, 1974.
150. Ogden, J. A.; Southwick, W. Osgood-Schlatter's disease and development of the tibial tuberosity. Clin Orthop 116:180, 1976.
151. Ogden, J. A.; Tross, R. B.; Murphy, M. J. Fractures of the tibial tuberosity in adolescents. J Bone Joint Surg 62-A:205, 1980.
152. Ogilvie, J. Epiphysiodesis: evaluation of a new technique. J Pediatr Orthop 6:174, 1986.
153. Olin, A.; Creasman, C.; Shapiro, F. Free physeal transplantation in the rabbit: an experimental approach to focal lesions. J Bone Joint Surg 66-A:7, 1984.
154. Paley, D. Current techniques of limb lengthening. J Pediatr Orthop 8:73, 1988.
155. Papavasiliou, V.; Neonpoulos, S.; Venturis, T. Fractures of the medial condyle of the humerus in childhood. J Pediatr Orthop 7:421, 1987.
156. Pappas, A. M. Elbow problems associated with baseball during childhood and adolescence. Clin Orthop 164:30, 1982.
157. Pappas, A. M.; Anas, P.; Toczylowski, H. M., Jr. Asymmetrical arrest of the proximal tibial physis and genu recurvatum deformity. J Bone Joint Surg 66-A:515, 1989.
158. Pauwels, F. Biomechanics of the Locomotor Apparatus. Berlin, Springer-Verlag, 1980.
159. Peterson, H. A. Partial growth plate arrest. In: Morrissy, R. T., ed. Lovell and Winter's Pediatric Orthopaedics, 3rd ed. Philadelphia, J. B. Lippincott, 1990.
160. Peterson, H. A. Partial growth plate arrest and its treatment. J Pediatr Orthop 4:246, 1984.
161. Peterson, H. A. Triplane fracture of the distal humeral epiphysis. J Pediatr Orthop 3:81, 1983.
162. Peterson, H. A.; Burkhart, S. S. Compression injury of the epiphyseal growth plate: fact or fiction? J Pediatr Orthop 1:377, 1981.
163. Poland, J. Traumatic Separation of the Epiphyses. London, Smith Elder, 1898.
164. Pritchett, J. W. Growth and predictions of growth in the upper extremity. J Bone Joint Surg 70-A:520, 1988.
165. Rang, M. The Growth Plate and Its Disorders. Baltimore, Williams & Wilkins, 1969.
166. Rinaldi, E.; Mazzarella, F. Isolated fracture avulsions of the tibial insertions of the cruciate ligaments of the knee. Ital J Orthop Traumatol 6:77, 1980.
167. Riseborough, E. J.; Barrett, I. R.; Shapiro, F. Growth disturbances following distal femoral epiphyseal fracture-separations. J Bone Joint Surg 65-A:885, 1983.
168. Robert, M.; Khouri, N.; Carlioz, H.; et al. Fractures of the proximal metaphysis in children: review of a series of 25 cases. J Pediatr Orthop 7:444, 1987.
169. Roberts, J. M.; Lovell, W. W. Fractures of the intercondylar eminence of the tibia. J Bone Joint Surg 52-A:827, 1970.
170. Robinson, S. C.; Driscoll, F. E. Simultaneous osteochondral avulsion of the femoral and tibial insertions of the anterior cruciate ligament. J Bone Joint Surg 63-A:1342, 1981.

171. Rosenberg, L. C. The physis as an interface between basic research and clinical knowledge. Editorial. J Bone Joint Surg 66-A:815, 1984.
172. Rutherford, A. Fractures of the lateral humeral condyle in children. J Bone Joint Surg 67-A:851, 1985.
173. Ryöppy, S.; Karaharju, E. O. Alteration of epiphyseal growth by an experimentally produced angular deformity. Acta Orthop Scand 45:290, 1974.
174. Salter, R. B.; Best, T. The pathogenesis and prevention of valgus deformity following fractures of the proximal metaphyseal region of the tibia in children. J Bone Joint Surg 55-A:1324, 1973.
175. Salter, R. B.; Harris, W. R. Injuries involving the epiphyseal plate. J Bone Joint Surg 45-A:587, 1963.
176. Schlonsky, J.; Olix, M. L. Functional disability following avulsion fracture of the ischial epiphysis. J Bone Joint Surg 54-A:641, 1972.
177. Schmidt, T. L.; Kalamchi, A. The fate of the capital femoral physis and acetabular development in developmental coxa vara. J Pediatr Orthop 2:534, 1982.
178. Scuderi, G.; Bronson, M. J. Triradiate cartilage injury: report of two cases and review of the literature. Clin Orthop 217:179, 1987.
179. Sever, J. I. Apophysitis of the os calcis. NY Med J, May 1, 1912.
180. Shannak, A. Tibial fractures in children: follow-up study. J Pediatr Orthop 8:306, 1988.
181. Shapiro, F.; Holtrop, M. E.; Glimcher, M. J. Organization and cellular biology of the perichondral ossification groove of Ranvier. J Bone Joint Surg 59-A:703, 1977.
182. Shelton, W. R.; Canale, S. T. Fractures of the tibia through the proximal tibial epiphyseal cartilage. J Bone Joint Surg 61-A:167, 1979.
183. Shopfner, C. E.; Coin, C. G. Effect of weightbearing on appearance and development of secondary calcaneal epiphysis. Radiology 86:201, 1966.
184. Silberstein, J. J.; Brodeur, A. E.; Graviss, E. R. Some vagaries of the lateral epicondyle. J Bone Joint Surg 64-A:444, 1982.
185. Silberstein, J. J.; Brodeur, A. E.; Gravvis, E. R. Some vagaries of the medial epicondyle. J Bone Joint Surg 63-A:524, 1981.
186. Skak, S. V. Valgus deformity following proximal tibial metaphyseal fracture in children. Acta Orthop Scand 53:141, 1982.
187. Speer, D. P. Collagenous architecture of the growth plate and perichondrial ossification groove. J Bone Joint Surg 64-A:399, 1982.
188. Staheli, L. T.; Williamson, V. Partial physeal growth arrest and treatment by bridge resection and fat interposition. J Pediatr Orthop 10:769, 1990.
189. Stirling, R. I. Complications of Osgood-Schlatter's disease. Abstract. J Bone Joint Surg 34-B:149, 1952.
190. Sward, L.; Hellstrom, M.; Jacobsson, B.; et al. Acute injury of the vertebral ring apophysis and intervertebral disc in adolescent gymnasts. Spine 15:144, 1990.
191. Trickey, E. L. Rupture of the posterior cruciate ligament of the knee. J Bone Joint Surg 50-B:334, 1968.
192. Tullos, H. S.; King, J. W. Lesions of the pitching arm in adolescents. JAMA 220:264, 1972.
193. Turz, A.; Crost, M. Sports-related injuries in children: a study of their characteristics, frequency, and severity, with comparison to other types of accidental injuries. Am J Sports Med 14:294, 1986.
194. Varma, B. P.; Srivastava, T. P. Fractures of the medial condyle of the humerus in children: a report of 4 cases, including the late sequelae. Injury 4:171, 1972.
195. Vostal, O. Fracture of the neck of the radius in children. Acta Chir Traumatol Cech 37:294, 1970.
196. Watson-Jones, R. Fractures and Joint Injuries. Baltimore, Williams & Wilkins, 1946.
197. Weber, B. G. Fibrous interposition causing valgus deformity after fracture of the upper tibial metaphysis in children. J Bone Joint Surg 59-B:290, 1977.
198. Weber, B. G.; Brunner, C.; Freuler, F. Treatment of Fractures in Children and Adolescents. New York, Springer-Verlag, 1980.
199. Wiley, J. J.; Galey, J. P. Monteggia injuries in children. J Bone Joint Surg 67-B:728, 1985.
200. Wilkins, K. E. Fractures and dislocations of the elbow region. In: Rockwood, C. A., Jr.; Wilkins, K. E.; King, R. E., eds. Fractures in Children. Philadelphia, J. B. Lippincott, 1984.
201. Wilkins, K. E. The uniqueness of the young athlete: musculoskeletal injuries. Am J Sports Med 8:377, 1980.
202. Williams, D. J. The mechanisms producing fracture-separation of the proximal humeral epiphysis. J Bone Joint Surg 63-B:102, 1981.
203. Wong-Chung, J.; O'Brien, T. Salter-Harris type III fracture of the proximal humeral physis. Injury 19:453, 1988.
204. Wood, V. E. Fractures of the hand in children. Orthop Clin North Am 7:527, 1976.
205. Woods, G. M.; Tullos, H. G. Elbow instability and medial epicondyle fracture. Am J Sports Med 5:23, 1977.
206. Wooton, J. R.; Cross, M. J.; Holt, K. W. G. Avulsion of the ischial apophysis: the case for open reduction and internal fixation. J Bone Joint Surg 72-B:625, 1990.
207. Yong-Hing, K.; Wedge, J. H.; Bowen, C. V. A. Chronic injury to the distal ulnar and radial growth plates in an adolescent gymnast: a case report. J Bone Joint Surg 70-A:1087, 1988.
208. Young, J. W. R.; Bright, R. W.; Whitley, N. O. Computed tomography in the evaluation of partial growth plate arrest in children. Skeletal Radiol 15:530, 1986.
209. Zaricznyj, B.; Shattuck, L. J.; Mast, T. A.; et al. Sports related injuries in school age children. Am J Sports Med 8:318, 1980.
210. Zehntner, M. K.; Jakob, R. P.; McGanity, P. L. J. Case report. Growth disturbance of the distal radial epiphysis after trauma: operative treatment by corrective radial osteotomy. J Pediatr Orthop 10:411, 1990.
211. Zimbler, S.; Merkow, S. Genu recurvatum: a possible complication after Osgood-Schlatter disease: case report. J Bone Joint Surg 66-A:1129, 1984.
212. Zionts, L. E.; Harcke, H. T.; Brooks, K. M.; et al. Posttraumatic tibial valga: a case demonstrating asymmetric activity at the proximal growth plate on technetium bone scan. J Pediatr Orthop 7:458, 1987.

William W. Robertson, Jr., M.D.

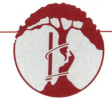

3

Pathologic Fractures and Tumors

A pathologic fracture occurs in bone that is weak or that lacks normal biomechanical properties. This fault can be intrinsic to bone, e.g., the osteopenia of rickets or disuse or the brittleness of osteopetrosis. On the other hand, the weakness can be caused by something extrinsic to normal constituents that lessens the inherent structural integrity of bone. Replacement of bone with tumor or iatrogenic intrusion (biopsy or internal fixation) can cause such an extrinsic defect. This abnormal weakness allows the bone to fail under stresses that it should normally tolerate or in anatomic areas where it would not fail under normal loads.

A normal child's bone is more plastic than that of an adult. Therefore, a greater loss of normal mineral content or architecture may be necessary for a given force to produce a fracture than in the corresponding adult bone.

A variant of the pathologic fracture is the stress fracture.[5] A stress fracture occurs when exceptional repetitive force is exerted on bone that has not had a chance to remodel physiologically to accommodate these forces. The "march" fracture of metatarsal bone of the military recruit is the classic example.

Presentation

Frequently the pain of a pathologic fracture is the first symptom of a pathologic process in bone. A 5-year-old girl tripped over an ottoman. Her pain on attempted weight bearing led her physician to x-ray her leg (Fig. 3–1). Reevaluation of her leg revealed significant bowing and subtle overgrowth. These signs completely corroborated the diagnosis of fibrous dysplasia.

Physicians must be mindful that fractures may present with pain (and in the insensate or neurologically compromised patient, with swelling and fever) without deformity. They must also ask themselves if any fracture is through normal bone.[3] This is especially important when the fracture site or mechanism of injury is inappropriate to the fracture pattern.

Mechanism

Pathologic bone fails in two ways. The energy required to produce a pathologic fracture may be as little as the repeated loading of weight bearing, generating a spontaneous fracture. Microfractures may occur in the bone substance—especially in areas of largely trabecular bone, the metaphysis of long bones, and the vertebral body. Frequently these microfractures are undisplaced, go unrecognized, and heal without consequence.

Figure 3–2 shows a nondisplaced fracture of the femoral neck in a child with osteopetrosis. The fracture presented with hip pain without a history of trauma. Because it was not complete, treatment consisted of rest and relief of weight bearing. If the fracture had been complete but still nondisplaced, consideration would have been given to cast immobilization. Although this situation is similar to a spontaneous fracture in the femoral neck of an osteoporotic adult, the child's relative tolerance of immobility obviates the necessity of internal fixation.

Multiple microfractures may, however, result in bony deformation. The "shepherd's crook" deformity of fibrous dysplasia or the kyphosis from seg-

57

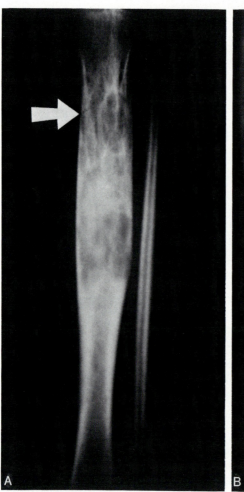 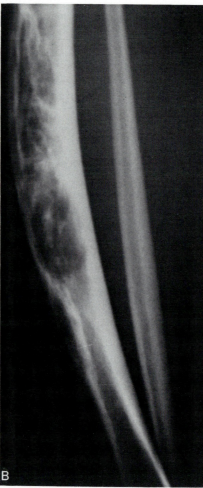

Figure 3–1

Anteroposterior (A) and lateral (B) views of the tibia of a 5-year-old female. The arrow points to cortical interruption in a nondisplaced fracture in fibrodysplastic bone.

mental vertebral wedging are examples of "chronic" fracture modeling of bone. Osteogenesis imperfecta fractures frequently produce deformities that because of the changed biomechanical tension-compression lead to recurrent fractures. Figure 3–3 demonstrates this phenomenon. Realignment of the abnormal bone was necessary to minimize the risk of refracture.

The second mode of fracture comes from greater forces. Higher energy trauma also may result in pathologic fracture. In this case it is the site of the fracture that is determined by the faulty bone. Usually these fractures are symptomatic, with inability to move the injured extremity or inability to bear weight, and they are frequently displaced. A 12-year-old boy who was known to have a fibrous cortical defect in his distal tibia (Fig. 3–4A) twisted his leg playing football (Fig. 3–4B). The fracture might have occurred whether the lesion was present or not, but the site of the fracture was clearly related to the stress riser in the cortical bone at the site of the defect. X-ray of the area 1 year later (Fig. 3–4C) shows healing of the fracture and partial remodeling-healing of the cyst.

Differential Diagnosis

Although the initial presenting sign of generalized bone disease in children may be fracture, the most common of these conditions (osteogenesis imperfecta, osteopetrosis, and rickets) are confirmed early either by diagnostic radiographs (see Figs. 3–2 and 3–3) or by conclusive laboratory findings. Generalized osteopenia secondary to chronic drug therapy (steroid or anticonvulsant) or to neural disuse also may become evident through pathologic fracture. In these cases the differential diagnosis is not a problem.

Osteomyelitis may weaken bone sufficiently for fracture (Fig. 3–5); however, systemic signs usually point to the infectious nature of the lesion. A greater problem may lie in the underlying diagnosis of focal disease of bone causing fracture. Enneking believes

Figure 3–2

A nondisplaced stress type fracture arises from the superior aspect of the lower femoral neck *(arrow)* in a patient with osteopetrosis.

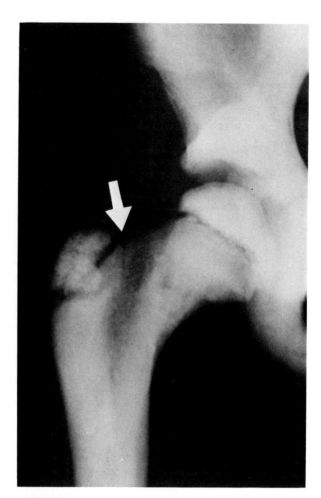

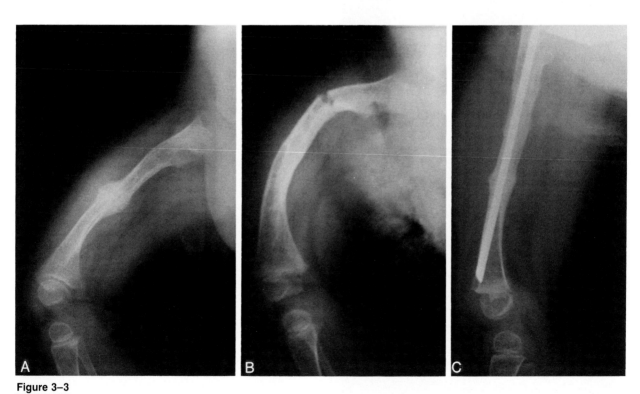

Figure 3–3

Sequential lateral views of the femur of a child with osteogenesis imperfecta show deformity from sequential fractures and healing *(A)*, refracture *(B)*, and healing post *shish-kebob* realignment osteotomies of the femur *(C)*.

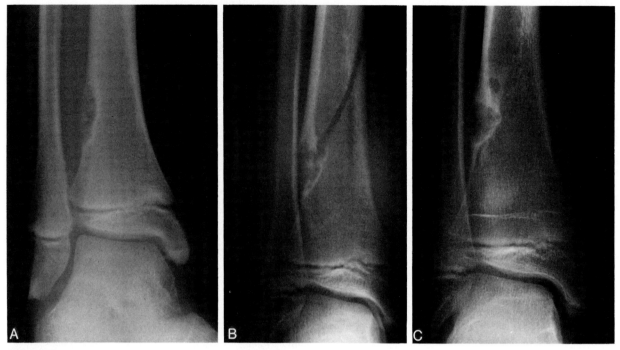

Figure 3–4

A fibrous cortical defect (A), which was identified as an incidental finding, becomes a stress riser when torsional force is applied (B). Healing of the fracture and remodeling have partially obliterated the lesion (C).

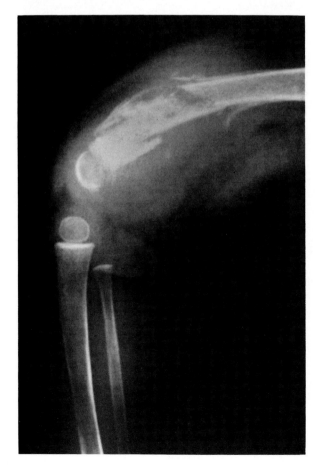

Figure 3–5

A pathologic fracture is evident in the distal femur of a 1-year-old child with osteomyelitis.

that approximately 75% of tumors are recognizable by x-ray appearance.[2] When fracture and its aftermath intrude, the diagnosis may not be so apparent. The lesion of the proximal fibula shown in Figure 3–6A presented with pain following a fall. Although the plain film shows a well-defined intraosseous margin, periosteal new bone is present. No fracture line can be seen. The technetium bone scan (Fig. 3–6B) shows marked increased uptake in the area of the lesion. Computed tomography (Fig. 3–6C) demonstrates marked bone formation, again without evidence of cortical interruption. This lesion proved to be a fracture through a nonossifying fibroma.

As with some "virginal" tumors, biopsy is the only recourse. After bone fractures, the surgeon must ensure that biopsy is done on representative areas of the bony lesion, not callus.[7] Anecdotes abound of the so-called osteosarcoma that was really a healing fracture.

Management

Management principles of pathologic fractures are altered frequently by the abnormal condition responsible for the fracture. The ultimate treatment plan must address the confluence of two goals: to treat the fracture and to treat the underlying cause of the fracture.

Fractures through bone that has been iatrogenically weakened by stress-raising implants or by biopsy or drill holes may be treated like any other fracture at that site in normal bone. If the fracture is in a high-stress area, such as the proximal femur, internal fixation must protect all weakened bone. A few benign lesions will heal spontaneously with the healing of the fracture. Treat the fracture, and one has treated the precipitating pathology. Conversely, the nondisplaced infractions accompanying metabolic diseases and certain marrow lesions (metastatic neuroblastoma and leukemia) will heal with treatment of the primary disease. Some fractures through benign tumors must be reduced closed and allowed to heal before the underlying problem can be treated. This approach may obviate the risk of instability at the time of curettage and grafting as well as ultimate deformity or shortening.

Consideration of the underlying pathology may change the criteria for an "acceptable" reduction. Fractures in dysplastic bone frequently heal well but heal with the same dysplastic problems that caused the fracture. In Figure 3–7A the displaced subtrochanteric femoral fracture (the opposite leg of the child shown in Fig. 3–2 two years later) was immo-

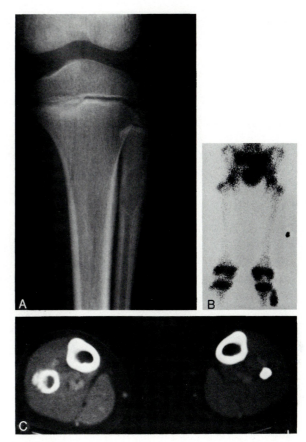

Figure 3–6

A lytic lesion of the proximal fibula exhibits good intraosseous margination but poorly defined periosteal new bone on plain film (A), marked increased uptake on technetium bone scan (B), and abundant new ossification by computed tomography (C). Biopsy proved the tumor to be a healing fracture through a nonossifying fibroma.

bilized in a spica cast with "appropriate" bayonet position of the fragments. In spite of excellent healing (Fig. 3–7B), little remodeling can be expected. Such is the nature of the underlying osteopetrosis.

Other circumstances require tandem treatment of the pathologic condition and the fracture. The requirements of the specific fracture may determine the course of treatment. The boy whose tibia appears in Figure 3–3 continued to be active in sports for the next 3 years. When he complained of pain in his distal arm, x-rays were obtained (Fig. 3–8A). The results were not reported before the next day's football game. After a fall on the field, he suffered an obvious fracture (Fig. 3–8B). A bone scan within 12 hours of the injury (Fig. 3–8C) showed uptake in the area of the fracture but no other lesions. Because of the question of diagnosis of the underlying lesion a biopsy was performed. The tissue

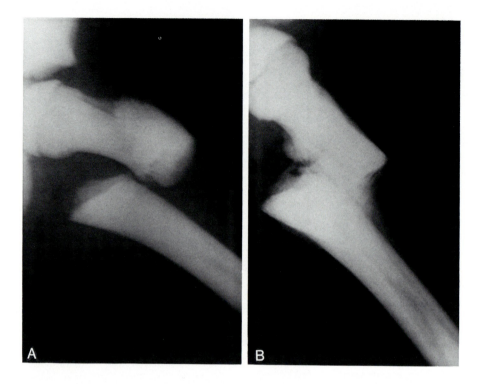

Figure 3–7
Initial films of a pathologic fracture of the femur of a child with osteopetrosis (A). The healed fracture shows little remodeling (B).

diagnosis was eosinophilic granuloma. Although this pathologic process required no further treatment, curettage of the lesion, grafting, and internal fixation lessened both the pain and the risk of significant shortening and deformity.

Other concurrent treatment plans may be driven by the histologic aspects of the underlying lesion. Aggressive benign bone lesions and malignancies may dictate aggressive approaches not required by the specific fracture pattern. Fractures through malignant bone tumors have traditionally been treated with amputation. While widely displaced fractures through malignant bone lesions continue to contraindicate limb salvage surgery,[2] certain nondisplaced fractures through chemosensitive tumors may heal during inductive adjuvant therapy.[4] The chemotherapy causes shrinkage of the reactive zone surrounding the tumor and fracture hematoma, making curative wide resection feasible. Bone-forming tumor cells may differentiate during inductive therapy, may accelerate ossification, and therefore may promote fracture healing. In this approach, all tissue that was contaminated by fracture hematoma must be removed at the time of definitive surgery.

Following this line of thought, Table 3–1 shows the common approaches required for pathologic fractures of specific tumors and tumor-like conditions. For those lesions that are likely to heal spontaneously with any type of intrusion (e.g., eosinophilic granuloma), the priority is to gain fracture healing. Benign pathologic processes that are less likely (e.g., aneurysmal bone cyst) or unlikely (e.g., chondromyxoid fibroma) to heal spontaneously may still require fracture healing to precede treatment

Table 3–1

Treatment for Fractures Associated with Tumors and Tumor-like Lesions

Priority for Treatment	Tumor/Tumor-like Lesion
Fracture (lesion may heal spontaneously)	Fibrous cortical defect Unicameral bone cyst Eosinophilic granuloma
Fracture—then *Lesion* (if necessary)	Unicameral bone cyst Aneurysmal bone cyst Eosinophilic granuloma Nonossifying fibroma Fibrous dysplasia Enchondroma Chondromyxoid fibroma
Fracture and *Lesion* (simultaneous)	Angiomas of bone Giant cell tumor Malignant bone tumors
Lesion (fracture may heal with lesional treatment)	Metastatic neuroblastoma Leukemia Selected malignant bone tumors (chemosensitive)

Figure 3–8

The same young man as in Figure 3–4 developed an unrelated lesion of the distal humerus (A). This lesion is purely lytic, with no obvious fracture but with periosteal new bone. Following a fracture through this lesion (B), an early bone scan (C) shows increased activity. Bone graft and internal fixation (D) led to good fracture and lesional healing of this eosinophilic granuloma.

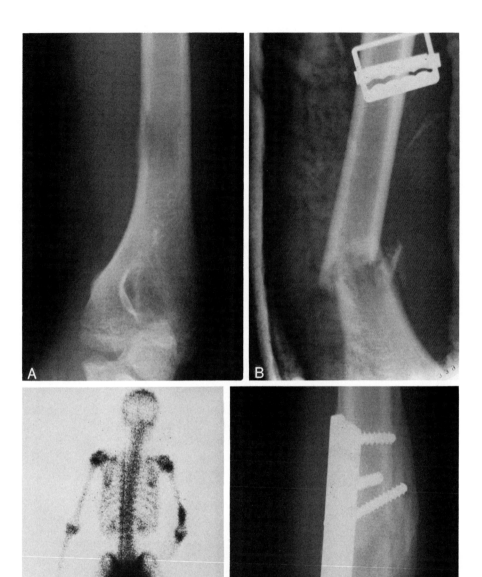

of the lesion. The potential problems of shortening and instability at the time of curettage and grafting have been mentioned. Aggressive lesions (e.g., giant cell tumors) will only grow larger while one waits for the natural process of fracture stabilization. These lesions require simultaneous treatment of the lesion (curettage/cementation/grafting) and of the fracture (grafting/internal fixation). The fourth group is limited to those nondisplaced fractures through lesions that have medical therapies (e.g., leukemias). These fractures heal well with only rest, symptomatic pain relief, and minimal splinting so long as the underlying pathology is effectively handled pharmacologically.

Prophylaxis

Pathologic fracture secondary to therapeutic interventions should be prevented by appropriate use of internal fixation; by protection of internal fixation by cast or brace, if indicated; and by the use of rounded edges of biopsy sites. Another measure is avoidance of unnecessary cortical penetration with drills and guide pins.

Once a fracture has occurred secondary to a previously unrecognized condition, prophylaxis can be employed to prevent subsequent fracture. This type of prophylaxis can extend from treatment of a primary systemic cause, to physical therapy and mobilization to decrease bone mineral wasting, to bracing of dysplastic bone at risk, to grafting and internal fixation of lesions before they fracture.

Guidelines for the prophylactic treatment of recurrent lesions or primary lesions that have been found serendipitously have been based on a paper by Arata and co-workers.[1] In this series the 23 fractured nonossifying fibromas were found to occupy greater than one half the bone's diameter in two planes. The minimum standard of acceptable treatment for any lesion occupying 50% of the cross-sectional area of the bone should be activity restriction and careful observation with radiographic examinations every 3 months. Serious consideration should be given to appropriate interventional treatment for the underlying pathology before the bone breaks. This latter approach will lessen the risk of further complications of shortening and malposition.

Summary

Pathologic fractures differ from fractures in normal bone in that the etiology of the abnormality of the bone and the natural history and treatment of these processes must be factors in planning treatment. Careful determination of this underlying diagnosis is critical in the appropriate care of these fractures.

REFERENCES

1. Arata, M.A.; Peterson, H.A.; Dahlin, D.C. Pathological fractures through non-ossifying fibromas. J Bone Joint Surg 63-A:980–988, 1981.
2. Enneking, W.F. Musculoskeletal Tumor Surgery. New York, Churchill Livingstone, 1983.
3. Mendez, A.A.; Keret, D.; Robertson, W.; MacEwen, G.D. Massive osteolysis of the femur (Gorham's disease). J Pediatr Orthop 9:604–608, 1989.
4. Meyer, W.H.; Malawer, M.M. Osteosarcoma. Pediatr Clin North Am 38:317–348, 1991.
5. Mirra, J.M. Bone Tumors. Philadelphia, Lea & Febiger, 1989.
6. Springfield, D.S. Musculoskeletal tumors. In: Canale, S.T.; Beaty, J.H., eds. Pediatric Operative Orthopaedics. St. Louis, Mosby-Year Book, 1991, pp. 1073–1113.
7. Springfield, D.S.; Brower T.D. Pathologic fractures. In: Rockwood, C.A.; Green, D.P., eds. Fractures in Adults. Philadelphia, J.B. Lippincott, 1984, pp. 295–312.

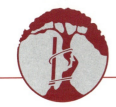

John H. Wilber, M.D.
George H. Thompson, M.D.

4

The Multiply Injured Child

Children who are victims of severe trauma usually sustain musculoskeletal injuries. However, they also may suffer injuries to other areas of the body that can be severe and even life-threatening. Although severe trauma is a major cause of morbidity and death in this age group, children and young adolescents are better able to survive it and often respond to treatment better than adults. Long-term morbidity or disability is due predominantly to injuries to the central nervous system (CNS) and musculoskeletal system. Careful, coordinated, and integrated management is mandatory to minimize morbidity and mortality. This chapter deals with the assessment of the child who has sustained injuries to multiple body or organ systems, which may or may not include injuries to the musculoskeletal system. It is not our intent to discuss in detail specific isolated injuries or their treatment, since this information is presented in other chapters. The focus is on evaluation and prioritization of treatment of the multiply injured child, with special consideration of aspects of care that may differ from those of an isolated injury.

Pathology

ANATOMY

It has been well documented in both the adult and the pediatric literature that a person who sustains multiple injuries must be managed differently than if similar injuries had occurred in isolation.[5, 41, 44, 49, 59, 99, 142, 150, 172] Concomitantly, it must be appreciated that the assessment and management of the multiply injured child differ from those for the adult. There are anatomic, biomechanical, and physiologic differences between injured adults and injured children.[35, 127, 144, 145, 156]

Anatomic Differences

The anatomic differences in the pediatric skeleton include the presence of preosseous cartilage, physes, and thicker, stronger periosteum that produces callus more rapidly and in greater amounts. Owing to the effects of growth and age, children also vary in body size.

The size of the child is important not only in the response to trauma but also in the type of injuries. Being variably smaller, the child will sustain a different complex of injuries than does an adult in a similar traumatic situation. An example is the pedestrian struck by a motor vehicle. In an adult, an injury to the tibia or knee is common because these bones are at the level of the car's bumper. In the child, depending on the height, the bumper will usually cause a fracture of the femur or pelvis or, in a toddler, a chest or head injury. Since the mass of the child's body is proportionately less, he or she is much more likely to become a projectile when struck, causing further injuries from secondary contact with the ground or another object. A classic example is Waddell's triad, consisting of an ipsilateral femoral shaft fracture, chest contusion, and a contralateral head injury (Fig. 4–1).[144] Owing to their smaller size, children are also more likely to be trapped beneath a moving object, such as a motor vehicle, sustaining crush injuries, fractures, and soft tissue damage. Crush injuries are relatively common in children, often result in severe soft tissue loss, and have a poor prognosis.[93]

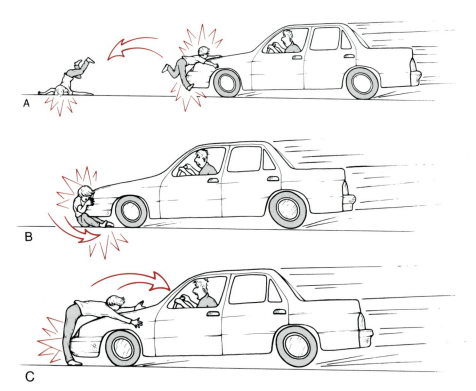

Figure 4–1

Different injury patterns resulting from a similar car vs. pedestrian mechanism. *A*, A typical Waddell's triad, in which the child sustains an ipsilateral femur and chest injury from the initial impact of the car and is then thrown forward, striking the contralateral side of the head on the ground. *B*, A smaller child being struck by the car, sustaining chest and head injuries from a direct blow on the bumper, and then sustaining lower extremity crush injuries from being dragged underneath the car. *C*, An adolescent being struck, sustaining tibia or knee injuries from the bumper, and then being thrown forward, sustaining chest, head, and neck injuries from impact on the windshield.

The child's body proportions, being quite different from those of the adult, can produce a different spectrum of injuries. The child's head is larger in proportion to the body, and the younger the child the more extreme this disproportion becomes.[72] This makes the head and neck much more vulnerable to injury, especially with falls from a height, since the weight of the head will often cause it to strike the ground first. In contrast, adults are more likely to protect themselves with their extremities. In addition to larger head size, the relative shortness of the extremities, especially the arms, as well as a lack of strength prevents children from adequately protecting themselves during a fall. This theory is well supported by the high incidence of head injuries suffered by children from falls (Fig. 4–2).[111]

Biomechanical Differences

The material properties, or composition, of bone in children is quite different from adult bone. Children, including those who are victims of multiple trauma, demonstrate unique fracture patterns. These include (1) compression (torus), (2) incomplete tension-compression (greenstick), (3) plastic or bend deformities,[100] (4) complete, and (5) epiphyseal fractures. Complete fractures occur more commonly in children with multiple trauma, as these are associated with high-velocity injuries. These fracture patterns are due to the presence of the physes, the thicker periosteum, and the material properties of the bone itself. Biomechanically, the pediatric skeletal system can absorb more energy prior to fracture than adult bone can. Pediatric bone has a lower ash content and increased porosity, which indicates less mineralization.[35] This results in more plasticity and less energy needed for bone failure.

Bending is the most common mode for failure in long bones. Stress on the tension side of a bone with a low-yield stress initiates a fracture that is followed by compression on the opposite side. As bending continues the fracture line eventually travels the entire width of the bone. Currey and Butler[35] demonstrated that although pediatric bone is weaker, it has a greater capacity to undergo plastic deformation than adult bone does. Because the pediatric bone yields at a lower force, the stress in the bone is less and the energy to propagate the fracture is less. These factors account for compression, greenstick, and plastic deformation fracture patterns. The increased porosity of pediatric bone that was previously felt to play a major role in the different fracture patterns is no longer accepted as a theory. Currey[34] studied impact energy absorption in 39 human femora ranging from 3 to 95 years. He found no relationship between porosity and the impact energy absorbed.

Ligaments frequently insert into the epiphyses.

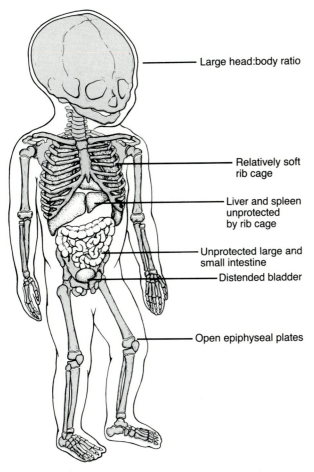

Figure 4–2
Anatomic differences predispose the child to injuries different from those of the adult. These differences include disproportionately large head, pliable rib cage with exposed liver and spleen below its margin, unprotected large and small bowel, distended bladder above the pelvic brim, and open physis.

As a consequence, traumatic forces applied to an extremity may be transmitted to the physis. The strength of the physis is enhanced by the perichondrial ring and in some cases by interdigitating mamillary bodies. However, the physis is not as strong biomechanically as the ligaments or the metaphyseal or diaphyseal bone. As a consequence, physeal fractures are relatively common in multiply injured children and ligamentous injuries less common than in the adult.

Since pediatric bone fractures with less force, it also affords less protection to the internal organs and other structures. The plasticity of bones can allow internal injuries without obvious external injuries. This is reflected in the increased incidence of cardiac and pulmonary injury without apparent damage to the thoracic cage and a high incidence of abdominal injuries without significant injury to the pelvis, abdomen, or lower ribs.[45, 163] Injuries to the liver and spleen are more common owing to less rib coverage of these structures as well as to the greater pliability of the ribs. The child also has less soft tissue coverage and muscle mass to protect the skeletal system from trauma. The lower mass of soft tissue may also contribute to injury of the internal organs.

Physiologic Differences

The child responds differently from the adult to the metabolic and physiologic stresses of trauma. Since the total blood volume is smaller, depending on the size of the child, less blood loss can be tolerated before signs of hypovolemic shock develop. This is because the smaller volumes lost represent a larger percentage of the total.[101] The higher ratio of surface area to volume also makes the child more vulnerable to hypothermia.[152] Klein and Marcus[88] have shown that there is a significant difference in the metabolic response between the adult and the child. Whereas the adult has a significant increase in metabolic rate resulting from the stresses of trauma, the child has minimal or no change. This is believed to be due to the child's significantly higher metabolic rate, which needs to be increased only a small amount to accommodate the increased metabolic demands. The accelerated metabolic rate response together with the ability to metabolize lipid stores provides a possible explanation for the increased survival rates seen in children after severe trauma.

Physiologically, pediatric fractures have the capacity to heal rapidly, remodel, overgrow, and develop a progressive deformity or shortening if the physis is injured. For these reasons, pediatric fractures secondary to severe trauma require careful management. Musculoskeletal morbidity is a common sequela of multiple trauma.[104]

Incidence

Trauma is the leading cause of death in the age group 14 years and under, accounting for approximately 50% of all deaths in children.[59] This is in contrast to 10% of deaths in the overall population of the United States. Fifteen thousand children 14 years or less die from accidental injuries each year in the United States, and an additional 19 million are injured severely enough to seek medical care or to have their activities restricted.[1, 5, 123] Haller[66] reported that more than 100,000 children are permanently crippled each year as a result of accidents. Marcus and co-workers[104] in a study of multiple injury in children found that long-term morbidity was directly related to the severity of the head and musculoskeletal injuries. Fortunately, most injuries in children are minor, the most common being due to falls with single extremity injury, usually the upper extremity. Chan and associates[30] in 1989 showed that approximately 13% of the children being evaluated in the emergency department of an urban teaching hospital had serious injuries. Gallagher and colleagues[54] in 1984 and Tsai[176] in 1987 showed a bimodal age distribution of traumatic injuries in children, the first being in the first year of life and the second being an increase through the adolescent years. Chan and co-workers[30] showed a steady increase in the number of age-associated injuries with respect to both total number and severity. Although the exact incidence and rate of severe traumatic injuries are not truly known, it has been shown in multiple studies that the incidence increases as the child begins to interact with the adult world, especially with motor vehicles.[30, 59, 77, 80] The vast majority of injuries occur where the child spends the most time, usually in or about the home. This changes as a child gets older, spending more time away from the home and beginning to enter the adult world.

Mechanism of Injury

As in adults, the severity of the injury sustained by children is directly related to the ultimate force applied. The two most common mechanisms of injury in children are falls and motor vehicle accidents.

FALLS

Gratz[59] has reported that most pediatric injuries are due to simple falls, accounting for 46% of injuries overall. According to Hall and associates,[65] falls account for 46% of all childhood deaths due to trauma. In spite of this, falls are only the seventh leading cause of death in children from all causes. Falls have an increasing importance in the younger child, since they are the third leading cause of mortality in children aged 1 to 4 years. Even simple falls in the infant or young child can be significant. According to these investigators,[65] falls contributed to 41% of the deaths in this age group. Musemeche and co-workers[120] showed that falls occur predominantly in the younger population, with a mean age of 5 years and a 68% male preponderance. Seventy-eight percent of the falls occurred from a height of two stories or less and occurred at or near the home. The majority of patients sustained a single major injury that usually involved the head or skeletal system. Fortunately, children have been shown to survive falls from a significant height, though significant injuries do occur[29, 186] As would be expected, morbidity and mortality increase with the height of the fall, the latter usually being related to falls of a distance exceeding 10 feet.

MOTOR VEHICLE ACCIDENTS

By far, the most common cause of multiple injury to children is motor vehicle accidents—both as riders and pedestrians. This is well documented in publications on multiply injured children (Table 4–1).[85, 99, 104] In the series by Kaufmann and co-workers[85] of 376 multiply injured children, motor vehicle–related accidents accounted for 58% of the overall injuries and 76% of the severely injured children. In the series by Marcus and associates[104] and Loder[99] there was, respectively, a 91% and a 96% incidence of motor vehicle–related mechanism of injury. Although the mechanism of injury was not analyzed by age, the incidence of motor vehicle–related injuries increases with age. According to the Injury Mortality Atlas, deaths from motor vehicle accidents are lowest from birth to 14 years (5.9 to 10 per 100,000 population) with the peak occurring in the 15- to 24-year age group (25.5 to 44.7 per 100,000).[78] Males in this age group have twice the mortality rate of females.

Table 4–1
Mechanism of Injury (From Published Series)

Mechanism	Marcus et al.[104] (N = 74) (%)	Loder[99] (N = 78) (%)	Kaufmann et al.[85] (N = 376) (%)
Motor vehicle accidents			
Occupant	9	35	18
Pedestrian	76	33	23
Bicycle	3	18	17
Motorcycle	3	5	0
Train	6	1	0
Falls	3	4	24
Other	0	4	19

Associated Injuries

By definition, the multiply injured child has injuries involving more than one organ system. It is critical to recognize all injuries sustained. Although many injuries occur in isolation or in combination, many others have been shown to occur in an associated pattern. One of the most common groups of associated injuries is that described as Waddell's triad.[144] The history of a child being struck by a car and the diagnosis of any one of the triad injuries should alert the physician to evaluate the other associated areas.

SPINAL INJURIES

The presence of facial injuries, including lacerations and fractures, has been shown to be associated with an increased incidence of cervical spine injury in both the child and the adult.[95] The presence of a spinal fracture at any level in a multiple-trauma patient is associated with a greater incidence (5 to 10%) of noncontiguous fractures at other levels of the spine.[60, 121, 139] Thus, the patient presenting with head, facial, or spinal injury at any level should alert the physician to carefully evaluate the entire spinal column. This is especially true in the head-injured child who is either comatose or unable to cooperate in the examination. In the multiply injured child, a spinal injury must be assumed to be present until proven otherwise by physical examination and radiographic evaluation.

FIRST RIB FRACTURES

The presence of a first rib fracture as a marker for severe trauma is well documented in the adult literature.[3] Harris and Soper[69] in 1990 demonstrated the same association in the pediatric multiple-trauma patient. First rib fractures are associated with a high incidence of other injuries, including fractured clavicles, additional rib fractures, head injuries, great vessel injuries, and pneumothoraces as well as lung and cardiac contusions. Multiple rib fractures are also a marker of severe trauma in a pediatric patient. Garcia and associates[56] reported a 42% mortality in the pediatric patient with multiple rib fractures; the risk of mortality increases with the number of ribs fractured. They found that a head injury with multiple rib fractures signified an even worse prognosis, with 71% mortality. Since head injuries are associated with a higher incidence of mortality and long-term disability, it is critical to recognize this relationship. Multiple rib fractures in the child under 3 years of age also should alert the physician to the possibility of child abuse, since 63% of patients in this age group in this series[56] were victims of child abuse. Multiple fractures in different stages of healing are also a sign of child abuse and should raise the physician's suspicion accordingly (see Chapter 15).

PELVIC FRACTURES

Pelvic fractures in children are an uncommon injury and, as in adults, are usually the result of a high-velocity force.[18, 25, 115, 119, 148] Simple or isolated pelvic fractures have been shown by Bond and co-workers[18] to have low morbidity and mortality and not to be associated with other injuries (Fig. 4–3). The vast majority of pelvic injuries in children are simple nondisplaced fractures. Conversely, complex pelvic fractures have an 80% incidence of gastrointestinal and genitourinary injuries, and these should be carefully evaluated.[18, 119] Complex pelvic fractures are associated with high-velocity injuries, and thus multiple injuries are expected. Unstable fractures, such as vertical shear or wide pelvic diastasis, are often associated with significant blood loss secondary to retroperitoneal bleeding (see Chapter 10).[155]

LAP BELT INJURIES

In an automobile accident, the use of a lap belt may produce a constellation of injuries referred to as the seat belt syndrome.[2] These injuries include flexion-distraction injury to the lumbar spine (Chance fracture) and small bowel disruption or contusion. Head and extremity injuries are unusual but can occur. This is in sharp contrast to the unrestrained passenger, who usually sustains severe head and solid organ injuries.[74, 149]

OTHER INJURY PATTERNS

Understanding injury patterns and the types of associated injury can be helpful in evaluating the multiply injured patient. However, almost any combination can occur in the child, and the injury patterns are most closely related to the mechanism, the total force applied, and the age of the patient. According to Peclet and associates,[133] head injuries are most common among child abuse victims, riders in vehicular crashes, and following falls; nearly 40% of abused children suffer injuries to the head and

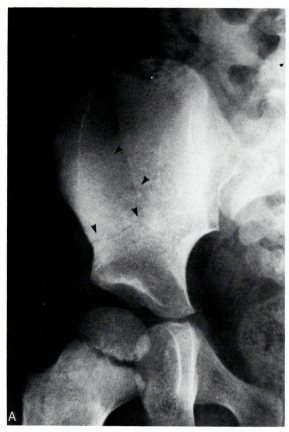
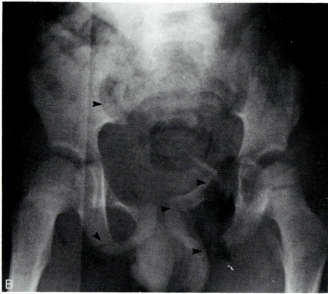

Figure 4–3

A, Anteroposterior radiograph of a 4-year-old child demonstrating a nondisplaced stable fracture of the iliac wing with no associated intrapelvic or infraabdominal injuries. *B,* Anteroposterior pelvic radiograph of a 5-year-old who was run over by a truck and sustained multiple pelvic injuries and multiple associated injuries, including proximal femur fractures, degloving soft tissue injuries, rectal perforation, and bladder ruptures.

face. In this study, thoracic and abdominal injuries were most common among children with penetrating injuries (gunshot wounds and stabs), while extremity injuries predominated among bicyclists and pedestrians. These investigators also showed that the types of injuries changed with age: Burns and foreign bodies accounted for the majority of injuries to children aged 1 to 2 years, compared with the median age of 7 years for pedestrian-bicycle injuries and 12 years for gunshot and stab wounds. Falls and traffic-related injuries predominated among children 5 to 10 years of age. Children who sustained injuries from falls were significantly younger than those with traffic-related injuries. Since the mechanisms of injury change with age, injury patterns and associated injuries also vary accordingly.

Classification

It is obvious that the multiply injured child presents with a spectrum of injuries of varying degrees of severity. The need for an objective measure of trauma is well recognized, both to assist in management and as a predictor of outcome in injuries of comparable severity. This requires the development and use of a severity of injury scale. This need has been documented in the adult trauma patient, and multiple systems have been advocated.[8–10] Similar systems have been recommended for the pediatric patient; the most widely used and accepted is the Modified Injury Severity Scale (MISS) introduced by Mayer and associates.[109, 110] More recently, the Pediatric Trauma Score has been introduced.[169, 170]

MODIFIED INJURY SEVERITY SCALE (MISS)

The MISS represents an adaptation of the American Medical Association's abbreviated scale for tissue damage and the Abbreviated Injury Severity Scale, which have been utilized in the assessment of the adult trauma patient.[9, 10, 32] The pediatric MISS categorizes the injuries into five body areas, which include (1) neural systems, (2) face and neck, (3) chest, (4) abdomen and pelvic contents, and (5) extremities and pelvic girdle (Table 4–2).[109, 110] The severity of each injury is rated on a scale of 1 to 5, with 1 point for minor injuries, 2 points for moderate injury, 3 points for severe but not life-threatening injury, 4 points for severe injury but probable survival, and 5 points for critical injuries with uncertain

Table 4–2
The Modified Injury Severity Scale (MISS) for Multiple-Injury Children

Body Area	1—Minor	2—Moderate	3—Severe, Not Life-Threatening	4—Severe, Life-Threatening	5—Critical, Survival Uncertain
Neural	GSC 13–14	GSC 9–12	GSC 9–12	GSC 5–8	GSC 4
Face and neck	Abrasion or contusions of ocular apparatus or lid Vitreous or conjunctival hemorrhage Fractured teeth	Undisplaced facial bone fracture Laceration of eye, disfiguring laceration Retinal detachment	Loss of eye, avulsion of optic nerve Displaced facial fracture "Blow-out" fracture of orbit	Bone or soft tissue injury with minor destruction	Injuries with airway obstruction
Chest	Muscle ache or chest wall stiffness	Simple rib or sternal fracture	Multiple rib fractures Hemothorax or pneumothorax Diaphragmatic rupture Pulmonary contusion	Open chest wounds Pneumomediastinum Myocardial contusion	Lacerations, tracheal hemomediastinum Aortic laceration Myocardial laceration or rupture
Abdomen	Muscle ache, seat belt abrasion	Major abdominal wall contusion	Contusion of abdominal organs Retroperitoneal hematoma Extraperitoneal bladder rupture Thoracic or lumbar spine fractures	Minor laceration of abdominal organs Intraperitoneal bladder rupture Spine fractures with paraplegia	Rupture or severe laceration of abdominal vessels or organs
Extremities and pelvic girdle	Minor sprains Simple fractures and dislocations	Open fractures of digits Nondisplaced long bone or pelvic fractures	Displaced long bone or multiple hand or foot fractures Single open long bone fracture Pelvic fractures with displacement Laceration of major nerves or vessels	Multiple closed long bone fractures Amputation of limbs	Multiple open long bone fractures

Adapted from Mayer T.; Matlak, M.E.; Johnson, D.G.; Walker, M.L. The Modified Injury Severity Scale in pediatric multiple trauma patients. J Pediatr Surg 15:719–726, 1980.

survival. The Glasgow Coma Scale is used for grading neurologic injuries (Table 4–3).[167] The usefulness of the Glasgow Coma Scale has been well established in head injuries in both adult and pediatric populations.

The MISS score is determined by the sum of the squares of the three most severely injured body areas. The MISS has been shown to be an accurate predictor of morbidity and mortality in pediatric trauma. Mayer and associates[109] found that scores of 25 points or more were associated with an increased risk of permanent disability. A score of more than 40 points was usually predictive of death. In their initial study a score of 25 points or more was associated with 40% mortality and 30% disability, whereas scores of 24 points and less had no deaths and only a 1% disability rate. Their mean MISS score for death was 33.4 points, and for permanent disability 30.2 points.

Marcus and colleagues[104] used the MISS in their series of 34 multiply injured children and showed a progressive increase in disability and mortality with increasing scores. The mean score was 22 points, with a range of 10 to 34 points. Children with a score of 25 points or less had a 30% incidence of impairment; children with a score of 26 to 40 points, a 33% incidence of impairment; and children with a score of more than 40 points, a 100% incidence of impairment. Contrary to the findings of Mayer and co-workers,[109] children with a score of over 40 points were able to survive but not without significant disability.

Loder[99] also confirmed the relationship of increasing MISS scores with increasing mortality and morbidity in his series of 78 multiply injured children. He reported a mean MISS score of 28 points (range, 10 to 57 points). There were no deaths among children with an MISS score of less than 40 points. The mortality rate for those with an MISS score above 40 points was 50%, and above 50 points it increased to 75%. Thus, the effectiveness of the MISS score in predicting both morbidity and mortality is well documented in several studies, although the absolute percentages seem to vary.

PEDIATRIC TRAUMA SCORE (PTS)

Another index used to predict injury severity and mortality for the pediatric population is the Pediatric Trauma Score (PTS).[169, 170] This score is based on

Table 4–3
Glasgow Coma Scale

Eye Opening
4, Spontaneous
3, To speech
2, To pain
1, None
Best Verbal Response
5, Oriented
4, Confused
3, Inappropriate
2, Incomprehensible
1, None
Best Motor Response
6, Obeys commands
5, Localizes pain
4, Withdraws
3, Flexes to pain
2, Extends to pain
1, None

From Teasdale, G.; Jennett, B. Assessment of coma and impaired consciousness: A practical scale. Lancet 2:81–84, 1974.

six components, including (1) size, (2) airway, (3) systolic blood pressure, (4) CNS injury, (5) skeletal injury, and (6) cutaneous injury. Each category is given a score of +2 (minimal or no injury), +1 (minor or potentially major injury), or −1 (major or immediate life-threatening injury) points, depending on the severity, and these scores are added (Table 4–4). One major advantage of this system is that it is based on criteria that can be easily obtained either in the field at the scene of the accident or in the emergency room, and thus it can be used for triage purposes. Tepas and associates[170] in 1988 demonstrated a direct linear relationship between PTS and Injury Severity Scale (ISS) and felt that PTS was an effective predictor of both morbidity and mortality. There were no deaths in children with a PTS greater than 8 points, compared with those having a PTS below zero, who had 100% mortality. The PTS allows for rapid assessment of trauma severity in a multiply injured child, which assists in appropriate field triage, transport, and early emergent treatment of these patients. It is recommended that children with a PTS of 8 points or less be transported to a pediatric trauma center for management.

Consequences of Injury

MORTALITY

Mortality rates in children vary greatly owing to differences in the mechanism, severity of injury, and age of the patient. Unlike adults, who have a trimodal distribution of mortality from trauma, children follow a bimodal curve. Peclet and associates[133] in 1990 demonstrated that the majority of deaths in children occurred within the first hour after injury, with another peak occurring at approximately 48 hours. In their series, 74% of deaths occurred within the first 48 hours. Overall, there was a 2.2% mortality for all patients admitted to the trauma service. Not all the patients in this series were multiply injured, thus explaining the low mortality rate. In series dealing only with multiply injured children, Mayer and colleagues,[109] Wesson and co-workers,[183] and Loder[99] reported mortality rates of 15, 13, and 9%, respectively. These series did not include those children who were dead on arrival in the emergency department.

The fact that mortality rates are closely associated with the severity of injury is not surprising. The higher the MISS or the lower the PTS, the greater the rate of mortality. In spite of obvious differences from adults, children tend to have similar outcomes from trauma when similar injuries are compared. This was supported by the work of Eichelberger and associates,[47] who used a statistical method based on trauma score, MISS, and age. These investigators were unable to show statistically significant differences between the various pediatric age groups and the adult population. Other studies have documented greater survival rates in the more severely injured child than has been shown in the adult population.[99, 104] This concept is accepted by many but may not be true, as is shown by Eichelberger and associates[46, 47] and Nakayama and co-workers.[122] Head injuries have been consistently associated with higher mortality rates than have other types of injuries.

Table 4–4
Pediatric Trauma Score (PTS)*

Component	Severity Points		
	+2	+1	−1
Size	>20 kg	10–20 kg	<10 kg
Airway	Normal	Maintainable	Unmaintainable
CNS	Normal	Obtunded	Comatose
Systolic BP	>90 mm Hg	90–50 mm Hg	<50 mm Hg
Open wounds	None	Minor	Major or penetrating
Skeletal	None	Closed fracture	Open or multiple fractures

*PTS ≤8 = Referral to pediatric trauma center.
Adapted from Tepas, J.J., III; Ramenofsky, M.L.; Moll, H.D.L.; et al. The Pediatric Trauma Score as a predictor of injury severity: An objective assessment. J Trauma 28:425–429, 1988.

MORBIDITY

Unlike the child with an isolated injury, which is usually associated with rapid healing, good function, and minimal residual disability, the multiply injured child has a significantly higher risk for residual disability. Morbidity in children is usually related to injuries of the CNS and musculoskeletal system.[104, 183] At a 6-month follow-up in the study by Wesson and associates[183] of severely injured children, 54% still had one or more functional limitations, with 4% in a vegetative state, 11% severely disabled, 32% moderately disabled, and 53% healthy. The cause of the disability at 6 months in 44% was head injury and in 32% was due to musculoskeletal injury. This is consistent with other reported series. In the series by Marcus and co-workers,[104] 10 of the 32 survivors had residual disabilities. Five were related to head injury with residual seizures and spasticity. The remainder were from musculoskeletal injuries, which included nonunions, malunions, and growth disturbances. The incidence and severity of the residual disability increase with the severity of the overall injury as reflected in a higher MISS score. In the child, disability can often present late and be progressive owing to the fact that the child is still growing and normal growth patterns have been disrupted.

Trauma Evaluation and Management

FIELD MANAGEMENT PRIOR TO TRANSPORT

The successful management of a multiply injured child requires a rapid systematic assessment with early emphasis on the treatment of life-threatening conditions. Treatment is initiated in the field with advance life support techniques. The importance of treatment in the field, or prehospital phase, is well documented.[5, 75, 130, 143, 157] Since mortality follows a bimodal distribution in the pediatric multiple-trauma patient, with most deaths occurring shortly after the accident, an efficient and effective system of prehospital care is mandatory.[54, 176] Delays in treatment have been shown by Seelig and associates[158] as well as by Holmes and Reyes[75] to significantly increase mortality. If necessary surgery for life-threatening conditions was delayed more than 4 hours after injury, mortality was approximately 90%, whereas if surgery was performed 4 hours or earlier the mortality was reduced to 30%. Functional recovery was also improved with more rapid surgical care. Delay in diagnosis and treatment has been shown to be particularly detrimental to head injury. The goal of field treatment is to rapidly evaluate the patient, stabilize life-threatening conditions, prepare the patient for transport by immobilizing injured areas, and deliver the patient to a center equipped for the resuscitation and definitive treatment of the multiply injured child.

The early resuscitation and stabilization of the pediatric trauma patient require specialized equipment, including small-diameter airway tubes, small-bore intravenous needles, modified backboards, hard collars, and splints of appropriate size to fit the smaller patient. As in the adult, it is critical to appropriately immobilize the patient prior to transport to avoid further damage to injured parts. This is especially true when dealing with spine injuries and extremity fractures. Preventable deaths in the multiply injured child have been placed into three major categories by Dykes and associates[41]: (1) respiratory failure, (2) intracranial hematoma, and (3) inadequately treated hemorrhage. Treatment of respiratory failure and hemorrhage can be initiated in the field. The optimal treatment of an intracranial hematoma, however, requires rapid field triage and transport for immediate surgical decompression. Ramenofsky and associates[142] showed a 53% incidence of preventable deaths, with field treatment errors occurring in 36% and transport errors in 23%. The importance of appropriate field treatment cannot be overemphasized.

PEDIATRIC TRAUMA CENTERS

Since most children sustaining multiple injuries will require specialized care, they should be rapidly transported to a center that is able to institute the necessary treatment. The American College of Surgeons has set standards categorizing the level of trauma care that an institution can provide in both adult and pediatric trauma victims.[5] It has also set guidelines regarding when a patient should be transferred to a pediatric trauma center. These are presented in Table 4–5. The inappropriate transport of an injured child to a facility lacking the capacity to adequately handle these injuries will significantly delay appropriate treatment and may allow inappropriate treatment to be initiated by a well-intentioned but inexperienced physician or staff. Improved outcomes for trauma victims treated at trauma centers is well documented in both the pediatric and the adult literature.[23, 41, 82, 85, 130, 142, 184, 185]

Table 4–5
Guidelines for Pediatric Trauma Center Referral
More than one body system injury
Injuries that require pediatric ICU care
Shock that requires more than one blood transfusion
Fractures with neurovascular injuries
Fractures of the axial skeleton
Two or more major long bone fractures
Potential replantation of an amputated extremity
Suspected or actual spinal cord injury
Head injuries with any of the following: Orbital or facial bone fractures   Altered state of consciousness   Cerebrospinal fluid leaks   Changing neurologic status   Open head injuries   Depressed skull fractures   Requirements of intracranial pressure monitoring
Ventilatory support required

From American College of Surgeons Committee on Trauma. Advanced Trauma Life Support Course. Instructor's Manual. Chicago, American College of Surgeons, 1984.

TRAUMA TEAM

The complexity and number of the injuries of the multiply injured child mandate a team approach. The need for a multidisciplinary approach with members of specialties working as equal partners has been advocated by Peters.[135] In the majority of cases the team leader should be a pediatric surgeon who specializes in the care of the multiply injured child. This person should take primary responsibility for supervising the resuscitation effort, coordinating team members, and making critical decisions regarding priorities in treatment. The members of the team are drawn from the pediatric surgical subspecialties and include a thoracic surgeon, cardiovascular surgeon, orthopaedic surgeon, neurosurgeon, urologist, and plastic surgeon. Additional members include emergency department physicians and nurses, pediatric intensive care physicians and nurses, respiratory therapists, and physicians and nurses from rehabilitation services. Social workers and counselors also have an important role in the treatment of these patients.

PRIMARY SURVEY AND RESUSCITATION

The principles of evaluation and stabilization of the pediatric trauma patient have been established as guidelines and protocols by the American College of Surgeons as Advanced Trauma Life Support.[5] Although these guidelines are similar to those for the adult, the pediatric patient does require special consideration owing to unique anatomic, physiologic, and pathophysiologic differences.[43] The initial treatment consists of basic resuscitative measures, with the major focus on diagnosis and treatment of life-threatening injuries. This is considered the primary survey, with attention directed toward the treatment of problems with the airway, breathing, and circulation (the ABCs of initial resuscitation). The primary survey concludes with a brief neurologic examination and complete exposure of the patient for further assessment.

Airway and Breathing

The assessment of the airway is a primary consideration in all trauma patients. The patency of the airway must be assessed from the oral pharynx to the trachea. Evaluation, treatment, and maintenance of the airway must be performed with control and stabilization of the neck, since there is an increased incidence of cervical spine injuries in these children. There is considerable variation in the anatomy of the upper airway in a child depending upon his or her size and age. In spite of age, the jaw thrust maneuver is best for restoring airway patency; debris can be cleared from the mouth manually or with suction, if available. The neck is stabilized with in-line cervical traction. It is important to realize that infants are obligatory nasal breathers and that any injury that occludes the nasal passages will also occlude the upper airway. These injuries include nasal fractures, foreign material in the nostrils, and bleeding within the nasal passages. Iatrogenically inserted tubes, such as nasogastric tubes, can also contribute to nasal occlusion. Thus, in the infant, both the oral pharynx and the nasal passage need to be cleared to restore the airway.

If a patent airway cannot be guaranteed with these maneuvers, an airway must be established with the use of an endotracheal tube. An oral airway is not recommended in children. Since the child's trachea varies in length and diameter according to size and age, the diameter of the endotracheal tube chosen will also vary. There are two useful rules for choosing an endotracheal tube. The first is to gauge it on the size of the external nares or the size of the child's little finger.[129] The other is the following formula[6, 42, 91]:

$$\text{Endotracheal tube (internal diameter in millimeters)} = \frac{16 + \text{Patient's age}}{4}$$

A full complement of endotracheal tube sizes needs to be available for dealing with the multiply injured child. These tubes should be uncuffed, which allows for a loose fit in the trachea to prevent subglottic edema, ulceration, and eventual stenosis.

The passage of an endotracheal tube in a child is complicated by several factors, including the inability of the child to cooperate, the flexed position of the head because of the large occiput, and the cephalic position of the larynx and glottis. The short length of the trachea in young children also increases the potential for bronchial intubation; this needs to be evaluated clinically by auscultation of breath sounds and with a postintubation anteroposterior (AP) radiograph of the chest.[31] Since the child's trachea is not calcified and is soft, the tip of the endotracheal tube may often be palpated to confirm its position. A pulse oximeter (oxygen saturation monitor) may be helpful in documenting tracheal versus esophageal intubation.

If there is acute obstruction of the upper airway in a child and an adequate nasotracheal or endotracheal airway cannot be established, a surgical airway must be urgently established. A needle cricothyrotomy can quickly and safely be performed to establish a temporary airway and is the treatment of choice.[22, 125, 165] Surgical cricothyrotomy is rarely indicated because of its association with subglottic tracheal stenosis. A large-bore needle (14 or 16 gauge) can be directly inserted percutaneously into the trachea through the cricothyroid membrane, temporarily achieving an airway.[165]

Considerations for emergency needle cricothyrotomy include laryngeal fracture, major foreign bodies that cannot to be removed manually, severe oropharyngeal bleeding prohibiting intubation, edema of the glottis, and facial or mandibular fractures. Since needle cricothyrotomy with the use of jet insufflation is a *temporary* airway, if it is deemed that an oral or nasal airway cannot be achieved rapidly, provision must be made to convert the needle cricothyrotomy into a surgical cricothyrotomy. This should be done in the operating room under controlled conditions to decrease the risk of subglottic tracheal stenosis. Surgical cricothyrotomy is not recommended in children under 12 years of age because of this potential complication.

As previously mentioned, the airway must be established with care taken to stabilize the neck. *All patients should be considered to have a cervical spine injury until proven otherwise.* Temporary stabilization of the neck using sandbags and a backboard can be used, though these should be replaced by a rigid cervical collar as soon as possible. A modified backboard should be used for young children and infants because of the large size of the child's head in relation to the trunk. Herzenberg and associates[72] demonstrated that the neck is flexed when the child is placed on a standard backboard, thus potentially displacing an unstable cervical spine injury (Fig. 4–4). A backboard with an occipital

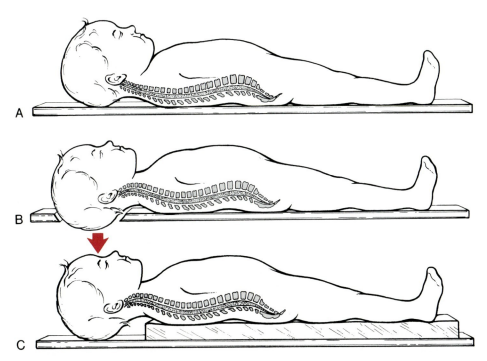

Figure 4–4

Standard adult backboard: *A,* The enlarged occiput causes the child to flex the head forward. *B–C,* Appropriate positioning on a modified board either with the occipital area cut out or with a pad under the thorax to prevent flexion of the cervical spine.

cutout or a pad under the trunk should be used to prevent flexion of the cervical spine. In-line traction should be used in all patients when trying to establish the airway. A lateral radiograph of the cervical spine should always be obtained following the primary survey. Major head and facial injuries should increase the physician's suspicion of potential cervical spine injuries.[95] In a comatose or uncooperative patient, a normal lateral radiograph of the cervical spine is inadequate evidence to rule out spinal injuries. The neck should be protected until a full radiographic series (AP, oblique, and odontoid views) and a clinical evaluation can be performed.

Once an airway has been established, adequate ventilation needs to be maintained. The adequacy of ventilation is evaluated both clinically and with arterial blood gas values. A pulse oximeter is also a rapid, noninvasive, and effective means of monitoring ventilation. Symmetric movement of the chest, auscultation for symmetric breath sounds, and palpation for equal chest expansion is necessary to assure adequate ventilation. A posteroanterior (PA) or AP radiograph of the chest needs to be obtained to evaluate the position of the endotracheal tube as well as to assess for injuries to the thorax (rib fractures), heart, lungs, and great vessels. Since the thoracic cage in the child is very compliant, the pediatric patient can have significant lung and cardiac injuries without obvious external damage to the chest and without rib fractures.[45, 163] The presence of first rib fractures and multiple rib fractures indicates severe trauma.[69]

Life-Threatening Ventilating Abnormalities. Injuries that may have a life-threatening effect on ventilation include tension pneumothorax, open pneumothorax, massive hemothorax, and flail chest. Since infants and small children ventilate primarily with the diaphragm, anything that compromises diaphragmatic excursion will restrict ventilation. Potential injuries that affect diaphragmatic excursion include diaphragmatic ruptures and intraabdominal injuries.

Gastric Distention. Severe gastric distention can severely decrease diaphragmatic excursion. Gastric decompression should be performed on all children with signs of ventilatory compromise. This can be achieved easily with the passage of a small nasogastric or orogastric tube. Because of particulate matter, a tube smaller than a No. 10 French will not adequately aspirate the gastric fluids and stomach contents and should not be used.

Tension Pneumothorax. A pneumothorax under pressure may initially be managed by the insertion of a large-caliber intravenous catheter, such as an 14- or 16-gauge Angiocath, into an intercostal space. This relieves the pressure and converts it into a simple pneumothorax, which can be managed with the use of a chest tube. Large penetrating chest wounds are initially treated with an occlusive dressing and positive-pressure ventilation. A flail chest is diagnosed by the observation of paradoxical motion with respirations.[39] If the child also has signs of inadequate ventilation, this should be treated with endotracheal intubation and mechanical ventilation.

Circulation and Resuscitation

Shock. It is critical to recognize and treat shock in the immediate phases of the primary survey. A child's response to shock is different than that of an adult. The child is often able to maintain a normal blood pressure by increasing heart rate and significant peripheral constriction while in the supine position. The signs of shock in children include tachycardia, tachypnea, poor peripheral perfusion (cool extremities), diminished responsiveness, decreased urine output, and a systolic blood pressure less than 70 mm Hg.[5]

A decrease in blood pressure is usually not seen or is a very late finding; absence of hypotension does not rule out shock. A child can often compensate for a 15 to 20% blood volume loss without a decline in blood pressure. The absolute blood pressure is not critical, and the American College of Surgeons guidelines state that it is unwise and time-consuming to obtain blood pressure readings during the acute resuscitative phase.[5] Blood pressure measurement can be performed once the child has been stabilized. A guide for normal blood pressures in children is a systolic pressure of 80 mm Hg plus twice the child's age in years, with the diastolic pressure being two-thirds the systolic pressure. Since infants are relatively incapable of increasing their cardiac stroke volume, their only way to increase cardiac output is by increasing heart rate. Thus, heart rate must be monitored closely. The normal vital signs by age are presented in Table 4–6.

Cardiac Tamponade. Tamponade occurs when the pericardial space surrounding the heart fills with fluid, preventing normal distention and contractility of the heart. This results in progressive decrease in cardiac output and ultimate failure. The clinical findings of cardiac tamponade include Beck's triad: muffled heart sounds, distended neck veins, and pulsus paradoxus. Initial emergent management consists of pericardiocentesis with the use of a long, plastic-sheathed needle that is attached to an electrocardiogram monitor and is inserted through a subxiphoid route. The need for emergency surgical drainage of the pericardium can be temporarily

Table 4–6
Approximate Weight, Blood Volume, Vital Signs, and Maintenance Fluids, by Age

Age	Approximate Weight (kg)	Blood Volume (ml/kg)	Pulse	Systolic BP (mm Hg)	Respiration	Maintenance Fluid/24 Hr (DR 1/4 NS)
Birth	3.5	90	140–160	80	40	100 ml/kg
6 Months	6.0	90	140–160	80	40	100 ml/kg
1 Year	12.0	85	120–160	90	30	1000 ml + 50 ml/kg over 10 kg
4 Years	16.0	80	120–140	90	30	1000 ml + 50 ml/kg over 10 kg
10 Years	35.0	75	100–120	100	20	1500 ml + 20 ml/kg over 20 kg
15 Years	55	70	80–100	110	20	1500 ml + 20 ml/kg over 20 kg

Modified from American College of Surgeons Committee on Trauma. Advanced Trauma Life Support Course. Instructor's Manual. Chicago, American College of Surgeons, 1984; and from Mayer, B.W. Pediatric Anesthesia—A Guide to Its Administration. Philadelphia, J.B. Lippincott, 1981, pp. 51–64, 251.

delayed by leaving the plastic sheath in place for continued drainage.

Hemorrhage. Severe exsanguinating hemorrhage requires prompt identification and treatment, usually by direct pressure. It is not wise to probe wounds and use clamps, since further damage can be caused. If direct pressure does not stop bleeding, the use of a temporary tourniquet is recommended. It is important to note the time of tourniquet application and to plan definitive treatment so that the tourniquet can be removed before permanent ischemic damage occurs. The treatment of shock should proceed concomitantly with the evaluation to determine its cause. If an obvious external source of blood loss is not found, one must assume that there is bleeding into a major body cavity. The presence of a head injury or multiple extremity fractures does not account for blood loss causing signs of shock, and thus other causes should be investigated.[11] An unstable pelvic fracture can cause significant blood loss and requires urgent reduction and stabilization.[155] This can be done with the temporary use of a MAST suit, an anterior external fixator, or open fixation with a plate. A simple anterior external fixation frame can be safely and rapidly applied using a single pin (4.0 or 5.0 mm depending on the size of the child) into each anterior iliac crest at the level of the gluteal ridge. These are then connected with a single anterior bar that adequately holds the pelvis closed. If emergency laparotomy is needed, a pubic diastasis can be plated through this incision using a two-hole plate. A trauma clamp has recently been developed and used.[55]

Resuscitation. As in the adult, two peripheral percutaneous intravenous lines should be inserted during the initial survey. These should be placed in the upper extremity, although the lower extremities can be used if venous access is inadequate or cannot be achieved. If percutaneous intravenous lines cannot be inserted, cutdowns must be performed. The most common sites for cutdowns are the greater saphenous vein on the medial aspect of the ankle, the cephalic vein at the elbow, and the external jugular vein of the neck. The use of percutaneous subclavian vein central lines is not routinely recommended in children, especially those under 2 years of age, owing to the difficulty of insertion and the potential for complications. They can be used in older children, although they are usually not necessary except for monitoring purposes. After adequate venous access has been achieved, other resuscitative measures can be instituted.

The primary objective of the initial resuscitation of the pediatric patient is to determine the degree of blood loss and the subsequent blood replacement. Fluid or blood replacement must be rapid enough to maintain stable vital signs and adequate urinary output. In the child with signs of shock, a bolus of Ringer's lactate with 5% dextrose solution should be given, calculating approximately 20 mL per kg body weight. A positive response includes a decrease in heart rate, an increase in blood pressure, improved peripheral circulation, increased urine output, and improved sensorium. If there are no signs of improvement, a second bolus of the same volume should be given.[5, 44, 101, 160] If there is still no obvious improvement after the second bolus, type-specific blood at 20 ml per kg body weight, or type O Rh-packed red blood cells at 10 ml per kg, should be administered. Blood less than 5 days old is recommended for transfusion, since it has higher levels of 2,3 diphosphoglycerate, which improves delivery of oxygen to the tissues.[134] When large volumes are required, the blood should be passed through a warming device to avoid hypothermia. Blood loss replacement in the child is based on the 3 for 1 rule: 3 ml of Ringer's lactate with 5% dextrose for 1 ml of blood loss. In the child with severe head injury, fluid administration should be adequate but judicious to avoid overhydration and increased intracranial pressure.

Acid-Base Balance. During resuscitation the pediatric patient may have acid-base complications. Most will resolve with adequate ventilation and perfusion. If the pH falls below 7.2, sodium bicarbonate ($NaHCO_3$) should be administered using the following formula[5]:

$$\text{Body weight (kg)} \times 0.3 \times \text{base deficit} = \text{total } NaHCO_3$$

One half may be given as a bolus, with the remainder given at a rate of 3 to 5 mEq per minute after adequate ventilation has been established. If carbon dioxide cannot be excreted, $NaHCO_3$ will not correct the acidosis.

Following resuscitation, maintenance fluids must be administered (Table 4–6).

Hypothermia. Hypothermia can be a significant problem in the child owing to the volume of fluids needed for resuscitation and the high ratio of body surface area to body mass. Every attempt should be made to use warmed fluids. Other means of maintaining body temperature include keeping the child covered, increasing the room temperature, and using overhead heaters and heating blankets. Hypothermia in the small child and infant can significantly complicate resuscitation, since it may render the patient refractory to the usual therapy for shock.[152] Hypothermia stimulates catecholamine secretion and muscle shivering, resulting in metabolic acidosis. The child may also develop coagulation disorders, which aggravate the condition. The child's temperature should be maintained at 36 or 37°C.

SECONDARY SURVEY

In the secondary survey, the history is completed and a complete physical examination performed. A trauma radiographic series is obtained concomitantly. The examination proceeds systematically with evaluation of the head, spine, chest, abdomen, and extremities to seek the extent of the injuries and prioritize subsequent treatment. The secondary survey is followed by definitive management of the injuries.

Trauma Radiographic Series

During the primary survey, plans should be made for obtaining a radiographic trauma series—a lateral view of the cervical spine, a supine AP view of the chest, and an AP view of the pelvis. These radiographs do not take precedence over the treatment of immediate life-threatening injuries. Depending on the size of the child the chest and pelvic radiographs may be obtained on a single cassette, thus saving time and reducing the need for movement of the child. These radiographs are obtained during the secondary survey.

Lateral Cervical Spine Radiograph. As mentioned previously, the lateral radiograph of the neck is used to screen for cervical spine injuries. Though it is useful as a screen, it cannot be used as the sole measure for determining cervical spine injury in the uncooperative or unresponsive child. Lateral neck radiographs in a young child can be difficult to interpret. It is not unusual to find a slight subluxation in the upper cervical spine, especially at the C2–C3 level. This is normal and is called pseudosubluxation of childhood.[28] A full cervical spine radiographic series in addition to a clinical evaluation is necessary to determine the presence of a cervical spine injury. The child should be treated with external support by in-line traction or sandbags or be placed in a rigid collar and assumed to have a cervical spine injury until it is proved otherwise.

Anteroposterior Chest Radiograph. The supine AP chest radiograph is extremely useful in evaluating for the presence of suspected injuries noted during the primary survey, to check on the response to any treatment rendered for these conditions, and to assess for more subtle injuries not suspected. Injuries that can be diagnosed on a chest radiograph include (1) pneumothoraces, (2) hemopneumothoraces, (3) pulmonary contusion, (4) aortic arch injury (mediastinal widening), (5) disruption of the trachea or a bronchus, (6) diaphragmatic ruptures, (7) rib fractures, and (8) thoracic spine injuries. As stated previously, because of the compliance of the ribs, the child can sustain significant internal injury without obvious damage to the chest.[45, 163] The diagnosis of a first rib fracture or multiple rib fractures is a marker of severe trauma in the child and warrants further evaluation.[56, 69]

Anteroposterior Pelvic Radiograph. This radiograph is useful in evaluating injuries to the pelvis. Though minor nondisplaced pelvic fractures may not be associated with significant complications, complex pelvic fractures, especially those that are displaced, have an increased risk for associated injuries and therefore a much worse prognosis.[18, 119] The presence of severe pelvic fractures should alert the physician to genitourinary injuries, such as urethral and bladder injuries, as well as to injuries of the abdominal and pelvic contents. These may include lacerations of the small or large intestine and visceral ruptures of the liver, spleen, and kidneys. Blood at the urethral meatus, a high-riding or nonpalpable prostate gland on a rectal examination, and blood in the scrotum are indications of potential damage to the genitourinary system and should alert the surgeon to evaluate this before inserting a Foley catheter.[51] If a pelvic fracture is diagnosed and if it is necessary to perform a peritoneal lavage, a supraumbilical approach is recommended instead of the routine infraumbilical approach. This is to avoid false-positive findings secondary to pelvic bleeding.

Fractures and dislocations of the hip and proximal femurs can also be assessed on the routine AP pelvic radiograph. A pelvic computed tomography (CT) scan is indicated if an injury of the sacrum, sacroiliac joint, or acetabulum is suspected clinically or by standard radiographs (see Chapter 10). Posterior pelvic injuries are not well visualized on standard radiographs; CT scan has been shown to be the best radiographic modality for evaluating these types of injuries.

Other Radiographs. Radiographs of the extremities should be obtained based on the clinical evaluation of the extremities, including palpation of the extremities. These radiographs are of lower priority and should not take precedence over the assessment and treatment of any life-threatening conditions. When radiographs are obtained, they should be orthogonal, with two views 90 degrees apart (AP or PA and lateral). They should include the joint above and below if a fracture is present. Comparison views are only occasionally necessary in the child. Appropriately placing the child or infant on a large plate will often give a single AP view of the entire body (babygram), which can be an extremely helpful screening technique.

Head Injuries

Head injuries in the child have a poor prognosis with a high incidence of morbidity and mortality.[15, 20, 168] Rapid evaluation and treatment are therefore indicated. Signs of external injury, including scalp lacerations, hematomas, and facial lacerations or fractures should increase suspicion of potential severe intracranial injury. The eyes should be evaluated both with regard to pupil size and reactivity and for evidence of increased intracranial pressure by funduscopic examination. A neurologic evaluation, including evaluation of the cranial nerves, motor function, strength, sensation, deep tendon reflexes, and rectal sphincter tone, should be performed and adequately documented. The Glasgow Coma Scale score should be determined and recorded (see Table 4–3).[167] A CT scan is indicated in any child sustaining a head injury, especially if he or she is unconscious or semiconscious. If surgery, and thus anesthesia, are necessary, the CT scan is required to clear the child for surgery. In the hemodynamically unstable child who warrants emergent surgery to control hemorrhage, the CT scan may need to be delayed until the patient has become stabilized and then performed before surgical treatment is continued. Herniation syndromes and expanding mass lesions must be decompressed urgently. Children with signs of increased intracranial pressure should have direct intracranial pressure measurements monitored routinely.[26] This can be done safely and greatly aids the treatment of this condition.

It is important to remember that uncorrected hypovolemic shock may further compromise a severe brain injury. Hypoxemia due to shock may result in a secondary brain injury. Hypoxemia must be corrected by intubation, adequate ventilation with supplemental oxygen, and fluid or blood replacement. Restriction of fluids to minimize cerebral edema is not appropriate until after hemodynamic stabilization.

Spine and Spinal Cord Injuries

Vertebral injuries may be present with or without spinal cord injury. In a child who is a victim of multiple trauma, a spinal column injury should be presumed until ruled out by physical and radiographic evaluation. Information regarding the mechanism of injury, the use of restraints or seat belts (motor vehicle accidents), the neurologic status at the scene of the accident, and any change in neurologic status is important to obtain during the initial evaluation. Any child sustaining an injury above the clavicle or a head injury resulting in loss or alteration of consciousness should be suspected of having a cervical spine injury. Injuries produced by high-velocity accidents should also arouse suspicion of vertebral column injuries.

Examination of a child with a suspected spinal injury is carried out with the patient supine, in a neutral position, and with stabilization of the head and neck. In small children it is appropriate to place a pad beneath the trunk to avoid hyperflexion of the neck due to the disproportion in head size.[72] The child should be thus protected until definitive radiographs have been obtained. A careful physical examination is performed with particular attention to the presence of prominent spinous processes, local tenderness, pain with attempted motion, edema, ecchymoses, visible deformities, and muscle spasms. In suspected cervical spine injuries it is also important to assess for tracheal tenderness or deviation and the presence of retropharyngeal hematoma. A careful neurologic examination must be performed and accurately recorded. This must include muscle strength, sensory changes, deep tendon reflex changes, and autonomic dysfunction. The last is identified by lack of bladder and rectal control.

In spinal cord injuries it is important to determine whether the lesion is complete or incomplete. The presence of superficial (pinprick) and deep pain discrimination indicates an incomplete lesion and intact lateral column function. Posterior column function is assessed by position and vibratory sensation. Because of the phenomenon of sacral spearing it is important that sensation to the anal, perianal, and scrotal areas be tested. Evaluation for sacral spearing should include sensory perception and voluntary contraction of the rectum. The presence of sacral spearing indicates that paralysis is not complete and is a good prognostic sign with respect to neurologic recovery. The evaluation of muscle function and sensation will determine the level of spinal cord injury.

Spinal shock may occur after spinal cord injury. The pulse rate is usually not increased with this type of shock, and the blood pressure typically falls to approximately 80 mm Hg systolic as blood pools from the dilated visceral vessels. Flaccid muscle paralysis, flaccid sphincters, and absent deep tendon reflexes are associated with spinal shock. The presence of a bulbocavernosus reflex may be important in distinguishing spinal shock from true spinal cord injury. After completion of a careful neurologic evaluation, spinal radiographs must be obtained.

The lateral cervical spine and AP chest radiographs are obtained on every patient sustaining multiple trauma. In the lateral radiograph of the cervical spine it is important that all seven vertebrae be identified. Occasionally, the patient's shoulders must be pulled down in order to visualize C6 and C7. Other cervical radiographs include anteroposterior, oblique, and odontoid views. Occasionally, tomograms may be necessary to confirm the cervical spine injury and to determine its stability. Lateral flexion and extension radiographs are dangerous and must be performed under appropriate supervision. When injuries of the thoracic and lumbar spine are suspected, AP and lateral radiographs are obtained. Occasionally, oblique radiographs of the lumbar spine may be useful.

The treatment of any vertebral column and associated spinal cord injury is under the direction of the orthopaedic surgeon and neurosurgeon (see Chapter 5). This is preferably performed at a pediatric trauma center. In unstable cervical spine fractures or fracture-dislocations, stabilization by the application of tongs and traction may be appropriate. However, traction should be used cautiously to avoid distraction. Traction weights should be applied sequentially and assessed by repeat lateral radiographs. The use of steroids in acute spinal cord injuries has recently been shown to be effective in improving neurologic recovery when these agents are given in the first 8 hours following injury.[21] Steroid use is controversial and has not been selectively studied in children or adolescents.

Chest Injuries

The child's chest, as stated previously, is very compliant, allowing significant intrathoracic injury without obvious external trauma.[45, 163] The chest should be evaluated by palpation, percussion, and auscultation in addition to the AP chest radiograph. The presence of a first rib or multiple rib fracture is an indicator of severe injury, and other associated injuries must be sought.[56, 69] Conditions previously stabilized in the primary survey should have definitive treatment during the secondary survey. This may include the insertion of a chest tube for a pneumothorax or drainage of a hemopneumothorax.

Though ruptures of the aorta are very rare in children, a widened mediastinum warrants an aortogram. Bronchial injuries and diaphragmatic ruptures occur more commonly. Pulmonary contusions are quite common with blunt chest trauma in children and are often complicated by the aspiration of gastric contents.[163]

Abdominal Injuries

The vast majority of serious abdominal injuries in children are the result of blunt trauma, although penetrating trauma has an increasing incidence in the inner city population, especially in adolescent males.[78] Serious injuries to the abdominal contents can be inflicted with less force than in an adult owing to the anatomic differences in the child. The costal margin is higher than in an adult, thus affording less protection to the upper abdominal viscera. There is also less abdominal musculature and a more compliant pelvis.

Routine examination of the injured child's abdomen may be difficult because of the patient's fear, inability to cooperate, and generalized response to pain. In addition, a child's typical response of aerophagia, which results in gastric distention, increases the difficulty of an examination. In an attempt to reduce this problem, all children sustaining blunt abdominal trauma should have a nasogastric tube inserted and the gastric contents aspirated. The bladder in infants and small children in the distended state can extend up to the umbilicus, and it is helpful to pass a Foley catheter, provided there is no evidence of pelvic fracture or genitourinary injuries, to decompress the bladder. Serial abdominal examinations in an injured child in the absence of pelvic or genitourinary injuries are critical.

The child who presents with signs of peritoneal irritation, a distended abdomen, or signs of hypovolemia without obvious external blood loss needs further urgent diagnostic studies. The child with peritoneal irritation and unstable vital signs requires emergency laparotomy. Those with stable vital signs may undergo further evaluation by peritoneal lavage, CT scan, or both, in combination with serial clinical examinations and assessment of vital signs. Peritoneal lavage is a very sensitive study for demonstrating intraabdominal bleeding.[38, 40, 140] Peritoneal lavage in a child may be difficult because of lack of cooperation, because of distention of the stomach or bladder (or both), and because the abdominal wall is thin, which allows sudden penetrations. The recommended technique is similar to that for an adult. After insertion of a nasogastric tube and Foley catheter, the catheter is inserted using an open technique, and 10 ml per kg body weight (up to 1 L) of Ringer's lactate solution is infused into the abdominal cavity over 10 minutes. It is then reaccumulated by gravity drainage, with

TABLE 4–7
Criteria for Positive Peritoneal Lavage in Children

Test	Positive	Intermediate	Negative
RBC count (mm³)	>100,000	50,000–100,000	<540,000
WBC count (mm³)	>500	100–500	<100
Amylase (units/dl)	>175	75–175	<75
Bile	+		
Bacteria	+		

Aspiration of 10 ml gross blood is considered positive, and lavage is not necessary.

Modified from Joyce, M. Initial management of pediatric trauma. In: Marcus, R.E., ed. Trauma in Children. Rockville, MD, Aspen Publishers, 1986, pp. 13–38; and from Eichelberger, M.R.; Randolph, J.G. Pediatric trauma—initial resuscitation. In: Moore, E.E.; Eisenman, B.; Van Way, C.E., eds. Critical Decisions in Trauma. St. Louis, C.V. Mosby, 1984, p. 344.

Table 4–8
Indications for Peritoneal Lavage vs. Abdominal CT Scan

Peritoneal Lavage	Abdominal CT Scan
CNS trauma unresponsive	Stable vital signs
Unexplained shock	Suspected intraabdominal injury
Penetrating chest injury below nipple	Slowly declining hematocrit
Major thoracic injury	Neurologic injuries
Major orthopaedic injury above and below diaphragm	Multiple injuries requiring general anesthesia
Worsening physical examination	Multiple bleeding sources
Patient going to operating room for other system injury	Blood in urine
Abdominal signs or symptoms	

Data from Drew, R.; Perry, J.F., Jr.; Fischer, R.P. The expediency of peritoneal lavage for blunt trauma in children. Surg Gynecol Obstet 145:885, 1977; and from Meissner, M.; Paun, M.; Johansen, K. Duplex scanning for arterial trauma. Am J Surg 161:552–555, 1991.

the empty intravenous bag being lowered to the floor and analyzed.[5] Criteria for a positive lavage are similar to those for the adult and are presented in Table 4–7.

An abdominal CT scan is frequently necessary to evaluate abdominal injury in children.[33, 83] This is especially true for assessing possible splenic, hepatic, and renal injuries. The CT scan has the advantages of being noninvasive and enabling more specific evaluation of solid visceral injuries. Its disadvantages include the added time needed for scanning, radiation exposure, expense, and its lesser specificity in evaluating perforations and injuries to the small or large bowel. There is controversy as to when to use peritoneal lavage or CT, or both.[58, 105] In general, the CT scan has replaced the peritoneal lavage in evaluating the traumatized patient who has stable vital signs and does not require immediate surgery for other associated injuries. The peritoneal lavage remains the test of choice in the patient with multiple injuries requiring immediate surgical intervention. The relative indications for peritoneal lavage versus CT are listed in Table 4–8. Initial screening with peritoneal lavage followed by serial CT scans in the stable child has been recommended by Rothenberg and associates.[154]

The spleen is the most commonly injured intraabdominal organ in children, but treatment is quite different than for adults. Unlike the case in the adult, the treatment of splenic injuries in the child is initially nonoperative to try and salvage the organ.[37, 48, 77] Several considerations influence this nonoperative approach. First, the incidence of late malignant sepsis following splenectomy in children is well documented.[52] Second, the capsule of the pediatric spleen is thicker than that in the adult, which allows for surgical repair. Third, the child's spleen will often stop bleeding spontaneously. The spleen is best evaluated with the use of serial CT scans or radioisotope imaging. Children who present with evidence of massive bleeding require emergent operative treatment, with every attempt made to repair and salvage the spleen. Patients with stable vital signs and hematocrits can be monitored in the pediatric or surgical intensive care unit and followed with a repeat CT scan in 5 to 7 days. Surgical intervention is indicated during that time if the patient shows signs of continued bleeding, such as a progressive decline in the hematocrit, or signs of increasing peritoneal irritation.

Hepatic injuries (the liver is the second most commonly injured abdominal organ in children) are also managed nonoperatively, if possible. Close serial clinical examinations and monitoring, in addition to initial and follow-up CT scans, are indicated.[12, 84]

Penetrating abdominal injuries, such as gunshot or stab wounds, should not be treated conservatively and require mandatory laparotomy.[114] CT scans and peritoneal lavage are not considered necessary in penetrating trauma.

Extremity Injuries

Definitive evaluation and management of extremity injuries, in general, have a low priority during both the primary and the secondary surveys. Extremity injuries are rarely life-threatening and should never take precedence over the evaluation and treatment of serious injuries. Initial treatment of extremity injuries should include covering all wounds with a sterile dressing, realigning deformed extremities, and splinting all potentially injured extremities. A neurovascular examination both before and after splinting is essential. Open wounds of the extremity require antibiotics and possibly tetanus prophylaxis (see Table 4–12). Wounds should never be left uncovered, and multiple inspections of the wounds should be avoided. Inappropriate handling of wounds has been shown to significantly increase the rate of infection.[177] The resulting infections are usually with nosocomial organisms, with the added problem of multiple-drug resistance. All wounds in proximity to a fracture should be considered as communicating, and the fracture treated as an open fracture.

The evaluation for extremity injuries includes visual inspection of the entire extremity, which mandates the removal of all clothing. All extremities should be palpated for evidence of tenderness, swelling, crepitus, and instability and all joints inspected both visually and manually for signs of swelling, effusion, and deformity. The range of motion and ligamentous stability should be assessed. All major joints are examined, with special attention to the knees. Ligamentous injury to the knee is commonly associated with other injuries, such as femoral shaft fractures and posterior hip dislocation, and the knee injury is often missed[87]; instability on examination may represent a physeal injury.

Knee dislocation or multiple ligamentous injury has a high association with injuries to the popliteal artery and warrants further evaluation. This can include arteriography, duplex sonography, and use of the Doppler systolic arterial pressure index.[81, 112] In the last, described by Johansen and associates[81] in 1991, the Doppler arterial pressure in the injured extremity is divided by the pressure in the uninjured extremity. A value of <0.90 was found to have a sensitivity and specificity of 95% and 97%, respectively, for a major arterial injury. The negative predictive value for an index >0.90 was 99%. This was confirmed in a clinical trial, and these authors now recommend using this noninvasive test for exclusion arteriography in patients at risk for silent extremity arterial injuries. This test is rapid as well as cost-effective and can save valuable time during the secondary survey. However, it will not disclose injuries to the profunda femoris, profunda brachii, and peroneal arteries. It also will not recognize lesions that do not reduce blood flow to the extremity, such as intimal flaps and small pseudoaneurysms. Doppler measurements are not useful in venous injuries.

Vascular Injuries. Injuries to major arteries in association with extremity fractures are uncommon in children.[53, 159, 162, 181] Most are due to supracondylar fractures of the distal humerus. Approximately 5 to 10% of open fractures (type IIIC by definition; see Table 4–10) have an associated vascular injury.[38, 53, 124] Prompt clinical recognition, radiographic evaluation, and repair or reconstruction are necessary for limb salvage. The cardinal signs of arterial injury include (1) pulselessness, (2) pain, (3) pallor, (4) paresthesias, and (5) paralysis.[117, 181] However, the presence of palpable pulses or Doppler-documented flow does not rule out an arterial injury.

When an arterial injury is suspected or diagnosed clinically, an arteriogram is necessary. Common indications for arteriographic evaluation of the extremities include dislocation of the knee, absent or asymmetric distal pulses, signs of peripheral ischemia, and severe open fractures. A formal arteriogram can be obtained if there is not significant ischemia of the injured extremity. A single-plane, single-bolus arteriogram in the operating room should be performed when there is ischemia of the extremity and prompt revascularization is essential. In the older child or adolescent, the technique is the same as that used in the adult.[128] In the infant and small child, a cutdown is usually necessary for vascular access to avoid iatrogenic injury to the vessels. Compartment syndromes can occur following vascular repair, and fasciotomies at the time of repair are recommended.[153]

Radiographs should be obtained of all extremities with a suspected injury. Initial radiographs in a single plane can be used for screening assessment, although orthogonal views are recommended before definitive treatment is planned. In an infant or small child a single cassette can be used to obtain a radiograph of the whole body, including extremities. This is used purely for screening purposes, and additional specific views will need to be obtained based on evaluation.

Compartment Syndromes. Compartment syndromes do occur in children and are related to the severity of the trauma (see Chapter 13).[106, 107, 153] Careful evaluation of injured extremities, looking for signs of compartment syndrome, should be made. The most important findings include swelling and tenseness of the compartment and exaggerated pain with passive stretch of the distal joints. Paresthesias, pulselessness, and paralysis are late findings, and the absence of these signs does not rule out this diagnosis. Compartment pressures should be measured in all children with signs consistent with compartment syndrome. Uncooperative children or those with head injuries need to be evaluated very carefully, since they will lack the usual symptoms. Rapid surgical treatment with the release of all involved compartments is critical to reduce potential complications.[57, 106, 107, 116, 117, 153] In the forearm, separate incisions are used to decompress the volar or extensor compartment (Fig. 4–5).[153] The Henry approach, with division of the lacertus fibrosus, allows excellent exposure and decompression. In the lower leg, the double-incision technique is recommended to decompress the four compartments (Fig. 4–6).[153]

Fracture Management of the Multiply Injured Child

Once the injuries of the extremities have been defined during the secondary survey, definitive treatment needs to be prioritized and planned. Extremity injuries that hold a high priority include major joint dislocations, open joint injuries, open fractures, fractures associated with vascular injury, and unstable pelvic injuries in children who are hemodynamically unstable. The need for stabilization of long bone fractures, especially the femoral shaft, is well documented in the adult victim of multiple trauma and is probably equally important in the adolescent.[19, 87, 150] Its importance is not as clear in the child and infant, although stabilization of these fractures can certainly aid in nursing care, mobility of the child, and decreased pain and blood loss. Loder[99] showed that early stabilization reduces the number of days in an intensive care unit as well as in the hospital. It also decreases the duration of ventilatory support and the overall complication rate in comparison with children with delayed skeletal stabilization. It is important to reemphasize that extremity injuries are not life-threatening injuries and should not supersede the latter. They can, however, be limb-threatening and should not be neglected. Long-term morbidity is most frequently associated with inadequate treatment of extremity injuries.[99, 104] Since children's fractures tend to heal more rapidly than similar fractures in adults, plans for surgical intervention need to be completed at an earlier time in the hospital course; otherwise, the option for fracture reduction surgery may be lost and osteotomies required.

INDICATIONS FOR SURGICAL MANAGEMENT

It has been well established that most pediatric fractures and dislocations can be managed satisfac-

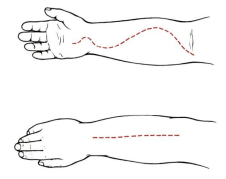

Figure 4–5

Standard fasciotomy sites for the forearm. Henry's approach is utilized for the volar surface, and a straight dorsal incision is made.

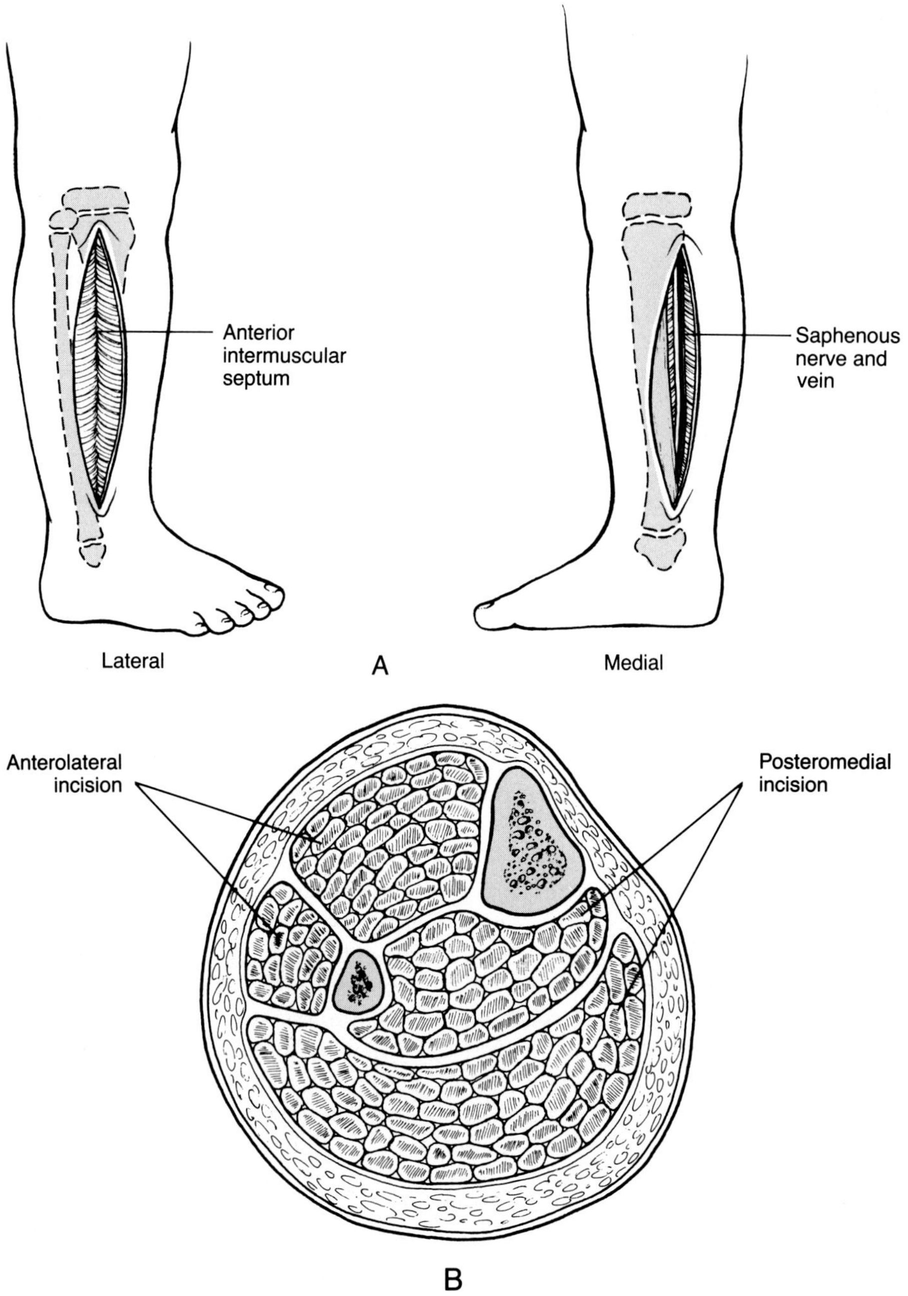

Figure 4–6

A, Double-incision fasciotomies of the lower leg allow access to all four compartments. Care must be taken on the medial side to avoid injuries to the saphenous nerve and vein. *B*, Cross section of the lower leg demonstrating access to the four compartments through the double incisions.

torily by closed reduction and cast immobilization or traction using skin or skeletal techniques.[17, 67, 127, 138, 144, 145, 151, 166, 182] However, there are specific situations in which surgical management may be more advantageous and result in decreased morbidity and better functional results.[172, 173] The multiply injured child and skeletally immature adolescent are major examples. The indications for operative treatment of pediatric fractures have been outlined by Thompson and co-workers.[173] These include (1) displaced epiphyseal fractures, (2) displaced intraarticular fractures, (3) unstable fractures, (4) multiple injuries, and (5) open fractures. The last frequently are present in the multiply injured child. The common fractures in each of the five categories are presented in Table 4–9.

In deciding on early and definitive management, several important factors must be considered: (1) the prognosis for survival and residual disability; (2) whether standard closed methods of treatment will adversely affect the management of other body area injuries; and (3) whether other body area

Table 4–9
Common Indications for Operative Management and Internal Fixation of Fractures in Children

Indication	Common Location
Displaced epiphyseal fractures (especially types III and IV)	Lateral condyle Radial head Phalanx Distal femur Proximal tibia Distal tibia
Displaced intraarticular fractures	Olecranon Radial neck Femoral neck Patella
Unstable fractures	Distal humerus (supracondylar) Radius/ulna diaphysis Phalanx Spine
Multiply injured children (especially with head injury)	Femoral diaphysis Tibial diaphysis Pelvis Spine
Open fractures	Severe soft tissue loss

From Thompson, G.H.; Wilber, J.H. Fracture management in the multiply injured child. In: Marcus, R.E., ed. Trauma in Children. Rockville, MD, Aspen Publishers, 1986, pp. 99–146.

injuries have a potentially deleterious effect on the musculoskeletal injuries if the latter are managed closed. If the prognosis is favorable and either of the last two factors is positive, the surgical option may be advantageous in the overall management of the child.[172] Possible examples include a child with a flail chest and a closed femoral shaft fracture. The femur fracture should not be treated in skeletal traction because this may compromise the care of the chest. Likewise, a child with a head injury who is combative or spastic may not be a candidate for conservative fracture management, especially of long bone fractures, because of the difficulty in maintaining satisfactory alignment. In both situations it would be more appropriate to surgically stabilize the fractures. It must be remembered that children tend to survive more serious injury than do adults, and thus, in all but the most extreme cases, survival should be expected.

TIMING OF FRACTURE MANAGEMENT

It has been well documented that severely injured children as well as adults are in their best physiologic state immediately after resuscitation. Delaying definitive treatment frequently allows secondary complications—pulmonary atelectasis, fat emboli, contamination of abrasions and wounds, fluid and electrolyte imbalances, deep venous thrombosis, and others—to occur, which may preclude surgical management for several weeks. This delay may result in subsequent musculoskeletal complications, such as nonunion, malunion, and others.[94, 104] If the musculoskeletal injuries are closed, if the other body area injuries do not require surgery, and if the child's condition is critical, closed management may be the most appropriate initial method even if less than optimal alignment is achieved. Definitive management may be delayed several days pending survival of the child. If surgery for other body areas must be performed the day of injury, operative fracture management should be performed concomitantly, if possible. Loder[99] showed that children undergoing immediate surgical stabilization of fractures had fewer complications than those whose stabilization was delayed. Since fractures heal rapidly in children, delays in treatment may significantly increase the difficulty of operative repair, if needed.

EPIPHYSEAL FRACTURES

Fractures involving the epiphysis and physeal growth plate are common injuries in children who are victims of multiple trauma. Peterson and Peterson[136] found that upper extremity physeal injuries had a higher incidence than those of the lower extremities (1.6:1). The physis of the distal radius was the most frequently injured physis followed by the distal tibia and finger phalangeal physes. Distal physes of long bones were found to be injured more often than proximal physes, except for the humerus. The peak age of incidence of physeal injuries is 12 to 13 years, with males predominating.

The most widely used classification of epiphyseal plate fractures is that of Salter and Harris (Fig. 4–7),[156] which has been demonstrated to be simple, accurate, and prognostically significant. A more complex classification has been proposed by Ogden.[126] The Salter-Harris classification has five types of epiphyseal fractures: (1) type I—complete separation of the epiphysis from the metaphysis without any bone fracture; type II—the fracture extends partially along the physis and then exits through a portion of the metaphysis, producing the Thurston-Holland sign; type III—the fracture extends partially through the physis and then extends through the epiphysis into the joint; type IV—the fracture extends obliquely across the metaphysis, the physis, and the epiphysis and enters the joint; and type V—

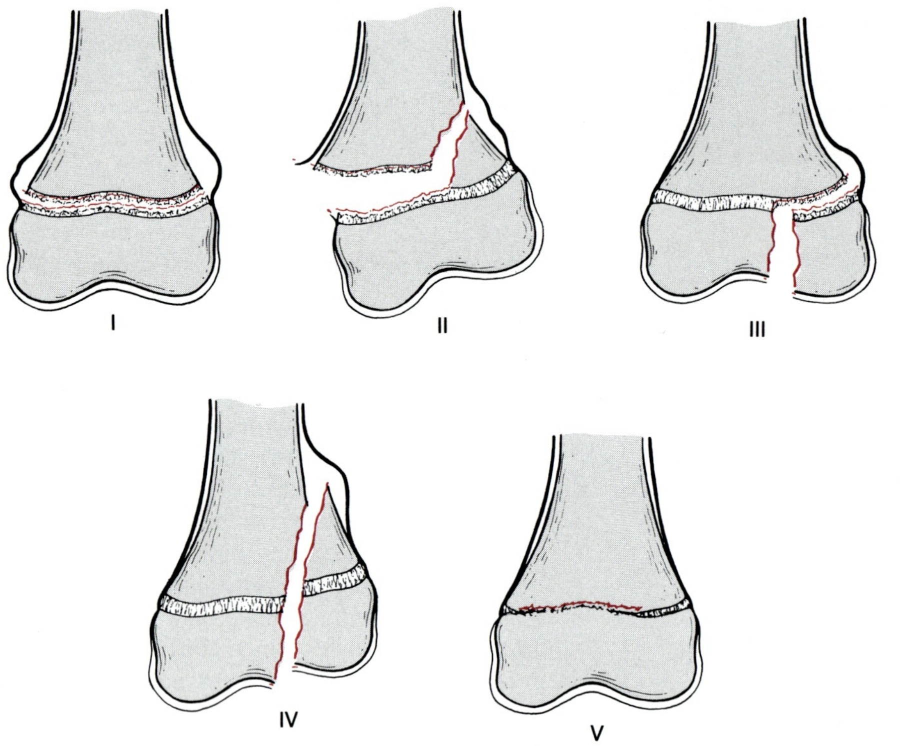

Figure 4–7

The Salter-Harris classification of epiphyseal fractures.

a nondisplaced crush injury to the physis without a definite fracture line visible radiographically.

Type I and type II fractures do not disturb the germinal layer of the physis and therefore usually have an excellent prognosis following closed reduction and cast immobilization. Displaced type III and type IV fractures require anatomic reduction, usually by open reduction and internal fixation, to restore alignment to the physis as well as to the articular surface of the joint. The prognosis is usually good provided the vascularity to the fracture fragment remains intact and the reduction is anatomic. If anatomic alignment of these fractures is not achieved, an osseous bridge may form across the physeal plate, resulting in premature physeal closure or asymmetric growth; central bridges result in shortening, and peripheral bridges tend to produce angular deformities. These bony bridges can occasionally be resected and fat or Silastic interposed to prevent re-formation. These techniques can be effective in restoring longitudinal growth.[24, 89, 137] The type V fracture has a poor prognosis because of the inherent damage to the physis, which subsequently leads to a growth disturbance. This injury is typically recognizable only in retrospect and is usually not amenable to resection.

PRINCIPLES OF SURGICAL MANAGEMENT

The principles of surgical management of fractures in the multiply injured child and skeletally immature adolescent are distinctly different from those in the mature adolescent and adult. Spiegel and Mast[164] have listed five general principles applicable to the operative management of pediatric fractures; these apply to multiple injuries as well as to isolated fractures requiring surgical intervention. (1) Multiple closed reductions of an epiphyseal fracture are contraindicated, as they may cause repetitive damage to the germinal cells of the physis, thereby predisposing to premature closure and late deformity. (2) At surgery, anatomic alignment is mandatory, especially for displaced intraarticular and epiphyseal fractures. (3) Internal fixation devices, when used, should be simple, such as Kirschner wires, and should be removed as soon as the fracture is healed. (4) Rigid fixation to allow immediate mobilization of the extremity is usually not the goal, but rather, stability sufficient to hold the fragments in anatomic alignment with a supplemental cast. (5) External fixators, when used, are removed as soon as possible and cast immobilization substituted when soft tissue problems have been corrected or when the fracture is stable. However, in the multiply injured patient the internal or external fixation must be of sufficient strength to allow for mobilization of the child. Thus, planning for appropriate surgical procedures is based on the age and size of the child, the bone fractured, and the extent and severity of other injuries.

SURGICAL TECHNIQUES

Three basic surgical techniques are utilized in the management of pediatric fractures, including cases of multiple trauma: (1) open reduction and internal fixation (ORIF); (2) closed reduction with internal fixation (CRIF); and (3) external fixation.[172]

Open Reduction and Internal Fixation

Displaced epiphyseal fractures, especially Salter-Harris types III and IV intraarticular fractures,[156] and unstable fractures, such as those involving the forearm diaphysis and the spine as well as and ipsilateral fractures of the femur and tibia ("floating knee"),[92] may require ORIF. Indications in the multiply injured child include closed fractures with neurovascular injuries requiring repair. Fractures are usually stabilized prior to vascular repair provided this does not significantly prolong ischemia time or take precedence over vascular repair if warm ischemia time is approaching 6 hours.[151, 156, 188] Occasionally, open fractures, especially of the femur or tibia, may be candidates for internal fixation.[68, 96]

Internal Fixation Devices. The type of internal fixation used during open reduction depends on the goals of management and the age of the patient. As stated by Spiegel and Mast[164] and others, the goal of fracture surgery in children is not usually rigid internal fixation, but rather, attainment and maintenance of anatomic alignment. Thus, most fractures can be managed by simple internal fixation devices such as Kirschner wires, Steinmann pins, cortical screws, and cannulated screws.[164, 172, 173] The fractured extremity is protected postoperatively with external immobilization, typically a plaster cast, until satisfactory union is obtained. This type of management usually allows the child sufficient mobilization to enhance his or her overall care. Occasionally, compression plates and closed intramedullary nailing are necessary for unstable diaphyseal fractures (especially in the lower extremity) in the older child and skeletally immature adolescent in order to achieve satisfactory mobilization. In children, internal fixation devices are removed soon after fracture union to minimize the risk of physeal injury and prevent incorporation of the device into the growing bone.

Closed Reduction and Internal Fixation

Closed reduction and internal fixation are indicated for certain displaced epiphyseal, intraarticular, and unstable metaphyseal or diaphyseal fractures. In children, this generally refers to percutaneous fixation with Kirschner wires or Steinmann pins. Pediatric fractures amenable to closed reduction and percutaneous internal fixation include humeral supracondylar, phalangeal, and femoral neck fractures. Anatomic alignment must be attainable by closed reduction before this method can be utilized. Failure to obtain anatomic alignment is an indication for open reduction.

The recent literature has suggested that certain pediatric fractures, especially those involving the femoral shaft, be managed by closed intramedullary nailing. With the exception of the femoral shaft, intramedullary nailing in pediatric fractures is uncommon as well as controversial.[171] There are no prospective studies contrasting the results of intramedullary nailing and closed management of fractures involving the humerus, radius and ulna, or tibia. Nailing of upper extremity and tibial shaft fractures is uncommon, although small series have been reported from Europe and Israel.[7, 90, 178, 179] The most common indication for intramedullary nailing in children is the femoral shaft fracture, especially in victims of multiple trauma.[50, 68, 70, 71, 87, 97, 98, 102, 135, 146, 178, 180, 189] These implants are inserted under fluoroscopic control, and prophylactic antibiotics are used in all cases. The results are superior to those of closed management. There are two basic techniques—reamed and unreamed nails. Reamed nails, including those that can be locked proximally or distally, or both, are used predominantly in the adolescent femur with the same technique as in adults.[187] Because of anatomic considerations and the risk for distal femoral physeal and greater trochanteric apophyseal injuries, reamed nails are not used in children younger than 10 years. Multiple flexible (Ender or Rush) nails are used in these children.

Internal Fixation Devices. Steinmann pins, Kirschner wires, and cannulated screws are the most commonly used devices in CRIF.[173] They are inserted percutaneously following closed reduction and can either traverse the fracture or be placed above and below the fracture and secured with an external fixation clamp or incorporated into a plaster cast. Smooth pins or wires may be placed across a physis if necessary for fracture fixation. These devices are usually removed as soon as the fracture is healed.

Unreamed and reamed intramedullary nails may be used in selected cases. As stated previously, reamed nails are used almost exclusively for the adolescent femoral shaft. The unreamed rods used for younger children include Rush rods, Ender rods, and small-diameter (2.5 to 4.0 mm) flexible rods of stainless steel.[171] Rush rods usually do not provide rigid fixation, and the extremity must be supported by a cast.[135, 189] Ender and flexible rods, however, can provide both alignment and length as well as rotationally stable fixation.[50, 70, 97, 98, 102, 178] These nails are prebent to conform to the anatomic curves of the involved bone, inserted to provide three-point fixation, and then anchored in the proximal and distal metaphyses. This allows end-to-end contact and maintenance of normal bone curvatures. The secondary muscles provide additional support. Slight movement occurs at the fracture site, thereby stimulating callus formation.

External Fixation

The accepted indications for external fixation of pediatric fractures include (1) severe grade II and grade III open fractures; (2) fractures associated with severe burns; (3) fractures with bone or extensive soft tissue loss that may require reconstructive procedures, such as free vascularized grafts, skin grafts, or others; (4) fractures requiring distraction, such as those with significant bone loss; (5) unstable pelvic fractures; (6) fractures in children with associated head injuries and spasticity; and (7) fractures associated with vascular or nerve repairs or reconstruction.[16, 93, 141, 147, 174, 175]

The advantages of external fixation include (1) rigid immobilization of fractures; (2) direct surveillance of the limb and associated wounds; (3) facilitation of wound dressings and management; (4) patient mobilization for treatment of other injuries and transportation for diagnostic and therapeutic procedures; and (5) possible insertion with local anesthesia in severely injured patients. The major complications of external fixation are pin tract infections and refracture following removal.[174]

External Fixation Devices. There are a multitude of commercially available external fixators, and newer multiplane devices are continually being developed. The use of half-pins is preferred to minimize additional muscle and soft tissue damage and possible neurovascular injury. During insertion, care must be taken to avoid the epiphysis and physis. Meticulous daily pin care is mandatory to minimize the risk of infection. It is recommended that the fixator be removed once satisfactory skin coverage has been obtained or when sufficient callus formation to provide fracture stability is demonstrated radiographically. Protection in a plaster cast following removal of the external fixator is suggested. Tolo reported refracture of 3 of 14 tibial fractures (21%) 5 to 10 months after removal of a Hoffmann device.[174] Whether refracture was secondary to stress shielding or to relative ischemia from the severe local trauma at the site of injury is not known.

OPEN FRACTURES

Open fractures are one of the most serious injuries to the pediatric musculoskeletal system. They are usually the result of high-velocity trauma and as such are increasing in frequency, especially in multiply injured children. In the series of multiply injured children reported by Marcus and co-workers,[104] 10% of fractures were open. Approximately 25 to 50% of children with open fractures have other body area injuries. The objectives of treatment of open fractures in children are the same as for adults: (1) preventing wound sepsis, (2) healing soft tissue injuries, (3) achieving bony union, and (4) returning the patient to optimal function.[61, 63, 64]

All open fractures must be graded as to the size of the wound, the extent of the soft tissue injury, and the degree of contamination, as these factors affect the prognosis. The most widely used classification was developed by Gustilo and associates (Table 4–10).[61, 63, 64] In the type I open fracture, the wound is less than 1 cm long. It is usually a clean puncture wound from a spike of bone that has pierced the skin. The fracture is usually simple, transverse, or short oblique with minimal comminution and soft tissue damage. In the type II open fracture, the wound is more than 1 cm in length, but there is no extensive soft tissue damage. There may be slight or moderate crushing injury, moderate comminution of the fracture site, and moderate contamination. Type III injuries are characterized by extensive damage to the skin and soft tissue, including muscle and possibly the neurovascular structures. There is a significant degree of contamination. This type of injury is usually caused by high-velocity trauma, resulting in considerable fracture comminution and instability.

Table 4–10
Classification of Open Fractures

Type I
Wound 1.0 cm or less (frequently from inside to outside)
Minimal muscle contusion
Simple transverse or short oblique fractures

Type II
Wound greater than 1 cm
Soft tissue damage, flaps, or avulsion
Minimal to moderate crushing component
Simple transverse or short oblique fractures with minimal comminution

Type III
Extensive soft tissue damage—muscles, skin, and neurovascular structures
Frequently a high-velocity injury with severe crushing component
    IIIA: Adequate bone coverage
          Segmental fractures
          Gunshot injuries
    IIIB: Periosteal stripping and bone exposure
    IIIC: Usually associated with massive contamination
          Associated with vascular injury requiring repair

Modified from Gustilo, R.B.; Mendoza, R.M.; Williams, D.N. Problems in the management of Type III (severe) open fractures: A new classification of Type III open fractures. J Trauma 24:742–746, 1984.

The type III open fracture may be subdivided into three additional groups.[63] In type IIIA, soft tissue coverage of the fracture bone is adequate despite the extensive soft tissue injury. This group includes segmental or severely comminuted fractures from high-energy trauma regardless of the size of the wound. In type IIIB, there is extensive injury to or loss of soft tissue, with periosteal stripping and exposure of bone. Massive contamination and comminution of these fractures are common. After debridement and irrigation is completed a segment of bone is exposed, and a local or free flap is needed for coverage. The type IIIC injury includes any open fractures associated with arterial injury that must be repaired regardless of the degree of soft tissue injury. The incidence of wound infection, delayed union, nonunion, amputation, and residual disability is directly related to the classification of the open fracture.

The methods of achieving the goals as described by Gustilo and associates[61, 63, 64] include (1) emergent initial care; (2) thorough initial evaluation to diagnose other life-threatening injuries; (3) appropriate antibiotic therapy; (4) extensive and possible repeat wound debridement; (5) fracture stabilization; (6) local wound care; (7) rarely, autogenous cancellous bone graft; and (8) rehabilitation. Each of these modalities is discussed in greater detail in Chapter 13, since the tibia and fibula are the most common bones to sustain an open fracture in pediatric multiple trauma.

Initial Care

Open fractures in children are surgical emergencies.[16, 61, 63, 64] At the scene of injury, the open wound is covered with a sterile dressing, the fractures are aligned through gentle manipulation, and the extremity is splinted for transport. Profuse bleeding is controlled by local compression.

Initial Evaluation

In the emergency room, the primary and secondary surveys are completed. If wound dressings are removed, mask and gloves are required. As stated previously, multiple inspections of the wound should be avoided. Tetanus prophylaxis (Tables 4–11 and 4–12)[27] and the first dose of intravenous antibiotics[132] are then given.

Antibiotic Therapy

Antibiotic therapy has been demonstrated to be effective in decreasing the risk of infection in open fractures.[36, 62, 132] Patzakis and Wilkins[132] found the infection rate to be 13.9% in 79 patients who received no antibiotics as compared with 5.5% in 815 patients who were treated with broad-spectrum antibiotics (cephalothin alone or cefamandole plus tobramycin). Approximately 70% of open fractures are contaminated with bacteria at the time of injury. Both gram-negative and aerobic gram-positive bacteria are pathogens for infections associated with open fractures. Because of the nature of the infecting organisms, combined antibiotic therapy is recommended for treatment of open fractures. However, hospital-acquired infections may also be a problem. For this reason, limiting the duration of initial antibiotic therapy to 2 or 3 days is important in order to minimize the development of resistant nosocomial bacterial infection.[132]

A first-generation cephalosporin is currently recommended for patients with an open fracture. For type I open fractures this is continued for 48 to 72 hours. In type II or III open fractures, combined therapy (first-generation cephalosporin plus an aminoglycoside) is necessary to cover both gram-positive and gram-negative organisms. This combination therapy also is continued for 72 hours. Penicillin is added if the patient sustained an injury on a farm,

Table 4-11
Schedule of Active Immunization Against Tetanus[10]

Dose	Age/Interval	Vaccine
Age less than 7 yr		
Primary 1	Age 6 wk or older	DPT
Primary 2	4–8 wk after the first dose	DPT
Primary 3	4–8 wk after the second dose	DPT
Primary 4	About 1 yr after the third dose	DPT
Booster	4–6 yr of age	DPT
Additional boosters	Every 10 yr after the last dose	Td
Age 7 yr and older		
Primary 1	First visit	Td
Primary 2	4–6 wk after the first dose	Td
Primary 3	6 mo–1 yr after the last dose	Td
Boosters	Every 10 yr after the last dose	Td

Abbreviations: DPT = Diphtheria and tetanus toxoids and pertussis vaccine absorbed; Td = tetanus and reduced-dose diphtheria toxoids absorbed (for adults only).
From Cates, T.R. Clostridium tetani (tetanus). In: Mandell, G.L.; Douglas, R.G., Jr.; Bennett, J.E., eds. Principles and Practice of Infectious Diseases. New York, Churchill Livingstone, 1990, pp. 1946–1982.

where animal excretion may be associated with spore-forming gram-positive bacilli (clostridia). Antibiotics are repeated when another major operation, such as delayed primary or secondary closure of a wound, elective open reduction and internal fixation, or bone grafting, is performed. Prolonged antibiotic therapy (more than 3 days) has not been shown to be efficacious in preventing the development of infection in wounds.

Debridement and Irrigation

The most important aspect of management of an open fracture is the debridement. This is a carefully planned and systematic process that removes all foreign and dead material from the wound. The wound edges are excised and the skin incisions liberally extended to allow unobstructed access to the entire injury zone. All dead and necrotic skin is resected to a bleeding edge, and necrotic or contaminated subcutaneous tissue and fat are sharply debrided. Contaminated fascia is resected, and prophylactic fasciotomies and epimysiotomies are performed to allow the injured tissue to swell and avoid secondary vascular compromise and tissue necrosis. Ischemic muscle is the principal nidus for bacteria; it is radically resected where compromised. The four "C's," consistency, contractility, color, and capacity to bleed, are classic guides to viability but, unfortunately, are not always reliable. Arteriolar bleeding and the capacity of tissue to contract after a gentle pinch with the forceps seem to be the best signs of viability.

When dealing with diaphyseal fractures, the medullary canal of the proximal and distal fracture fragments should be visualized and any contaminated material removed. Small devitalized and contaminated pieces of cortical bone are discarded. Although large nonviable cortical fragments are often retained in adults, they should be discarded in children, as whose capacity for bony regeneration is so much greater. Major neurovascular structures need to be carefully identified and protected.

Debridement is completed when all contaminated, dead, and ischemic tissue has been resected and the remaining wound cavity is lined by viable and bleeding tissue. Following debridement, pulsed irrigation with 5000 to 10,000 ml of normal saline

Table 4-12
Guide to Tetanus Prophylaxis

History of Tetanus Immunization (Doses)	Clean, Minor Wounds		All Other Wounds	
	Td[a]	TIG[b]	Td[a]	TIG[b]
Uncertain or less than 2	Yes	No	Yes	Yes
2	Yes	No	Yes	No[c]
3 or more	No[d]	No	No[e]	No

[a]Tetanus toxoid.
[b]Tetanus immune globulin.
[c]Yes, if wound > 24 hr old.
[d]Yes, if > 10 yr since last dose.
[e]Yes, if > 5 yr since last dose. (More frequent boosters are not needed and can accentuate side effects.)
From Cates, T.R. Clostridium tetani (tetanus). In: Mandell, G.L.; Douglas, R.G., Jr.; Bennett, J.E., eds. Principles and Practice of Infectious Diseases. New York, Churchill Livingstone, 1990, pp. 1946–1982.

solution is recommended. For final irrigation, 2000 ml of bacitracin-polymyxin solution is used. At the completion of the debridement and irrigation, additional aerobic and anaerobic wound cultures are obtained. When positive, these are more likely to identify the infecting organism.

Nerves, vessels, tendons, and denuded cortical bone are covered with local soft tissue, and the wound cavity is dressed with a bandage soaked in isotonic saline or an antiseptic. Despite meticulous care the extent of tissue necrosis is easily underestimated; the wound should be left open after the initial debridement. The wound should be reevaluated in the operating room within 48 to 72 hours. At that time it may be necessary to do more debridement. The process of debridement is repeated at intervals of 2 to 3 days or less, until the wound is clean, is viable, and can be closed or covered without the risk of infection.

Fracture Stabilization

Fixation of the principal fracture fragments reduces pain, prevents additional injuries to surrounding soft tissues, decreases the spread of bacteria, and allows for early soft tissue and bony repair.[118] The method of stabilization must allow for wound and limb access to carry out repeated debridements and to assess limb viability. Later, the fixation must be sufficiently rigid to permit weight bearing without interfering with range-of-motion exercises in adjacent joints.

Splints and Cast Immobilization. Plaster splints reinforcing soft cotton or wool dressings (Robert Jones dressings) are often adequate for the early care of stable open fractures of type I and some type II severity.[68] Once the tissue edema has subsided and the soft tissues are closed, more rigid fixation of the bony fragments is needed. In most instances, further immobilization of the fracture can be achieved with a well-padded cast.

External Fixation. For most unstable open fractures, cast treatment is not ideal.[4, 68] The more severe lesions (type II and all type III open fractures) often require repeated debridements with unobstructed wound access. These situations may be managed with an external fixator.[4, 13, 16, 68, 86, 147] The devices should allow free access to the wound for initial debridements and, if necessary, secondary flap procedures or bone grafts.[16] They should be of sufficient rigidity to prevent further injuries to the soft tissues, preserve length, and allow mobilization of the patient and possible full weight bearing.

With the exception of the athletic or obese teenager, simple one-plane unilateral frames afford sufficient rigidity for early unsupported weight bearing. Hansen[68] recommends an anterior half-pin device with dual bars for stability as the best method of treatment for type III open pediatric tibia fractures. Ring fixators (Ilizarov), using wires under tension, which can be ideal for pediatric leg length discrepancies, malalignments, or soft tissue contractures, are rarely used in treating an open tibial fracture in a child.[16] These devices tend to obstruct the wound, bind the soft tissues, and impale neurovascular structures.

Internal Fixation. Wires, pins, and screws, although common internal fixation devices in children, usually do not provide sufficient stabilization for open fractures. Occasionally, they may be used for the approximation of metaphyseal fragments, generally in conjunction with an external fixator, in order to neutralize the effects of bending and axial forces on the fracture zone.[16] Internal fixation of type I and some type II fractures with compression plates and screws or intramedullary rods has been successfully used in selected pediatric cases, especially for lower extremity fractures. However, deep late infections have been reported following the use of internal fixation in children.[73]

Wound Care

Appropriate soft tissue coverage is necessary for wound healing in the more extensive open fracture. Proper planning is facilitated if the wound is reassessed during the first or second debridement, in consultation with an expert in soft tissue and microvascular techniques.[76] The goal is to provide soft tissue coverage within 5 to 7 days after injury, before the wound is secondarily colonized or infected.[130] Prior to soft tissue coverage the wound must be kept damp with moist saline dressings. In children with degloving injuries of the lower leg, Letts has recommended that the skin be defatted and grafted to the extremity.[93] In severe cases the skin can be properly stored and reapplied several days later. External fixation is beneficial in stabilizing the fracture during wound care. Additional split-thickness skin grafts are usually necessary for complete wound coverage.

Most open fractures from type I to type IIIA can easily be covered by delayed primary wound closure. Occasionally a split-thickness skin graft is needed to cover a large cutaneous defect overlying muscle or fascia covered with healthy granulation tissue. For larger defects, particularly over the knee and the proximal anteromedial aspect of the tibia, the medial gastrocnemius or other muscle flaps are ideal for children.[76] The soleus muscle flap can be used to provide coverage of the middle one third of the tibia and microvascular free flaps for large distal-one-third defects.[76] Muscle and composite free flaps are useful for massive soft tissue and bony defects.[76, 79, 113] In addition to giving excellent coverage, these free flaps eliminate low-grade bacterial colonization in the recipient bed and facilitate union of the associated fractures.

Early Autogenous Cancellous Bone Grafting

The incidence of nonunion in pediatric fractures is low and usually is limited to situations with major soft tissue compromise and bone loss. Planned autogenous bone grafting is indicated in all fractures with partial bone loss exceeding more than half the bone diameter. If there is combined soft tissue and bone loss, placement of a muscle flap generally precedes autogenous bone grafting by 4 to 8 weeks. A large segmental defect in a very young child may simply reconstitute if there is retained periosteum, whereas in the older child a large cancellous bone graft may be needed. In adolescents the microvascular transfer of free bone segment, such as the fibula, is one effective method. Behrens[16] recommends autogenous bone grafting if no significant callus is visible 10 to 12 weeks after injury. Stabilization of these unstable fractures during the healing process is generally accomplished with an external fixator. Fixators usually can remain in place until the lesions are healed. If large bone defects occur, bone transport using a ring fixator system and callotasis technique is an option.[131]

Rehabilitation

Once the soft tissue and body cavity injuries have healed and bone union has been obtained, rehabilitation of the child is important. This typically consists of range-of-motion exercises followed by strengthening of the musculature. It is important that these children undergo long-term follow-up to determine ultimate outcome with respect to function and growth of the injured extremities. Follow-up should continue until skeletal maturity, to monitor growth development of the injured extremities.

Formal physical therapy and rehabilitation are generally not necessary for the majority of injured children. This is due to the fact that most of these injuries are simple, low-velocity injuries that heal rapidly as well as to the resiliency of the child. In the multiply injured child, however, this is usually not the case. Owing to the severity and complexity of the injuries, long hospitalization and multiple surgeries are often required. Although it has been shown that a child can tolerate prolonged immobilization without the usual complications seen in an adult, such as joint stiffness, severe muscular atrophy, and disuse osteoporosis, complications can and do occur, and a good result cannot always be assumed. As has been discussed previously, significant long-term disability, most often related to injuries to the CNS and musculoskeletal system, can occur in children. Aggressive treatment has been shown to decrease these complications and improve the overall results.[99]

PHYSICAL THERAPY

Physical therapy should be initiated as soon as the child's medical condition permits. Early physical therapy consists of gentle range-of-motion exercises of the noninjured or stabilized extremities to avoid soft tissue contractures and joint stiffness. This is especially important in the head-injured or spine-injured patient. More physical therapy can be instituted as the child's condition allows, including transfer training, resistive strengthening, and eventually ambulation. Each case must be dealt with separately, since the spectrum and severity of injuries will dictate the type and level of therapy. Close communication and cooperation between physicians and therapist is extremely important. The majority of physical therapy can be initiated while the child is still in the trauma center. Once the child's condition no longer requires that level of specialization, transfer to a different facility can be considered. This might be to another acute care facility that is not a trauma center but is more accessible to the family, or to a long-term rehabilitation facility if acute care is no longer necessary. Since children are often transferred long distances to be treated at trauma centers and these distances can potentially become a burden for families, attempts should be made for a transfer to a closer facility when the child's condition improves. Some trauma centers are equipped with facilities for both acute care and long-term rehabilitation services. This enables transfer from acute care to long-term care status while maintaining continuity of treatment by many of the same physicians and therapists. This is very desirable, since children do develop important relationships with, and dependencies on, the treating physicians and therapists, and severing these relationships can be extremely traumatic to the patient.

Children with severe head, spinal, and musculoskeletal injuries are most often in need of prolonged rehabilitation and are more likely to have permanent disabilities.[99, 104, 108, 109] Severe head injuries account for the majority of long-term rehabilitations as well as long-term disabilities. Children with head injuries require specialized facilities equipped for long-term rehabilitation. Not only physical rehabilitation is needed but also rehabilitation of cognitive capacities, including speech and learning. Multiple fractures in the absence of CNS injury can also result in long-term disability requiring prolonged rehabilitation. In addition to the usual modalities, specialized treatment with orthoses, prostheses, and appliances is often necessary for appropriate rehabilitation to optimal function. The fitting and use of orthoses and prostheses in children are very specialized, since the child continues to grow, and close monitoring and frequent modifications are often necessary. The appropriate use of physical therapy can significantly improve the outcome in these children.

PSYCHOLOGIC REHABILITATION

The psychologic rehabilitation of the injured child is equally important as the physical rehabilitation.[103] The physical trauma often creates severe psychologic trauma that in many cases is overlooked. Following the initial traumatic event the patient is faced with continued pain from the injury and multiple, often painful surgical procedures; disfigurement and loss of body image; and prolonged separation from parents, siblings, family, friends, and home. This psychologic trauma is not limited to the child but affects the parents and family and often the person who feels responsible for the injury. Dysfunctional behavior is seen frequently in children after trauma and includes phobias, scholastic difficulties, depression, and rage attacks.[14] This is manifested not only by children with head injuries but also by those with severe injuries without CNS involvement. Delays in the normal developmental processes are common, and in many cases the child is noted to regress. Such reactions can be considered normal, though they can at times become extreme.

These psychologic problems cannot be avoided completely, but they certainly can be lessened by the appropriate intervention with the patient and the family from the very beginning. The physicians and staff must be aware of these problems and try to be as supportive as possible. It is important to spend time with the patient and family, informing them of the injuries sustained, what is to be expected, the types of procedures to be performed, and the prognosis. Painful procedures should be explained in detail and their importance stressed. Children should be allowed to express their fears and concerns and made to feel a part of the process. They must be given assurances that they have not lost total control over their environment. The family should be allowed to be with the child as much as is physically possible. It is often desirable to allow one of the family members to remain in the patient's room. Many rooms are equipped with extra beds so that parents may sleep in the room with their child. Social as well as psychologic counseling is often necessary, especially when the child or family appears to have problems coping with the situation. Marcus[104] has generalized the child's normal and abnormal psychologic responses to trauma; these are presented in Table 4–13.

EDUCATION

Since many children will require prolonged hospitalization and rehabilitation, their schooling will be interrupted, in many cases for a extended period. This may put them significantly behind the level of

---

Table 4–13

Normal and Abnormal Psychologic Responses of Children to Trauma

1. **Impact Phase**—Crying, screaming, panic
2. **Rebound Phase**—Defensive response
   Avoidance of feelings and thoughts regarding the situation
   Behavioral withdrawal and regression
   Increased dependency
   Nightmares; increased startle responses
3. **Reintegration and Recovery Phase**
   Preoccupation with the traumatic experience (thoughts, feelings, play activities)
   Possible continued sleep problems and disturbing dreams
4. **Posttraumatic Phase**
   Intensity of experiences diminished (thoughts, feelings)
   Normal sleep
   Return to pretrauma personality function
   Return to self-confidence and self-esteem
5. **Pathologic Responses**
   Prolongation of phases 1 to 3 beyond expected
   Phase 4 impaired
      (chronic anxiety, depression, behavioral problems, sleep disturbances, nightmares, guilt, withdrawal, excessive hostility)
   Low self-confidence and self-esteem
   Obsession with trauma
   Neurotic symptoms
      (tics, neuroses, encopresis, or other regressive patterns)

From Marcus, I.M. Emotional and psychological implications of trauma in children. In: Marcus, R.E., ed. Trauma in Children. Rockville, MD, Aspen Publishers, 1986, pp. 245–257.

their peers, which will give them an added problem when they are ready to return to school. It is important to initiate schooling and tutoring in the hospital as soon as the patient's condition allows, recognizing that the duration of tutoring may be lengthy. The child with a severe head injury faces another spectrum of problems, since he or she may require a specialized educational program as part of the rehabilitation process.

REFERENCES

1. Accidental Death and Disability. The Neglected Disease of Modern Society. Washington, D.C., National Academy of Sciences–National Research Council, 1966.
2. Agram, P.F.; Donkle, D.E.; Winn, D.G. Injuries to a sample of seatbelted children evaluated and treated in a hospital emergency room. J Trauma 27:58–64, 1987.
3. Albers, J.E.; Rath, R.K.; Glaser, R.S.; et al. Severity of intrathoracic injuries associated with first rib fractures. Ann Thorac Surg 33:614–618, 1982.
4. Alonso, J.E.; Horowitz, M. Use of the AO/ASIF external fixator in children. J Pediatr Orthop 7:594–600, 1987.
5. American College of Surgeons Committee on Trauma. Advanced Trauma Life Support Course. Instructor's Manual. Chicago, American College of Surgeons, 1984.
6. American National Standards Institute Z 79.1. Tracheal Tubes and Cuffs. New York, American National Standards Institute, 1974.
7. Amit, Y.; Salai, M.; Chechik, A.; et al. Closing intramedullary nailing for the treatment of diaphyseal forearm fractures in adolescence: a preliminary report. J Pediatr Orthop 5:143–146, 1985.
8. Baker, C.C.; Oppenheimer, L.; Stephens, B.; et al. Epidemiology of traumatic deaths. Am J Surg 140:144, 1980.
9. Baker, S.P.; O'Neill, B. The Injury Severity Score: An update. J Trauma 16:882–885, 1976.
10. Baker, S.P.; O'Neill, B.; Hadden, W., Jr.; et al. The Injury Severity Score: A method of describing patients with multiple injuries and evaluating emergency care. J Trauma 14:187–196, 1974.
11. Barlow, B.; Niemirska, M.; Gandhi, R.; Shelton, M. Response to injury in children with closed femur fractures. J Trauma 27:429–430, 1987.
12. Bass, B.; Eichelberger, M.R.; Schisgall, R.; et al. Hazards of nonoperative therapy of hepatic injury in children. J Trauma 24:978–982, 1984.
13. Bassey, L.O. The Use of P.O.P. integrated pins as an improvisation on the Hoffmann's apparatus: contribution to open fracture management in the tropics. J Trauma 29:59–64, 1989.
14. Basson, M.D.; Guinn, J.E.; McElligott, J.; et al. Behavior disturbances in children after trauma. J Trauma 31:1363–1368, 1991.
15. Becker, D.P.; Miller, J.D.; Ward, J.D.; et al. The outcome from severe head injury with early diagnosis and intensive management. J Neurosurg 47:491–502, 1977.
16. Behrens, F. External fixation in children: lower extremity. Inst Course Lect 39:205–208, 1990.
17. Blount, W.P. Fractures in Children. Baltimore, Williams & Wilkins, 1954.
18. Bond, S.J.; Gotschall, C.S.; Eichelberger, M.R. Predictors of abdominal injury in children with pelvic fractures. J Trauma 31:1169–1173, 1991.
19. Bone, L.B.; Johnson, K.D.; Weigett, S.; et al. Early vs. delayed stabilization of femoral fracture. A preoperative randomized study. J Bone Joint Surg 71-A:336–340, 1989.
20. Bowers, S.A.; Marshall, L.F. Outcome in 200 consecutive cases of severe head injury in San Diego County: a prospective analysis. Neurosurgery 6:237–242, 1980.
21. Bracken, M.B.; Shephard, M.J.; Collins, W.F.; et al. A randomized, controlled trial of methyl prednisolone or naloxone in the treatment of acute spinal-cord injury. N Engl J Med 322:1405–1411, 1990.
22. Brantigan, C.O.; Grow, J.B. Cricothyroidotomy—elective use in respiratory problems requiring tracheotomy. J Thorac Cardiovasc Surg 71:72, 1976.
23. Breaux, C.W.; Smith, G.; Georgeson, K.E. The first two years' experience with major trauma at a pediatric trauma center. J Trauma 30:37–43, 1990.
24. Bright, R.W. Operative correction of partial epiphyseal plate closure by osseous-bridge resection. J Bone Joint Surg 56-A:655–664, 1974.
25. Bryan, W.J.; Tallos, H.S. Pediatric pelvic fractures: a review of 52 patients. J Trauma 19:799–805, 1979.
26. Caniano, D.A.; Nugent, S.K.; Rogers, M.C.; et al. Intracranial pressure monitoring in the management of the pediatric trauma patient. J Pediatr Surg 15:537–542, 1980.
27. Cates, T.R. Clostridium tetani (tetanus). In: Mandell, G.L.; Douglas, R.G., Jr.; Bennett, J.E., eds. Principles and Practice of Infectious Diseases. New York, Churchill Livingstone, 1990, pp. 1946–1982.
28. Cattell, H.S.; Filtser, D.L. Pseudosubluxation and other normal variation in the cervical spine in children. J Bone Joint Surg 47-A:1295–1298, 1985.
29. Chadwick, D.L.; Chin, S.; Salerno, C.; et al. Death from falls in children: How far is fatal? J Trauma 31:1353–1355, 1991.
30. Chan, B.S.H.; Walker, P.J.; Cass, D.T. Urban trauma: an analysis of 1,116 pediatric cases. J Trauma 29:1540–1547, 1989.
31. Coldiron, J.S. Estimation of nasotracheal tube length in neonates. Pediatrics 41:823, 1968.
32. Committee on Medical Aspects of Automotive Safety. Rating the severity of tissue damage. I. The abbreviated scale. JAMA 215:277–280, 1971.
33. Cooney, D.R. Splenic and hepatic trauma in children. Surg Clin North Am 61:1165–1180, 1981.
34. Currey, J.D. Changes in the impact energy absorption of bone with age. J Biomech 12:459–469, 1979.
35. Currey, J.D.; Butler, G. The mechanical properties of bone tissue in children. J Bone Joint Surg 57-A:810–814, 1975.
36. Dellinger, E.P.; Miller, S.D.; Wertz, M.J.; et al. Risk of infection after open fracture of the arm or leg. Arch Surg 123:1320–1327, 1987.
37. Douglas, G.L.; Simpson, J.S. The conservative management of splenic trauma. J Pediatr Surg 6:565, 1971.
38. Drew, R.; Perry, J.F., Jr.; Fischer, R.P. The expediency of peritoneal lavage for blunt trauma in children. Surg Gynecol Obstet 145:885, 1977.
39. Duff, J.H.; Goldstein, M.; McLean, A.P.H.; et al. Flail chest: A clinical review and physiological study. J Trauma 8:63, 1968.
40. DuPriest, R.W., Jr.; Rodriguez, A.; Shatney, G.H. Peritoneal lavage in children and adolescents with blunt abdominal trauma. Am Surg 48:460, 1982.
41. Dykes, E.H.; Spence, L.J.; Bohn, D.J.; Wesson, D.E.

Evaluation of pediatric trauma care in Ontario. J Trauma 29:724–729, 1989.
42. Eckenhoff, J. Some anatomic considerations of infant larynx influencing endotracheal anesthesia. Anesthesiology 12:401, 1951.
43. Eichelberger, M.R.; Randolph, J.G. Pediatric trauma—initial resuscitation. In: Moore, E.E.; Eiseman, B.; Van Way, C.E., eds. Critical Decisions in Trauma. St. Louis, C.V. Mosby, 1984, p. 344.
44. Eichelberger, M.R.; Randolph, J.G. Pediatric trauma. An algorithm for diagnosis and therapy. J Trauma 23:91–97, 1983.
45. Eichelberger, M.R.; Randolph, J.G. Thoracic trauma in children. Surg Clin North Am 61:1181–1197, 1981.
46. Eichelberger, M.R.; Mangubat, E.A.; Sacco, W.J.; et al. Outcome analysis of blunt injury in children. J Trauma 28:1109–1117, 1988.
47. Eichelberger, M.R.; Mangubat, E.A.; Sacco, W.S.; et al. Comparative outcomes of children and adults suffering blunt trauma. J Trauma 28:430–434, 1988.
48. Ein, S.J.; Shandling, B.; Simpson, J.S.; et al. Nonoperative management of traumatized spleen in children. How and why. J Pediatr Surg 12:117, 1978.
49. Faist, E.; Baue, A.E.; Dittmer, H.; et al. Multiple organ failure in polytrauma patients. J Trauma 23:775–785, 1983.
50. Fein, L.H.; Pankovich, A.M.; Spero, C.M.; Baruch, H.M. Closed flexible intramedullary nailing of adolescent femoral shaft fractures. J Orthop Trauma 3:133–141, 1989.
51. Flaherty, J.J.; Kelley, R.; Burnett, B.; et al. Relationship of pelvic bone fracture patterns to injuries of urethra and bladder. J Urol 99:297–300, 1968.
52. Francke, E.L.; Neu, H.C. Postsplenectomy infection. Surg Clin North Am 61:135, 1981.
53. Friedman, R.J.; Jupiter, J.B. Vascular injuries and closed extremity fractures in children. Clin Orthop 188:112–119, 1984.
54. Gallagher, S.S.; Finison, K.; Guyer, B.; et al. The incidence of injuries among 87,000 Massachusetts children and adolescents: Results of the 1980–81 State-Wide Children Injury Prevention Surveillance System. Am J Public Health 74:1340–1347, 1984.
55. Ganz, R.; Krushell, R.J.; Jakob, R.P.; Kuffer, J. The antishock pelvic clamp. Clin Orthop Rel Res 267:71–78, 1991.
56. Garcia, V.F.; Gotschall, C.S.; Eichelberger, M.R.; Bowman, L.M. Rib fractures in children: A marker of severe trauma. J Trauma 30:695–700, 1990.
57. Gilberman, R.H.; Zakaib, G.S.; Murbarak, S.J.; et al. Decompression of forearm compartment syndromes. Clin Orthop 134:225–229, 1978.
58. Goldstein, A.S.; Sclafani, S.J.; Kupferstein, N.H.; et al. The diagnostic superiority of computerized tomography. J Trauma 25:938–946, 1985.
59. Gratz, R.R. Accidental injury in childhood: A literature review on pediatric trauma. J Trauma 19:551–555, 1979.
60. Gupta, A.; El Masri, W.S. Multilevel spinal injuries: incidence, distribution, and neurologic patterns. J Bone Joint Surg 71-B:692–695, 1989.
61. Gustilo, R.B. Principles of the management of open fractures. In: Gustilo, R.B., ed. Management of Open Fractures and their Complications. Philadelphia, W.B. Saunders, 1982.
62. Gustilo, R.B.; Anderson, J.T. Prevention of infection in treatment of 1025 open fractures of long bones: Retrospective and prospective analysis. J Bone Joint Surg 58-A:453–458, 1976.
63. Gustilo, R.B.; Mendoza, R.M.; Williams, D.N. Problems in the management of type III (severe) open fractures: A new classification of type III open fractures. J Trauma 24:742–746, 1984.
64. Gustilo, R.B.; Merkow, R.L.; Templeman, D. Current concepts review. The management of open fractures. J Bone Joint Surg 72-A:299–304, 1990.
65. Hall, J.R.; Reyes, H.M.; Horvat, M.; et al. The mortality of childhood falls. J Trauma 29:1273–1275, 1989.
66. Haller, J.A. Pediatric trauma, the No. 1 killer of children—commentary. JAMA 249:47, 1983.
67. Handelsman, J.R. Management of fractures in children. Surg Clin North Am 63:629–670, 1983.
68. Hansen, S.T. Internal fixation of children's fractures of the lower extremities. Orthop Clin North Am 21:353–363, 1990.
69. Harris, G.J.; Soper, R.T. Pediatric first rib fractures. J Trauma 30:343–345, 1990.
70. Heinrich, S.D.; Drvaric, D.M.; Darr, K.; MacEwen, G.D. The operative stabilization of pediatric diaphyseal femur fractures with flexible intramedullary nails. Presented at the Annual Meeting of the Pediatric Orthopaedic Society of North America. Dallas, May 12–15, 1991.
71. Herndon, W.A.; Mahnken, R.F.; Ynrgve, D.A.; Sullivan, J.A. Management of femoral shaft fractures in the adolescent. J Pediatr Orthop 9:29–32, 1989.
72. Herzenberg, J.E.; Hensinger, R.N.; Dedrick, B.K.; Phillips, W.A. Emergency transport and positioning of young children who have an injury to the cervical spine. J Bone Joint Surg 71-A:15–22, 1989.
73. Highland, T.R.; LaMont, R.L. Deep, late infections associated with internal fixation in children. J Pediatr Orthop 5:59–64, 1985.
74. Hoffman, M.A.; Spence, L.J.; Wesson, D.E.; et al. The pediatric passenger: Trends in seatbelt use and injury patterns. J Trauma 27:974–976, 1987.
75. Holmes, M.J.; Reyes, H.M. A critical review of urban pediatric trauma. J Trauma 24:253–255, 1984.
76. Horowitz, J.H.; Nichter, L.S.; Kenney, J.G.; Morgan, R.F. Lawnmower injuries in children: Lower extremity reconstruction. J Trauma 25:1138–1146, 1985.
77. Howman-Giles, R.; Gilday, D.W.; Venagopal, S.; et al. Splenic trauma—Nonoperative management and long term follow up by scintiscan. J Pediatr Surg 12:121, 1978.
78. Injury Mortality Atlas of the United States, 1979–1987. Washington, D.C., U.S. Department of Health and Human Services, 1987.
79. Iwaya, T.; Kiyonori, H.; Yamada, A. Microvascular free flaps for the treatment of avulsion injuries of the feet in children. J Trauma 22:15–19, 1982.
80. Izant, R.J.; Hubay, C.A. The annual injury of 15,000,000 children. A limited study of childhood accidental injury and death. J Trauma 6:65–74, 1966.
81. Johansen, K.; Lynch, K.; Paun, M.; Copass, M. Noninvasive vascular tests reliability exclude occult arterial trauma in injured extremities. J Trauma 31:515–522, 1991.
82. Joyce, M. Initial management of pediatric trauma. In: Marcus, R.E., ed. Trauma in Children. Rockville, MD, Aspen Publications, 1986, pp. 13–38.
83. Karp, M.P.; Cooney, D.R.; Berger, P.E.; et al. The role of computed tomography in the evaluation of blunt abdominal trauma in children. J Pediatr Surg 16:316, 1981.
84. Karp, M.P.; Cooney, D.R.; Pros, G.A.; et al. The non-

operative management of pediatric hepatic trauma. J Pediatr Surg 18:512–518, 1983.
85. Kaufmann, C.R.; Rivara, F.P.; Maier, R.V. Pediatric trauma: Need for surgical management. J Trauma 29:1120–1126, 1989.
86. Kendra, J.C.; Price, C.T.; Songer, J.E.; Scott, D.S. Pediatric applications of dynamic axial external fixation. Contemp Orthop 19:477–486, 1989.
87. Kirby, R.M.; Winquist, R.A.; Hansen, S.T., Jr. Femoral shaft fractures in adolescents: A comparison between traction plus cast treatment and closed intramedullary nailing. J Pediatr Orthop 1:193–197, 1981.
88. Klein, L.; Marcus, R.E. Trauma in children: Management, prognosis and metabolism. In: Marcus, R.E., ed. Trauma in Children. Rockville, MD, Aspen Publications, 1986, pp. 1–12.
89. Langenskiöld, A.; Osterman, K. Surgical elimination of post-traumatic partial fusion of the growth plate. In: Houghton, G.R.; Thompson, G.H., eds. Problematic Musculoskeletal Injuries in Children. London, Buttersworth, 1983, pp. 14–31.
90. Lascombes, P.; Prèvot, J.; Ligier, J.N.; et al. Elastic stable intramedullary nailing in forearm shaft fractures in children: 85 cases. J Pediatr Orthop 10:167–171, 1990.
91. Lee, K.W.; Dougal, R.M.; Templeton, J.J.; et al. Selection of endotracheal tubes in infants and children. Abstract. American Academy of Pediatrics Annual Spring Meeting, Section of Anesthesiology, Las Vegas, 1980, p. 15.
92. Letts, M.; Vincent, N.; Gouw, G. The "floating knee" in children. J Bone Joint Surg 68-B:442–446, 1986.
93. Letts, R.M. Degloving injuries in children. J Pediatr Orthop 6:193–197, 1987.
94. LeWallen, R.P.; Peterson, H.A. Non-union of long bone fractures in children: A review of 30 cases. J Pediatr Orthop 5:135–142, 1985.
95. Lewis, V.L.; Manson, P.N.; Morgan, R.F.; et al. Facial injuries associated with cervical fractures: Recognition patterns and management. J Trauma 25:90–93, 1985.
96. Lhowe, D.W.; Hansen, S.T. Immediate nailing of open fractures of the femoral shaft. J Bone Joint Surg 70-A:812–820, 1988.
97. Ligier, J.N.; Metaizeau, J.P.; Prèvot, J.; Lascombes, P. Elastic stable intramedullary pinning of long bone shaft fractures in children. Z Kinderchir 40:209–212, 1985.
98. Ligier, J.N., Metaizeau, J.P., Prèvot, J.; Lascombes, P. Elastic intramedullary nailing of femoral shaft fractures in children. J Bone Joint Surg 70-B:74–77, 1988.
99. Loder, R.T. Pediatric polytrauma: Orthopaedic care in hospital course. J Orthop. Trauma 1:48–54, 1987.
100. Mabrey, J.D.; Fitch, R.D. Plastic deformation in pediatric fractures: Mechanism and treatment. J Pediatr Orthop 9:310–314, 1989.
101. Mangubat, E.; Eichelberger, M. Hypovolemia shock in pediatric patients: A physiologic approach to diagnosis and treatment. Trauma Clin Update Surg 2:1–8, 1985.
102. Mann, D.C.; Weddington, J.; Davenport, K. Closed Ender nailing of femoral shaft fractures in adolescents. J Pediatr Orthop 6:651–655, 1986.
103. Marcus, I.M. Emotional and psychological inplications of trauma. In Marcus, R.E., ed. Trauma in Children. Rockville, MD, Aspen Publications, 1986, pp. 245–257.
104. Marcus, R.E.; Mills, M.; Thompson, G.H. Multiple injury in children. J Bone Joint Surg 65-A:1290–1294, 1983.
105. Marx, J.A.; Moore, E.E.; Jordan, R.C.; et al. Limitations of computed tomography in the evaluation of acute abdominal trauma: A prospective comparison with diagnostic peritoneal lavage. J Trauma 25:933–937, 1985.
106. Matsen, F.A.; Veith, R.G. Compartmental syndromes in children. J Pediatr Orthop 1:33–41, 1981.
107. Matsen, F.A.; Winquist, R.A.; Krugmire, R.B. Diagnosis and management of compartmental syndromes. J Bone Joint Surg 62-A:286–291, 1980.
108. Mayer, B.W. Pediatric Anesthesia—A Guide to Its Administration. Philadelphia, J.B. Lippincott, 1981, pp. 51–64, 251.
109. Mayer, T.; Matlak, M.E.; Johnson, D.G.; Walker, M.L. The Modified Injury Severity Scale in pediatric multiple trauma patients. J Pediatr Surg 15:719–726, 1980.
110. Mayer, T.; Walker, M.L.; Clark, P. Further experience with the Modified Abbreviated Injury Severity Scale. J Trauma 24:31–34, 1984.
111. Mayer, T.; Walker, M.L.; Johnson, D.G.; Matlak, M.E. Causes of morbidity and mortality in severe pediatric trauma. JAMA 245:719–721, 1981.
112. Meissner, M.; Paun, M.; Johansen, K. Duplex scanning for arterial trauma. Am J Surg 161:552–555, 1991.
113. Meland, N.B.; Fisher, J.; Irons, G.B.; et al. Experience with 80 rectus abdominis free-tissue transfers. Plast Reconstr Surg 83:481–487, 1989.
114. Moore, E.E.; Moore, J.B.; VanDuzer-Moore, S.; et al. Mandatory laparotomy for gunshot wounds penetrating the abdomen. Am J Surg 140:847, 1980.
115. Morden, M.L. Pelvic fractures in children. In: Houghton, G.R.; Thompson, G.H., eds. Problematic Musculoskeletal Injuries in Children. London, Butterworth, 1983, pp. 159–177.
116. Mubarak, S.J.; Carroll, N.C. Volkmann's contracture in children: Aetiology and prevention. J Bone Joint Surg 61-B:285–293, 1979.
117. Mubarak, S.J.; Owens, C.A.; Hargens, A.R.; et al. Acute compartment syndromes: Diagnosis and treatment with the aid of the Wick catheter. J Bone Joint Surg 60-A:1091–1095, 1978.
118. Mueller, M.E.; Allgower, M.; Schneider, R.; Willenegger, H. Manual of Internal Fixation, ed. 2. New York, Springer Verlag, 1979.
119. Murr, P.C.; Moore, E.E.; Lipscomb, R.; et al. Abdominal trauma associated with pelvic fracture. J Trauma 20:919–923, 1980.
120. Musemeche, C.A.; Barthel, M.; Cosentino, C.; Reynolds, M. Pediatric falls from height. J Trauma 31:1347–1349, 1991.
121. Myer, P.R., Jr. Surgery of Spine Trauma. New York, Churchill Livingstone, 1989, pp. 197–198.
122. Nakayama, D.K.; Copes, W.S.; Sacco, W.J. The effect of patient age upon survival in pediatric trauma. J Trauma 31:1521–1526, 1991.
123. National Safey Council. Accident Facts. Chicago, National Safety Council, 1982.
124. Navarre, J.R.; Cardillo, P.J.; Gorman, J.F.; et al. Vascular trauma in children and adolescents. Am J Surg 143:229–231, 1982.
125. Neff, C.C.; Pfister, R.C.; VanSonnenberg, E. Percutaneous transtracheal ventilation: Experimental and practical aspects. J Trauma 23:84–90, 1983.
126. Ogden, J.A. Skeletal growth mechanism injury patterns. J Pediatr Orthop 2:371–377, 1982.
127. Ogden, J.A. Skeletal Injury in the Child, ed. 2. Philadelphia, W.B. Saunders, 1990.

128. O'Gorman, R.B.; Feliciano, D.V. Arteriography performed in the emergency center. Am J Surg 152:323, 1986.
129. O'Neill, J.A. Special pediatric emergencies. In: Boswick, J.A., ed.. Emergency Care. Philadelphia, W.B. Saunders, 1981, p. 13.
130. Ornato, J.H.P.; Crasen, M.A.; Nelson, N.M.; et al. Impact of improved emergency medical services and emergency trauma care on the reduction in mortality from trauma. J Trauma 25:575–578, 1985.
131. Paley, D.; Catagni, M.A.; Argnani, F.; et al. Ilizarov treatment of tibial nonunions with bone loss. Clin. Orthop 241:146–165, 1989.
132. Patzakis, M.J.; Wilkins, J. Factors influencing infection rate in open fracture wounds. Clin Orthop 243:36–40, 1989.
133. Peclet, M.H.; Newman, K.D.; Eichelberger, M.R.; et al. Patterns of injury in children, J Pediatr Surg 25:85–90, 1990.
134. Pediatric transfusions practice. In: Snyder E.L. (ed.). Blood Tranfusion Therapy. Arlington, VA, American Association of Blood Banks, 1983, p. 49.
135. Peters, R. Trauma centers. Editorial. J Trauma 25:538–540, 1985.
136. Peterson, C.A.; Peterson, H.A. Analysis of the incidence of injuries to the epiphyseal growth plate. J Trauma 12:275–281, 1972.
137. Peterson, H.A. Partial growth plate arrest and its treatment. J Pediatr Orthop 4:246–258, 1984.
138. Pollen, A.G. Fractures and Dislocations in Children. Baltimore, Williams & Wilkins, 1973.
139. Powell, J.N.; Waddell, J.P.; Tucker, W.S.; Tranfeldt, E.E. Multiple-level noncontiguous spinal fractures. J Trauma 29:1146–1151, 1989.
140. Powell, R.W.; Smith, D.E.; Sarins, C.K.; et al. Peritoneal lavage in children with blunt abdominal trauma. J Pediatr Surg 11:973, 1976.
141. Quinten, J. External fixation in child traumatology. Orthopaedics 7:463–470, 1984.
142. Ramenofsky, M.L.; Luterman, A.; Quindlen, E.; et al. Maximum survival in pediatric trauma: The ideal system. J Trauma 24:818–823, 1984.
143. Ramenofsky, M.L.; Luterman, A.; Currer, P.W.; et al. EMS for pediatrics: Optimal treatment or unnecessary delay? J Pediatr Surg 18:498–504, 1983.
144. Rang, M. Children's Fractures, 2nd ed. Philadelphia, J.B. Lippincott, 1983.
145. Rang, M.; Thompson, G.H. Children's fractures: Principles and management. Reconstr Surg Traumatol 17:2–15, 1979.
146. Reeves, R.B.; Ballard, R.I.; Hughes, J.L. Internal fixation versus traction and casting of adolescent femoral shaft fractures. J Pediatr Orthop 10:592–595, 1990.
147. Reff, R.B. The use of external fixation devices in the management of severe lower extremity and pelvic injuries in children. Clin Orthop 188:21–33, 1984.
148. Reichard, S.A.; Helikson, M.A.; Shorter, N.; et al. Pelvic fractures in children—review of 120 patients with a new look at general management. Pediatr Surg 15:727–734, 1980.
149. Reid, A.B.; Letts, R.M.; Black, G.B. Pediatric Chance fractures: Association with intra-abdominal injuries and seatbelt use. J Trauma 30:384–391, 1990.
150. Riska, E.B.; von Bonsdorff, H.; Hakkinen, S.; et al. Prevention of fat embolism by early internal fixation of fractures in patients with multiple injuries. Injury, 8:110–116, 1976.
151. Rockwood, C.A., Jr.; Wilkens, K.E.; King, R.E. (eds.). Fractures in Children, Vol. 3. Philadelphia, J.B. Lippincott, 1984.
152. Roe, C.F.; Santulli, T.V.; Blair, C.S. Heat loss in infants during general anesthesia and operations. J Pediatr Surg 1:266, 1966.
153. Rorabeck, C.H. A practical approach to compartmental syndromes. Part III. Treatment. Instr Course Lect 32:102–113, 1983.
154. Rothenberg, S.; Moore, E.E.; Maxx, J.A.; et al. Selective management of blunt abdominal trauma in children. The triage role of peritoneal lavage. J Trauma 27:1101–1106, 1987.
155. Rothenberger, D.A.; Fischer, R.P.; Perry, J.D., Jr. Major vascular injuries secondary to pelvic fractures: An unsolved clinical problem. Am J Surg 136:660, 1978.
156. Salter, R.B.; Harris, W.R. Injuries involving the epiphyseal growth plate. J Bone Joint Surg 45-A:587–622, 1963.
157. Schwab, C.W.; Peelet, M.; Zachnowski, S.W.; et al. The impact of an air ambulance system on an established trauma center. J Trauma 25:580–586, 1985.
158. Seelig, J.M.; Becker, D.P.; Miller, J.D.; et al. Traumatic acute subdural hematoma. N Engl J Med 304:1511, 1981.
159. Shaker, I.J.; White, J.J.; Signer, R.D.; et al. Special problems of vascular injuries in children. J Trauma 16:863–867, 1976.
160. Shires, G.T.; Canizaro, P.C. Fluid resuscitation in the severely injured. Surg Clin North Am 53:1341–1365, 1973.
161. Siemens, R.A.; Fulton, R.L. Gastric ruptures as a result of blunt trauma. Am Surg 43:229, 1977.
162. Smith, C.; Green, R. Pediatric vascular injuries. Surgery 90:20–31, 1981.
163. Smyth, B.T. Chest trauma in children. J Pediatr Surg 14:41, 1979.
164. Spiegel, P.G.; Mast, J.W. Internal and external fixation of fractures in children. Orthop Clin North Am 11:405–421, 1980.
165. Spoerel, W.E.; Narayanan, P.S.; Singh, N.P. Transtracheal ventilation. Br J Anaesth 43:932, 1971.
166. Tachdjian, M.O. Pediatric Orthopedics, 2nd ed., Vol. 4. Philadelphia, W.B. Saunders, 1990.
167. Teasdale, G.; Bennett, B. Assessment of coma and impaired consciousness: A practical scale. Lancet 2:81–84, 1974.
168. Tepas, J.J., III; DiScala, C.; Ramenofsky, M.L.; et al. Mortality and head injury: The pediatric perspective. J Pediatr Surg 25:92, 1990.
169. Tepas, J.J., III; Molitt, D.L.; Talbert, J.L.; Bryant, M. The Pediatric Trauma Score as a predictor of injury severity in the injured child. J Pediatr Surg 22:14–18, 1987.
170. Tepas, J.J.; Ramenofsky, M.L.; Mollitt, D.L.; et al. The Pediatric Trauma Score as a predictor of injury severity: An objective assessment. J Trauma 28:425–429, 1988.
171. Thompson, G.H. Nailing children's fractures. Perspect Orthop Surg 2:40–54, 1992.
172. Thompson, G.H.; Wilber, J.H. Fracture management in the multiply injured child. In: Marcus, R.E., ed. Trauma in Children. Rockville, MD, Aspen Publishers, 1986 pp. 99–146.
173. Thompson, G.H.; Wilber, J.H.; Marcus, R.E. Internal fixation of fractures in children and adolescents. A comparative analysis. Clin Orthop 188:10–20, 1984.
174. Tolo, V.T. External skeletal fixation in children's fractures. J Pediatr Orthop 3:435–442, 1983.
175. Torode, I.; Zieg, D. Pelvic fractures in children. J Pediatr Orthop 5:76–84, 1985.

176. Tsai, A. Epidemiology of pediatric prehospital case. Ann Emerg Med 16:284–292, 1987.
177. Tscherne, H.; Gotzen, L. Fractures with Soft Tissue Injuries. Berlin, Springer-Verlag, 1984.
178. Verstreken, L.; Delronge, G.; Lamoureaux, J. Orthopaedic treatment of pediatric multiple trauma patients. A new technique. Int Surg 73:177–179, 1988.
179. Verstreken, L.; Delronge, G.; Lamoureaux, J. Shaft forearm fractures in children. Intramedullary nailing with immediate motion: A preliminary report. J Pediatr Orthop 8:450–453, 1988.
180. Viljanto, J.; Linna, M.I.; Kiviluoto, H.; Paananen, M. Indications and results of operative treatment of femoral shaft fractures in children. Acta Chir Scand 141:366–369, 1975.
181. Voto, S.J.; Pigott, J.; Riley, P.; Donovan, D. Arterial injuries associated with lower extremity fractures. Orthopaedics 11:357–360, 1988.
182. Weber, B.G.; Brunner, C.; Freuler, F., eds. Treatment of Fractures in Children and Adolescents. Berlin, Springer-Verlag, 1980.
183. Wesson, D.E.; Williams, J.I.; Spence, L.J.; et al. Functional outcome in pediatric trauma. J Trauma 29:589–592, 1989.
184. Wesson, D.E.; Williams, J.I.; Salmi, L.R.; et al. Evaluating a pediatric trauma program: Effectiveness versus preventable death. J Trauma 28:1226–1231, 1988.
185. West, J.G.; Trunkey, D.D.; Lim, R.C. Systems of trauma care: A study of two counties. Arch Surg 114:455–460, 1979.
186. Williams, R.A. Injuries in infants and small children resulting from witnessed and corroborated free falls. J Trauma 31:1350–1352, 1991.
187. Winquist, R.A.; Hansen, S.T., Jr.; Clawson, D.K. Closed intramedullary nailing of femoral fractures. A report of five hundred and twenty cases. J Bone Joint Surg 66-A:529–539, 1984.
188. Wolma, F.J.; Larrieu, A.J.; Alsop, G.C. Arterial injuries of the legs associated with fractures and dislocations. Am J Surg 140:806–809, 1980.
189. Ziv, I.; Rang, M. Treatment of femoral fractures in the child with head injury. J Bone Joint Surg 65-B:276–278, 1983.
190. Ziv, I.; Blackburn, N.; Rang, M. Femoral intramedullary nailing in the growing child. J Trauma 24:432–434, 1984.

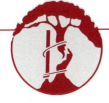

Robert N. Hensinger, M.D.

5

Complications of Fractures in Children

Vascular Injuries

ARTERIAL INJURIES

Penetrating trauma is the most common cause (51%) of arterial injuries in children; the remainder are due to polytrauma from vehicular accidents (30%) and falls (19%). Only 18% of arterial injuries are associated with fractures, usually crush injuries and segmental fractures.[10, 16] Importantly, 45% of patients have injuries to peripheral nerves owing to their close association within the neurovascular bundle.[11, 16]

Typically, the artery involved is near the fracture; for example, the common femoral artery is often associated with intertrochanteric fractures of the hip and hip dislocation and the superficial and profunda femoral arteries with subtrochanteric and midshaft fractures.[5, 8] The femoral artery can be injured at the adductor hiatus by a supracondylar femur fracture.[5] Injury to the popliteal artery or a combination of the anterior and posterior tibial arteries is usually associated with fracture of the distal femoral (Fig. 5–1) or proximal tibial epiphysis or a knee dislocation (32 to 64%).[7, 8, 11, 17]

The usual signs of vascular compromise are absent distal pulse, lower skin temperature, and poor skin circulation with diminished capillary and venous filling distal to the injury.[10] An angiogram should be considered whenever vascular injury is suspected.[7] The absolute indications for an angiogram are diminished or absent pulse, large or expanding hematoma, external bleeding, unexplained hypotension, a bruit, and a peripheral nerve injury.[5, 15] If the period of ischemia approaches 6 hours, operative exploration should proceed immediately, and it may be necessary to obtain an angiogram in the operating room.[9] Skeletal injury in the proximity of a major vessel accompanied by a pulse deficit was 100% predictive of a vascular injury in one study.[15] In another report, however, of those patients with documented arterial injuries, 68% had normal pulses.[11]

Pulses may be initially palpable and then disappear (delayed loss of pulse). This usually is due to damage to the intima with consequent development of a thrombosis.[11, 15] Damage to the popliteal artery from a knee dislocation is commonly limited to the intima.[5, 6, 8] In children, intimal damage is often more extensive than is apparent on simple inspection. Children are particularly prone to ischemia and gangrene due to arterial spasm, a rare problem in adults.[12, 13] Damron and McBeath recommend that any diminution of pulse, even if the pulse is detectable by Doppler testing, pressure, or palpation, should be considered abnormal.[5] The patient should be further evaluated if the pulse does not return following reduction of the fracture or dislocation (Fig. 5–2).[11] Observation only of a warm pulseless leg after dislocation of the knee is insufficient. Often there is good capillary flow in these patients because the amount of flow required to maintain viability of the skin and subcutaneous tissue is much less than is required by muscle.[8] In these circumstances, Green and Allen reported that 90% of the limbs either came to amputation or had claudication or incapacitating muscle fibrosis and contracture.[8]

Ninety percent of limbs can be salvaged if circulation is reestablished within 6 hours, whereas re-

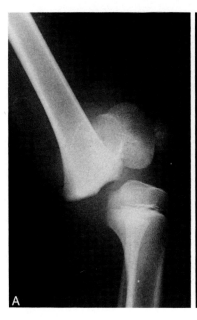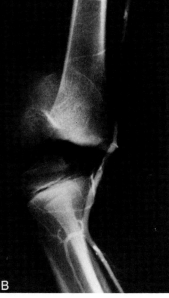

Figure 5–1

A, Supracondylar fracture of the femur in an 8-year-old male with complete displacement of the distal femoral epiphysis. Decreased pulses and this fracture pattern should make one suspicious of a vascular injury. B, Arteriogram demonstrates attenuation of the popliteal artery, but it is still intact. The fracture was reduced and fixed with crossed pins with subsequent premature growth arrest.

vascularization after 8 hours from the time of injury can result in an amputation rate of 72 to 90%.[6, 8] Stanford and colleagues found that the tissues of a child's limb, particularly the nerves and muscles, are at greater risk from prolonged periods of ischemia than adult tissue.[16] Thus, in children, a delay greater than 6 hours was associated with a poor result in 77%.[16] With massive crush injuries and collateral vessel damage, the 6-hour period of warm ischemia may be too long.[10] Distal compartment syndromes are common following late diagnosis or repair of vascular injuries. Fasciotomies are indicated in children, but not fibulectomy, as this can lead to a valgus deformity of the ankle.[7, 8]

All major arterial injuries should be repaired; however, repair of venous injuries remains controversial.[10, 14] Ligation of the popliteal artery leads to an alarmingly high rate of amputation—approximately 70 to 86%.[6, 8] In children, autogenous vein grafts are recommended rather than synthetic or bovine material.[17] Spatulation of the ends of the vessels allows for a longer suture line that will accommodate later increase in vessel size without stricture.[17] Surgical shortening of the bone may facilitate vascular repair, and the leg length discrepancy can be resolved at a later time.

Fracture stabilization can be accomplished by a variety of means. Ideally, if time permits, reduction

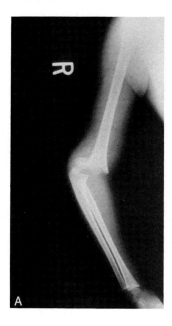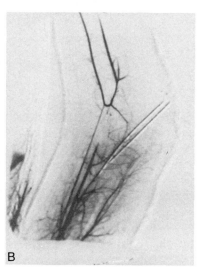

Figure 5–2

A, Supracondylar fracture of the humerus in a 7-year-old with absent pulses despite satisfactory reduction and pinning. B, Arteriogram demonstrates good collateral circulation but a complete block of the brachial artery. The artery was explored; an intimal flap was found that was resected, and a successful end-to-end anastomosis was performed.

and fixation of the fracture should precede vascular repair.[7] Initial bony fixation provides maximum skeletal stability and reduces further trauma to the soft tissues, nerves, and collateral blood vessels.[5] Similarly, surgical repair of nerve lacerations is facilitated with bony stabilization. If soft tissue coverage can be achieved, internal fixation is preferred.[4] External fixation, particularly in the severely traumatized limb, has many advantages, including a short operative time.[4] Indwelling arterial and venous shunts can be helpful in selected cases to reduce the risks of further vessel damage and compartment syndrome.[7,10] Similarly, temporary shunting can provide a satisfactory solution to the clinical problem of whether the ischemic limb should be revascularized prior to fracture fixation.[1,9]

In general, the indications for limb salvage are extended in children because of their greater capacity for healing, however, there are no data to establish the limits. One must consider the seriousness of associated polytrauma, the degree of damage to the ipsilateral foot, the time required to obtain soft tissue coverage and bone healing, and the potential for rehabilitation.[10] In children, a delay longer than 4 hours was associated with a 50% incidence of long-term severe disability and resulted in a late amputation in 30%.[10] Repair of a proximal artery may not result in saving the entire limb but may preserve the knee, which has important functional implications.[11] Navarre and co-authors found that the typical problem was undue optimism in regard to conservative treatment to obtain limb survival without due consideration of growth demands and potential social and career requirements.[11]

Early complications include wound infections, below-knee amputations, deep vein thrombosis, and motor and sensory deficits.[7] Revascularization does not eliminate the possibility of abnormal growth (overgrowth and undergrowth).[7,17] All children should be followed with scanograms until maturity.[17] Loss of normal pulse blood flow influences growth; as the child ages the collateral circulation may not be adequate to meet the increased physiologic demands, with the development of ischemia-like symptoms related to activity.[7]

VASCULAR INJURIES ASSOCIATED WITH SUPRACONDYLAR FRACTURES OF THE HUMERUS

Vascular injury is the most serious complication associated with supracondylar fracture; fortunately, it is uncommon. If the child has a pulseless extremity, the fracture should be reduced immediately in an attempt to restore blood supply and avoid compartmental ischemia (see Fig. 5–2).[2] Because children are uniquely susceptible to vasospasm a pulse may not be restored to normal, and a Doppler wave form analysis may be helpful.[17] There may be very good secondary capillary profusion, and this can lead to the false assumption that the vascularity is intact. The collateral circulation may be sufficient to maintain a pulse in the distal circulation but not sufficient to maintain profusion through specific muscle groups.[7] With more frequent use of fixation for supracondylar fractures, the incidence of vascular injury seems to have decreased, suggesting that some of the previous vascular problems were due to the flexed position required to maintain the reduction. If there is a doubt about the vascular status of the limb, arteriographic studies should be performed promptly.[2,7]

Compartment Syndromes

Compartment syndromes can occur in the multiply injured child with the same frequency as in the adult. The condition is due to swelling and increased pressure in a closed space, such as a fascial compartment, but can occur from tight skin or a circumferential cast. If not treated promptly it results in complete death of the structures within the compartment and Volkmann's ischemic contracture (Fig. 5–3). Compartment syndromes occur in the interosseous compartments of the hand and foot, the volar and dorsal compartments of the forearm, and the thigh and all four compartments of the leg.[25] Crush and wringer injuries are the classic causes,

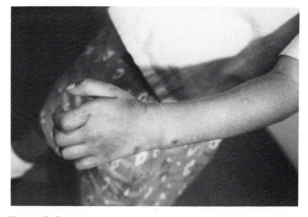

Figure 5–3

Volkmann's ischemic contracture of the forearm following treatment of a both-bones fracture and unrecognized compartment syndrome. Note the contracture of the fingers, which are partially insensitive.

but more commonly compartment syndromes are associated with fractures, severe contusion, drug overdose with limb compression, burns, and vigorous exercise.[26] In children, this can accompany a vascular injury or osteotomy of the bone, especially the proximal tibia.[25] Multiple trauma predisposes the child to a compartment syndrome because of additional high-risk factors such as hypotension, vascular injury, and high-energy blunt trauma, which increase tissue necrosis.[27] Compartment syndromes in the thigh have been reported in teenagers following blunt trauma, systemic hypertension, external compression using antishock trousers, and vascular injury with or without fracture of the femur.[23, 27]

The injury may be a simple Salter-Harris type I or II fracture of the distal radius or proximal tibia, and compartment syndrome may occur with both open and closed injuries. A common misconception is that an open injury will decompress the compartment. However, not all compartments are successfully relieved by an open injury.[27] Similarly, closed fractures treated with closed intramedullary fixation, such as femoral fractures, are susceptible to compartment ischemia. In restoring the femoral length, the muscles are pulled to length, the integrity of the compartments is restored, and a compartment syndrome can occur.[21, 27]

As the pressure increases within the space the first finding or complaint is a decrease in sensation, or paresthesias.[26] Pain, swelling, and tenseness of the compartment are found on physical examination. This may be difficult to recognize in children who are too young to cooperate with the examination or who have a head injury. If the process continues, there is a decrease in voluntary use of the muscles and finally complete paralysis. Pain on stretching the involved muscles is a common finding but is subjective and may be due to trauma. Early ischemia of the nerve may cause anesthesia and obscure this very sensitive finding.[26] An excellent example of this diagnostic dilemma is the loss of toe dorsiflexion after metaphyseal fracture of the proximal tibia, which may be due to a direct injury to the peroneal nerve or anterior tibial artery or to an anterior compartment syndrome.[25]

The compartment pressures seldom are high enough to occlude a major artery, so the peripheral pulses are often palpable and capillary filling is demonstrated routinely in the skin of the hand or foot.[26] With a tissue pressure exceeding 30 mm Hg, the capillary pressure is not sufficient to maintain blood flow to the muscles, resulting in necrosis.[26] With severe intercompartmental edema, the nerves show a gradual decline in the action potential amplitude.[20] Complete conduction block can be obtained with a pressure as low as 50 mm Hg, and after 6 to 8 hours of sustained pressure, of 30 or 40 mm Hg.[20]

The diagnosis or exclusion of compartment syndrome on clinical grounds alone may be impossible.[25] The easiest and quickest method to make the diagnosis is by measuring the compartment pressure. It is mandatory that anyone who is managing trauma in children be able to determine these values. Generally, a pressure greater than 30 mm Hg is considered abnormal and demands close observation; a pressure over 40 mm Hg warrants surgical decompression.[25, 26] Muscle damage is significant with intercompartmental pressures greater than 30 mm Hg of 6 to 8 hours' duration.[19, 20]

Decompression should be performed on anyone who has interruption of blood supply with an ischemic interval of more than 6 hours. Muscle ischemia exceeding 3 or 4 hours not only endangers muscle function and viability but also causes significant muscle swelling when circulation is reestablished.[25] Elevated tissue pressure appears to act synergistically with ischemia to produce more severe cellular deterioration than ischemia alone.[21] Children do not differ significantly from adults in that shock, hypoxia, and arterial occlusion may lower tissue pressure tolerances. Elevation of the limb may increase compartment pressures, and may be counterproductive if coupled with a decrease in perfusion; this may be the mechanism by which ischemic contractures occur following femur fractures in children.[24] Myoglobinuria may further complicate a compartment syndrome; thus adequate hydration and urinary output should be ensured after decompression is accomplished.[24]

The duration of the compartment syndrome, prior to definitive surgical decompression, is the most important factor in determining the functional outcome.[25] If the decompression is within 12 hours of the very first sign or symptom, the majority of patients will have normal function.[25] Late surgical decompression exposes devitalized muscle that requires debridement, and, in some instances, infection can ensue, requiring multiple debridements and antibiotics.

Fat Embolism

This is a syndrome associated with long bone fractures, in which fat emboli to the lungs lead to respiratory problems. It is believed to be due to dissolution of normal circulating fat; however, the exact mechanism is still unexplained.[29, 30] This may be a true leaking of fat into the blood stream or a metabolic change that allows the normal circulating fat to become free fatty acids. Many children have fat emboli following injury, but very few develop the clinical syndrome.[28, 29] Drummond and co-workers reported an incidence of 0.5% in 1800 children with pelvic and femoral fractures compared with a 5.0% incidence in adults with similar injuries.[29] Fat embolism more often is seen in teenagers and late adolescents, and the onset is usually shortly after the injury (within the first 2 to 3 days).[29] The pulmonary changes prevent exchange of oxygen across the aveolar-capillary membrane. In adults, this is referred to as adult respiratory distress syndrome.

With the full-blown syndrome, the children have respiratory distress, tachypnea, and a deterioration in blood gas values, particularly the O_2 saturation.[28] Clinically, the child may appear restless and confused; if untreated, stupor and coma may develop. Petechiae may develop in the skin and on the chest, axilla, and base of the neck but can be very transient and are frequently missed or overlooked.[30] The most significant laboratory finding is a decrease in arterial oxygen tension. Fat examination of urine and sputum is of little value in comparison with more modern diagnostic measures. The chest roentgenogram classically demonstrates interstitial edema and increased peripheral vascular markings.[30, 31]

If untreated, fat embolism can be lethal; however, early diagnosis and prompt management can usually sustain the patient until the problem clears. Treatment consists of supportive measures for the respiratory problem, which include improving oxygen saturation (>70 mm Hg) and may require endotracheal positive-pressure breathing. Blood volume should be restored and fluid and electrolyte balance maintained. Adequate oxygenation is the most important part of the treatment, as respiratory failure is the most common cause of death.[29] Treatment with steroids and heparin remains controversial.

Hypercalcemia of Immobilization

Many children exhibit hypercalcemia following immobilization for a fracture. Christofaro and Brink reported 7 of 20 children who demonstrated an increase in serum calcium levels of 10.7 to 13.2 dl (normal 8.5 to 10.5 dl).[33] Urinary excretion of calcium peaks approximately 4 weeks after immobilization begins and can be expected to return to normal levels with activity.[34, 35] This is believed to be part of the normal reparative process. In those who have preexisting metabolic bone disease, such as rickets or parathyroid disease, immobilization can further increase serum calcium levels.[35] Similarly, for unexplained reasons, some young patients, usually 9 to 14 years of age, may have very significant blood levels and systemic symptoms.[35]

Symptoms include anorexia, nausea, vomiting, and increased irritability; if severe generalized seizures, pain with movement, flaccid paralysis, muscle hypertonia, and blurred vision; and, if not controlled, renal calculi.[33, 34] The serum alkaline phosphatase level is usually normal, unlike the case with hyperparathyroidism, in which the serum level is generally high.[34] However, to definitely distinguish the two conditions, a parathyroid hormone assay should be done.[33]

Intravenous administration of fluids and corticosteroids has been reported to be successful in lowering the serum calcium level until mobilization can be accomplished.[34, 35] Usually a low-calcium diet is recommended. Mithramycin also effectively lowers calcium either by direct antagonism of bone resorption or by interference in the metabolism of parathyroid hormone.[34] Appropriate hydration and diuresis can help, as can immediate weight bearing and movement.[34, 35]

Another problem that is similar in nature is acute hypercalcemia following quadriplegia.[32] Particularly in young people, this can be troublesome and should be evaluated routinely during the first 6 weeks following the onset of paralysis.

Ectopic Bone Formation

Ectopic bone has been reported to appear around all major joints, most often the hip, elbow, and knee (Fig. 5–4).[37] The condition is more common in teenagers, but any age group is at risk. This is typically associated with head injury and burns.[37] The exact etiology is unknown. Mital and colleagues found that 15% of head-injured children developed heterotopic bone and that coma and spasticity were the most commonly related factors.[37]

The process is usually preceded by an inflammatory response and tenderness near the affected joint in an area of soft tissue and bone trauma. Elevated levels of serum alkaline phosphatase usually precede ossification and remain elevated during active bone formation.[37] Roentgenographic evidence will be apparent within 3 to 4 weeks after the injury.[37] There may be some resorption after joint movement has

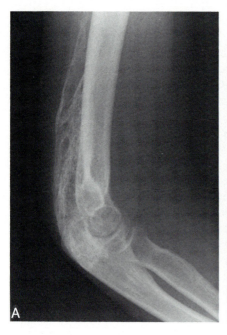 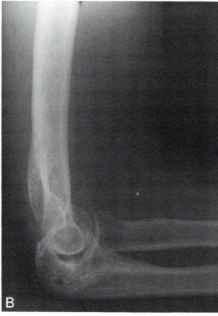

Figure 5–4

Ectopic bone formation leading to complete elbow ankylosis. Roentgenograms were obtained prior to surgery 6 months following a head injury *(A)* and 6 months after surgical excision *(B)*. (From Mital MA, Garber JE, Stinson JT: Ectopic bone formation in children and adolescents with head injuries: Its management. J Pediatr Orthop 7:83, 1987.)

begun. Attempts to excise the heterotopic bone should be delayed until the process is completely mature, usually about a year after injury.[38] There have been reports that pharmalogic agents can reduce the incidence of ectopic bone formation. Mital and associates found that in head-injured children salicylates can help minimize or eliminate the ectopic bone, particularly following excision.[37] Similarly, indomethacin has been reported to be helpful.[37] Diphosphonates have been used, but owing to problems with bone metabolism they are not currently recommended.[36] Most children can be managed successfully by observation and the condition allowed to run its course because few develop long-term problems.[36]

Cast Syndrome

The cast syndrome consists of acute gastric dilatation and vomiting. In the past, this was most often recognized in those treated with a hip spica or body cast, hence the name.[40, 42] However, in more recent times, it has been reported to occur in the absence of a cast, such as following traction for extended periods, spine surgery, and Harrington instrumentation, particularly in the treatment of Scheuermann's kyphosis.[39, 41] The problem is due to mechanical obstruction of the third portion of the duodenum by the superior mesenteric artery (Fig. 5–5).[39] This can come from hyperlordosis positioning in the cast, but more often it is associated with weight loss and a decrease in the fat protecting the superior mesenteric artery from the duodenum.[39, 40] The angle between the superior mesenteric artery and the aorta becomes more acute and compresses the duodenum.[42] Those with an asthenic body habitus and those who have an alteration of spinal curve are at greatest risk.[39] If this condition is not treated aggressively the problem becomes very difficult to manage, with progressive weight loss, hypokalemia, and life-threatening dehydration and electrolyte abnormalities.[40, 42]

The cast syndrome can be reversed by increasing the bulk of retroperitoneal fat. Treatment consists of passing a feeding tube beyond the obstruction or intravenous hyperalimentation plus repositioning (side-lying) to encourage appropriate duodenal drainage.[41] If the cast is hyperextending the spine, it should be modified. In extreme cases, which do not resolve with conservative treatment, a complete derotation of the duodenum and colon with stabilization of the mesenteric (Ladd procedure) can resolve the obstruction.[39]

Traction-Induced Hypertension

An uncommon event is hypertension associated with traction for a long bone fracture. This has also been described during limb lengthening as a result of the traction of the bone and its soft tissue surround.[43, 46] This may be due to tension on the sciatic nerve, activation of renin/angiotensin, or prolonged immobilization.[43, 45] Hamdan and co-workers found elevation of blood pressure in 68% of patients

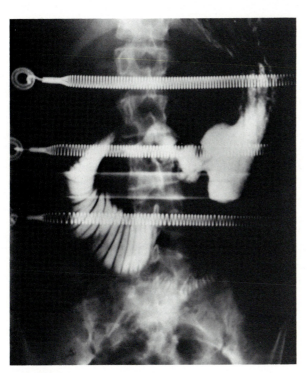

Figure 5–5

Upper gastrointestinal series in a patient with a cast syndrome demonstrating a compression of the fourth portion of the duodenum from the superior mesenteric artery. Complete resolution followed aggressive intravenous hyperalimentation.

undergoing traction, three of whom required treatment.[43] This problem can be controlled by modification of the traction and hypertension medication until the primary condition has been resolved.[43, 44]

Spontaneous Deep Vein Thrombosis

This is a very uncommon complication in childhood, with only scattered reports in the literature.[47–49] Generally, the clinical findings are similar to those found in the adult, with local discomfort, tenderness and warmth, and, often, swelling of the extremity. This should be confirmed by appropriate noninvasive testing and perhaps venograms.[47, 49] It is likely that many cases are unrecognized.[47, 48] Most children respond to routine treatment, similar to adults.[47] Initial treatment is with heparin followed by warfarin (Coumadin) over an appropriate period. There are no particular risk factors, although the problem occurs more often in older teenagers, the obese, and with local infection in the extremity.[47, 49] Acute pulmonary embolism is extremely rare but has been reported and should be managed with the same caution as for an adult.[47]

Malunion

The most common malunion experienced by children is in the supracondylar fracture of the humerus, usually cubitus varus (Fig. 5–6).[50] In the past, the deformity was attributed to a disturbance of elbow growth. However, clinical and experimental evidence indicates that the more common cause is an initial unsatisfactory reduction or early loss of reduction.[50] Unfortunately, the cross section of the proximal humeral fragment is narrow, and unless the distal fragment is reduced anatomically, it is easy for this fragment to rotate and tilt medially, leaving the cubitus varus deformity and limitation of elbow flexion.[59] The growth at the distal humerus

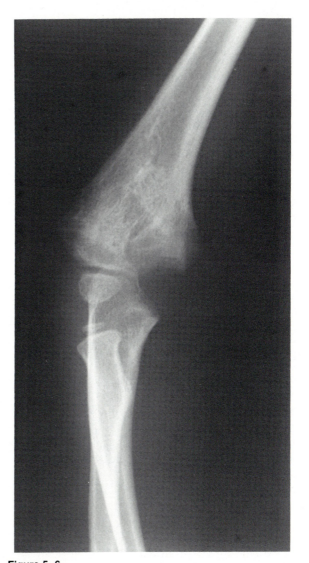

Figure 5–6

Supracondylar fracture of the humerus in a 4-year-old that healed with a cubitus varus deformity.

contributes only 10% of the length of the upper extremity, and, as a consequence, the potential for subsequent remodeling is limited. The recent popularity of closed reduction with exact anatomic alignment maintained by pin fixation has lessened the frequency of this complication.

Most children do not have a functional deficit but may have a significant cosmetic deformity.[59] If the deformity is present after 1 year and is posing problems, it may be managed by a corrective osteotomy. Several authors have described a variety of ways of achieving angular correction.[50, 52, 61] Correction of the rotation, however, is much more difficult but is usually adequately compensated by the shoulder.[61] Fixation of the osteotomy is a problem owing to the smallness and peculiar shape of the distal humerus, which does not lend itself to standard fixation methods.[50, 52, 61]

Another complication related to the elbow is interarticular entrapment of the medial humeral epicondyle after reduction of an elbow dislocation. This may be difficult to visualize roentgenographically. If not removed from the joint, the epicondyle will severely limit flexion and be painful. This should be recognized early and treated appropriately, as late treatment is difficult and can lead to ulnar neuropathy.[56]

Fractures of the forearm in children are a common cause of malunion, because the reduction can be easily lost and difficult to regain (Fig. 5-7).[53, 54] Young children can occasionally remodel the fracture dramatically; as a consequence, there is a tendency on the part of the physician to depend heavily on remodeling and accept a less than adequate reduction. Price and co-workers recommend acceptance up to 10 degrees of angulation, 45 degrees of malrotation, and complete displacement before attempting remanipulation or resorting to open reduction and internal fixation.[62] Although there is limited potential for the angulatory deformity to remodel, there is no potential for rotational deformities to improve, and initially they should be treated aggressively. Residual rotational deformity can compromise pronation and supination of the forearm, although the clinical significance of this limited rotation has not been clearly established.[62] Remodeling of angulatory deformity is better in the distal third of the radius and ulna than in the midshaft or proximal third and is better in the younger child.[53-55, 63] In general, midshaft fractures in children under 8 years tend to remodel almost completely; however, in children age 11 years and older (particularly females, who mature earlier), spontaneous correction cannot be anticipated.[55] Late correction is both difficult and embarrassing for the treating surgeon.

Length discrepancy, angulation, and encroachment on the interosseous space are unpredictable indicators of loss of motion. Loss of motion may be due to soft tissue scarring that produces tension on the interosseous membrane; a few patients with complete remodeling have failed to regain motion.[62] Similarly, anatomic restoration of alignment by open reduction and internal fixation does not always restore full range of motion. Price and colleagues suggest that the shortening due to fracture displacement allows for relaxation of the interosseous membrane, which preserves motion.[62] The combination of proximal fracture with angulation, malrotation, and encroachment carries the greatest risk for loss of motion.[62] Tredwell and Price and their co-workers recommend open reduction and internal fixation after a refracture, as there is a greater likelihood in this circumstance of losing forearm rotation.[62, 64]

In the lower extremity, malunion occurs frequently in the child with a head or spinal cord injury.[51, 57, 58] Ninety percent of head-injured children recover from coma in less than 48 hours. In long-term follow-up, 84% of children who initially were in deep coma (score 5 to 7 on the Glasgow Coma Scale) eventually are able to walk freely. Thus one must assume a full neurologic recovery.[57] If those with a Glasgow score over 5 do not recover in 3 days, the fracture should be fixed (if the child is over 5 years of age).[57, 60, 66] Rigid fixation of long bone fractures will aid in nursing care and rehabilitation efforts. Muscle spasticity in the first few days will often displace or angulate fractures immobilized in casts or lead to overriding of those in traction (Fig. 5-8).[51, 57] Nonoperative management of fractures in these children results in healing but with an unacceptable incidence of malunion, angulation, and shortening (Fig. 5-9).[57, 60] Skin insensitivity combined with disorientation may result in skin breakdown with the potential for secondary osteomyelitis.[57] If the child must be moved for special studies such as CT or MRI scans or requires extensive dressing changes or multiple debridements in the operating room or whirlpool for burns, the fracture should be stabilized, since manipulation of the fracture may increase the intracranial pressure. In children with acute quadriplegia or paraplegia, fracture fixation decreases the incidence of skin problems and pressure sores from cast immobilization and the need for external support, which may compromise nursing and rehabilitative efforts.

Bohn and Durbin have recently called attention

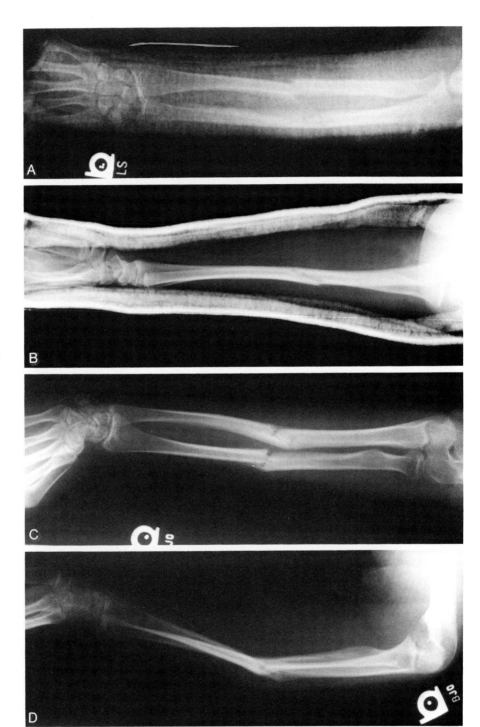

Figure 5–7

Fracture of the radius and ulna in a 12-year-old female. Anteroposterior (A) and lateral (B) views of the injury following satisfactory reduction and cast immobilization. C–D, Fracture reduction was lost owing to early removal of the cast, requiring open reduction and plate fixation to restore satisfactory alignment. In a female of this age, spontaneous correction cannot be expected.

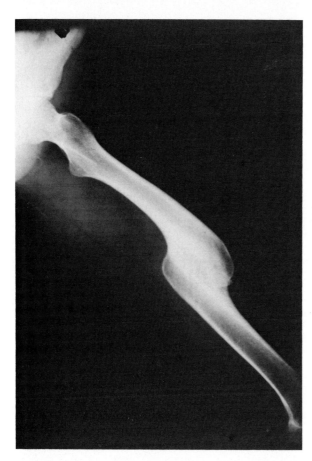

Figure 5–8

Fifteen-year-old male with serious head injury treated in traction for a femoral shaft fracture. Note the shortening and overriding. The patient has recovered and walks with a cane. The leg length discrepancy has caused numerous problems.

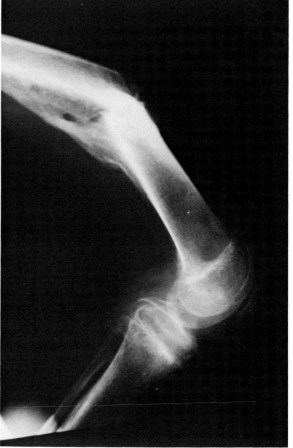

Figure 5–9

Angulation of a femoral shaft fracture in a 13-year-old head-injured patient who was treated with skeletal traction.

to the problem of the floating knee or ipsilateral fracture of the femur and tibia.[51] In general, younger patients (<10 years) with this injury respond well to closed treatment, femoral traction (90/90), and short leg cast followed by a hip spica.[51] However, in older children and adolescents whose femoral fractures were treated with traction, these investigators found an increased incidence of complications (40%), including malunion/nonunion, angulation, and refracture.[51] In this group, operative stabilization of the femoral fracture was associated with fewer complications and better results. Importantly, the incidence of tibial complications in this older group was 50% even in those treated with open reduction or external fixation.[51] The tibial problems may be related to severity of injury rather than to age.

Synostosis (Cross Union)

Cross union is a rare and serious complication of fractures of the forearm. Rotation of the forearm is impossible and may lead to a serious compromise of function. Cross union must be distinguished from myositis ossificans, which is more common and typically less disabling. Most cross unions are confined to the proximal third of the radius and ulna. They are often associated with excision of the radial head following displaced comminuted fracture, which is a significantly greater risk factor than open reduction alone.[65] Most authors recommend that if open reduction is required the surgery be performed through two incisions; however, this does not necessarily prevent cross union.[65] Other predisposing factors include severe initial displacement, residual displacement, periosteal interposition, delayed surgery, remanipulation, and fracture at the same level of the radius and ulna.[65]

Vince and Miller recommend that prior to excision of a cross union there be at least a 1-year interval.[65] A bone scan may be useful to establish that the healing reaction is complete and that the isotope uptake has returned to the same level as the that in the surrounding bone. When excising a synostosis it is important that the bone bridge and its periosteum be removed intact to lessen the chance of recurrence. Several authors suggest interposing fat or Silastic between the radius and ulna to prevent recurrence; however, follow-up data on the success or failure of these proposals are limited.[65] If surgery is delayed too long, soft tissue contractures may preclude gaining a maximum range of pronation and supination (Fig. 5–10).

The same problem can happen between the tibia and the fibula. A similar surgical recommendation could be considered to keep the fibula moving freely at the ankle joint. Another alternative is resection of a portion of the fibula and screw fixation of the distal fibula to the tibial epiphysis.

Late Angulation

This is a common problem with fractures of the proximal tibial metaphysis in the young child. Typically, this is a relatively nondisplaced or easily reducible fracture of the proximal tibial metaphysis.[68, 70] It heals uneventfully, but over the ensuing months, the limb develops a progressive valgus angulation that can be alarming in its appearance (Fig. 5–11).[68, 70] Many will improve spontaneously, and one should wait at least 18 months to 2 years to be confident that the maximum improvement has occurred (Fig. 5–12).[67, 72] Usually this condition is not associated with fracture of the fibula, but it has been reported with fracture of both bones. Although many theories have been advanced, the most likely mechanism is an increased vascular response leading to growth stimulation of the medial metaphysis of the proximal tibia.[68–70]

Interestingly, proximal metaphyseal osteotomy of the tibia and fibula for correction of the deformity can also initiate a progressive valgus deformity and an unacceptably high rate of recurrence.[67, 70] Thus, it is wise to delay the surgery until the child is older and less likely to experience this phenomenon.

Varus deformity of the elbow and loss of the carrying angle is a common sequela following lateral humeral condylar fractures.[71] Very few have functional problems, and the cosmetic appearance is usually acceptable. So found that the average angle was 10 degrees in the undisplaced fracture group and 9.6 degrees in the displaced fracture group treated with open reduction but was more severe in those who were not reduced. It is suggested that the increased vascularity on the lateral side of the elbow leads to overgrowth.[71]

Injury to Triradiate Cartilage

Traumatic disruption of the acetabular triradiate physeal cartilage occurs infrequently. However, if bone is fractured during the active growth phase,

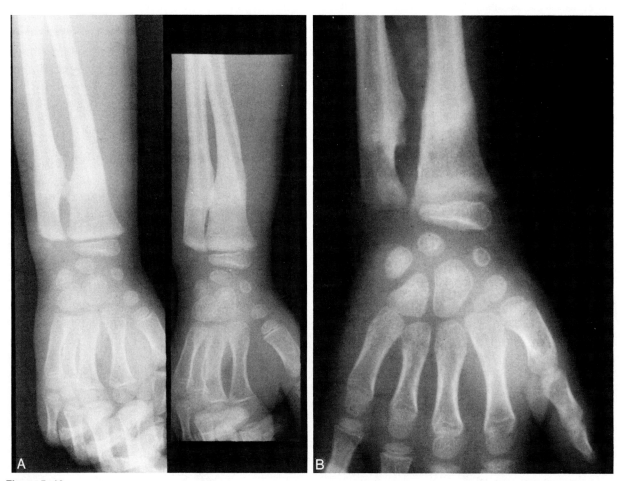

Figure 5–10

A, Anteroposterior and oblique views of the distal forearm and wrist of a 7-year-old boy who sustained a fracture of both bones of the forearm. The fracture healed in a malrotated and angulated position with subsequent synostosis that is easily seen on the oblique view that separates the radius and ulna. *B*, The traumatic synostosis was resected with interposition of fat. Preoperatively the patient had no forearm rotation, and postoperatively he regained 50 degrees of forearm rotation. (Courtesy of Neil E. Green, M.D.)

Figure 5–11

Clinical appearance of a 2½-year-old who developed valgus angulation secondary to a fracture of the proximal tibial metaphysis.

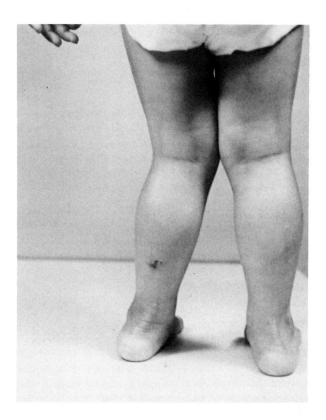

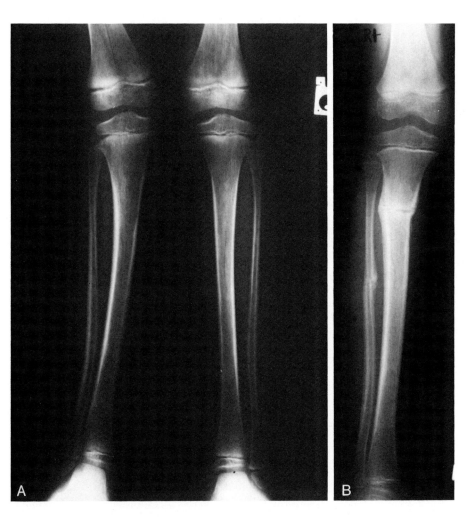

Figure 5–12

A, Fracture of the proximal tibial metaphysis in a 7-year-old; it was sustained approximately 3½ years before but has not undergone spontaneous remodeling, and the child continues to have a valgus deformity. *B,* Roentgenogram following a proximal tibial osteotomy to correct the deformity.

there is great potential for early closure and development of a shallow acetabulum.[73] This is more common in children under 10 years of age, and in this situation it can lead to incongruity of the hip joint and progressive subluxation, requiring acetabular reconstruction.[73] Simple displacements of the triradiate have a more favorable prognosis. In contrast, severe crushing of the triradiate frequently ends in early closure and the worst prognosis. The severe, more crushing type of injury may be difficult to detect on the initial roentgenograms, and CT scans are helpful.[73] In older children with less growth potential, this pattern is not as troublesome.

Irregularities of growth of the proximal femur may occur as well.[73] As the femoral head expands, it displaces laterally and superiorly. It increases pressure against the superior portion of the acetabulum, which can interfere with normal endochondral ossification, increasing the acetabular index similar to the developmental changes accompanying hip subluxation in cerebral palsy.[73] Experimentally induced closure in rabbits further supports this paradigm.[74] If a definite osseous bridge can be identified, resection with fat interposition is recommended.[73] However, the problem is often not discovered until complete closure of the triradiate has occurred.

CT scanning can be helpful in assessment of pelvic fractures, particularly in those patients who may have an osteochondral injury with a retained fragment.[75] If there is persistent joint widening, one must be very suspicious, even in the absence of a clear history of hip dislocation.[75] An arthrogram may not always be diagnostic.[75] The child may require a bone scan to assess the vascularity of the femoral capital epiphysis.[75]

Fractures of the Femoral Shaft: The Overgrowth Phenomenon

It is well known that a fracture of the femur leads to overgrowth averaging 1 cm (range 0.4 to 2.7 cm). Shapiro found that this was independent of age, level of fracture, or position of the fracture at the time of healing (shortened, lengthened, or distracted).[80] Overgrowth occurs in the entire limb, and, interestingly, overgrowth of the ipsilateral tibia averaged 0.29 cm (range 0 to 0.5 cm). The phenomenon occurred in 82% of patients; 78% of overgrowth occurs in the first 18 months following fracture.[80] In 9%, overgrowth continues throughout the period of remaining growth, although at a slower rate. Staheli has noted slightly greater overgrowth in children 4 to 8 years of age.[76] Available evidence suggests that this is due to an increase in vascularity to the bone as a result of the healing reaction.[80] It is an obligatory phenomenon rather than a compensating mechanism for shortening.[80] This has led to the clinical suggestion to leave the fracture fragments overlapped approximately 1 to 1.5 cm in the young child with the expectation that this will lessen the problem of overgrowth.[79] This may become more troublesome as more femoral shaft fractures are managed by intramedullary fixation or external fixation, which restores the fracture to length.

Hunter and Hensinger reported the problem of complete closure of the epiphyses following fracture of the femur that did not involve the growth plates.[78] In their report, the patient spontaneously closed all growth plates of the lower extremity, leading to considerable shortening. Similar cases have been reported sporadically.[76a, 77, 79]

Growth Disturbances

PHYSEAL FRACTURES

Owing to the cross-sectional area of the distal femoral physeal plate, there is great potential for a growth injury following simple types I and II Salter-Harris fractures that rarely occurs in smaller physes, such as the distal radius. Riseborough and co-workers found an alarmingly high rate of complications: 56% developed a growth arrest and a limb length discrepancy greater than 2.4 cm, and 26% developed angular deformities of more than 5 degrees, requiring osteotomy (see Fig. 5–1A).[89] Growth problems correlate well with the injury severity and were seen in all the Salter-Harris types. Fractures in the young child (<11 years) are invariably due to severe trauma and have the poorest prognosis, with 83% of these children developing growth problems. Riseborough and associates believed that the problem was due to interruption of the blood supply to this area[89]; however, there is no proof for this conclusion. The distal femoral physis has a very complex geometric configuration; as a consequence, the damage is not uniform across the physeal cartilage, a circumstance that encourages osseous bridging.

Immobilization in a hip spica cast provides the best result owing to a more consistent maintenance of reduction than that afforded by a long leg cast. Riseborough and associates recommend anatomic reduction and greater use of internal fixation[89]; however, there is no guarantee that this will restore normal growth if there has been a severe injury to the growth plate. With a type II fracture-separation, internal fixation of the large metaphyseal fragment will provide better results.[89] As the potential for growth arrest is so high, children should be followed closely over the period of remaining growth. Tomograms or CT with reconstructions are of great value in delineating the presence and extent of the bone bridge. If the resultant bridge is of moderate size, less than 40% of the surface, and surgically accessible it can be excised. However, if the projected leg length discrepancy is less than 4.8 cm, Riseborough and colleagues advise contralateral distal femoral arrest.[89] Importantly, this does not correct any existing discrepancy but serves only to further limit leg length inequality. With greater differences, limb lengthening will have to be considered.

Changes in the tibiofibular relationship due to growth disturbances following ankle fractures in children are frequent.[83] Fortunately, most occur near the end of growth and, as a consequence, cause only minor problems. Growth arrest of the distal fibula and continued growth of the tibia may be compensated initially by distal sliding of the fibula as the result of traction from the ankle ligaments. If the deformity is of long duration, a valgus deformity will occur (Fig. 5–13). Growth arrest of the distal tibia may cause a varus deformity if the fibula continues to grow (Fig. 5–14). However, the fibula may slide proximally to compensate for tibial overgrowth, with the fibular head becoming more prominent at the knee. An arrest of the distal fibula may be necessary.

PARTIAL GROWTH ARREST: DIAGNOSIS, ASSESSMENT, AND TREATMENT

One of the unique complications of epiphyseal injuries is the interruption of the normal growth of the physis. This poses a wide range of problems,

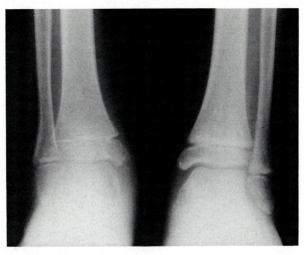

Figure 5–13

An 11-year-old male developed complete closure of the right distal tibial epiphyseal plate following a direct impact from a fall. Note that the distal fibular growth plate has not closed and that further growth may pose a problem at the ankle.

from complete arrest with no further growth to partial arrest and gradual slowing or progressive angulation. Typically, the injury results in a bridge of bone from the metaphysis to the epiphysis, commonly referred to as a bony bar. If the injury is at the periphery, the bar acts as a tether, leading to an angular deformity with some decreased growth. If allowed to persist, it will eventually result in complete closure (Fig. 5–15). A central arrest leads to slowing of growth; roentgenographically it appears as tenting of the epiphyseal plate with cupping of the epiphysis by the metaphysis. The epiphysis appears to be sucked up into the metaphysis (Fig. 5–16). This situation is more commonly associated with a vascular injury, infection such as meningococcemia, or thermal injury such as frostbite.

Figure 5–14

A, A 12-year-old sustained a Salter-Harris type III fracture of the medial malleolus and a type I fracture of the distal fibula. *B*, Development of a bony bar with progressive deformity of the ankle mortise. (From Kling TF, Bright RW, Hensinger RN: Distal tibial physeal fractures in children that may require open reduction. J Bone Joint Surg 66-A:647, 1984.)

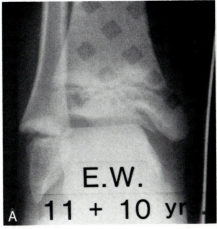 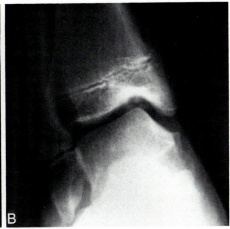

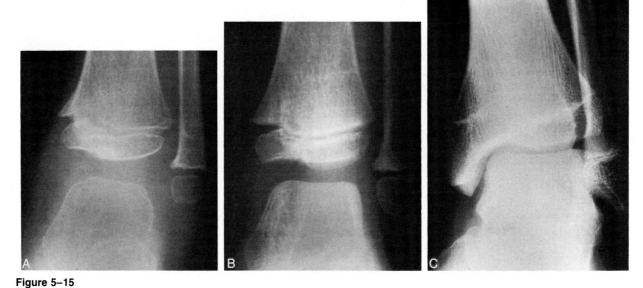

Figure 5–15

A 4-year-old sustained a distal tibial fracture, Salter-Harris type IV. *A,* Six months following initial healing. *B,* Two years following injury. *C,* Follow-up at 12 years of age. Note the development of angulation and deformity of the ankle joint with overgrowth of the fibula. (Roentgenograms provided by Herman D. Hoeksema, M.D.)

The majority of bony bars occur in fracture patterns that traverse the physis, such as Salter-Harris type IV, but they have been reported following all types of physeal injuries. Certain ones are very typical; type III injury of the medial malleolus (see Fig. 5–14), and type IV at the distal tibia (see Fig. 5–15) or distal femur have been reported in considerable detail.[84, 87, 90] With the exception of iatrogenic damage from pins or screws across the physis, most cannot be prevented. There is evidence that with exact anatomic reduction, some problems can be avoided, or at least minimized, and treatment facilitated. Those who treat these injuries should be cognizant of the potential for bar formation. The children should be followed closely to detect early bridging. Early diagnosis will allow one to deal with the bar much more effectively than with one that is discovered late.

The size of the epiphyseal plate, its rate of growth, the age of the patient, and the contour of the physis all play a role in the development of the bar.[87, 90] The distal femoral physis is particularly noteworthy, as its extreme size and irregularity render it more susceptible to irreversible changes and premature closure.[89] In contrast, the distal radius, although more frequently injured, is less prone to bar formation. Injuries to the distal tibia are particularly subject to bar formation; however, those who sustain such injuries are usually near the end of growth, and, as a consequence, the growth disturbance poses fewer problems.[87, 90] The femur is the most common location for growth arrest, followed by the distal

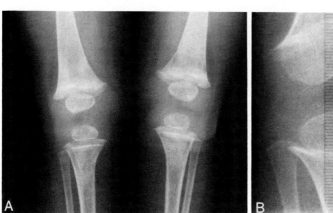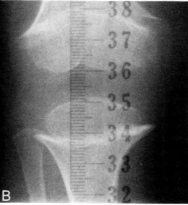

Figure 5–16

Central growth arrest following severe meningococcemia at age 2 years. *A,* Initial normal appearance of knees. *B,* Two years later, demonstrating central growth arrest of right distal femur and proximal tibia. Note that the metaphysis appears to cup the epiphysis and that the epiphyseal plate is tented.

tibia and proximal tibia, radius, and humerus.[90] The proximal tibia and distal femur account for only 3% of all physeal injuries but are responsible for a majority of bony bars. This is particularly troublesome as they account for 60 to 70% of the growth of the respective bones.[87]

The mechanism of injury and its pathomechanics are important parts of the evaluation, inasmuch as many are predictable. The polytomogram or laminagram has been the standard for determining the size and position of the bar. Very thin cuts (anteroposterior and lateral) are used to demonstrate the extent of the formation over the surface of the epiphyseal plate. An excellent paper by Carlson and Wenger provides a detailed description of the tech-

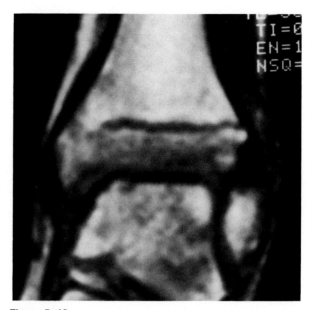

Figure 5–18

An MRI of the distal tibia demonstrating a medial growth arrest.

nique for mapping the partial physeal arrest using laminagrams, preparatory to its surgical excision (Fig. 5–17).[82]

Recently, computed tomography (thin cut) with reconstructions has proved helpful but has not reached the same level of quality as polytomograms.[88] The use of MRI has been suggested; however, it has not proved to be superior in localizing the extent of the lesion (Fig. 5–18). Scanograms should be taken to determine the precise length of the extremities and to evaluate hand and wrist for bone age prior to planning surgical resection.

The decision will be whether to resect the bar or to arrest the remaining growth in the physis. The determination is based on the potential of the bar to cause further length discrepancy or angular deformity and the technical problems involved in removing it.[87] The general recommendation is that if less than 50% of the growth plate is involved and the child has 2 years of remaining growth, resection should be considered.[87, 90] In general, a leg-length discrepancy of 1 inch or less represents little functional impairment, and many discrepancies up to 2 inches can be adequately compensated by growth arrest of the opposite physis. It is further dependent upon the percentage of growth contribution of the individual physis to the length of the lower extremity. For example, the distal tibial epiphysis accounts for only 18%, so complete arrest in a teenager is less of a problem; a contralateral epiphysiodesis may be appropriate, which would not be the case in

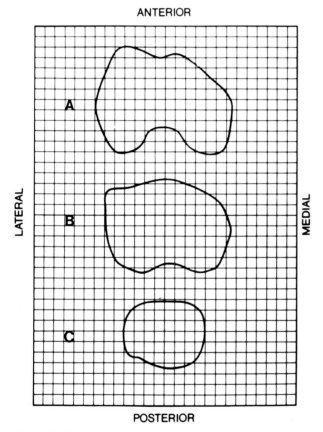

Figure 5–17

Outlines that can be used for mapping of a physeal bar. *A,* Distal femoral physis. *B,* Proximal tibial physis. *C,* Distal tibial physis. With the use of anterior posterior and lateral tomograms, the extent of the bony bridge is analyzed on each cut, proceeding from the lowest to the highest, making certain to maintain the orientation. The extent of the bony bridge is determined at each level and plotted as a thick straight line on the outline. Both anteroposterior and lateral views are plotted on the same graph. This will determine the exact cross-sectional anatomy of the physeal bar. (From Carlson WO, Wenger DR: Mapping methods for partial physeal arrest. J Pediatr Orthop 4:232, 1984.)

a young child. The decision is much less problematic in the upper extremity, as length discrepancy seldom causes functional impairment; many authors recommend that discrepancies of 4 inches or less are best left untreated.

If the bar is to be resected, it is important to prevent re-formation. A number of methods that employ interposing material to block the healing reaction have been described. Materials include fat, bone wax, Silastic, and Cranioplast. Langenskiöld first popularized bar excision in the 1960s, when he resected the bar and filled the space with autogenous fat.[85] He subsequently reported that over the long term the fat functions as a very satisfactory material; it generally prevented bar reformation and continued to grow with the patient.[86] Silastic was popular but is a controlled substance that cannot be used without investigational permission from the FDA and has come under criticism recently related to its use as a breast implant. Cranioplast has been popularized by Peterson; it is helpful in the larger resections, particularly when the bone is structurally weakened, as it is a solid substance that fills the cavity, aids in hemostasis, and decreases the need for postoperative protection.[87] It is important that whatever material is interposed remain in the area of the resection to prevent late bar re-formation.

Peripherally located bars are approached directly, and the periosteum is excised to prevent re-formation (Fig. 5–19). The bar is removed under direct

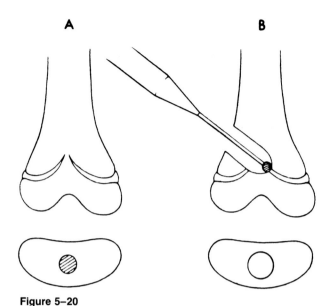

Figure 5–20

A, Central bar with growth peripherally results in tenting of the physis. B, Excision of the central bone through a window in the metaphysis. (From Peterson HA: Partial growth plate arrest and its treatment. J Pediatr Orthop 4:246, 1984.)

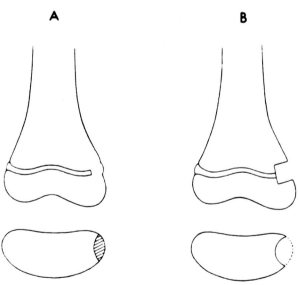

Figure 5–19

Drawing of a peripheral growth arrest, shown in an anteroposterior view and transverse section through the physis below. A, With map of bar composed from tomograms. B, Bar excised by direct approach. (From Peterson HA: Partial growth plate arrest and its treatment. J Pediatr Orthop 4:246, 1984.)

vision using a motorized bur, as the bony bar is extraordinarily hard. Magnification may be helpful. Curettes are used as one nears the normal physis. It is important to undermine both the metaphysis and the epiphysis, so that the physis is well exposed to prevent bar formation but not so much as to jeopardize its vascularity.[87]

Centrally located bars are difficult to resect (Fig. 5–20). They are approached through the metaphysis and generally require a wide metaphyseal window. These bars can be anatomically confusing, as they have a volcanic appearance and resecting the interior can be difficult. The entire circumference of the physis must be visualized to adequately remove the bar. Dental mirrors and the arthroscope have been used to better visualize the normal physis. To prevent migration, the material may be stabilized with a pin or the resection designed to create a cavity in the epiphysis so that the material is held within the substance of the epiphysis as the child grows (Fig. 5–21). An innovative suggestion is to use the Ilizarov apparatus to distract the epiphysis and cause epiphysiolysis, resecting the bony bridge and filling it with methylmethacrylate, and correcting an angular deformity at the same time.[81] These preliminary results are encouraging but will need further investigation.[90] It is common to use metal markers for both the epiphysis and the metaphysis to facilitate documentation of continued growth in the postoperative period.

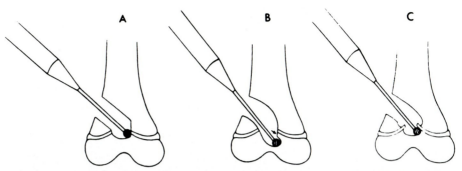

Figure 5–21

Contour of cavity. *A,* As normal, physis is exposed. The adjacent metaphyseal bone surface should be smooth to help prevent the plug from staying with metaphysis. *B,* Bone in the epiphysis is undermined in an attempt to allow the plug to stay with the epiphysis. A small rim of epiphyseal bone should be preserved to maintain viability of the physis *(arrow). C,* Undermining bone away from the physis should be avoided because the protruding physis would be deprived of its blood supply and prevented from growing inward over the plug as the physis grows distally. (From Peterson HA: Partial growth plate arrest and its treatment. J Pediatr Orthop 4:246, 1984.)

Angular deformity of up to 9 degrees may correct spontaneously as a result of "catch-up" growth following bar resection.[87, 90] An accompanying corrective osteotomy is recommended when angular deformities are greater than 10 degrees and whenever there is a significant deformity and the area of the bar is greater than 25%.[90] Near-normal longitudinal growth and correction of moderate angular deformities can be expected when the bridge is less than 25%; most poor results occur in those with very large growth arrests.[90] Williamson and Staheli recommend that resection be considered in all young children who have considerable growth remaining, even if the bar is large.[90] They reported a 48% resection in a 2-year-old and another of 54% that obtained excellent growth for 2 years before they recurred.

The children should be followed until maturity with scanograms; wire markers are helpful to assess growth. Successful results in resections as great as 50% have been reported, with 84% of anticipated growth achieved.[87, 90] All grow vigorously in the beginning, but some close prematurely and may require epiphysiodesis of the contralateral physis toward the end of growth.[87] Reporting on growth disturbances of the distal radial epiphysis after trauma, Zehntner and co-workers noted that corrective osteotomies work quite well.[91]

Nonunion

Nonunion of fractures of long bones is rare in children (Fig. 5–22).[95] In a large series from the Mayo Clinic, the tibia was involved most often (50%) and the femur, ulna, humerus, radius, and fibula less commonly.[95] Generally, nonunion is associated with high-energy trauma and open fractures with extensive soft tissue disruption and infection.[95] Open reduction and internal fixation may contribute if the fixation is inadequate or holds the fracture fragments apart. Nonunion is more likely in the older child who is approaching maturation.

The same treatment techniques that have been successful in adults can be used here. To improve the endosteal response, the dense fibrous tissue and subchondral bone should be resected so that the marrow spaces are communicating. Internal fixation and an autogenous bone graft are recommended.[95] The Ilizarov fixator may improve results in the lower extremities in addition to treating the pseudarthrosis, and the discrepancy in length or angulation can be corrected at the same time.

Nonunion of a displaced fracture of the lateral humeral condyle (Fig. 5–23) is a common problem. Initially, this may show only minimal separation; yet if the cartilage hinge is broken, the fracture fragments easily displace in the early period of cast immobilization. The fracture must be watched closely for displacement if nonoperative treatment is elected. If the fracture displaces, it has a great propensity for nonunion, as the fracture surface of the condyle rotates away from the metaphysis. Flynn recommended that when the distance is 2 mm or greater, these fractures should be surgically reduced and pinned to prevent further displacement and nonunion.[93]

Early recognition of the nonunion leads to salvage by early stabilization and bone grafting if the fragment is in an acceptable position and the growth plate of the condyle is open.[93] Procrastination may allow the physis of the condylar fragment to close prematurely with the loss of a golden opportunity to salvage the elbow. If the fragment is not too rotated or displaced, removal of the fibrous tissue and bone grafting usually suffice.[93] Greater displacement will require pinning the fragments together with a screw or threaded pin. Every effort should

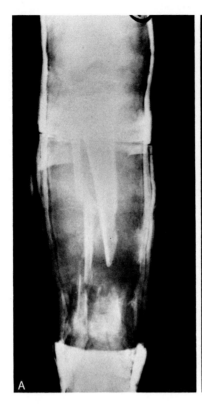
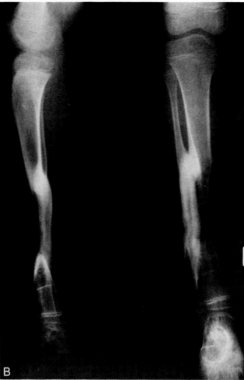

Figure 5–22

A, Nonunion of the tibia following a lawn mower injury with extensive soft tissue loss and infection. *B*, After the soft tissue problems and infection were resolved, adequate skin coverage was obtained and a bone graft from the fibula to the proximal and distal tibia was performed to achieve stability of the leg.

Figure 5–23

Nonunion of a the lateral humeral condyle. The fracture fragment will easily displace if the cartilage hinge is broken. If cast immobilization is used, this fracture must be watched closely for displacement. Early recognition leads to salvage by early stabilization. This nonunion healed after bone grafting.

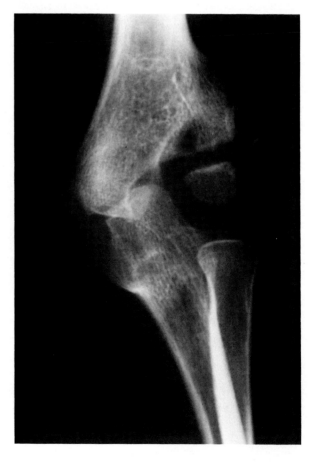

be made to avoid further stripping of soft tissue in order to prevent avascular necrosis of the fragment. It is imperative to reduce the fragment, as reduction may prevent a valgus unstable elbow and subsequent ulnar nerve palsy.[93]

The pediatric carpal scaphoid nonunion is similar to that seen in the adult; usually this occurs in adolescents in whom the injury was initially unrecognized. If the fracture is treated initially with cast immobilization, nonunion is rare. The treatment of the nonunion is similar to that in the adult.[96]

Traumatic loss, sepsis, or resection of the distal fibula may lead to valgus of the ankle, the result of loss of the buttressing effect of the fibula. It is possible for the ankle ligaments to pull the fibular shaft down to compensate for fibular shortening of about 1 cm. If growth arrest occurs more than 2 years before skeletal maturity, distal movement of the fibula will be insufficient to compensate, and the talus will displace laterally into a valgus position.[93] In a gap that is small, treatment with reduction and bone grafting has been helpful. If the gap is large, the fibula can be osteotomized and the distal fragment repositioned and fixed to the distal tibial epiphysis. This should be done routinely if the fibula is used for a graft.[93] It has been reported that distal tibial growth arrest may retard the growth of the distal fibula, but this has not been a consistent finding.

Refracture

Refracture is most common in young boys, suggesting accidental repetition of the original injury—probably a combination of fragile union and reckless physical activity.[92] As healing is rapid in children, immobilization is often discontinued early. Refracture can occur as late as 12 months after the original injury. There is a significant increase in deformity after refracture. The fractures tend to be sticky and difficult to reduce by closed methods, and most authors feel that open reduction is indicated.[92] Children who have osteopenic conditions, such as osteogenesis imperfecta, myelodysplasia, paraplegia, or quadriplegia, are at great risk of secondary fractures in the extremity that has been immobilized. In this group, immobilization should be of short duration and as little as necessary to keep the bone aligned, such as splints and soft dressings. Typically, there is exuberant callus formation, which splints the fracture and allows early removal of the cast.

Ligamentous Instability

Although ligamentous injury can occur in any joint in children, certain problems are often undetected at the time of injury, particularly in the cervical spine and knee. In the cervical spine, the teenager seems to be particularly susceptible to soft tissue and ligamentous disruption between the posterior elements.[97] This frequently follows a hyperflexion injury. Typically, the initial roentgenograms appear satisfactory; however, with the resolution of the pain and swelling, flexion views reveal posterior widening between the spinous process. This is commonly associated with injuries in the lower portion (C4–5, C5–6, and C6–7).[97] The lesion will not heal spontaneously, and the loose segments should be stabilized by a simple one C-level, or occasionally two-level, posterior spine fusion.

Ligamentous injuries about the knee are frequently not recognized, particularly when there is associated fracture of the femur or tibia, or both (the floating knee). Injuries can be to the collateral ligaments or the anterior cruciate and, less commonly, the posterior cruciate. Whether there is an increasing incidence of this injury or improved recognition of it is difficult to determine; however, it emphasizes the importance of early assessment of ligamentous integrity. When there is an adjacent long bone fracture, examination of the knee may be difficult. If traction for a femur fracture is planned after insertion of the femoral pin, the knee can usually be examined adequately. Similarly, if there is an effusion present, aspiration and inspection of the fluid for blood and fat can be helpful, and stress roentgenograms can be obtained (Fig. 5–24). Traction through the knee with the proximal tibial pin is contraindicated if a knee ligament injury is suspected. Similarly, if the ligamentous injury is reparable, the femur should be stabilized. Most authors recommend that the tibia be stabilized as well to facilitate knee ligament repair and subsequent rehabilitation. Although teenagers are the age group most often involved, these recommendations would be the same for a young child.

Nerve Injuries

Late development of neuropathy is often associated with fractures about the elbow, particularly the ulnar nerve. The ulnar nerve can be injured in the initial trauma, during the reduction, or later as the result

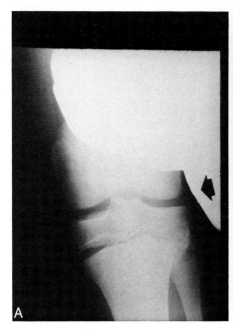 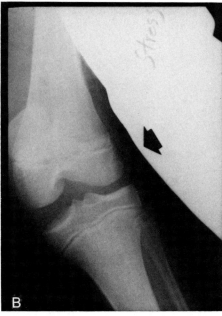

Figure 5–24

Two children who have sustained injuries at the knee. *A*, A 13-year-old male whose stress roentgenogram demonstrates a fracture of the proximal tibial epiphyseal plate. *B*, A 14-year-old male whose stress roentgenogram demonstrates torn medial collateral ligaments and possible disruption of the anterior cruciate ligament.

of progressive elbow deformity.[102] Childhood elbow injuries are believed to be responsible for up to half of all ulnar nerve palsies in adults. The ulnar nerve is often damaged acutely by posterior dislocation of the elbow, particularly if associated with a medial epicondylar fracture.[102] However, ulnar nerve damage has been reported with supracondylar, epicondylar, and condylar fractures.[102]

Valgus deformity that occurs after a lateral condylar fracture can lead to ulnar nerve problems. Varus deformity has also been reported, but less frequently, as a cause of ulnar nerve palsy due to impingement by the triceps tendon. Late ulnar nerve lesions at the elbow have been divided into three main categories: compression within the limited space of the cubital tunnel, traction such as occurs in a valgus deformity, and friction from bone fragments or osteophytes in close proximity to the nerve.[102] This condition is usually associated with ulnar nerve distribution symptoms, including paresthesias, intrinsic muscle weakness, and wasting.[102] An electromyelogram can be helpful in establishing the diagnosis.

Treatment usually consists of surgical decompression of the nerve or correction of the angulatory deformity of the elbow, or both. Transposition is recommended if the ulnar nerve appears normal, if the symptoms are intractable, or if there is a valgus deformity of the elbow. If the condition has been long-standing, the pain and paresthesias should resolve, but weakness and muscle wasting may persist.[102]

Nerve injury is associated with approximately 12 to 16% of supracondylar fractures, most commonly of the ulnar and radial nerves and less often of the median nerve.[100] If the injury is closed and the reduction satisfactory, the child can be treated expectantly, and most will recover, usually in the first 2 months.[100] One of the more subtle median nerve injuries is to the anterior interosseous branch. Physical findings are inability to flex the distal phalanges of the thumb and index finger without associated sensory deficits (Fig. 5–25). This condition can be treated expectantly and usually resolves within 6 to 10 weeks.[100]

Under very unusual circumstances, the median and ulnar nerves can become entrapped following dislocation of the elbow.[98, 101] When this occurs, there is often a delay in diagnosis. Early signs of entrapment are the presence of a lesion of the median nerve and pain greater than expected following reduction of the elbow dislocation.[98, 99] Later signs include a severe elbow flexion contracture and roentgenographically a bony depression in the distal medial humeral cortex corresponding to the location at which the median nerve travels posterior to the humerus and enters the elbow joint.[98, 99] In most children with median nerve injuries, the medial epicondyle has been avulsed.[98] Green claims that every median nerve injury associated with an elbow dislocation should be viewed as representing a probable nerve entrapment, particularly if more than mild hypoesthesia is present.[98] Pain is a guideline if the neurologic deficit progresses; it should not be

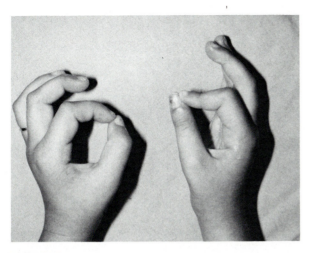

Figure 5–25

Supracondylar fracture in an 8-year-old female that resulted in an anterior interosseous nerve palsy. Note the physical findings—inability to flex the distal phalanges of the thumb and index finger. The patient did not have an associated sensory deficit. She was treated expectantly, and the neurapraxia resolved in 6 weeks.

severe once the dislocation has been reduced. The presence of intense pain should alert one to the possibility of entrapment of the median nerve. The brachial artery and vein and the median nerve can be trapped between the fracture fragments with a widely displaced supracondylar fracture. Attempts at closed reduction usually lead to vascular compromise and necessitate surgical reduction.

Secondary nerve injuries can result from simple positioning, particularly in children who are in coma or following head injury.[99, 101] The ulnar nerve is very susceptible to compression at the elbow and the radial nerve at the mid portion of the humerus if the arm is not properly positioned. If recognized early, these neurapraxias have good potential for recovery. The peroneal nerve may be compressed as it passes over the neck of the fibula. Frequent checks of the extremity for neurovascular status are essential, particularly in the immediate postinjury and early recovery periods or until the child is alert enough to report any changes. Obviously, in children with head injuries, casts should be well padded over these susceptible areas.

Reflex Sympathetic Dystrophy

This condition is believed to be due to dysfunction of the anatomic nervous system, usually following an injury to the ankle and foot, knee, or shoulder and hand.[103] Many terms have been used in the past to describe the condition, including causalgia, post-traumatic pain syndrome, shoulder-hand syndrome, and Sudeck atrophy. The onset is heralded by severe pain and exquisite tenderness to light touch, including that of clothing.[103] Symptoms are intensified by weight bearing and relieved by keeping the involved areas as motionless as possible.[103] The extremity is usually swollen and exhibits vasomotor instability, including skin discoloration, swelling with dependency, and decreased peripheral pulses; the skin temperature is usually colder with increased sweating. The onset of symptoms may follow a trivial injury, such as a simple twisted ankle or sprain, or may not be associated with a definite event.[103] Reflex sympathetic dystrophy is usually seen in adolescents but has been described in those as young as 10 years of age. There are a variety of theories but no satisfactory explanation for its onset.[106]

Typically, the condition is present for an extended period before the diagnosis is made (average 8 to 16 weeks, range 1 week to 26 months). Differential diagnoses include juvenile rheumatoid arthritis, polymyositis, rheumatic fever, systemic lupus erythematosus, neoplasia, gout, and thrombophlebitis.[110] Results of laboratory studies are usually within normal limits.[103] Roentgenograms may reveal a diffuse osteoporosis of the involved part. Bone scan findings have been inconsistent, showing both increased uptake when there is a strong vasomotor phase and decreased uptake with marked osteoporosis.[103, 108]

Most of the pediatric patients are found to have psychologic problems, usually a pronounced indifference to the implications of the illness.[103] The children have a tendency to accept responsibility beyond their years and are very involved in school and extracurricular activities, sports, or social functions.[103, 109] They have difficulty expressing anger or being assertive on their own behalf.[103, 109] Their strength is in doing rather than saying; this is a manner of expression consistent with how these children best approach their environment.[109] Typically, the condition serves a functional role by allowing them to slow down gracefully and affords a safe means of frustrating their parents' demands for performance without having to take responsibility for their behavior.[103] All have emotional problems, and treatment must take these psychologic factors into account.[109] Marital discord was present in about half the families of these patients, and the child often had the burden of keeping peace in the household. Many families show inappropriately high levels of enmeshment between parents and child;

because of high levels of stress in the parental relationship, the child consciously or unconsciously attempts to alleviate the problem.

The primary emphasis in management is to make the diagnosis and rule out other potential problems. Prompt diagnosis and therapy are directed at alleviating the symptoms quickly, significantly improving the chance for permanent relief.[105] Most authors suggest narcotic analgesics be avoided in children.[106] Vigorous active exercises, weight-bearing activities, and direct stimulation of the skin are usually successful. Corticosteroid therapy and sympathetic blockade are seldom necessary in children; most respond to continued positive reinforcement by a multidisciplinary team.[103,104] Recovery occurs in 8 weeks.[107]

The condition is more benign in children than in adults.[103,107] Children seldom develop the chronic atrophic changes that are found in adults.[103,107] In follow-up, few children have long-term problems; most continue to function normally.[103,107] Long-term problems are related to shortness of the limb or foot due to prolonged immobilization and osteoporosis.[108]

REFERENCES

Vascular Injuries

1. Bach, A.; Johansen, K. Limb salvage using temporary arterial shunt following traumatic near-amputation of the thigh. J Pediatr Orthop 2:187–190, 1982.
2. Clement, D. A.; Phil, D. Assessment of a treatment plan for managing acute vascular complications associated with supracondylar fractures of the humerus in children. J Pediatr Orthop 10:97–100, 1990.
3. Cole, W. G. Arterial injuries associated with fractures of the lower limbs in childhood. Injury 12:460–463, 1981.
4. Connolly, J. Management of fractures associated with arterial injuries. Am J Surg 120:331, 1970.
5. Damron, T.; McBeath, A. Diagnosis and management of vascular injuries associated with skeletal trauma. Orthop Rev 19:1063–1070, 1990.
6. Fabian, T. C.; Turkleson, M. L.; Connelly, T. L.; Stone, H. H. Injury to the popliteal artery. Am J Surg 143:225–228, 1982.
7. Friedman, R. J.; Jupiter, J. B. Vascular injuries and closed extremity fractures in children. Clin Orthop 188:112–119, 1984.
8. Green, N. E.; Allen, B. L. Vascular injuries associated with dislocation of the knee. J Bone Joint Surg 59-A:236–239, 1977.
9. Johansen, K.; Bandyk, D.; Thiele, B.; Hansen, S. T. Temporary intraluminal shunts: Resolution of a management dilemma in complex vascular injuries. J Trauma 22:395–402, 1982.
10. Lange, R. H.; Bach, A. W.; Hansen, S. T.; Johansen, K. H. Open tibial fractures with associated vascular injuries: Prognosis for limb salvage. J Trauma 25:203–208, 1985.
11. Navarre, J. R.; Cardillo, P. J.; Gorman, J. F.; et al. Vascular trauma in children and adolescents. Am J Surg 143:229–231, 1982.
12. Russo, V. J. Traumatic arterial spasm resulting in gangrene. J Pediatr Orthop 5:486–488, 1985.
13. Samson, R.; Pasternak, B. M. Traumatic arterial spasm—rarity or nonentity? J Trauma 20:607–609, 1980.
14. Shaker, I. J.; White, J. J.; Signer, R. D.; et al. Special problems of vascular injuries in children. J Trauma 16:863–867, 1976.
15. Smith, P. L.; Lim, W. N.; Ferris, E. J.; Casali, R. E. Emergency arteriography in extremity trauma: Assessment of indications. AJR 137:803–807, 1981.
16. Stanford, J. R.; Evans, W. E.; Morse, T. S. Pediatric arterial injuries. J Vasc Dis 27:1–7, 1976.
17. Vasli, L. P. Diagnosis of vascular injury in children with supracondylar fractures of the humerus. Injury 19:11–13, 1988.
18. Whitehouse, W. M.; Coran, A. G.; Stanley, J. C.; et al. Pediatric vascular trauma. Manifestations, management and sequelae of extremity arterial injury in patients undergoing surgical treatment. Arch Surg 111:1269–1275, 1976.

Compartment Syndromes

19. Hargens, A. R.; Akeson, W. H.; Mubarak, S. J.; et al. Fluid balance within the canine anterolateral compartment and its relationship to compartment syndromes. J Bone Joint Surg 60-A:499–505, 1978.
20. Hargens, A. R.; Romine, J. S.; Sipe, J. C.; et al. Peripheral nerve-conduction block by high muscle-compartment pressure. J Bone Joint Surg 61-A:192–200, 1979.
21. Clancey, G. J. Acute posterior compartment syndrome in the thigh. A case report. J Bone Joint Surg 67-A:1278–1280, 1985.
22. Heppenstall, R. B.; Scott, R.; Sapega, A.; et al. A comparative study of the tolerance of skeletal muscle to ischemia. Tourniquet application compared with acute compartment syndrome. J Bone Joint Surg 68-A:820–828, 1986.
23. Langen, R. P.; Ruggieri, R. Acute compartment syndrome in the thigh complicated by a pseudoaneurysm. A case report. J Bone Joint Surg 71-A:762–763, 1989.
24. Matsen, F. A., III. Compartment syndrome: A unified concept. Clin Orthop 113:8–14, 1975.
25. Matsen, F. A., III; Veith, R. G. Compartmental syndromes in children. J Pediatr Orthop 1:33–41, 1981.
26. Mubarak, S. J.; Owen, C. A.; Hargens, A. R.; et al. Compartment syndromes: Diagnosis and treatment with the aid of the Wick catheter. J Bone Joint Surg 60-A:1091–1095, 1978.
27. Schwartz, J. T.; Brumback, R. J.; Lakatos, R.; et al. Acute compartment syndrome of the thigh. A spectrum of injury. J Bone Joint Surg 71-A:392–400, 1989.

Fat Embolism

28. Carty, J. B. Fat embolism in childhood. Review and case report. Am J Surg 94:970–973, 1957.
29. Drummond, D. S.; Salter, R. B.; Boone, J. Fat embolism in children: Its frequency and relationships to collagen disease. Can Med Assoc J 101:200–203, 1969.
30. Limbird, T. J.; Ruderman, R. J. Fat embolism in children. Clin Orthop 136:267–268, 1978.
31. Shulman, S. T.; Grossman, B. J. Fat embolism in childhood. Review with report of a fatal case related to physical therapy in a child with dermatomyositis. Am J Dis Child 120:480–484, 1970.

Hypercalcemia of Immobilization

32. Claus-Walker, J.; Carter, R. D.; Campos, R. J.; Spencer, W. A. Hypercalcemia in early traumatic quadriplegia. J Chron Dis 28:81–90, 1975.
33. Cristofaro, R. L.; Brink, J. D. Hypercalcemia of immobilization in neurologically injured children: A prospective study. Orthopaedics 2:485–491, 1979.
34. Henke, J. A.; Thompson, N. W.; Kaufer, H. Immobilization hypercalcemia crisis. Arch Surg 110:321–323, 1975.
35. Winters, J. L.; Kleinschmidt, A. G.; Frehsilli, J. J.; Sutton, M. Hypercalcemia complicating immobilization in the treatment of fractures. J Bone Joint Surg 48-A:1182–1184, 1966.

Ectopic Bone Formation

36. Carlson, W. O.; Klassen, R. A. Myositis ossificans of the upper extremity: A long-term follow-up. J Pediatr Orthop 4:693–696, 1984.
37. Mital, M. A.; Garber, J. E.; Stinson, J. T. Ectopic bone formation in children and adolescents with head injuries: Its management. J Pediatr Orthop 7:83–90, 1987.
38. Thompson, H. G.; Garcia, A. Myositis ossificans: Aftermath of elbow injuries. Clin Orthop 50:129–134, 1967.

Cast Syndrome

39. Amy, B. W.; Priebe, C. J.; King, A. Superior mesenteric artery syndrome associated with scoliosis treated by a modified Ladd procedure. J Pediatr Orthop 5:361–363, 1985.
40. Berk, R. N.; Coulson, D. B. The body cast syndrome. Radiology 94:303–305, 1970.
41. Walker, C.; Kahanovitz, N. Recurrent superior mesenteric artery syndrome complicating staged reconstructive spinal surgery: Alternative methods of conservative treatment. J Pediatr Orthop 3:77–80, 1983.
42. Warner, T. F. C. S.; Shorter, R. G.; McIlrath, D. C.; Dupree, E. L., Jr. The cast syndrome. An unusually severe case. J Bone Joint Surg 56-A:1263–1266, 1974.

Traction-Induced Hypertension

43. Hamdan, J. A.; Taleb, Y. A.; Ahmed, M. S. Traction-induced hypertension in children. Clin Orthop 185:87–89, 1984.
44. Linshaw, M. A.; Stapleton, F. B.; Gruskin, A. B.; et al. Traction-related hypertension in children. J Pediatr 95:994–996, 1979.
45. Talab, Y. A.; Hamdan, J. A.; Ahmed, M. S. Orthopaedic causes of hypertension in pediatric patients. Case report and review of the literature. J Bone Joint Surg 64-A:291–292, 1982.
46. Turner, M. C.; Ruley, E. J.; Buckley, K. M.; Strife, C. F. Blood pressure elevation with orthopaedic immobilization. J Pediatr 95:989–992, 1979.

Spontaneous Deep Vein Thrombosis

47. Horwitz, J.; Shenker, I. R. Spontaneous deep vein thrombosis in adolescence. Clin Pediatr 16:787–790, 1977.
48. Joffe, S. Postoperative deep vein thrombosis in children. J Pediatr Surg 10:539–540, 1975.
49. Wise, R. C.; Todd, J. K. Spontaneous, lower-extremity venous thrombosis in children. Am J Dis Child 126:766–769, 1973.

Malunion—Synostosis

50. Bellemore, M. C.; Barrett, I. R.; Middleton, R. W. D.; et al. Supracondylar osteotomy of the humerus for correction of cubitus varus. J Bone Joint Surg 66-B:566–572, 1984.
51. Bohn, W. W.; Durbin, R. A. Ipsilateral fractures of the femur and tibia in children and adolescents. J Bone Joint Surg 73-A:429–439, 1991.
52. Carlson, C. S.; Rosman, M. A. Cubitus varus: A new and simple technique for correction. J Pediatr Orthop 2:199–201, 1982.
53. Creasman, C.; Zaleske, D. J.; Ehrlich, M. G. Analyzing forearm fractures in children. The more subtle signs of impending problems. Clin Orthop 188:40–53, 1984.
54. Davis, D. R.; Green, D. P. Forearm fractures in children. Pitfalls and complications. Clin Orthop 120:172–184, 1976.
55. Fuller, D. J.; McCullough, C. J. Malunited fractures of the forearm in children. J Bone Joint Surg 64-B:364–367, 1982.
56. Fowles, J. V.; Kassab, M. T.; Moula, T. Untreated intra-articular entrapment of the medial humeral epicondyle. J Bone Joint Surg 66-B:562–565, 1984.
57. Hoffer, M. M.; Garrett, A.; Brink, J.; et al. The orthopaedic management of brain-injured children. J Bone Joint Surg 53-A:567–577, 1971.
58. Kirby, R. M.; Winquist, R. A.; Hansen, S. T. Femoral shaft fractures in adolescents: A comparison between traction plus cast treatment and closed intramedullary nailing. J Pediatr Orthop 1:193–197, 1981.
59. Labelle, H.; Bunnell, W. P.; Duhaime, M.; Poitras, B. Cubitus varus deformity following supracondylar fractures of the humerus in children. J Pediatr Orthop 2:539–546, 1982.
60. Loder, R. T. Pediatric polytrauma: Orthopaedic care and hospital course. J Orthop Trauma 1:48–54, 1987.
61. Oppenheim W. L.; Clader, T. J.; Smith, C.; Bayer, M. Supracondylar humeral osteotomy for traumatic childhood cubitus varus deformity. Clin Orthop 188:34–39, 1984.
62. Price, C. T.; Scott, D. S.; Kurzner, M. E.; Flynn, J. C. Malunited forearm fractures in children. J Pediatr Orthop 10:705–712, 1990.
63. Thomas, E. W.; Tuson, K. W. R.; Browne, P. S. H. Fractures of the radius and ulna in children. Injury 7:120–124, 1979.
64. Tredwell, S. S.; Peteghen, K. V.; Clough, M.: Pattern of forearm fractures in children. J Pediatr Orthop 4:604–608, 1984.
65. Vince, K. G.; Miller, J. E. Cross-union complicating fracture of the forearm. Part II: Children. J Bone Joint Surg 69A:654–661, 1987.
66. Ziv, I.; Rang, M.: Treatment of femoral fracture in the child with head injury. J Bone Joint Surg 65B:276–278, 1983.

Late Angulation

67. Balthazar, D. A.; Pappas, A. M. Acquired valgus deformity of the tibia in children. J Pediatr Orthop 4:538–541, 1984.
68. Green, N. E. Tibia valga caused by asymmetrical overgrowth following a nondisplaced fracture of the proximal tibial metaphysis. J Pediatr Orthop 3:235–237, 1983.
69. Jordan, S. E.; Alonso, J. E.; Cook, F. F. The etiology of valgus angulation after metaphyseal fractures of the tibia in children. J Pediatr Orthop 7:450–457, 1987.
70. Robert, M.; Khouri, N.; Carlioz, H.; Alain, J. L. Fractures of the proximal tibial metaphysis in children: Review of a series of 25 cases. J Pediatr Orthop 7:444–449, 1987.

71. So, Y. C.; Fang, D.; Leong, J. C. Y.; Bong, S. C. Varus deformity following lateral humeral condylar fractures in children. J Pediatr Orthop 5:569–572, 1985.
72. Zionts, L. E.; Harcke, H. T.; Brooks, K. M.; MacEwen, G. D. Posttraumatic tibial valga: A case demonstrating asymmetric activity at the proximal growth plate on technetium bone scan. J Pediatr Orthop 7:458–462, 1987.

Injury to Triradiate Cartilage

73. Bucholz, R. W.; Ezaki, M.; Ogden, J. A. Injury to the acetabular triradiate physeal cartilage. J Bone Joint Surg 64-A:600–609, 1982.
74. Hallel, T.; Salvati, E. A. Premature closure of the triradiate cartilage. A case report and animal experiment. Clin Orthop 124:278–281, 1977.
75. Harder, J. A.; Bobechko, W. P.; Sullivan, R.; Daneman, A. Computerized axial tomography to demonstrate occult fractures of the acetabulum in children. Can J Surg 24:409–411, 1981.

Overgrowth and Undergrowth

76. Beals, R. K. Premature closure of the physis following diaphyseal fractures. J Pediatr Orthop 10:717–720, 1990.
77. Bowler, J. R.; Mubarak, S. J.; Wenger, D. R. Tibial physeal closure and genu recurvatum after femoral fracture: Occurrence without a tibial traction pin. J Pediatr Orthop 10:653–657, 1990.
78. Hunter, L. Y.; Hensinger, R. N. Premature monomelic growth arrest following fracture of the femoral shaft. A case report. J Bone Joint Surg 60-A:850–852, 1978.
79. Kohan, L.; Cumming, W. J. Femoral shaft fractures in children: The effect of initial shortening on subsequent limb overgrowth. Aust NZ J Surg 52:141–144, 1982.
80. Shapiro, F. Fractures of the femoral shaft in children. The overgrowth phenomenon. Acta Orthop Scand 52:649–655, 1981.
81. Staheli, L. T.: Femoral and tibial growth following femoral shaft fracture in childhood. Clin Orthop 55:159, 1967.

Growth Disturbances

81. Bollini, G.; Tallet, J. M.; Jacquemier, M.; Bouyala, J. M. New procedure to remove a centrally located bone bar. J Pediatr Orthop 10:662–666, 1990.
82. Carlson, W. O.; Wenger, D. R. A mapping method to prepare for surgical excision of a partial physeal arrest. J Pediatr Orthop 4:232–238, 1984.
83. Karrholm, J.; Hansson, L. I.; Selvik, G. Changes in tibiofibular relationships due to growth disturbances after ankle fractures in children. J Bone Joint Surg 66-A:1198–1210, 1984.
84. Kling, T. F.; Bright, R. W.; Hensinger, R. N. Distal tibial physeal fractures in children that may require open reduction. J Bone Joint Surg 66-A:647–657, 1984.
85. Langenskiöld, A. Surgical treatment of partial closure of the growth plate. J Pediatr Orthop 1:3–11, 1981.
86. Langenskiöld, A.; Österman, K.; Valle, M. Growth of fat grafts after operation for partial bone growth arrest: Demonstration by computed tomography scanning. J Pediatr Orthop 7:389–394, 1987.
87. Peterson, H. A. Partial growth plate arrest and its treatment. J Pediatr Orthop 4:246–258, 1984.
88. Porat, S.; Nyska, M.; Nyska, A.; Fields, S. Assessment of bony bridge by computed tomography: Experimental model in the rabbit and clinical application. J Pediatr Orthop 7:155–160, 1987.
89. Riseborough, E. J.; Barrett, I. R.; Shapiro, F. Growth disturbances following distal femoral physeal fracture-separations. J Bone Joint Surg 65-A:885–893, 1983.
90. Williamson, R. V.; Staheli, L. T. Partial physeal growth arrest: Treatment by bridge resection and fat interposition. J Pediatr Orthop 10:769–776, 1990.
91. Zehntner, M. K.; Jakob, R. P.; McGanity, P. L. J. Growth disturbance of the distal radial epiphysis after trauma: Operative treatment by corrective radial osteotomy. J Pediatr Orthop 10:411–415, 1990.

Nonunion and Refracture

92. Arunachalam, V. S. P.; Griffiths, J. C. Fracture recurrence in children. Injury 7:37–40, 1975.
93. Flynn, J. A. Nonunion of slightly displaced fractures of the lateral humeral condyle in children: An update. J Pediatr Orthop 9:691–696, 1989.
94. Hsu, L. C. S.; O'Brien, J. P.; Hodgson, A. R. Valgus deformity of the ankle in children with fibular pseudarthrosis. J Bone Joint Surg 56-A:503–510, 1974.
95. Lewallen, R. P.; Peterson, H. A. Nonunion of long bone fractures in children: A review of 30 cases. J Pediatr Orthop 5:135–142, 1985.
96. Maxted, M. J.; Owen, R. Two cases of non-union of carpal scaphoid fractures in children. Injury 13:441–443, 1982.

Ligamentous Instability

97. Pennecot, G. F.; Leonard, P.; Peyrot Des Gachons, S.; et al. Traumatic ligamentous instability of the cervical spine in children. J Pediatr Orthop 4:339–345, 1984.

Nerve Injuries

98. Green, N. E. Entrapment of the median nerve following elbow dislocation. J Pediatr Orthop 3:384–386, 1983.
99. Hallett, J. Entrapment of the median nerve after dislocation of the elbow. A case report. J Bone Joint Surg 63-B:408–412, 1981.
100. McGraw, J. J.; Akbarnia, B. A.; Hanel, D. P.; et al. Neurological complications resulting from supracondylar fractures of the humerus in children. J Pediatr Orthop 6:647–650, 1986.
101. Pritchett, J. W. Entrapment of the median nerve after dislocation of the elbow. J Pediatr Orthop 4:752–753, 1984.
102. Royle, S. G.; Burke, D. Ulna neuropathy after elbow injury in children. J Pediatr Orthop 10:495–496, 1990.

Reflex Sympathetic Dystrophy

103. Bernstein, B. H.; Singsen, B. H.; Kent, J. T.; et al. Reflex neurovascular dystrophy in childhood. J Pediatr 93:211–215, 1978.
104. Doolan, L. A.; Brown, T. C. K. Reflex sympathetic dystrophy in a child. Anaesth Intensive Care 12:70–72, 1984.
105. Fermaglich, D. R. Reflex sympathetic dystrophy in children. Pediatrics 60:881–883, 1977.
106. Forster, R. S.; Fu, F. H. Reflex sympathetic dystrophy in children. A case report and review of literature. Orthopaedics 8:475–477, 1985.

107. Ruggeri, S. B.; Athreya, B. H.; Doughty, R.; et al. Reflex sympathetic dystrophy in children. Clin Orthop 163:225–230, 1982.
108. Rush, P. J.; Wilmot, D.; Saunders, N.; et al. Severe reflex neurovascular dystrophy in childhood. Arthritis Rheum 25:952–956, 1985.
109. Sherry, D. D.; Weisman, R. Psychologic aspects of childhood reflex neurovascular dystrophy. Pediatrics 81:572–578, 1988.
110. Wotring, K.; Mehn, J.; Stengem, C. Evaluation and treatment of the pediatric reflex neurovascular dystrophy patient. Arthritis Rheum 28:S143, 1985.

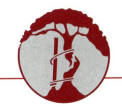

Peter F. Armstrong, M.D., F.R.C.S.C., F.A.C.S.
V. Elaine Joughin, M.D., F.R.C.S.C.
Howard M. Clarke, M.D., Ph.D., F.R.C.S.C.

6

Pediatric Fractures of the Forearm, Wrist, and Hand

Fractures of the Forearm

Forearm fractures are very common injuries in childhood. They account for 45% of all fractures in children and for 62% of upper limb fractures. The vast majority (81%) occur in children who are more than 5 years of age.[26]

The most common cause of forearm fractures is a fall in or around the home. Sports-related injuries are next in frequency.[99] There is a peak incidence of these fractures from April through September, the good weather months in which children are more likely to play outdoors.[26]

Approximately 75 to 84% of forearm fractures occur in the distal third, 15 to 18% in the middle third, and 1 to 7% in the proximal third.[8, 26] A small percentage are bilateral, and as many as 13% have an associated supracondylar fracture.[8, 26, 83] Just over 50% of these fractures are greenstick fractures.[99] Injuries to the distal growth plate of the radius occur in 14 to 18% of forearm fractures.[26, 99]

Historically it has been the standard to treat most of these fractures in children by closed reduction and immobilization in a cast. It was thought that remodeling with growth would correct residual deformity even if anatomic reduction could not be achieved or maintained. Although this is true in many instances, several studies have shown that complete remodeling does not always occur. This is especially so in children who are older than 8 to 10 years. These children have insufficient growth and remodeling potential remaining to provide correction of significant residual deformity.[15, 17, 36, 52]

Rotation of the forearm is the motion most frequently lost after these fractures.[52] Residual rotational losses of greater than 20 degrees have been found in 60% of patients who were treated for forearm fractures.[17, 19] Subjective results, however, are usually excellent, and a decreased range of motion is often detectable only by special goniometric testing.[15, 17] Mild limitations of rotation are not noticeable to the patient because abduction and internal rotation at the shoulder adequately compensate for any loss in pronation, and adduction and external rotation of the shoulder may partially compensate for limitation in supination.[39] Therefore, even with stringent criteria, 85% of patients with displaced fractures achieve satisfactory results from closed reduction of the forearm.[15, 17]

Nevertheless, we believe that there are a number of very important principles that should be followed to achieve the ideal goal of fracture healing without deformity or dysfunction. It is very important that every effort be made to achieve an adequate, but not necessarily anatomic, reduction. In certain instances this may require an open reduction and internal fixation.

GENERAL PRINCIPLES

As with all fractures, the basic principle is to accurately align, both axially and rotationally, the distal fracture fragments with the proximal fragments and to maintain this position until the fracture is healed. Managing fractures of the forearm in children requires an understanding of several factors: (1) anatomy of the forearm, (2) deforming muscular forces, (3) mechanism of injury, and (4) remodeling potential.

Anatomy

To accurately align fractures in the forearm, there must be an understanding of the basic anatomy of the forearm, including the normal shape of the forearm bones; of the normal shape and importance of the interosseous space; and of the anatomy of the proximal and distal radioulnar articulations. Children's fractures are different from fractures in adults, as growth and remodeling continue after the fracture has healed. This growth potential exists until the epiphyseal plates close at maturity. Thus, it is important to be aware of the timing of plate closure to determine the extent of remodeling capacity.

Development. The radius and ulna ossify from primary ossification centers in the eighth week of gestation. At the wrist, the secondary ossification center of the distal radial epiphysis appears within the first year of age in girls, and at just over 1 year of age in boys. There may be a separate ossification center in the tip of the radial styloid process that may be confused with a fracture. The distal ulnar epiphysis begins to ossify at 6 years in both girls and boys and often develops from two centers. Closure of the distal radial physis occurs at approximately age 17 years in girls and at age 18 to 19 years in boys. The distal ulnar epiphysis closes at between ages 16 and 17 years in girls and ages 17 and 18 years in boys.[28, 37, 61]

At the elbow, the proximal radial epiphysis appears in the fifth to seventh year, while the proximal ulnar epiphysis appears in the ninth to tenth year. Both these epiphyses unite with the shaft between the ages of 16 and 18 years (Fig. 6–1).[37]

Osteology. The radius is a curved bone that is cylindrical in the proximal third, is triangular in the middle third, and flattens out in the lower end. The interosseous membrane attaches to the apex of the triangle on the radius. The bicipital tuberosity, which is the insertion point for the biceps tendon, is located just below the neck of the radius. In the supinated position, the shaft normally bows laterally distal to the bicipital tuberosity. In addition, there is a mild posterior bow with the apex in the midshaft region. Distally and laterally the radial styloid forms the insertion point for the brachioradialis.

The ulna has a triangular shape throughout the shaft, and the interosseous membrane attaches at its sharp lateral border. Like the radius, the ulna

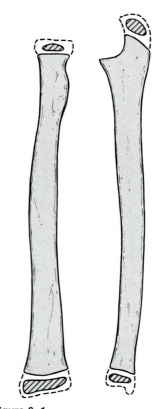

Figure 6–1

Ossification centers of the radius and ulna.

has a bow, but its apex is located posteriorly in the proximal third (Fig. 6–2). In the accurate reduction of fractures in the forearm, the anatomic contour of these bones must be restored to fully regain pronation and supination. Rotational malalignment can be recognized when the widths of the proximal and distal fragments do not match at the fracture site or if there is discontinuity in the normally smooth curvature of the bone (Fig. 6–3).

Radioulnar Articulations. The radius is connected to the ulna throughout its length via the proximal radioulnar articulation, the interosseous membrane, and the distal radioulnar articulation. Because the forearm is a two-bone complex, injury usually results in a fracture of both bones or a fracture of one bone associated with injury to one of the radioulnar articulations.

Proximally the radial head articulates with the capitellum and proximal ulna. The annular ligament is the major structure responsible for maintaining the stability of the proximal radioulnar joint. This joint is most stable in supination. In supination the broadest portion of the articular surface of the radial head comes into contact with the proximal notch of the ulna; the interosseous membrane is most taut;

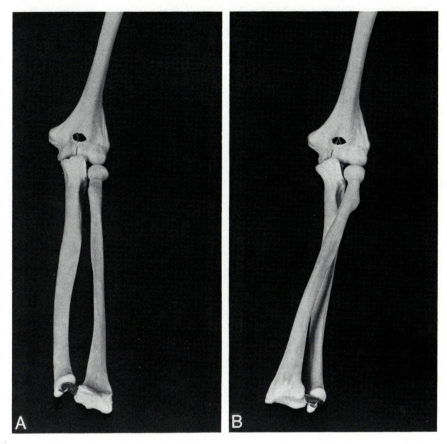

Figure 6–2

The appearance of the radius and ulna in supination *(A)* and pronation *(B)*.

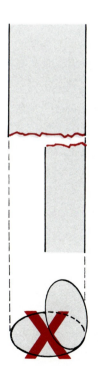
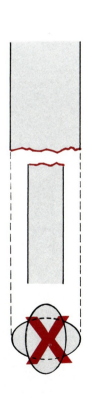
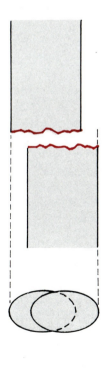

Figure 6–3

Matching of the width and shape of the fracture fragments on x-ray is essential to ensure correct rotational alignment. (From King, R.E.: Fractures of the shafts of the radius and ulna. *In*: Rockwood, C.A.J.; Wilkins, J.E.; King, R.E., eds. Fractures in Children, Vol 3. Philadelphia, J.B. Lippincott, 1984.)

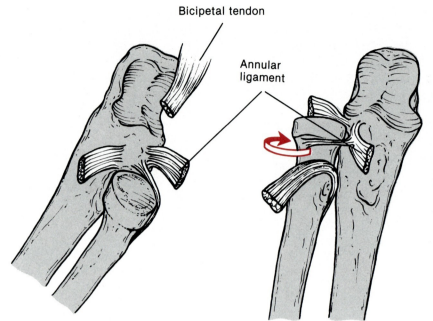

Figure 6–4

The annular ligament is the major stabilizing structure of the proximal radioulnar articulation. When the forearm is supinated, the anterior border of the quadrate ligament becomes taut and draws the radial head snugly against the radial notch of the ulna. (From Spinner, M.; Kaplan, E.B. The quadrate ligament of the elbow—Its relationship to the stability of the proximal radio-ulnar joint. Acta Orthop Scand 41:632, 1970.)

and the anterior fibers of the quadrate ligament stabilize the radial head strongly into the proximal radioulnar joint.[82] In pronation and supination the head of the radius pivots within the annular ligament while the lower end of the radius swings around the head of the ulna, contained by the triangular fibrocartilage complex (Fig. 6–4).

Distally the triangular fibrocartilage complex is composed of an articular disk that is joined by the volar and dorsal radiocarpal ligaments and by fibers of the ulnar collateral ligament at the wrist (Fig. 6–5). The disk is attached to the margin of the radius, separating the ulnar notch from the carpal articular surface. Its apex is fixed in the fossa at the base of the styloid process of the ulna. The disk measures about 1 cm and is thickest at the circumference, where it is connected with the articular capsule. It firmly unites the distal ends of the bones. In addition, it limits the rotational movements of the radius and ulna and maintains congruity of the radioulnar joint against the torsional stresses of rotation of the forearm.[53, 73, 76] The distal radioulnar joint is stabilized by the ulnar collateral ligament, which originates from the distal portion of the styloid; the anterior and posterior radioulnar ligaments; and the pronator quadratus muscle.[53] The posterior distal radioulnar ligament has been shown to become taut in phase with pronation; the anterior becomes taut with supination.[76]

The distal and proximal radioulnar joints are interdependent for stability. With pronation and supination there is movement at each of these joints. Bado noted that with pronation the radius "short-ens" and that with supination it "lengthens" relative to the ulna.[4] This interdependence may be the reason for late dislocation of the radial head in children who have had shortening of the ulna following an injury to the distal ulna. Similarly, exces-

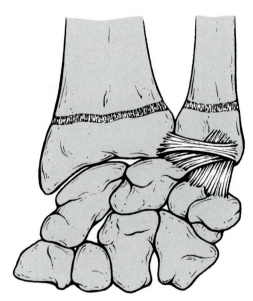

Figure 6–5

The triangular fibrocartilage complex consists of the triangular fibrocartilage and the ulnocarpal ligaments. This provides the articular surface for the carpus, provides a flexible mechanism for stable rotational movements of the radius and ulna, suspends the ulnar carpus from the radius, and cushions the forces transmitted through the ulnocarpal axis. (From Bowers, W.H. The distal radioulnar joint. In: Green, D.P., ed.: Operative Hand Surgery. Vol 2, 2nd ed. New York, Churchill Livingstone, 1988, pp. 939–989.)

sive resection of the radial head can cause posterior dislocation of the distal ulna.[76]

The radial and ulnar shafts are connected by the interosseous membrane (Fig. 6–6). With the forearm in supination the interosseous space forms an elongated ellipse that is widest in the middle third of the forearm. Narrowing of the interosseous space has been shown to restrict the rotation of the forearm. In a study of cadavers, it was shown that the interosseous distance depends on the position of the forearm. The narrowest distance was in pronation, and the greatest distance was in neutral to 30 degrees of supination. The interosseous membrane is taut in neutral to 30 degrees of supination but becomes increasingly relaxed with further supination or pronation.[13] From this, it appears that in treating fractures of the forearm, restoring the interosseous distance with the forearm in neutral to 30 degrees of supination would be ideal to regain full rotation.

Bicipital Tuberosity. Evans suggested that the bicipital tuberosity could be used as a landmark to determine the rotational position of the proximal fragment to which the distal fragment is aligned.[19] The "tuberosity view," an anteroposterior view of the elbow joint taken with the x-ray tube at an angle of 20 degrees cephalad, was recommended by Evans for determining the position of the bicipital tuberosity relative to the shaft of the radius.[19] In full supination, the bicipital tuberosity appears on the medial aspect of the radius. In midposition, it appears to be fully superimposed on the shaft of the radius. In full pronation, it lies in the lateral position (Fig. 6–7).[18]

Unfortunately, the bicipital tuberosity is not always well visualized on x-rays of the forearm in children, making this view less useful than would first appear.[15, 93] Other clues, such as the width and shape of the shaft at the fracture site, the contour of the bones after reduction, and the stability of the fracture in different positions of the forearm on trial reduction, are often more useful guides in determining the correct rotational alignment of the fracture.

Forearm Rotation. The forearm rotates through supination and pronation in an average range of 150 to 180 degrees.[4, 96] The mechanical axis of the forearm lies along a line connecting the rotational centers of the proximal radius and distal ulna (Fig. 6–8). Rotation of the radius about the ulna has been described as a half-cone.[4, 64]

Reduction of the interosseous space by any means results in a limitation of the amplitude of the arc through which the radius swings around the ulna. Experimental fractures produced in cadavers and plated in 10 degrees of malrotation create a limitation in rotation of 10 degrees. Ten degrees of angulation in the middle third of the shaft limits rotation by 20 to 27 degrees because it produces widening and narrowing of the interosseous membrane during rotatory movements.[52, 86] Bayonet apposition, or overlapping, does not limit rotation as long as the interosseous space is maintained. In proximal fractures, narrowing of the interosseous distance may restrict rotation by causing the bicipital tuberosity to impinge on the ulna. Malalignment of fractures of the distal ulnar metaphysis may increase the tension on the articular disk so that the head of the ulna does not rotate freely.[70] Soft tissue tension (especially of the interosseous membrane) may be an important contributing factor to the limitation of rotation.[86]

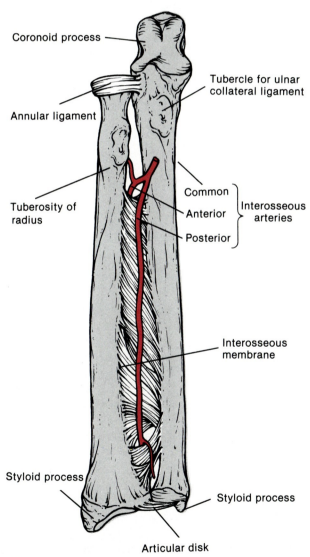

Figure 6–6

The interosseous membrane. (From Grant, J.C.B. An Atlas of Anatomy, 6th ed. Baltimore, Williams & Wilkins, 1972.)

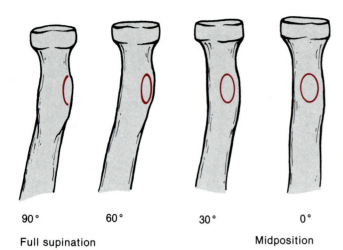

Figure 6–7

The radiologic position of the bicipital tuberosity from full supination (90 degrees) to midposition (0 degrees). (From Evans, E.M. Fractures of the radius and ulna. J Bone Joint Surg 33-B:548, 1951.)

These cadaver studies, of course, do not take into account any remodeling that may occur. Hogstrom and co-workers state that there is poor correlation between residual angulation of these fractures and range of motion of the involved extremity after healing.[32] Even with fractures that heal in perfect alignment, loss of forearm rotation can result.[60]

Repeated closed and open reductions are not without risk.[15] In children, fractures in the proximal third of the forearm treated with open reduction and internal fixation are likely to result in loss of rotation even with complete restoration to anatomic alignment.[89] The residual impairment of function is probably due to soft tissue scarring. This must be taken into account when surgical management of a fracture is considered. Mild angular and rotatory deformities resulting from closed management may produce limitations of motion that are, nevertheless, acceptable.[86]

One standard that is useful in assessing the results of fracture treatment is to compare the range of motion with that needed for most activities of daily living. Morrey and associates have established that 30 degrees to 130 degrees of flexion at the elbow, and 50 degrees of pronation to 50 degrees of supination, are needed for most activities of daily living.[55]

Rotation of the injured forearm is usually compared with that of the opposite normal forearm. Unfortunately, forearm rotation is one of the most difficult clinical measurements to assess accurately and reproducibly because the rotation of the carpus is difficult to exclude. Determining the total arc of forearm rotation rather than of pronation and supination separately is a more accurate method of measuring rotation.[55]

It is generally accepted that there is no remodeling potential for correction of rotational malalignment, although this has not been well studied. Although experimental studies have shown that 10 degrees of rotatory malalignment does not produce any significant clinical impairment, no studies have been able to clinically compare supination and pronation at the time of healing with range of motion after remodeling has occurred.

Periosteum. Children's bones have very thick pluripotential periosteum. In the event of a fracture, the periosteum is usually disrupted on the convex,

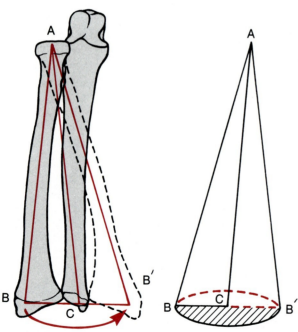

Figure 6–8

The rotation of the radius on the ulna has a mechanical axis from the center of the radial head to the ulnar styloid. (From Ogden, J.A. Radius and ulna. In: Ogden, J.A., ed.: Skeletal Injury in the Child, 2nd ed. Philadelphia, W.B. Saunders, 1990, pp. 451–526.)

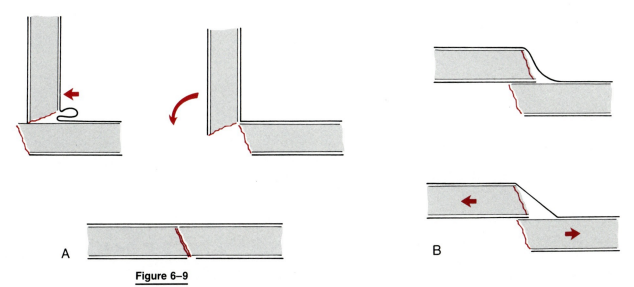

Figure 6–9

The technique of fracture reduction in children by opening of the periosteal hinge.

or tension, side at the fracture site. Thus a "hinge" of intact periosteum is present on the concave, or compression, side.

In a complete fracture with the fragments in bayonet apposition, applying traction to the forearm will tighten the periosteal sleeve, locking the fragments in their relative positions, thus preventing the reduction of the fracture. By increasing the deformity and unlocking the hinge, the fracture can be reduced (Fig. 6–9). Once the fracture is reduced, the intact periosteum can be used to stabilize the reduction by molding the cast appropriately using "three-point fixation" (Fig. 6–10).

Deforming Muscular Forces

The muscular attachments in the forearm are important to consider in the management of forearm fractures. Muscles influence the position of the proximal fragment and create deforming forces that affect the position of both the proximal and the distal fragments within the cast (Fig. 6–11). In the proximal third of the radius, the biceps and the supinator cause flexion and supination of the forearm. The pronator teres inserts into the middle third of the radius and pronates the forearm. In the distal third of the forearm, the brachioradialis, inserting on the lateral surface of the distal radius above the radial styloid process, pulls the forearm into neutral. The pronator quadratus, extensors of the wrist and thumb, the abductors of the thumb, and the flexor muscles of the forearm also contribute to fracture deformity; the magnitude of the deforming force depends on the configuration of the fracture.

It has been traditional to suggest that positioning of the reduced forearm be based on the location of the fracture in relation to the insertion of the pronator teres. Fractures of the proximal third should therefore be aligned in supination; in the middle third, the forearm should be in neutral; and in the distal third, the forearm should be pronated.[9] Evans disputed this idea, stating that fractures at a given location in the forearm do not necessarily present the same degree of rotational deformity. He found that in all cases, including fractures of the upper

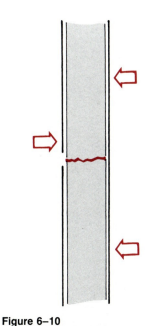

Figure 6–10

The technique of three-point fixation.

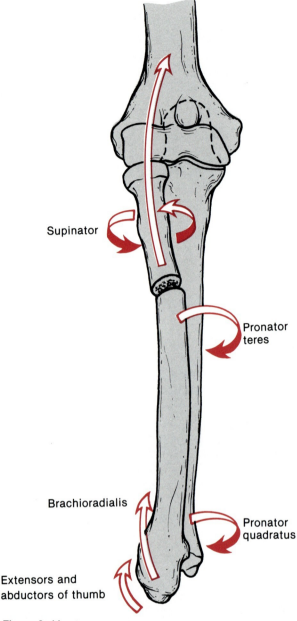

Figure 6–11

Main deforming muscular forces of the forearm. (Redrawn from Cruess, R.L. The management of forearm injuries. Orthop Clin North Am 4:969, 1973.)

and lower thirds, the proximal fragments were supinated. Other factors that may influence the rotational position of the fracture fragments include variations in the direction and leverage of muscle pull at varying degrees of angulation of the fragments, variations in the tension of the biceps tendon with flexion and extension of the elbow, and the effect of the interosseous membrane.[19] Therefore, each fracture must be evaluated on an individual basis to determine the position of the proximal fragments and, consequently, the best position in which to immobilize the forearm.

Mechanism of Injury

The most frequent mechanism of injury in forearm fractures is a fall on the outstretched hand.[46] The child automatically puts out the hand to break the fall, usually with the forearm pronated. On landing, the thenar eminence strikes first, creating a sudden, supinational force on the pronated forearm. The hand becomes fixed on the ground, and above it the momentum of the body continues to supinate the forearm. Although angular deformity is apparent on the radiographs, there is in reality rotational malalignment. Thus, reduction must be obtained by pronating the forearm in addition to correcting the angular deformity.[19]

Pronation and flexion are closely allied. A fracture occurring while the forearm is pronating is likely to develop posterior angulation at the fracture site. Supination and extension are similarly related, and supination fractures will angulate anteriorly (Fig. 6–12). In each case vertical compression supplies the fracturing force, but the rotational element determines the direction of angulation. With rotational forces, the fractures of the two bones are likely to occur at different levels.

Forced pronation injuries include (1) anterior dislocation of the head of the radius, (2) Galeazzi

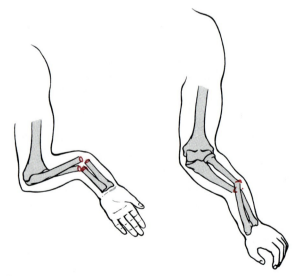

Figure 6–12

Relationship of pronation of posterior angulation and supination to anterior angulation. (From Rang, M. Children's Fractures, 2nd ed. Philadelphia, J.B. Lippincott, 1982, p. 197.)

fracture-dislocation with posterior dislocation of the lower end of the ulna, and (3) anterior Monteggia fracture-dislocation.[19]

Other mechanisms of injury include a direct blow to the forearm and trapping the forearm in between two objects (e.g., between the bars on a crib). The fracture pattern in these cases is more likely to be a true angular deformity, without a rotational component, so that the fractures of the two bones are usually at the same level. Frequently the mechanism of injury in children is not obtainable by history. In most cases, however, it can be deduced by observing the position of the forearm. The fracture is generally reduced by reversing the deformity.

Remodeling Potential

Forearm fractures in children can be managed differently from adult fractures because of continuing growth in both the radius and the ulna after the fracture has healed. As long as the physes are open, remodeling can occur. It is generally accepted that the amount of spontaneous correction is dependent on the age of the child, the amount of residual angulation at the fracture site, the distance between the fracture and the epiphyseal plate, and the relationship of the deformity to the plane of movement in an adjacent joint.[9]

The time between healing of the fracture and epiphyseal plate closure is an important factor in determining the potential for correction of a deformity. Remodeling at the fracture site occurs by resorption of bone on the convex side and apposition of new bone on the concave side. Correction of angulation is brought about by an alteration in the direction and the amount of longitudinal growth that occurs at the epiphyseal plate. The capacity for this correction is influenced by the degree of angulation of the fracture and the distance from the fracture to the epiphyseal plate (Fig. 6–13).[21, 22]

Friberg showed that fracture deformity at the distal end of the radius will correct at the rate of about 0.9 degree a month, or 10 degrees a year, as a result of epiphyseal growth. Volar and ulnar angulations result in a higher rate of correction than do dorsal angulations. This redistribution of growth in the epiphyseal plate induced by an abnormal inclination of the plate may be due to a change in the direction and amplitude of the biomechanical forces acting on the plate. The rate of correction follows an exponential course so that increased correction takes place when there is a greater deformity. Overcorrection by a few degrees has been shown to occur with remodeling.[21]

Unfortunately, although generalizations about the amount of remodeling potential can be made, only crude predictions on the amount of correction in a specific patient with a specific fracture are possible.[23] As discussed previously, it is generally believed that rotational deformities do not remodel.[15, 17] Fuller and McCullough are the only authors to report that in a long-term follow-up of malunited fractures, correction of malrotation did occur in younger children.[24] In the absence of definitive studies concerning the remodeling potential of rotational deformities, it is recommended that rotational malalignment be completely corrected at the time of reduction (Fig. 6–14).

Bayonet apposition is acceptable and will remodel in the child less than 8 to 10 years of age if rotation is correct, if the interosseous space is preserved, and if there is no angulation (Fig. 6–15).[70]

CLASSIFICATION

Fractures of the radius and ulna in children may be classified according to fracture type: (1) plastic deformation (Fig. 6–16); (2) buckle or torus or compression fracture (Fig. 6–17); (3) greenstick or incomplete (Fig. 6–18); and (4) complete.

They can also be classified according to the location of the fracture: Shaft fractures are of the distal one third, midshaft, or proximal one third. Growth plate injuries are to the distal or proximal growth plate. Other special fracture patterns include fracture-dislocations (Monteggia and Galeazzi and their variants) and combination (fractures of the humerus and forearm—"floating elbow").

Since the forearm is a two-bone complex, there is almost always an injury to both bones. A single-bone fracture should raise suspicion of an injury to the proximal or distal joint. The only exception is an injury caused by a direct blow to the forearm. Very commonly, the fracture type (e.g., plastic deformation, greenstick, buckle, or complete) in the radius and the ulna may be different. A frequent combination is a greenstick fracture of the ulna with a complete fracture of the radius (Fig. 6–19).[46]

DIAGNOSIS

The mechanism of injury, the age of the child, and the presence of any associated injuries should be determined first. In very small children the exact mechanism of injury may be unclear. On physical examination, the presence and location of swelling, deformity, and localized tenderness should be noted. The skin should be carefully inspected for

Text continued on page 141

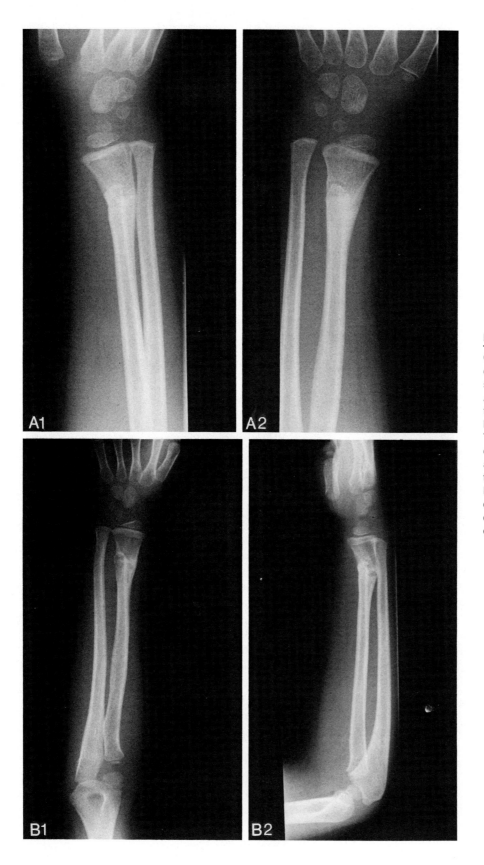

Figure 6–13

Complete fracture of the distal radius in association with a greenstick fracture of the distal ulna. *A,* A 6-year-old boy sustained a fracture of the right distal forearm that healed in bayonet apposition. *B,* Two months later he complained of wrist pain after a minor fall, and a new fracture line was seen at the site of the previous fracture. Note the change in the orientation of the growth plate as well as the cortical remodeling that has occurred.

Figure 6–14

Malunion with a residual rotational deformity after reduction. This 4½-year-old girl was treated for a distal radius and ulna fracture with a closed reduction. There was a recurrence of the deformity several weeks later that required re-reduction. These are her x-rays 6 months following the injury. Note that the proximal forearm appears pronated while the distal forearm appears supinated, indicating that the fracture has healed in a malrotated position. Clinically, she has 40 degrees of excessive supination and 30 degrees less pronation than in the opposite forearm.

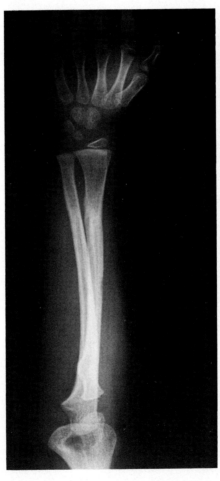
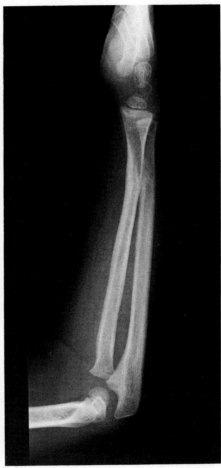

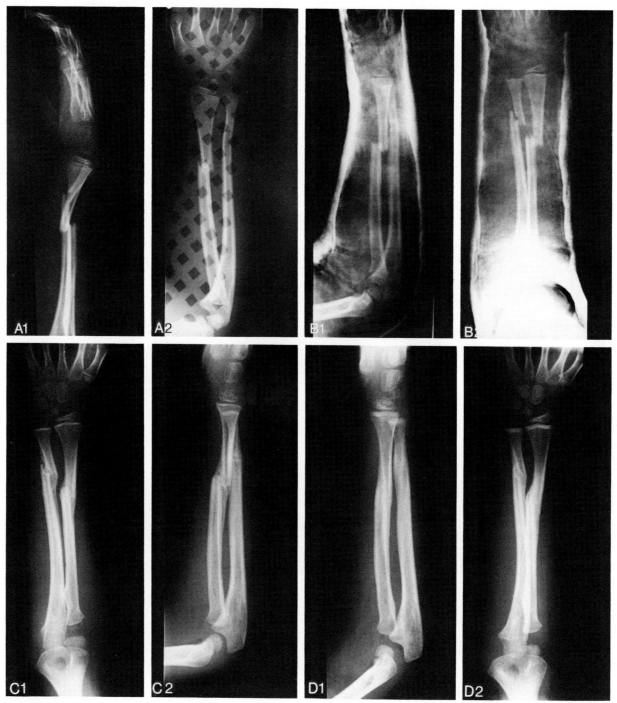

Figure 6–15

Bayonet apposition of the radius and ulna. *A,* A 6-year-old boy fell off a swing and sustained a complete fracture of the shaft of the radius and a greenstick fracture of the distal ulna. Note that the distal fragment is volar to the proximal fragment, which differs from the usual dorsal displacement seen with this injury. This appearance is consistent with continued rotation of the forearm after the fracture occurred. *B,* The radius was manipulated, with the patient under general anesthesia, so that the distal fragment was dorsal to the proximal fragment, and the usual reduction technique was then attempted. The greenstick fracture of the ulna was completed during the manipulation, increasing the instability of the fracture. An end-to-end reduction could not be obtained, and the fracture was casted in bayonet apposition. Note that the fracture ends of the distal and proximal fragments match in width and shape, indicating correct rotatory alignment. *C,* The cast was removed at 6 weeks. *D,* On follow-up 1 month later there was full supination and pronation, as in the normal left forearm.

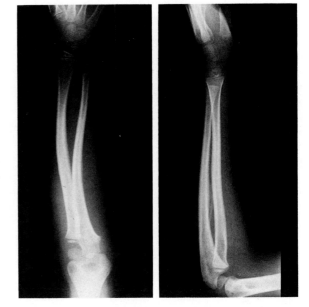

Figure 6–16
Plastic deformation of the radius and ulna in a 6-year-old boy.

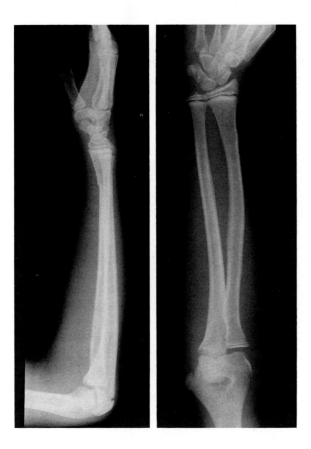

Figure 6–17
Buckle fracture of the distal radial metaphysis in a 12-year-old boy.

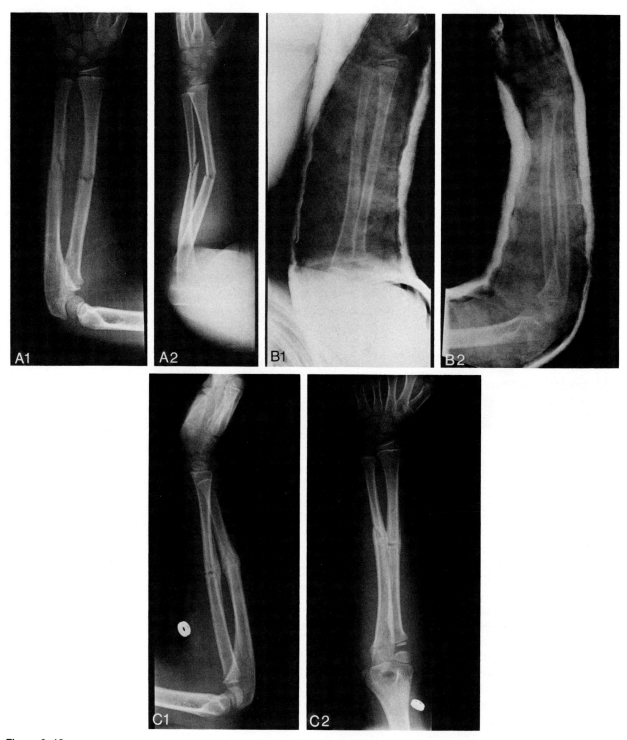

Figure 6–18

Greenstick fractures of the midshaft radius and ulna. *A,* A 6-year-old girl fell off the couch, resulting in greenstick fractures in the midshafts of both bones. *B,* Manipulation with patient under general anesthesia. On follow-up there was no displacement. *C,* One month after cast removal there was normal range of motion.

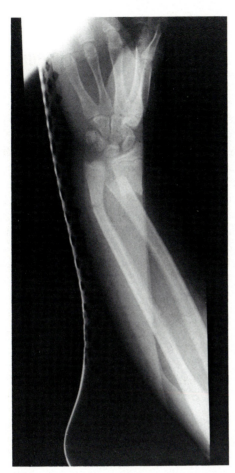

Figure 6–19

Complete fracture of the radius with a greenstick fracture of the ulna.

the presence of open wounds; this means that any splint or bandage must be removed to fully expose the arm. A careful neurologic and vascular examination must be performed. Injury to the anterior interosseous nerve should be differentiated from a median nerve injury; similarly, posterior interosseous nerve injury should be differentiated from a radial nerve injury. One of the subtle signs of neurologic injury is the absence of sweating, indicating sympathetic nerve disruption.

All fractured limbs should be examined for the presence of a compartment syndrome. Despite the high incidence of forearm fractures in children, compartment syndrome is rare; nevertheless, a high index of suspicion must be maintained. It is essential to examine the joints proximal and distal to the fracture clinically as well as radiographically to avoid missing associated dislocations or fractures. Roentgenographic studies should include adequate anteroposterior and lateral x-rays of the forearm as well as both views of the wrist and elbow. They should be taken by changing the position of the x-ray tube rather than by rotating the forearm. The latter technique frequently changes the position through the fracture site.

MANAGEMENT

When the child arrives in the emergency department, the extremity should be splinted for both pain relief and prevention of further injury once a thorough clinical examination has been performed. The splint should be in place when the x-rays are taken to prevent the radiology technician from inadvertently injuring the extremity further by moving the limb instead of the x-ray tube.

Most displaced fractures of the forearm in children can be treated with closed reduction and maintenance in a well-molded long arm cast. In some centers, a "sugar-tongs" type of immobilization is used. If there is concern about subsequent excessive swelling inside the cast, the cast can be split immediately to accommodate the soft tissue swelling while still controlling the fracture position. The extent and type of deformity and the age of the child are factors used to determine whether the reduction can be accomplished with sedation, local anesthesia, or general anesthesia. X-ray equipment or an image intensifier should be available to check the alignment of the fracture after the reduction is performed.

Undisplaced Fractures

Undisplaced fractures may be treated in a cast or splint, mainly for comfort, until the fracture site is no longer painful.

Plastic Deformation

Pediatric bone is able to absorb more energy prior to fracture than adult bone, primarily because it has a greater capacity to undergo plastic deformation. A material is said to have exceeded its elastic limit and undergone plastic deformation when it deforms under a load but does not recover its original length when the load is released. Plastic bowing results from changes occurring within the bone at a microscopic level caused by a combination of compressive and tensile forces (Fig. 6–20).[50]

Plastic deformation of the forearm occurs in children between the ages of 2 and 15 years. Bowing of the radius and ulna can encroach upon the interosseous space and cause limitation of pronation and

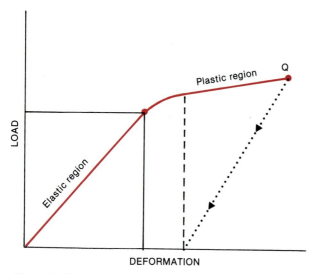

Figure 6–20

Load-deformation curve. If a load is applied in the elastic region and is then released, no permanent deformation will occur. If loading is continued past the yield point (Y) and the load is released, plastic deformation will result. If loading continues, ultimate failure of the bone occurs at the failure point (Q). (From Frankel, V.H.; Nordin, M. Basic Biomechanics of the Skeletal System. Philadelphia, Lea & Febiger, 1980, pp. 15–16.)

supination of the forearm. In children younger than 4 years, deformities of less than 20 degrees usually remodel. Mabrey and Fitch have stated that any plastic deformity that prevents the reduction of a concomitant fracture or dislocation, that prevents full rotation in children over the age of 4 years, or that exceeds 20 degrees should be corrected.[50]

This condition may be difficult to correct. Manipulation should always be done with use of general anesthesia because forces as great as 20 to 30 kg are usually necessary to correct the deformity.[50] The technique consists of placing the apex of the deformity over a wedge and applying a constant force at points proximal and distal to the apex of the bow over 2 to 3 minutes. Both rotational and angular components of the deformity must be corrected sequentially. Recurrence of the deformity is very common, but its incidence can be reduced through the use of a well-fitting and carefully molded long arm cast. An average correction of 13 degrees or 85% of the pre-reduction deformity can be expected.[50]

It is common for one bone to undergo plastic deformation while the other bone fractures. During reduction it is just as important to correct the plastic deformity as it is to reduce the fracture. Insufficient reduction may contribute to recurrent deformity or subsequent disruption of the distal radioulnar articulation. Unrecognized disruption of the distal radioulnar joint may result in long-term pain and disability.

Greenstick Fractures

Greenstick fractures can usually be managed with closed reduction. It has been traditionally thought that completing a greenstick fracture decreases the risk for recurrence of the deformity.[9] Since the deformity can also recur in complete fractures, and sometimes after completing the greenstick fracture, the difficulty of reduction can be magnified by increasing the displacement and instability of the fracture. Some authors have recommended reversing the deformity and maintaining the arm in a well-molded cast without fracture of the intact cortex. However, Ogden recommends that careful cracking of the intact cortex be routinely performed for these fractures.[64]

Complete Displacement

Complete fractures of the radius and ulna can be very challenging to manage. The potential for malunion in the forearm is significant, owing primarily to difficulties in obtaining and maintaining the reduction of two parallel bones that are subjected to angulatory and rotatory forces from muscular attachments. If the normal bow in a single bone is altered, its length relative to the other bone may decrease, causing disruption to either the proximal or the distal radioulnar joint. A change in bow angulation of greater than 10 degrees and shortening of greater than 3 to 4 mm at the distal radioulnar joint necessitate remanipulation and correction of position.[15]

Fractures in patients over 10 years of age, who have limited capacity for remodeling, and fractures in the proximal third of the forearm can be difficult to manage with closed manipulation and casting. Proximal fractures are challenging because the reduction is often difficult to maintain, resulting in frequent redisplacement. These injuries, therefore, have a disproportionate share of problems on long-term follow-up.[15] Knight and Purvis stated over 40 years ago that in order to obtain a satisfactory reduction it is necessary to regain length and achieve apposition, axial alignment, and normal rotation of the fracture fragments.[39]

Technique of Closed Reduction

Most completely displaced fractures of the forearm are best reduced with adequate muscle relaxation,

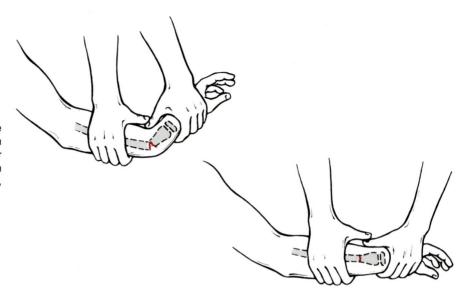

Figure 6–21

Technique of reduction of a complete fracture of the forearm. (Adapted from Levinthal, D.H. Fractures in the lower one-third of both bones of the forearm in children. Surg Gynecol Obstet 790, 1933.)

using heavy sedation, and regional or general anesthesia. An image intensifier should be available to check the alignment of the fracture during the reduction of the deformity.

The fracture deformity must first be increased to disengage the fracture fragments and to open the periosteal hinge. It is often necessary to increase the deformity to greater than 90 degrees to allow sufficient distraction of the fracture for reduction to be accomplished. The radius and ulna are each reduced separately. With the operator applying traction in line with the angulated distal segment, the distal fragment is pushed with the operator's thumb onto the end of the proximal fragment. At the same time the pronation or supination deformity is corrected. Once the reduction has been achieved, maintaining the pressure on the side of the intact periosteum will stabilize the reduction (Fig. 6–21).

The position of immobilization is determined by the position of the proximal fragment. The fracture should be immobilized in any position in which the alignment is correct and the reduction feels stable.[70] The reduction should be maintained in a well-molded circular cast with three-point fixation. The cast should be lightly and evenly padded (Fig. 6–22). The forearm portion should be oval with a straight ulnar border. Three-point molding is applied by pushing with the palm of one hand distal to the fracture site on the side of the intact periosteum, with the other hand proximal to the fracture site on the opposite side, and a third point more proximal on the arm on the same side as that of the operator's distal hand (Fig. 6–23). The elbow is immobilized at a right angle. The back of the arm portion should be flat to prevent the elbow from slipping inside the cast. A loop should be placed proximal to the site of the fracture to prevent "sagging" of the fracture fragments when the cast becomes loose from atrophy of the muscles in the proximal half of the forearm (Fig. 6–24).[39, 70]

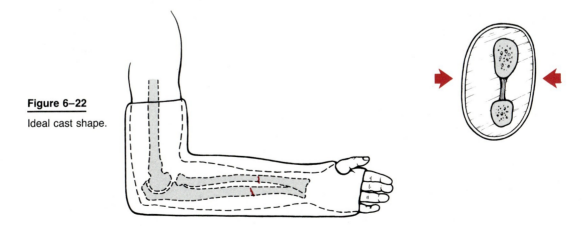

Figure 6–22

Ideal cast shape.

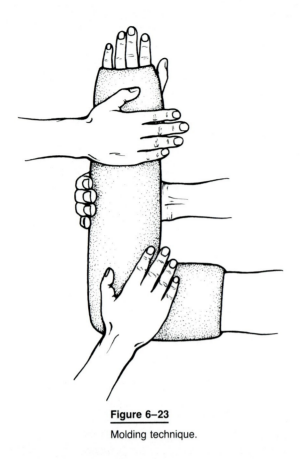

Figure 6–23

Molding technique.

Most displaced fractures of the forearm are best maintained in a long arm cast to immobilize the elbow and to neutralize the deforming forces of muscles that originate above the elbow. The above-elbow segment is usually applied after the forearm portion has been completed. To prevent the distal segment of the cast from digging into the forearm at the elbow, it is important to apply the padding in a continuous manner before either segment is applied. For this reason, some authors recommend that the above-elbow portion be applied first.

The fracture is followed carefully with weekly x-rays for the first 3 weeks following reduction. This usually allows redisplacement to be detected before consolidation of the fracture occurs. Redisplacement occurs in 7 to 13% of cases, most of the time within 2 weeks of the injury. As previously mentioned, greenstick fractures have a greater potential for redisplacement. There does not appear to be any correlation between the age of the patient or severity of initial displacement and the timing or severity of redisplacement.[92]

Recurrent deformity is frequently managed by applying a new, well-molded cast. In some instances in which the deformity is too great to allow for correction by cast molding, the fracture must be remanipulated and recasted. In patients less than 2 years of age, repeat manipulation is best performed within 1 week of the fracture because of the rapidity of fracture healing. In patients between 2 and 5 years of age, minor improvements can be made up to 2 weeks following the fracture. Generally, "good reductions last better than poor reductions, particularly in a well-molded cast."[70]

COMPLICATIONS

The potential complications of forearm injuries in children include malunion, refracture, nonunion, nerve and arterial injuries, compartment syndrome,

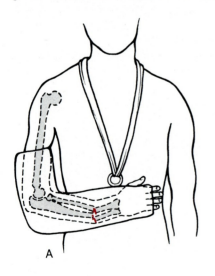
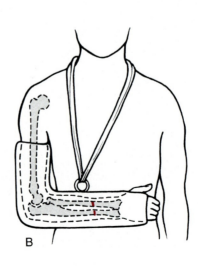

Figure 6–24

A, A loop placed distal to the fracture site will support the cast at the hand and not the elbow, allowing the cast to angle on the forearm and allowing the fracture to sag. *B*, A loop placed proximal to the fracture site will create support for the cast so that there is no deforming force at the fracture. (From Rang, M. Children's Fractures, 2nd ed. Philadelphia, J.B. Lippincott, 1982, p. 207.)

infection, and reflex sympathetic dystrophy. As each of the fractures is discussed the specific complications associated with that fracture will be presented in more detail. The following is a general discussion of complications that may be common to all.

Malunion

It is common for deformity to recur in any forearm fracture managed with closed manipulation. However, with careful follow-up, malunion is a potentially avoidable complication. Common causes of malunion are inadequate follow-up, improper positioning of the forearm in supination or pronation, failure to perform cast changes when appropriate, failure to correct an inadequate reduction, and delay in diagnosis until after the fracture is united.[26, 70]

In studies of malunited fractures, the only patients who complain of any disability are those in whom there is a severe restriction in forearm rotation.[17, 24, 60] Daruwalla found that loss of pronation was more common than loss of supination after forearm fractures in children.[17] In contrast, Knight and Purvis, in a study of adult fractures, found that supination was more frequently limited.[39] These authors agreed, however, that the main causes of limitation were residual angulatory deformity (especially if it resulted in narrowing of the interosseous space), residual posterior angulation of the ulnar fracture, residual rotational malalignment of the fracture fragments, and derangement of the inferior radioulnar joint due to relative shortening of the radius.[17, 39] It is interesting to note that inferior radioulnar instability is found infrequently in spite of the fact that slight radial shortening is common.[39]

If a fracture has achieved early consolidation in an unsatisfactory position but is not yet solid, manual osteoclasis can be attempted (Fig. 6–25). With the child under general anesthesia, the fracture is manipulated using steady pressure at the fracture site. A wooden block in the shape of a wedge is used as a fulcrum and is placed at the apex of the deformity. Once the fracture deformity is corrected, a long arm cast is applied with the forearm in the appropriate degree of rotation. The fracture is maintained in the cast for 4 to 6 weeks until the fracture is solid. In distal fractures, the cast can usually be changed at 4 weeks to a short arm cast that is worn for the final 2 weeks.

If the fracture callus is mature, drill osteoclasis is a good method for correcting angular deformities. An incision is made over the apex of the deformity sufficiently large to introduce a drill guide to protect the soft tissues and to retract superficial cutaneous nerves and vessels. Several holes are made in the bone with a drill, guided by the image intensifier. A second incision is made over the apex of the other bony deformity, and the procedure is repeated. The bones are then manipulated to correct the deformity. A long arm cast is applied for 6 weeks until the fracture is solidly united. Unlike angular deformity, rotational malalignment cannot be corrected with manual or percutaneous drill osteoclasis, and open techniques are necessary.

After the fracture is solidly united, a cosmetically poor result or malunion that restricts more than 50% of normal forearm rotation and causes functional impairment can be treated by osteotomy (Fig. 6–26). Because of the variability between children in range of forearm rotation, it is important to measure rotation by comparing the fractured forearm with the opposite, normal forearm.[75] It is worthwhile, especially in younger children, to wait for 1 to 2 years after the fracture has healed to allow for maximum remodeling to occur. Comparable x-rays of the opposite forearm are obtained for preoperative planning of the osteotomy. Two-dimensional angular deformity noted on radiographs is usually a combination of rotational and angular malposition.[15] Angular corrections are easier to plan and perform than is rotational correction. Trial reductions with intraoperative x-rays help guide restoration of the normal anatomic contour. By placing the forearm through a range of motion prior to permanently fixing the plate, one can assess the amount of motion that has been regained. The osteotomy is secured using standard compression plating techniques. For those late results with distal radioulnar disruption, pain, and loss of rotation, the Darrach procedure seems to give an excellent outcome, in terms of both restoring motion and abolishing pain.[15]

Refracture

Recurrent fractures occur in up to 12% of cases.[26, 42] Refracture probably takes place either because of failure of the original fracture to unite solidly or because of a similar mechanism of injury (Fig. 6–27). Osteoporosis secondary to immobilization can contribute to the risk of refracture. Unfortunately, little can be done to completely avoid this complication apart from recommending that the child refrain from participating in active sports for 1 month following the removal of the cast. Refracture can occur as late as 1 year following the initial injury, but it is not reasonable to protect every child for this length of time. Warning the family of the possibility of refracture can help relieve anxiety should this complication occur.

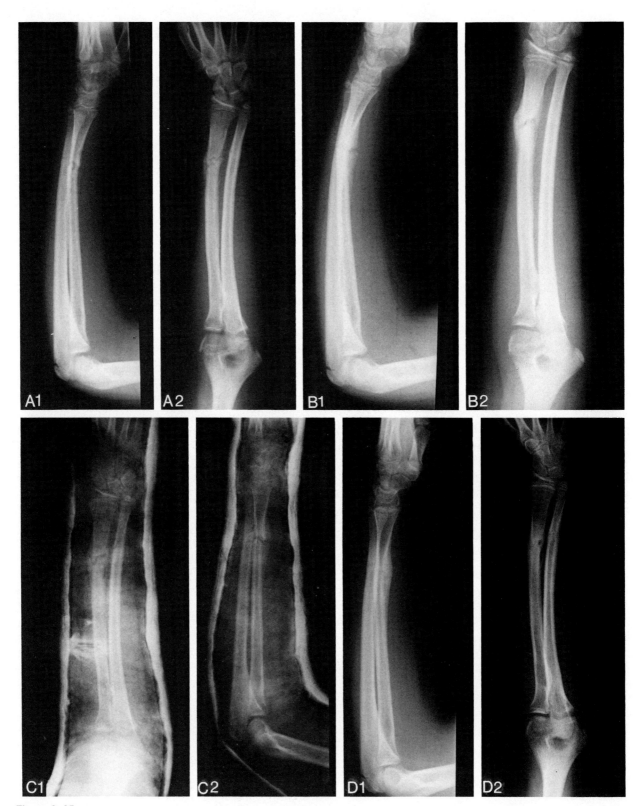

Figure 6–25

Closed osteoclasis. An 11-year-old girl had an open, completely displaced fracture of the distal radius and ulna that was initially treated with debridement and open reduction without internal fixation. *A,* The cast was removed prematurely, 3 weeks after the injury. *B,* At 7 weeks she developed an unacceptable deformity at the fracture site. *C,* A manual osteoclasis was performed with the patient under general anesthesia. The cast was removed 6 weeks later. *D,* On follow-up, the patient had a normal range of motion. There was no clinical evidence of infection. The radiolucency at the fracture site seen on this x-ray resolved on further follow-up.

Figure 6–26

Malunion treated by osteotomy of the radius. *A,* A 14-year-old boy had a malunited fracture in the proximal third of both bones of the forearm after conservative treatment. The arm lacked 45 degrees of pronation, preventing normal function. *B,* An osteotomy with plating of the radius was performed. *C,* Almost full motion was present 4 months postoperatively. The plate was removed 1 year after the osteotomy.

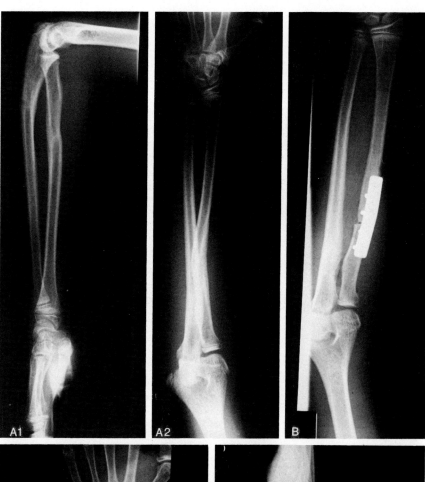
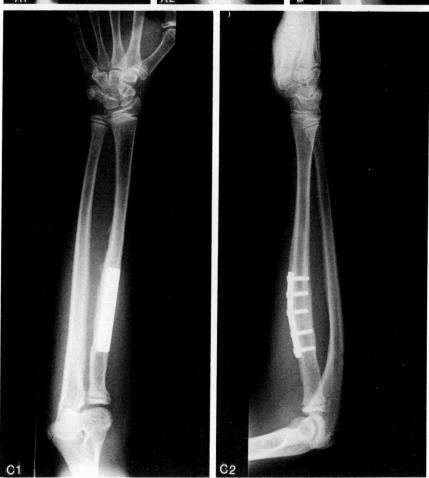

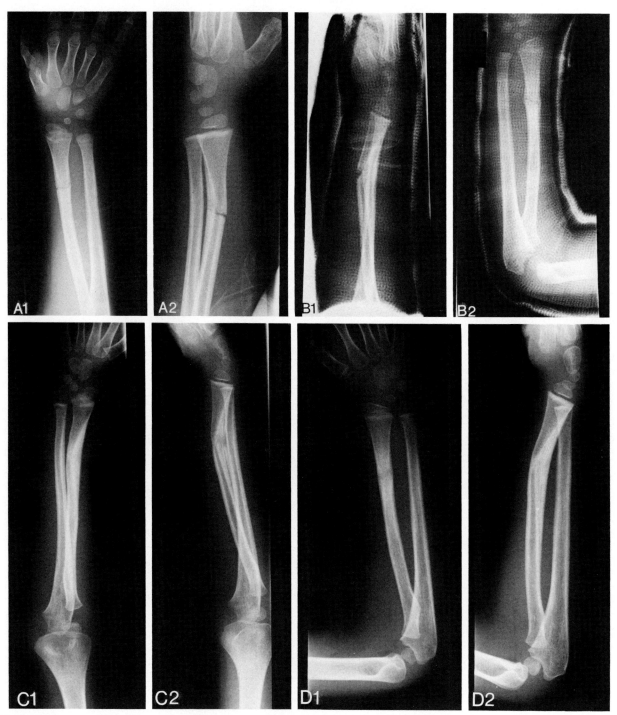

Figure 6–27

Remodeling after fracture. *A*, A 5-year-old boy refractured the radius 10 weeks after a previous fracture. *B*, The deformity was not reduced but was allowed to heal in the displaced position. *C*, Early remodeling with apposition of new bone along the deformity is seen. *D*, Subsequent x-rays show increased new bone in the metaphysis adjacent to the growth with early reorientation of the growth plate.

Nonunion

Nonunions in children are rare. They are more likely to occur as a result of high-energy trauma, after an open fracture, or in fractures associated with significant soft tissue loss or infection. Open reduction and internal fixation may contribute to nonunion, particularly when the fixation is inadequate or when it distracts the fracture fragments.[9, 47] One of the two bones usually unites.[47] The ulna is more prone to nonunion than the radius. Delayed union is more common than nonunion. With time and patience, most fractures will heal.

Nerve and Vessel Injuries

In closed forearm fractures, nerves and vessels are injured relatively infrequently. This is probably because the intervening layer of muscles surrounding the radius and ulna protects the nerves and vessels from injury.[70] However, injury to the anterior interosseous nerve secondary to a fracture of the radius has been reported[25, 95] as has entrapment of the median nerve within a greenstick fracture.[98] Injury to the posterior interosseous nerve may occur in Monteggia fractures, especially those with lateral dislocation of the radial head. Fractures of the distal forearm that are completely displaced may be associated with compression of the median nerve at the wrist.

Compartment Syndrome

Compartment syndrome is uncommon following fracture of the forearm. Although it is more likely to develop after crush injuries of the forearm or with an associated supracondylar fracture of the humerus, it can also occur after a simple fracture. Careful examination with monitoring while maintaining a high degree of suspicion is important to ensure that early treatment is initiated. This is essential for avoiding a potentially crippling result. Loss of reduction is insignificant when compared with the sequelae of an overlooked compartment syndrome.

The cardinal symptom of a compartment syndrome is pain that is frequently but not always out of proportion to the injury. It is usually aggravated by passive stretch of the muscles in the involved compartment. The pain is usually not relieved by splinting and tends to become progressively more severe. Other symptoms include numbness and tingling. Inability of the child to actively move the fingers and severe pain with gentle passive extension of the fingers are classic features of an impending problem. The earliest physical finding is tenseness of the affected compartment. It is important to be aware that, in the younger child with abundant subcutaneous fat, a tense compartment can be difficult to feel. Casts or splints must be removed for thorough examination. The hand is often held stiffly, with the fingers relatively extended at the metacarpophalangeal joints and the fingers flexed at the interphalangeal joints. The child is reluctant to move the hand. Loss of the radial pulse and pallor of the extremity occur late in the course of events and are generally not useful signs.

The first step in management of a suspected compartment syndrome is to remove constricting bandages and to widely split circular casts, including all the padding material under the cast. If the cast or bandage is the cause of the problem, there should be immediate relief of pain. If the diagnosis cannot be made clinically; if the child is very young, uncooperative, or unconscious; or if there is an associated nerve injury that confounds the diagnosis, compartment pressure measurements should be performed. The techniques of compartment pressure measurement are well described (Fig. 6–28).[95] If the compartment pressure is greater than 40 mm Hg, or 30 cm water, fasciotomy is indicated.[85] Fasciotomies of the forearm are performed with the patient under general anesthesia and require opening of skin, fascia, and epimysium. Generally two approaches are necessary, using dorsal and volar incisions (Fig. 6–29).

Technique of Forearm Decompression. The volar forearm decompression is performed using a curvilinear volar incision beginning 1 cm proximal and 2 cm lateral to the medial epicondyle proximal to the antecubital fossa. The incision is carried obliquely across the antecubital fossa and over the volar aspect of the mobile term. It is continued distally to the proximal wrist crease, just ulnar to the palmaris longus tendon, obliquely across the crease, and along the thenar crease to the midpalm at a level even with the base of the thumb-index web. The fascia is incised in line with the skin incision. The lacertus fibrosus of the biceps tendon is divided proximally. The carpal tunnel is released under direct vision to avoid injuring the palmar cutaneous branch of the median nerve. Other areas of possible nerve compression are the proximal edge of the pronator teres and the proximal edge of the flexor digitorum superficialis. The deep flexor musculature should be adequately inspected and decompressed, since it is frequently more severely involved. The dorsal compartment pressure is then remeasured. If

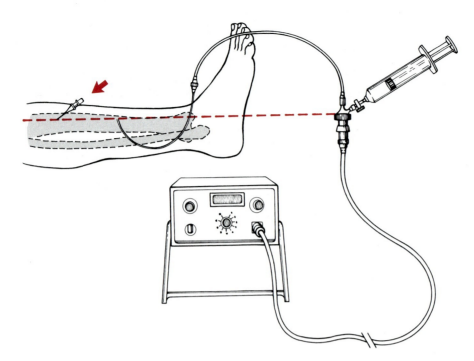

Figure 6–28

Slit catheter method of measuring compartment pressures.

this is still too high, the dorsal compartment must also be decompressed. The incision begins 2 cm lateral and 2 cm distal to the lateral epicondyle. It is extended straight distally toward the midline of the wrist. The dorsal fascia is incised in line with the skin incision.

In both instances, if the muscle appears necrotic, conservative debridement can be performed. If there is any doubt about muscle viability, it should be left and inspected again at a subsequent dressing change. The fascia and skin are left open, and a dressing is applied. Internal or external fixation techniques are often useful to stabilize the fracture for easier management of the soft tissue injury. Secondary closure or skin grafting is performed 7 to 10 days later.[85]

Infection

Infection is a potential complication of open fractures and open reduction of closed fractures of the forearm. The management of an open fracture should include (1) swabbing the open wound for culture and sensitivity studies; (2) covering the wound with a sterile dressing; (3) ensuring that tetanus immunization is up to date; (4) administering intravenous broad-spectrum antibiotics that cover penicillin-resistant *Staphylococcus aureus;* and (5) adequately debriding and irrigating the fracture wound within 8 hours of injury.

If the wound is grossly contaminated, an aminoglycoside and penicillin should be added to the antibiotic regimen. The duration of antibiotic coverage after debridement is controversial, but 2 to 3 days of coverage is generally adequate for most wounds that do not become grossly infected. Treatment of an infected fracture should include debridement of the fracture site and treatment with antibiotics effective against the organism that has been cultured. Internal fixation should not be removed until the fracture has united. Infection can occur after a closed fracture, but this is unusual.[12]

Reflex Sympathetic Dystrophy

Reflex sympathetic dystrophy is very uncommon in children. The syndrome consists of continuous burning or aching pain in the involved extremity, hyperesthesia, excessive sweating, purple or reddish discoloration, swelling, and joint stiffness. Radiographically, patchy osteopenia may be evident 6 to 8 weeks later.

The pathophysiology of this syndrome is not well understood. It is hypothesized that there is chronic and excessive activity in the autonomic nervous system, causing increased local blood flow to the affected limb. They may also be chronic irritation of a peripheral sensory nerve that leads to excessive autonomic nervous activity. The personalities of the child and his or her family are probably important

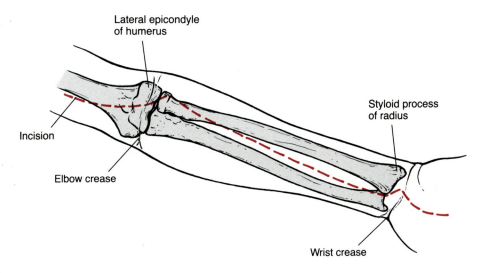

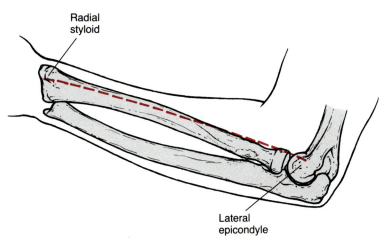

Figure 6–29

Incisions for forearm fasciotomy.

factors in determining the risk or likelihood of developing this complication.

Management of this condition usually consists of aggressive physical therapy with emotional and psychologic counseling. Transcutaneous nerve stimulation has also been used with good results.[62] Pharmacologic therapy with corticosteroids or narcotics is not usually necessary and should be avoided. The condition usually resolves with time, generally within 6 to 12 months after injury.[62]

Overgrowth

A broken bone will usually grow faster for the first 6 to 8 months after the fracture is healed. In the forearm, overgrowth of one or both bones is likely to average about 6 to 7 mm and is therefore insignificant.[2, 9, 59] Significant relative overgrowth of one bone may occur only after the other bone has sustained a physeal injury resulting in premature closure. Permanent growth plate injuries of both the radius and the ulna have been reported.[58, 69, 90]

MANAGEMENT OF SPECIFIC INJURIES

Growth Plate Injuries to the Distal Radius and Ulna

Fractures of the distal radial growth plate are the most common physeal plate injuries, accounting for 46% of all fractures of the physis. Of these, 75% occur in children between 10 and 16 years of age. Injuries to the distal radial growth plate are uncommon in children under age 5 years.[77, 99]

The Salter-Harris type II fracture is the most frequent type of physeal injury, accounting for 58% of fractures of the distal radial epiphysis. The next most common are type I fractures of the distal radius, which occur in 22% of cases. Types III, IV, and V fractures are rare, accounting for only 5% of cases.[43, 44]

Classification

Classification of growth plate injuries is presented in Chapter 1. The Salter-Harris classification will be used in this discussion (Fig. 6–30).[63, 77]

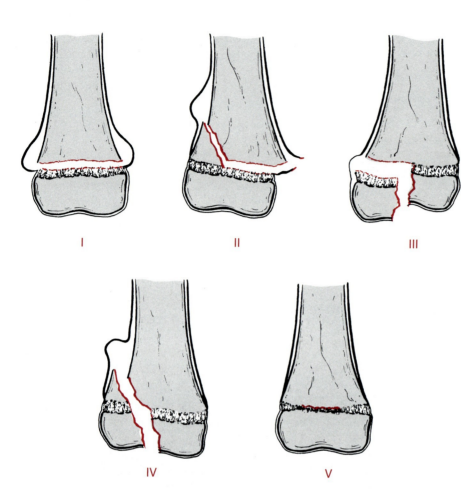

Figure 6–30

The Salter-Harris classification of growth plate injuries. (From Salter, R.B., Harris, W.R. Injuries involving the epiphyseal plate. J Bone Joint Surg 45-A:587, 1963.)

Fifty-five percent of distal radial epiphyseal injuries have an associated fracture of the distal ulna, usually a fracture of the ulnar styloid. A greenstick or complete fracture of the distal ulna or plastic deformation of the distal ulna may also occur.[43]

Mechanism of Injury

As with most forearm fractures, the usual mechanism of injury is a fall on the outstretched hand. The epiphyseal plate is weaker than the fibrous joint capsule, tendons, and ligaments in children.[77] Shearing or avulsion forces are capable of separating an epiphysis.

Diagnosis

As for all fractures of the forearm, clinical examination should include looking for evidence of deformity, localization of tenderness and swelling, determination of the neurological and vascular status of the forearm, and inspection of the skin. Finally, the examiner should check specifically for signs and symptoms suggestive of a compartment syndrome as these can occur despite the distal nature of the injury.

Type I injuries occur in younger children, are seldom very displaced, and are diagnosed on clinical suspicion.[24, 70, 77] In these fractures there is swelling and tenderness at the growth plate despite normal radiographs. The correct diagnosis is made on clinical grounds and can be confirmed by the presence of periosteal new bone on radiographs taken after the fracture is healed.

Management of Undisplaced Fractures

Undisplaced fractures are protected in a short arm cast for 2 weeks in children younger than age 2 years, and for 3 weeks in older children.

Management of Displaced Fractures

Salter-Harris Types I and II. These fractures are usually displaced dorsally. The principles of reduction are similar to those for other completely displaced fractures of the forearm. The reduction is performed gently so as to avoid further injury to the physis.[43] The intact hinge of periosteum on the dorsal aspect of the radius will usually prevent overcorrection with manipulation.[77] A long arm cast or a "sugar-tongs" splint with three-point molding is applied with the forearm pronated. Because the fracture occurs through the growth plate, healing is rapid,[77] and 3 weeks of immobilization is all that is usually necessary.

Some displaced Salter type II fractures may be difficult to reduce anatomically. Therefore, if 50% end-to-end apposition of the fracture fragments is achieved and angular and rotational malalignment has been corrected, repeated manipulation is not necessary (Fig. 6–31). This is especially true in children with epiphyseal remodeling potential of more than 2 years. Even with an incomplete reduction, remodeling proceeds with minimal risk of growth arrest.[43, 44] The best time to reduce an epiphyseal plate injury is the day of the injury. After 10 days, type I and type II injuries are difficult to shift without excessive force. It is wiser to accept an imperfect reduction than to risk damage to the growth plate due to either forceful manipulation or surgery.[77] In a study of fractures of the distal radial epiphysis in children, premature growth arrest was noted in 27% of patients who underwent two or more attempts at closed reduction under general anesthesia. In contrast, none of the patients who had had a single manipulation exhibited growth arrest. The remaining four patients who had a significant growth disturbance had experienced a compression type of injury that probably represented a Salter-Harris type V injury to the growth plate.[43]

Salter-Harris type II fractures have been encountered that were irreducible owing to an invaginated periosteal flap on the tension side of the fracture[44] or to displacement of the volar tendons, median nerve, and radial artery and veins.[51] These fractures require open reduction and, in some cases, internal fixation with smooth Kirschner wires (K-wires).

Abnormal growth of the distal radius is rare and occurs mainly after epiphyseal compression injuries or repeated forceful attempts at reduction.[43] Subsequent physeal growth is infrequently disturbed after fracture because the germinal layers of the physis remain attached to the epiphysis, and the epiphyseal circulation is usually intact.[77] Even if the metaphyseal circulation is interrupted, the circulation is reestablished within 4 weeks; vascular invasion of the hypertrophic zone of the physis is resumed, allowing ossification of the zone of provisional calcification.[44] Invaginated periosteum between the hypertrophied and provisionally calcified zones is likely to undergo fibrous degeneration and resorption. Subsequent remodeling of metaphyseal bone then allows for correction of the deformity.[44] The length of time after injury during which the physis remains open will limit the amount of growth and remodeling that can occur after a physeal fracture and must be taken into account when deciding how much deformity is acceptable.[21, 22]

A rare injury is a type II fracture that is displaced anteriorly. The most common mechanism of injury appears to be a fall on the palmar surface of the hand associated with high energy, or forced flexion of the wrist. The anterior part of the articular surface of the radius is thus submitted to axial compression while there is traction on the posterior part. These fractures are easily reduced by closed manipulation but are very unstable and tend to redisplace. Seriat-Gautier and Jouve recommend open reduction and fixation using a volar buttress plate that is attached to the metaphysis by screws, but without screws in the epiphysis; this maintains anatomic reduction and avoids injury to the growth plate.[79]

Salter-Harris Type III. In the child, type III fractures on the volar aspect of the distal radius are analogous to the Barton type of fracture in the adult. These must be anatomically reduced to restore articular congruity and to decrease the likelihood for growth arrest. As with a Barton fracture, open reduction may be necessary to achieve the desired position. Internal fixation using pins or screws parallel to the physis is desirable, but if the fragment is too small, a smooth transphyseal pin may be inserted to stabilize it. This should be removed approximately 3 weeks after injury, once the fragment is stable.

Salter-Harris Type IV. Type IV fractures of the distal radius are quite rare. Anatomic reduction must be achieved, and open reduction is usually required if there is displacement (Fig. 6–32). If anatomic reduction is not achieved, growth disturbance secondary to formation of a bony bridge is likely.[77]

Salter-Harris Type V. Type V fractures are frequently diagnosed retrospectively after a growth arrest has occurred. As no fracture or displacement is usually evident, the injured forearm is splinted or casted for pain relief for 3 weeks.

Follow-up

Deformity is likely to recur, and for this reason careful follow-up is important. Up to 10% of fractures redisplace during the healing phase.[43] Weekly follow-up with adequate anteroposterior and lateral x-rays is recommended until new periosteal bone is seen.

In Salter-Harris types I and II epiphyseal plate injuries, angulation of up to 30 degrees is acceptable in children less that 10 years of age. In children older than 10 years, up to 15 degrees of angulation is acceptable. However, injuries with angular de-

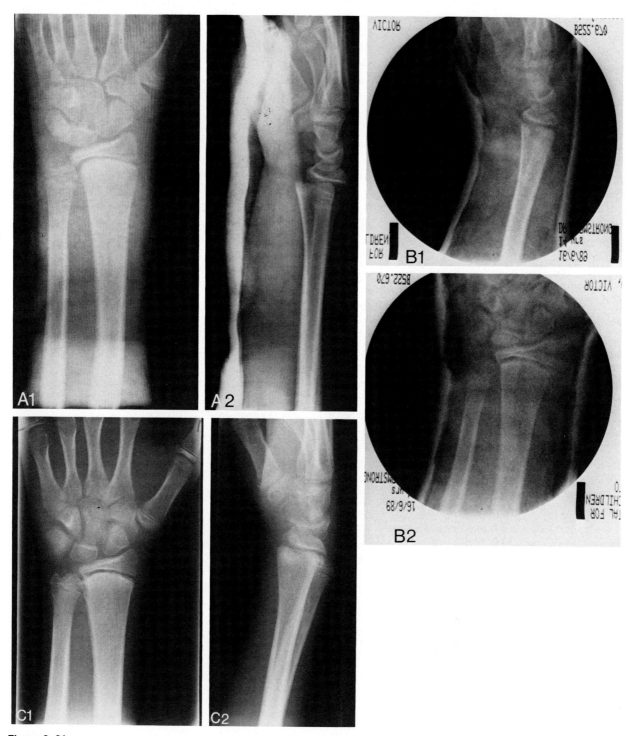

Figure 6–31

Salter-Harris type II fracture of the distal radius and plastic deformation of the distal ulna. *A,* A 14-year-old boy fell while jumping. His initial x-rays appeared to show a type I injury to the distal radial growth plate. Note the plastic deformation of the distal ulna. *B,* The fracture was reduced with the patient under general anesthesia. *C,* Follow-up x-rays show a small metaphyseal fragment, indicating that the injury was, in fact, a type II injury. The residual displacement did not need remanipulation since complete remodeling is expected.

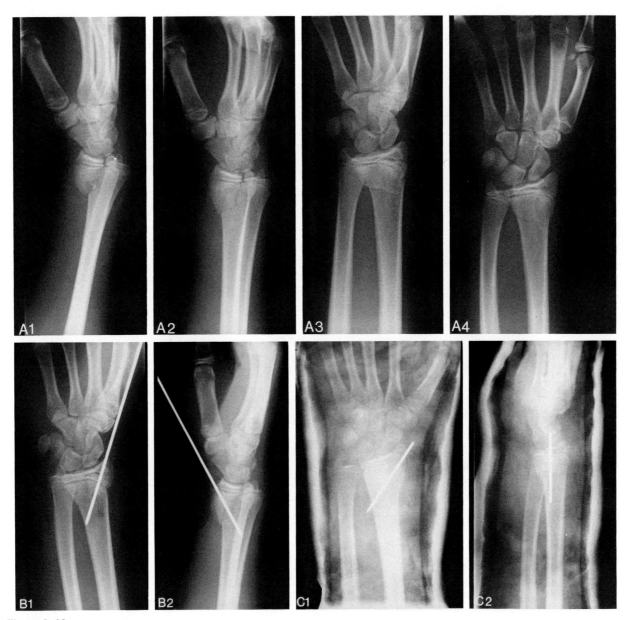

Figure 6–32

Salter-Harris type IV fracture of the distal radius. *A,* A 12-year-old girl fell on her arm while playing soccer, sustaining a type IV fracture of the distal radius. *B,* Closed reduction with the patient under general anesthesia failed, and open reduction and fixation with a smooth K-wire were performed. *C,* The arm was immobilized in a short arm cast. The fracture healed without subsequent displacement.

Illustration continued on following page

formity of up to 30 degrees will heal satisfactorily provided that the time to epiphyseal closure is greater than 2 years.[43]

Complications

The complications of forearm fractures have been discussed earlier. Growth disturbance is an additional complication of epiphyseal plate injury

Malunion. Unacceptable angular deformity may require corrective osteotomy. Malunion of Salter type III injuries can result in posttraumatic arthritis. Once union has occurred these are very difficult to correct. Reconstruction using osteotomy is indicated if there is gross deformity prior to the onset of symptoms. Malunion of Salter type IV injuries can result in growth disturbances secondary to formation of a bony bridge as well as in posttraumatic arthritis if there is significant joint incongruity.

Growth Disturbance. Significant growth disturbances occur in 7% of epiphyseal plate injuries and

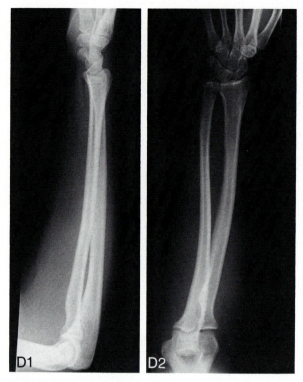

Figure 6–32 Continued
D, Follow-up radiograph at 2 years did not demonstrate any growth abnormality.

can result in progressive angulation or progressive shortening.[43] Premature closure of the growth plate is more common following epiphyseal compression injuries or repeated forceful attempts at reduction. The growth plate injury may be discovered only when deformity begins to appear. Children who have sustained an injury to the growth plate should be followed for a minimum of 1 year following the injury.[77] Prompt diagnosis can sometimes allow appropriate surgical intervention before a severe deformity develops.

After an epiphyseal plate injury, the severity of the clinical problem depends on the site of growth disturbance, the extent of involvement of the epiphyseal plate, and the expected amount of growth remaining in the involved plate.[77] Some of the wrist deformities resemble Madelung's deformity, with premature fusion of the medial half of the radial epiphysis, triangularization of the distal radial epiphysis with unequal growth of the epiphysis, and ulnar and volar angulation of the distal radial articular surface associated with dorsal subluxation of the ulna and enlargement and distortion of the ulnar head.[69] "Pseudo-Madelung" deformity, a rare occurrence, may cause limited painful wrist motion, wrist crepitus, decrease in grip strength, and permanent disability.[101] However, posttraumatic deformity can be variable, depending on the degree and location of the partial growth arrest at the distal radial physis. Gross deformity develops if the discrepancy between radial and ulnar lengths is more than 4 mm.[43]

Investigations to detect growth arrest should include tomograms and CT or MRI scanning to map the extent of the bony bridge. If the bone bridge is less than 50% of the physis, resection and interpositional grafting may be indicated. If there is a length discrepancy of the radius and ulna, this procedure should be accompanied by epiphysiodesis of the corresponding unaffected ulnar epiphysis. These techniques are discussed extensively in Chapter 7.

If there is significant deformity and the bone bridge is extensive, other reconstructive surgery must be considered. The Darrach procedure is unacceptable in very young patients because of the loss of power and function that frequently results from it.[101] Simultaneous ulnar shortening and radial osteotomy to correct the radiocarpal angle give consistently better clinical results than does ulnar epiphysiodesis or the Darrach procedure.[43] Tricortical iliac grafts can be interposed into the radial osteotomy to restore the radiocarpal and radioulnar angle (Fig. 6–33).[101] Newer techniques of correcting deformities, such as the Ilizarov technique, are being used more frequently.

Rarely, growth arrest of the distal ulnar epiphyseal plate may occur after injury. This is best managed by radial shortening or ulnar lengthening with reconstruction of the distal radioulnar joint.[6]

Distal Radius and Ulna Fractures

Distal radius and ulna fractures are most commonly seen in the age group from 11 to 13 years in girls and from 13 to 15 years in boys, when it is postulated that there is a temporary increase in the porosity of bone during the period of most rapid linear growth.[5] The incidence of fracture is lower in girls than in boys.[5]

A fracture of the ulnar styloid frequently accompanies a distal radial fracture. This may be because a distal radial fracture is usually due to a fall on a pronated hand, when the dorsal portion of the triangular fibrocartilage and the dorsal radiocarpal ligament tend to be taut.[64]

Diagnosis

The mechanisms of injury for forearm fractures in general also apply to fractures in the distal radius and ulna. A "dinner-fork" type of deformity, which is the appearance of a dorsally displaced fracture of the distal forearm, is seen after a supinatory force has been applied to the pronated hand. Dorsal

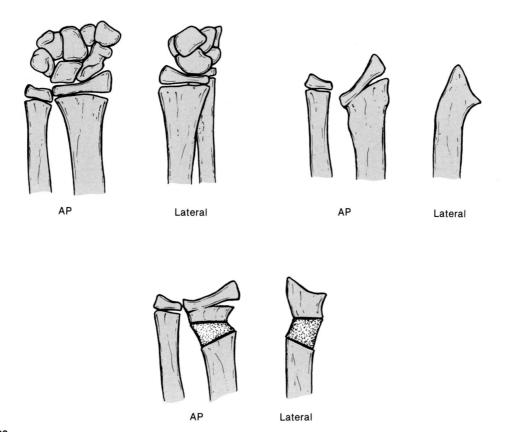

Figure 6–33
One method of correcting angular deformity of the distal radius that is secondary to growth disturbance. *A,* Comparison with normal wrist. *B,* X-ray appearance of the distal radius and ulna. *C,* Appearance after insertion of a tricortical iliac crest bone graft designed to normalize the radiocarpal angles. (From Zehntner, M.K.; Jakob, R.P.; McGanity, P.L. Growth disturbance of the distal radial epiphysis after trauma: operative treatment by corrective radial osteotomy. J Pediatr Orthop 10(3):411, 1990.)

angulation and volar displacement are seen after a pronation mechanism of injury.

Management

The key to successful closed treatment of distal forearm fractures is recognition of the deforming forces and reversal of the deformity. It is acknowledged that most residual deformities of the distal third of the forearm with angulation as great as 35 degrees will correct fully in 5 years in children who are still growing.[24, 26] Therefore, as with other fractures in the forearm, the length of time after fracture during which the physis remains open must be taken into account when deciding how much deformity is acceptable.

Buckle Fractures. Torus or buckle fractures can be immobilized in a short arm cast. These are stable injuries and need be immobilized only for comfort while the fracture is healing. A period of 2 to 3 weeks is usually sufficient.

Greenstick Fractures. Management of greenstick fractures of the forearm was discussed earlier. We recommend that well-molded long arm casts or sugar-tongs splints be used to limit pronation and supination. This cast is usually replaced after 3 to 4 weeks with a short arm cast for an additional 2 weeks, until the fracture is solid (Fig. 6–34).

Complete Fractures. These fractures can usually be reduced with closed manipulation (discussed under management of forearm fractures). For fractures of both radius and ulna, one fracture should be reduced first, and then the other. If the ulnar segment is very short, it may be difficult to achieve a perfect reduction of the ulna, but mild angulation will not be a problem (Fig. 6–35).

According to traditional teaching, the fracture of the distal third of the forearm should be immobilized in pronation. Rang, however, cautions that if the fracture is put in either full pronation or full supination, one fragment will angulate anteriorly while the other angulates posteriorly.[70] Placing the fracture in each of these positions can be done intraoperatively under image intensification to find the position in which it is most stable and in which reduction is optimal. The arm should be immobilized in that position, with a long arm cast.

The fracture should be followed weekly for 3 weeks after reduction while there is potential for

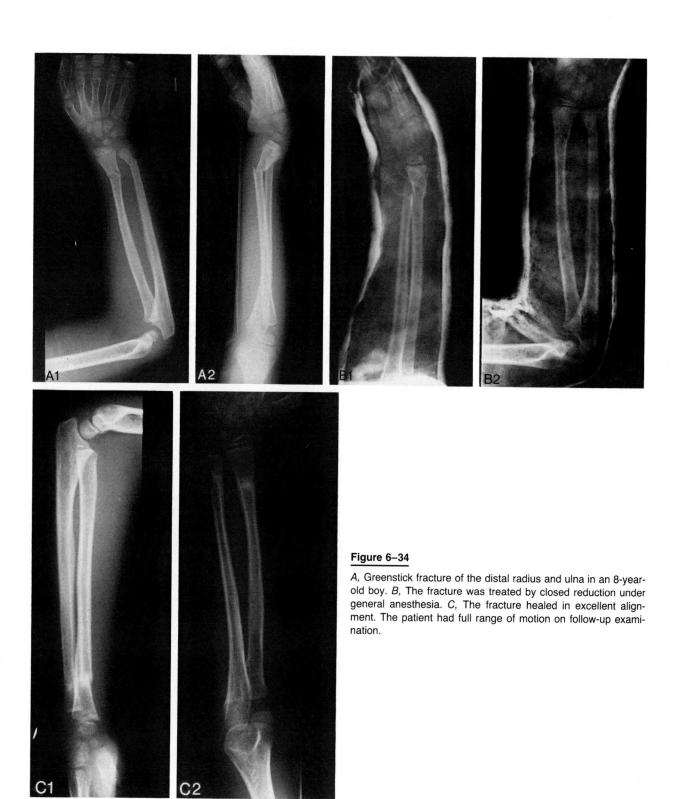

Figure 6–34

A, Greenstick fracture of the distal radius and ulna in an 8-year-old boy. *B*, The fracture was treated by closed reduction under general anesthesia. *C*, The fracture healed in excellent alignment. The patient had full range of motion on follow-up examination.

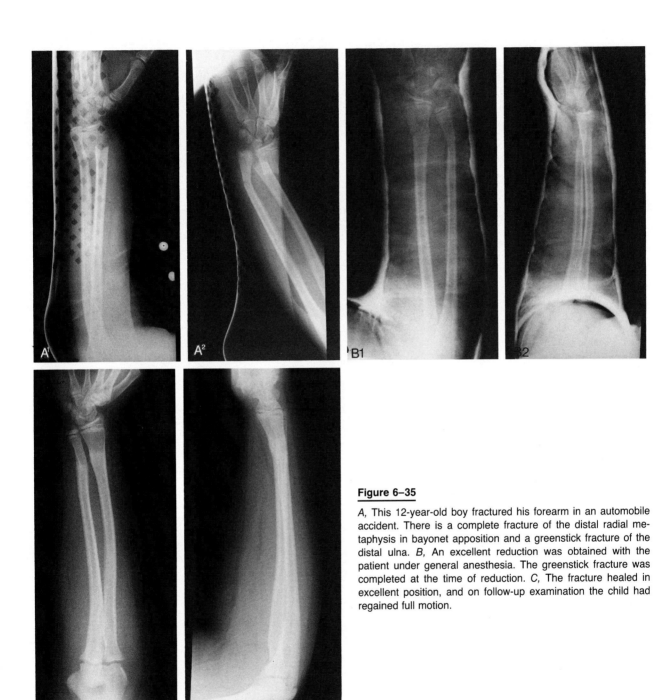

Figure 6–35

A, This 12-year-old boy fractured his forearm in an automobile accident. There is a complete fracture of the distal radial metaphysis in bayonet apposition and a greenstick fracture of the distal ulna. B, An excellent reduction was obtained with the patient under general anesthesia. The greenstick fracture was completed at the time of reduction. C, The fracture healed in excellent position, and on follow-up examination the child had regained full motion.

redisplacement. Angulation in the postoperative period may occur, but this is usually corrected relatively easily without anesthetic if the deformity is mild and detected before the fracture is solid.

Although there is wide disagreement in the literature as to the acceptable limits of reduction, the following guidelines have been recommended. In infants, up to 30 degrees of angulation in the coronal plane can be accepted. Between the ages of 5 and 10 years, a good result can be expected if the residual angulation is no greater than 15 to 20 degrees. In children over 10 years of age, the upper limit is 15 degrees in the coronal plane and 10 degrees of radial deviation.[17, 61, 64] Infrequently, an adequate reduction cannot be achieved, and one should proceed with open techniques.

Fractures of the Distal Third of the Radius

The fracture of the radius at the junction of the metaphysis and diaphysis with supinational deformity has been dubbed "the slipper" by Rang because of the tendency for angulation to recur after reduction (Fig. 6–36).[70] This should be differentiated from the Galeazzi fracture, which is associated with disruption of the radioulnar triangular fibrocartilage

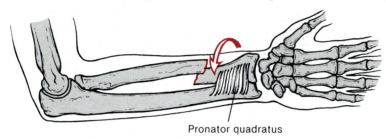
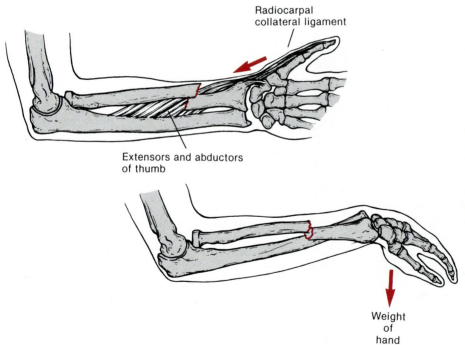
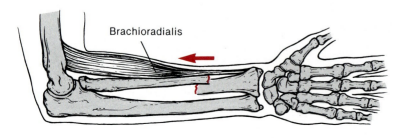

Figure 6–36

Deforming forces in fractures of the distal third of the radius. (From Hughston, J.C. Fracture of the distal radial shaft. Mistakes in management. J Bone Joint Surg 39-A:250, 1957.)

complex. The fracture of the distal third of the radius occurs more frequently in patients over 8 years of age. This is often an oblique fracture. The distal fragment is usually displaced medially secondary to the pull of the pronator quadratus, extensor pollicis longus, and abductor pollicis brevis. This fracture, alone or in association with a greenstick fracture or buckle fracture of the distal ulna, is unstable and can be tricky to manage.

The fracture is reduced in the usual manner by first increasing the deformity and hooking the distal fragment onto the proximal fragment. Once the traction on the arm is released, however, the fracture tends to again shorten and angulate owing to its obliquity. Even by including the thumb in the cast, shortening is difficult to prevent (Fig. 6–37).

According to traditional teaching, the fracture should be immobilized in pronation because it is distal to the insertion of the pronator teres. However, in pronation the pull of the brachioradialis displaces the fragment. The oblique thenar muscles and brachioradialis are relaxed in supination, stabilizing the reduction (Fig. 6–38).

Gupta and Danielsson reported a randomized trial of 60 patients with solitary fractures of the distal radius that were immobilized in a position of pronation, neutrality, or supination. Initially, minimally displaced and nondisplaced fractures tended to angulate even if immobilized in an above-elbow cast. When the wrist was immobilized in pronation, the incidence of recurrent angulation was greater in patients who had required closed reduction than in

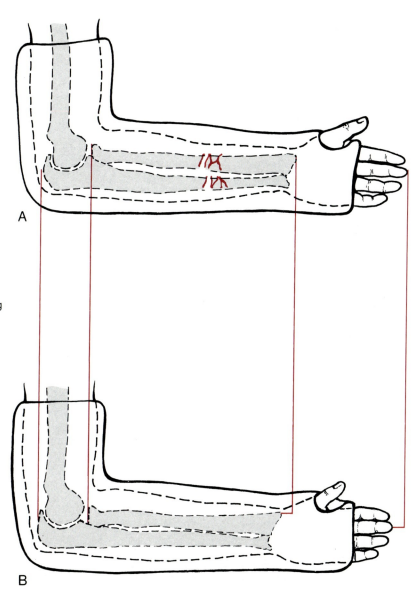

Figure 6–37

Shortening cannot be prevented by including the thumb in the cast.

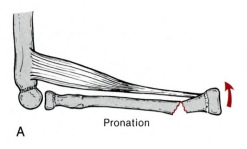
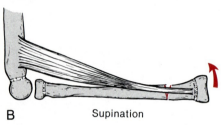

Figure 6–38
The role of the brachioradialis muscle, which tends to displace the fracture in pronation (A) and to "lock" the reduction in supination (B). (From Gupta, R.P.; Danielsson, L.G. Dorsally angulated solitary metaphyseal greenstick fractures in the distal radius: results after immobilization in pronated, neutral, and supinated positions. J Pediatr Orthop 10:90, 1990.)

the undisplaced fracture group. The mean increase of dorsal angulation after initial treatment was less in the fractures treated with the forearm in supination as compared with those treated in pronation and in a neutral position. These authors concluded that fractures of the distal radius should be immobilized in the supinated position.[29] It is recommended that the arm be immobilized in a long arm cast with the forearm in supination. The thumb should be included in the cast for additional rotational control. The fracture is followed carefully with weekly x-rays to detect early redisplacement, at which time cast changes or remanipulation can be performed. The cast should be removed at 6 weeks.

Some authors advocate pinning these frequently unstable fractures. A closed reduction is performed first. A K-wire is then inserted at the lateral distal metaphysis and across the fracture site through a small incision in the skin to prevent skewering of subcutaneous nerves or vessels. A long arm cast is applied for the first 4 weeks, followed by a short arm cast for another 2 weeks or until the fracture is healed. The pin is removed at approximately 6 weeks, when the radial fracture has healed.

Although reasonable alignment can usually be achieved with a closed reduction, frequently some shortening of the radius with respect to the ulna occurs. Angulation of up to 10 degrees and shortening of the radius of up to 5 mm are acceptable.[54] Slight displacement usually results in little or no functional disability as evidenced by the paucity of reports on long-term disability from this type of fracture. If a reasonable position cannot be achieved, open reduction and plating or pinning of the distal radius should be performed.

Fractures of the Shafts of the Radius and Ulna

Eighteen percent of all forearm fractures occur in the shafts of the radius and ulna. Whereas in older children the injury usually occurs in the metaphyseal region of the bone, in younger children it occurs in the diaphysis. Both bones of the forearm are usually injured unless the mechanism of injury is a direct blow to the arm, which may result in an isolated fracture of either the radius or the ulna. There may be a combination of complete fracture, greenstick fracture, or plastic deformation to the radius and ulna at any location in the forearm. If only one bone appears to be injured, careful clinical and radiologic evaluation must be performed to eliminate the possibility of a disruption at either the elbow or the wrist.

Classification

Fractures of the shaft of the radius and ulna are classified according to the fracture types: plastic deformation, greenstick, and complete fractures. Complete fractures may be classified according to fracture configurations: transverse, oblique, spiral, butterfly, and comminuted fractures.

Diagnosis

Careful examination of swelling, tenderness, and skin involvement must be undertaken and neurologic and vascular status ascertained. Radiologic assessment must include the wrist and the elbow in both anteroposterior and lateral views. The most commonly injured nerves are the median nerve at the wrist and the anterior interosseous nerve at the elbow.

Management

General principles in the management of fractures of the forearm were enumerated earlier. Further guidelines specific to shaft fractures will be presented next.

Plastic Deformation. Plastic deformation of both

bones of the forearm is more common in the child younger than 5 years. Provided that the angular deformity is less than 20 degrees, little disability will result even if the deformity is not corrected. In children older than age 10 years, correction of the angular and rotatory deformity is essential to restore forearm rotation. The technique for reducing plastic deformities was described earlier.

Greenstick Fractures. Both angular and rotational components of the injury must be reduced. A well-molded long arm cast should be applied with good three-point fixation.

Complete Displacement. If an anatomic reduction is achieved, the fracture usually becomes relatively stable. Greater than 50% end-on apposition is desirable to achieve adequate stability of the fracture during closed treatment. The position of immobilization is determined by the position of the proximal fragment. The fracture should be immobilized in any position in which the alignment is correct and the reduction feels stable. A well-fitting long arm cast should be applied. Some authors suggest that if the radius is comminuted or tends to shorten, the thumb may be included in the cast.[70] However, as mentioned previously, the addition of the thumb spica does little to prevent shortening. If the fracture remains unstable in an unsatisfactory position, either internal or external fixation should be considered.

In the proximal third of the forearm, the bones are surrounded by a thick mass of muscles that makes it difficult to attain a perfect reduction. As the muscles atrophy during the period of immobilization, the cast becomes loose, reducing the effect of the three-point fixation within the cast. Angulation of 10 degrees at this site is more likely to cause a restriction of motion than a similar angulation in more distal fractures.[17] Several authors have therefore recommended that fractures in the proximal one third of the forearm be immobilized with the elbow extended to avoid angulation of the fracture secondary to slippage inside a loose curved cast (Fig. 6–39).[25, 70] Rang has also suggested that all fractures of both bones of the forearm in children under 2 years be immobilized in extension, presumably because there is an increased chance for the cast to slip owing to the short upper extremity and increased body fat in children of this age.[70]

The child should be followed weekly for 3 weeks after reduction of the fracture, during the time of greatest risk for redisplacement. This period is dependent on the age of the child because of the speed of fracture healing. In children less than 2 years of age, remanipulation can correct angulation without excessive force within 1 week of the fracture. In patients between 1 and 5 years of age, minor improvements should be done within 2 weeks following the fracture.

Bayonet apposition in the forearm of a child under the age of 10 years is acceptable provided that the interosseous distance is maintained and there is no

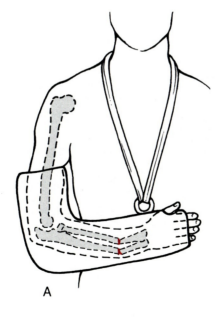
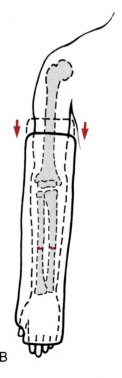

Figure 6–39

Slippage of the arm in a straight cast does not cause redisplacement of the fracture. (From Rang, M. Children's Fractures, 2nd ed. Philadelphia, J.B. Lippincott, 1982, p. 209.)

malrotation or angulation of the fracture. In children over 10 years, a fracture left in bayonet apposition will not remodel sufficiently to ensure maintenance of the interosseous distance, and permanent loss of motion will ensue (Fig. 6–40). For children younger than 8 years, injuries with 20 degrees of angulation will remodel sufficiently to obtain an excellent result. In children older than 8 years, 10 degrees of residual angulation at union will not result in a significant loss of pronation or supination. Difficulty arises when the immediate postreduction or 1-week radiographs show residual or secondary displacement. Kramhoft and Solgaard showed that 50% of fractures having 7 to 10 degrees of dorsal angulation displaced further during healing.[40] The aim in the treatment of diaphyseal fractures in children aged 8 years or more is the restoration of correct alignment and rotation, which may necessitate surgical intervention.[24]

Surgical Treatment

The indications for surgical treatment include (1) failure to achieve an adequate reduction in patients older than 10 years, (2) failure to maintain an adequate reduction after one or two manipulations, and (3) open fractures.

It has been previously acknowledged that although pediatric fractures heal well and have a great capacity for remodeling, good results are not always obtained with closed management in older children. If an adequate reduction cannot be obtained and maintained, it is mandatory that open reduction and internal or external fixation be performed. The method of choice for internal fixation depends on the configuration of the fracture and the experience of the surgeon. The two most common and accepted techniques are (1) AO techniques using plates and screws and (2) intramedullary fixation. The presence

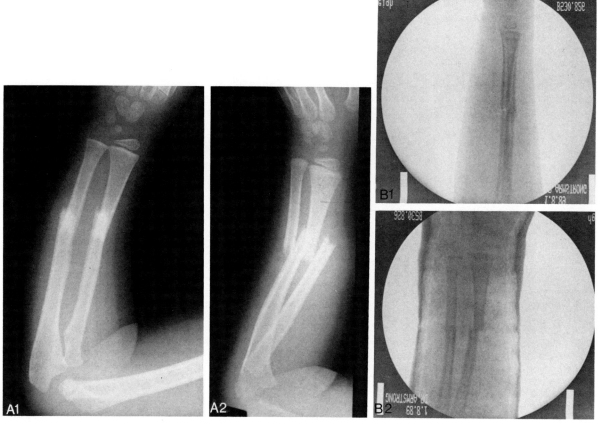

Figure 6–40

Complete midshaft fractures of the radius and ulna with bayonet apposition. *A*, A 5-year-old boy who fell at camp, fracturing the midshafts of both forearm bones. *B*, With the patient under general anesthesia the fractures were reduced. There was 50 percent cortical end-on apposition of the radius.

Illustration continued on facing page

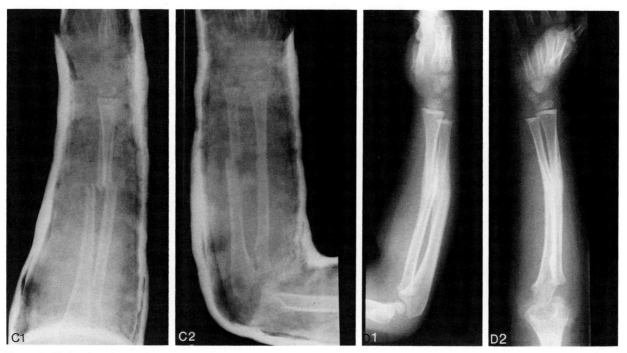

Figure 6–40 Continued

C, Subsequent displacement did occur, but the position was felt to be acceptable. *D,* The cast was removed 5 weeks later. After 1 month, the forearm lacked 30 degrees of supination and 15 degrees of pronation. At age 5 years, future remodeling is likely to result in improved motion.

of open physes is not a contraindication to good fracture management.

Intramedullary fixation is a very useful technique for unstable transverse fractures of the ulna and radius (Fig. 6–41). This method provides internal splintage, maintaining improved angular alignment of the fractures. End-to-end reduction ensures that overlapping cannot occur at the fracture site and that cortical contact will decrease the risk of malrotation during healing. The curvature of the rod and the anchorage in the upper and lower metaphyses produce a three-point pressure system. Some movement at the fracture site ensures optimal development of external callus by reducing shear and converting it into a compression or traction force.[42] This technique does not provide solid internal fixation, and thus rotatory alignment must be controlled postoperatively with a long arm cast.

The advantages of this technique are that removal of the intramedullary rods is a minor procedure and that no stress risers are created following removal, possibly increasing the risk of refracture. This technique should be used with caution, however, in children older than age 12 years, in whom anatomic reduction is desirable. Blunt-ended rods of high-quality steel, cold-hammered at 140°C, or of titanium with diameters of 1.5 to 2.5 mm are ideal. Steel rods should be precurved. Titanium rods are more flexible than standard stainless steel rods, are easier to introduce, and allow controlled motion to occur at the fracture site, which theoretically increases the speed and potential for healing.

The ulna, being subcutaneous and straighter than the radius, is more suited to intramedullary fixation.[39] With a smooth K-wire or Rush rod, the apophyseal plate of the olecranon process will not be damaged. Frequently reduction and closed intramedullary pinning of the ulna will improve the alignment of the radius and stabilize the fracture sufficiently that fixation of the radius is unnecessary.

Because of the curved contour of the radius, introduction of an intramedullary device through the metaphysis of the distal radius is technically more exacting. Although the pin should be bent to reproduce the normal curve of the radius, anatomic alignment may be difficult to achieve. Intramedullary pin fixation of the radius is suitable for children younger than 10 years, when anatomic reduction of the radius is less important. For fixation of the radius in the adolescent, open reduction with fixation using the AO dynamic compression plate or semitubular plate and screws is a better option.

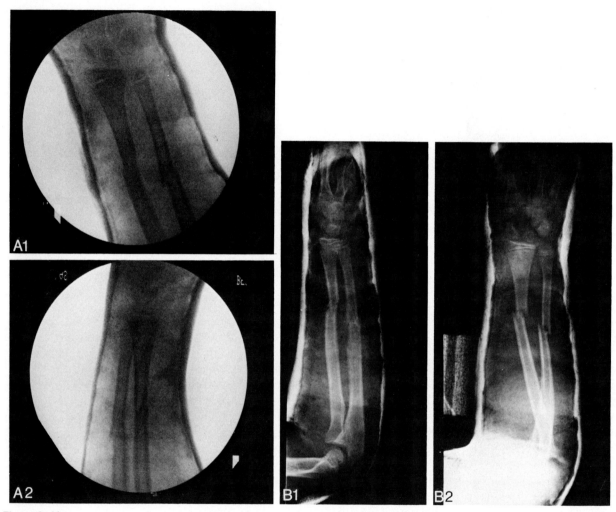

Figure 6–41

Ulnar intramedullary pin fixation for fractures of both bones of the forearm. *A,* A 10-year-old boy fell off his bicycle, fracturing the midshafts of both bones of the forearm. Initially, an excellent alignment was achieved by closed reduction with the patient under general anesthesia. Note the obliquity of the fractures, predisposing this fracture to redisplacement. *B,* The fracture started to displace 1 week later.

Illustration continued on facing page

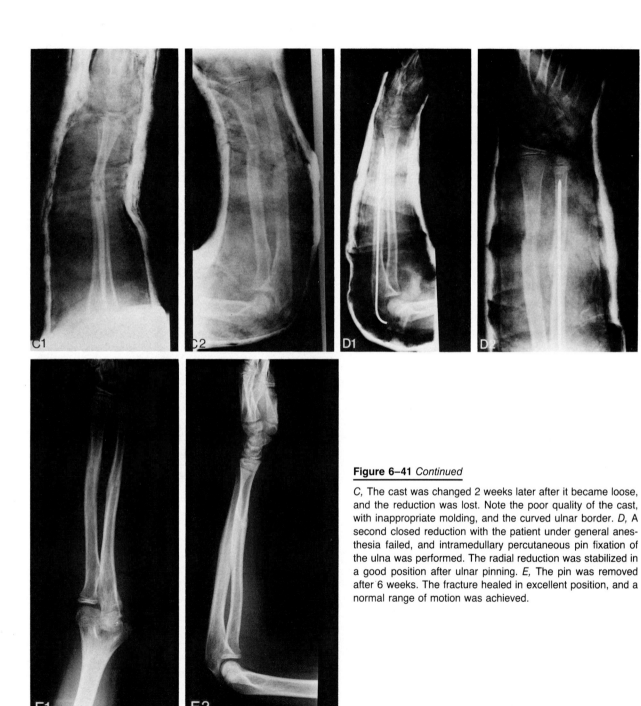

Figure 6–41 Continued

C, The cast was changed 2 weeks later after it became loose, and the reduction was lost. Note the poor quality of the cast, with inappropriate molding, and the curved ulnar border. *D,* A second closed reduction with the patient under general anesthesia failed, and intramedullary percutaneous pin fixation of the ulna was performed. The radial reduction was stabilized in a good position after ulnar pinning. *E,* The pin was removed after 6 weeks. The fracture healed in excellent position, and a normal range of motion was achieved.

Fixation including six cortices proximal and distal to the fracture is sufficient in the pediatric group (Fig. 6–42).

Other methods of fixation that have been reported include external fixation techniques, or pins and plaster,[93] which may be useful in extensive open injuries to the forearm or in comminuted fractures. These techniques are rarely necessary.

Closed Intramedullary Pinning of Both Bones of the Forearm (Fig. 6–43). The patient is placed supine on the operating table with the arm abducted and the elbow flexed to 90 degrees. A preliminary reduction is performed. Ideally, traction is applied to provide slight distraction at the fracture site to facilitate pin insertion. A 1 cm skin incision is made at the tip of the olecranon. A drill hole is made in the tip of the olecranon, and the ulnar medullary canal is drilled, guided by fluoroscopy. Either a smooth Steinmann pin or a Rush rod is inserted depending on the width of the medullary canal and the length of the ulna.

Once the ulna is pinned, a 2 cm skin incision is made 1 cm proximal to the distal radial epiphysis, guided by fluoroscopy. The radial vein and radial nerve are identified and retracted. An oblique hole angulated at 45 degrees in the horizontal plane is drilled in the lateral cortex of the metaphysis. A bend of approximately 15 to 45 degrees is made in the pin 1 cm from its tip, and a similar bend is made in the middle of the pin. If titanium rods are used, no prebending is needed. The first bend facilitates entrance into the radial medullary canal; the second bend enables it to conform to the curve in the radius as well as to provide internal three-point splinting of the fracture.[3] The nail must be curved over its entire length. After the tip of the nail is close to the fracture site, the fracture is reduced and the nail is advanced. The summit of the curve should lie at the level of the fracture. If the reduction is not perfect, the nail should be rotated until the angulation is corrected. The proximal end of the pin is bent at 90 degrees and cut 5 mm from the bone.[42]

Lascombes and co-workers reported on the results of 85 cases of closed intramedullary nailing without any postoperative immobilization.[42] Complications were seen in 14 cases (16%), including hypoesthesia secondary to injury to the sensory branches of the radial nerve, irritation of the skin over the end of

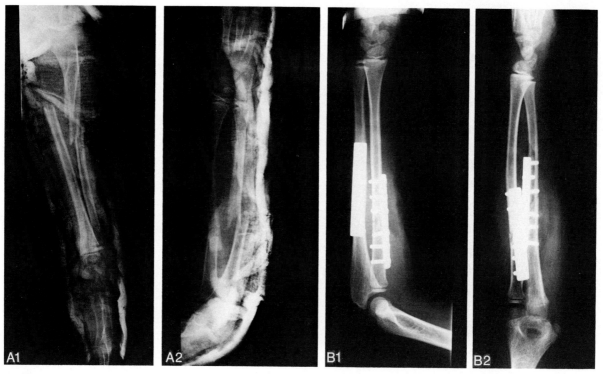

Figure 6–42

Open reduction and internal fixation using plates and screws. *A,* A 12-year-old boy was assaulted, and he sustained fractures of the radius and ulna. This fracture configuration may also be classified as a Monteggia equivalent. *B,* With the patient under general anesthesia the fractures were manipulated, but since a satisfactory position could not be achieved, an open reduction was performed using two separate incisions.

the nail, secondary displacement of the fracture of less than 10 degrees of angulation due to inadequate anchorage at the extremity of the nail, and delayed union. It is interesting to note that in six patients older than 10 years, the fracture remained malunited, with deficits in pronation and supination.[42]

Follow-up Care and Rehabilitation

Closed Reduction. The parents should be warned at the initiation of treatment that several cast changes may be necessary during its course to ensure that alignment is maintained. If a minor change in alignment is observed, a cast change to correct the position is recommended, with application of a well-fitting and well-molded cast.

In midshaft fractures of the forearm that are undisplaced, 6 weeks in a long arm cast is recommended. If the fracture site is still tender after 6 weeks, the child is treated in a short arm cast for an additional 2 weeks. In children less than 5 years of age who have an undisplaced fracture, 4 weeks in a long arm cast followed by 2 weeks in a short arm cast may be sufficient.

After removal of the cast, the child is encouraged to practice range-of-motion exercises of the elbow and forearm. The child is reviewed clinically and radiologically after 4 weeks. In most children, physiotherapy is not necessary. However, in the occasional child in whom the range of motion has not returned by 8 weeks following fracture and in whom a mechanical block is not suspected, physiotherapy can be initiated. The child is discouraged

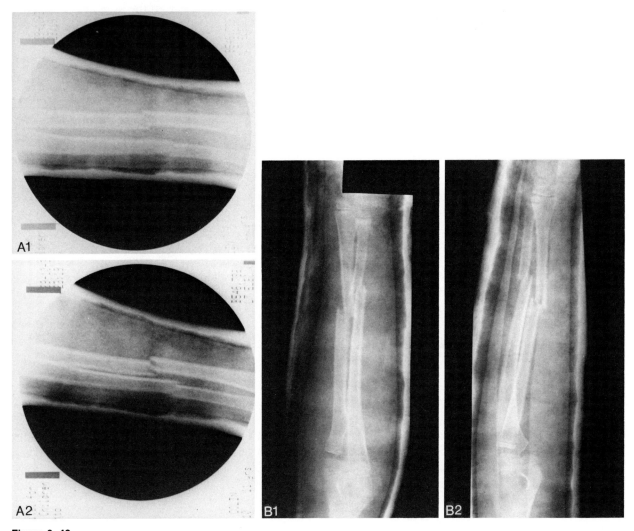

Figure 6-43

Intramedullary pinning of both radius and ulna after redisplacement of transverse shaft fractures. *A,* An 11-year-old boy fell from an all-terrain vehicle, fracturing both bones of the forearm. Initial reduction with the patient under general anesthesia was satisfactory, with 75 per cent end-on cortical apposition. *B,* After the swelling had subsided, the fractures redisplaced.

Illustration continued on following page

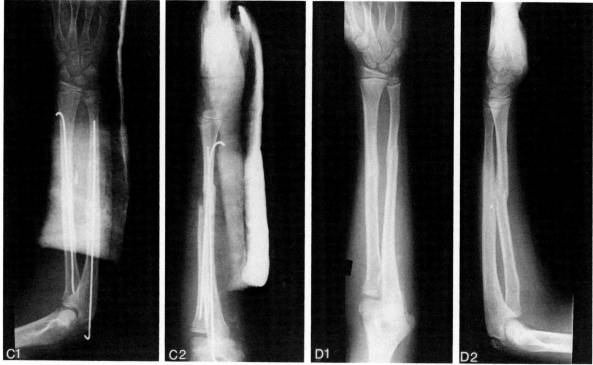

Figure 6–43 Continued

C, A second closed reduction with intramedullary pinning of both bones was performed. The cast was changed to a short arm cast 4 weeks later, and the fracture was immobilized for an additional 2 weeks. *D,* Four months later the patient had regained full range of motion.

from returning to contact sports for 1 month following removal of the cast because of the risk of refracture.

Surgical Treatment. If solid internal fixation, i.e., plates and screws, has been used, it is often useful to splint the forearm for comfort for 1 to 2 weeks postoperatively. Otherwise the child is allowed to move the elbow, forearm, and wrist. He or she is not permitted to return to any active sports requiring the use of the arm, except swimming, until the fracture is healed clinically and radiologically. Hardware removal is recommended in children 1 year after fracture healing. The forearm is protected for 6 to 8 weeks following removal of the hardware owing to the risk of refracture through the screw holes.

Many orthopaedic surgeons remove most internal fixation devices in children. Many reasons have been quoted to substantiate the case for a second operative procedure to remove hardware. These include the potential for plate corrosion during the child's long remaining life span, a decrease in bone strength due to the stress-shielding properties of plates, the potential for the plate to act as a stress riser during subsequent trauma, and stimulation of growth caused by the proximity of metal hardware to open physes. The long-term effects of changes in ionic composition secondary to metal are similarly unknown. On the other hand, some studies supply evidence that removal of hardware from critical areas, such as the proximal radius, exposes the child to the risk of damage to neurovascular structures that may be caught within the scar from the initial surgery.[41] Unfortunately, there are no definitive studies to support or advise against hardware removal in children with forearm fractures.

The forearm should be immobilized in a long arm cast after intramedullary fixation for 4 weeks, followed by 2 weeks in a short arm cast. Intramedullary rods can be removed 6 to 8 weeks after the fracture is healed. Lascombes and colleagues recommended removal of the rods 1 year after insertion because of the risk of refracture.[42] From this series, however, the refracture rate did not appear to be influenced by the presence of rods, and late removal did not alter the risk of refracture.[42]

Complications

The potential complications of shaft fractures of the forearm were discussed earlier. Following are some additional points that are specific to these fractures.

Malunion is the most frequent complication, resulting in loss of supination or pronation of the forearm. If there is less than 45 degrees of supination or pronation 2 years after union of the fracture, surgical correction may be considered. An osteotomy should be planned preoperatively by comparing the radiographic appearance of the radius and ulna with that of the normal side. Solid fixation with plates and screws is recommended to ensure that the intraoperative correction is maintained. Range-of-motion exercises are then initiated in the early postoperative period.

Nonunion is an infrequent problem in children. The majority of reported nonunions have either followed open fractures or followed open reduction and internal fixation in cases of severe comminution or bone loss. These are treated with bone grafting and solid compression and fixation with AO dynamic compression plate and screws (Fig. 6–44). Alternatively, external fixation techniques with compression can be used.

Cross union of the radius and ulna is a potential complication for fractures of the radius and ulna at the same level[68]; in the pediatric age group, this is rare. The risk of cross union is significantly increased following repeated manipulations, severe comminution and displacement of the fragments, surgical trauma, application of onlay bone grafts (especially with narrowing of the interosseous space), and closed head injury.[68] Although a single incision doubtless increases the likelihood of cross union, surgery through two incisions does not necessarily prevent it. Disabling loss of pronation and supination is an indication for excision of the cross union, which should await a bone scan confirmation that bone formation is quiescent. Interposed fat or Silastic is inserted to prevent recurrence of the cross union. However, the results after excision are not as good in children as in adults. This may be due to the growth potential of immature periosteum or soft tissue contractures that preclude regaining full motion.[91]

Ipsilateral Fractures of the Upper Extremity

In approximately 4 to 13% of elbow fractures in children, a fracture of the ipsilateral forearm may be present.[66] Some of the frequently seen combinations include (1) fracture of the forearm in association with a supracondylar fracture of the humerus; (2) fracture of the distal radial epiphysis with a supracondylar fracture of the humerus (Fig. 6–45); (3) dislocation of the elbow in association with a fracture of the forearm; (4) fracture of the olecranon with an epiphyseal plate injury to the distal radius; (5) fracture of the forearm in association with a lateral condylar fracture of the humerus[66]; and (6) fracture of the distal forearm in association with type I or equivalent Monteggia lesions.[4]

Ipsilateral fractures of the elbow and forearm have been called a floating elbow. They usually occur in children between the ages of 6 and 12 years. The mechanism of injury is frequently a fall from a height onto the outstretched hand. Less frequently, these fractures result from a traffic accident.[66] The segmental nature of the injuries increases the risk of significant compromise of arterial flow and venous return and therefore increases the potential for the development of a compartment syndrome.[83] Similar to the management of the "floating knee," it is recommended that one or both of these fractures be reduced and stabilized with internal fixation.

If there is an associated supracondylar fracture of the humerus, the first step consists of a closed reduction and percutaneous fixation of this fracture, thus providing a stable base for management of the associated forearm injury.[83] Similarly, lateral condylar fractures should be pinned, even if there is no initial displacement of the fracture, before dealing with the distal fracture.[66]

OPEN FRACTURES

Open fractures should always be treated with careful debridement of soft tissues and bones, copious irrigation of the wound, and then reduction of the fracture. Internal fixation is an option if there is extensive soft tissue damage or if instability of the fracture is present. In the event that internal fixation is required in a grossly contaminated wound, the actual fixation can be delayed until subsequent wound inspections and dressing changes have resulted in a clean wound.

MONTEGGIA FRACTURES

Giovanni Battista Monteggia in 1814 first described the injury consisting of a fracture of the proximal third of the ulna and an anterior dislocation of the proximal epiphysis of the radius. Bado redefined the Monteggia lesion as a group of traumatic lesions having in common a dislocation of the radiohumeroulnar joint, associated with a fracture of the ulna at various levels or with lesions at the wrist.[4] Although in 60 to 70% of cases the ulnar fracture is at the junction of the proximal and middle thirds, Bado included in his classification fractures at any location in the ulna.[4] Of all forearm fractures in children, 0.4% are Monteggia type.[26] The peak incidence occurs between the ages of 4 and 10 years.[65]

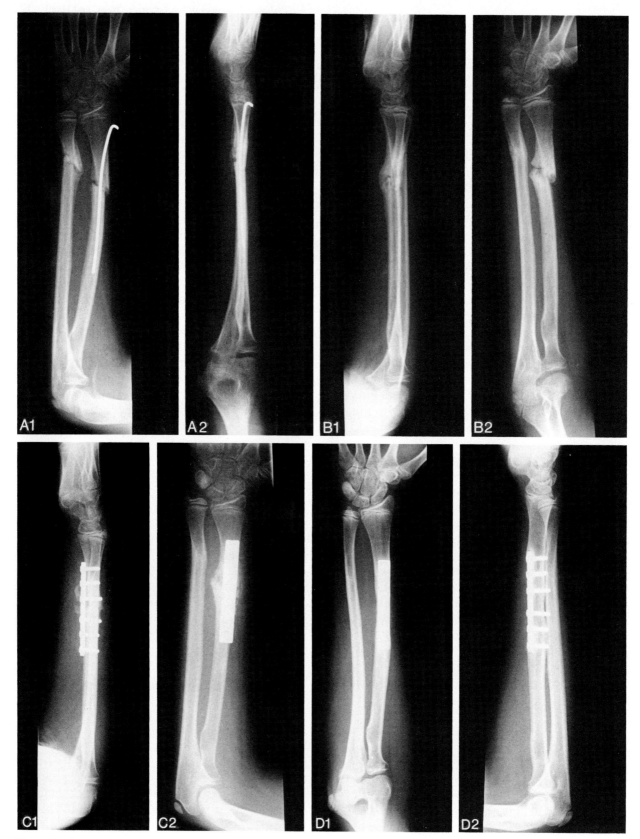

Figure 6–44

Nonunion of the radius. *A,* A 13-year-old boy who had grade I open fracture of the distal radius and ulna was treated with debridement and immobilization in a cast. After the reduction was lost, open reduction and fixation with an intramedullary pin were performed. *B,* The radial fracture did not unite. *C,* Bone grafting and compression plating of the radius were done 4 months after the fracture. *D,* The fracture united, and the plate was removed.

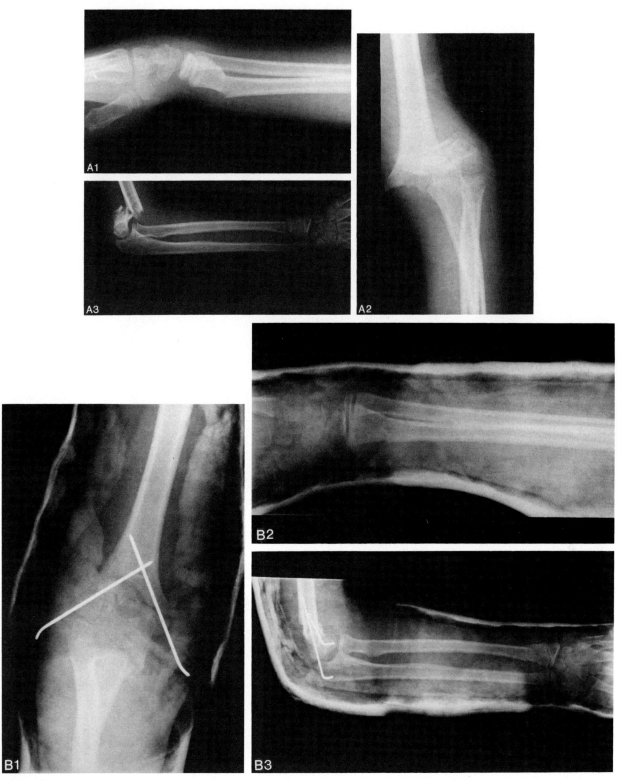

Figure 6–45

Supracondylar fracture of the humerus with ipsilateral fracture of the distal radius. *A,* An 8-year-old boy sustained a supracondylar fracture of the humerus and fracture of the distal radius and ulna. *B,* The supracondylar fracture was first reduced and pinned. The distal radius and ulna were then reduced, and the arm was immobilized in a long arm cast.

Illustration continued on following page

174   6 / Pediatric Fractures of the Forearm, Wrist, and Hand

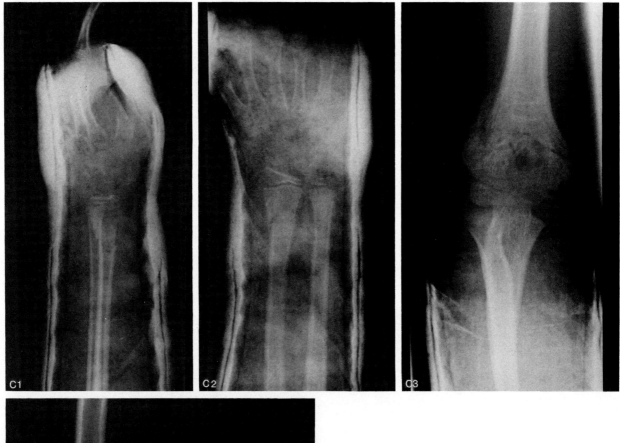

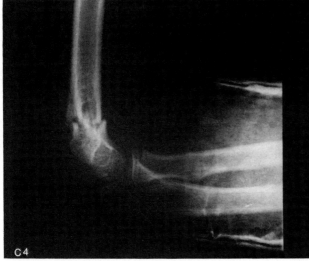

Figure 6–45 *Continued*
C, The long arm cast was removed at 3 weeks and the pins removed. A short arm cast was applied for another 3 weeks. The fracture healed in excellent position.

Classification

Bado's classification originally was devised to include lesions in both children and adults. Since the relative frequency of the various Monteggia fractures differs in children and adults, some authors dispute the usefulness of this classification in children.[45] However, since Bado's classification includes all the lesions that do occur in children, with modification, it is still useful (Fig. 6–46).

A. Monteggia lesion

Type I—Anterior dislocation of the radial head and fracture of the ulnar diaphysis at any level with anterior angulation. Most common fracture pattern.

Type II—Posterior or posterolateral dislocation of the radial head and fracture of the ulnar diaphysis with posterior angulation. Rare in children.

Type III—Lateral or anterolateral dislocation of the radial head with fracture of the ulnar metaphysis. More common in children than in adults.

Type IV—Anterior dislocation of the radial head with fracture of the proximal third of the radius and fracture of the ulna at the same level.

B. Monteggia equivalents

Type I (Fig. 6–47)

1. Anterior dislocation of the radial head with plastic deformation of the ulna.
2. Fracture of the ulnar diaphysis with fracture of the neck of the radius.
3. Fracture of the ulnar diaphysis with a fracture of the proximal third of the radius proximal to the ulnar fracture.
4. Fracture of the ulnar metaphysis with anterior dislocation of the radius (not included by Bado).
5. Fracture of the ulnar diaphysis with anterior dislocation of the radial head and fracture of the olecranon.

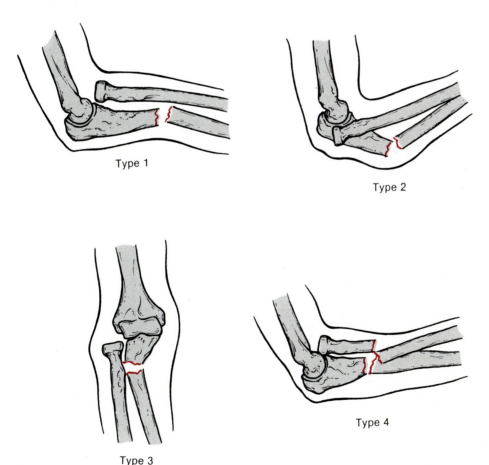

Figure 6–46

Monteggia fracture classification. (From Olney, B.W.; Menelaus, M.B. Monteggia and equivalent lesions in childhood. J Pediatr Orthop 9:219, 1989.)

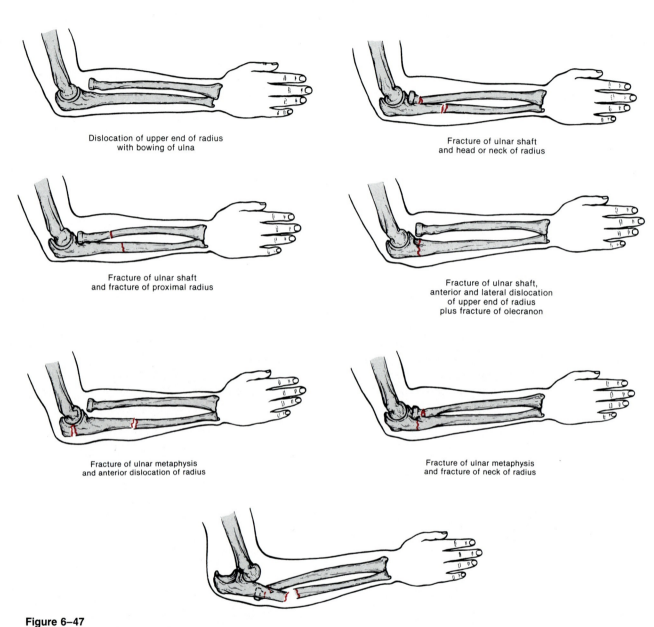

Figure 6–47
Monteggia type I–equivalent fractures. (From Olney, B.W.;. Menelaus, M.B. Monteggia and equivalent lesions in childhood. J Pediatr Orthop 9:219, 1989.)

6. Fracture of the ulnar metaphysis with fracture of the neck of the radius (not included by Bado).
7. Posterior dislocation of the elbow and fracture of the ulnar diaphysis, with or without fracture of the proximal radius.

Bado also included the "pulled elbow syndrome," simple anterior dislocation of the radial head (Fig. 6–48), and fracture of the neck of the radius in his classification, but these are not commonly accepted as Monteggia fractures. Most isolated traumatic dislocations of the radial head are probably Monteggia equivalents in which the ulna has undergone plastic deformation.[4, 45]

Type I fractures are the most common in both children and adults. Type II fractures occur rarely in children but are the second most frequent lesion in adults. Rarely seen in adults, type III fractures are the second most common Monteggia lesion in children, followed by Monteggia variants.[45] The most common Monteggia variant is a fracture of the ulnar diaphysis with a more proximal fracture in the radius,[67] although not all authors recognize this entity as a Monteggia variant.[65] The second most common Monteggia variant is the type I–equivalent injury associated with a proximal radius fracture.[65]

Mechanism of Injury

Type I. The classic type I Monteggia fracture may result from direct trauma, from a bending force as in hyperextension, or from forced hyperpronation.[72] Evans in 1949 experimentally reproduced the most common mechanism of injury—forced hyperpronation of the forearm due to a fall on the outstretched hand. After the hand strikes the ground a rotational force is added to the downward momentum of the falling body when a twisting of the trunk causes external rotation of the arm. If this force continues, the ulna fractures and the radius is forced into extreme pronation and is levered forward until the radial head dislocates. The radius crossing the ulna at the junction of the middle and proximal thirds acts as a fulcrum to force the radial head to dislocate anteriorly.[4]

Type II. This lesion is thought to be due to direct trauma with the forearm in supination or due to a rotational force in supination.[4, 73] Frequently the fracture is open. This injury is rare in children.

Type III. These injuries are unusual, and all reported cases have been in children.[57] The mechanism of injury may be direct trauma over the inner aspect of the elbow, with or without rotation.[73] This provides an adduction force, but both angulation

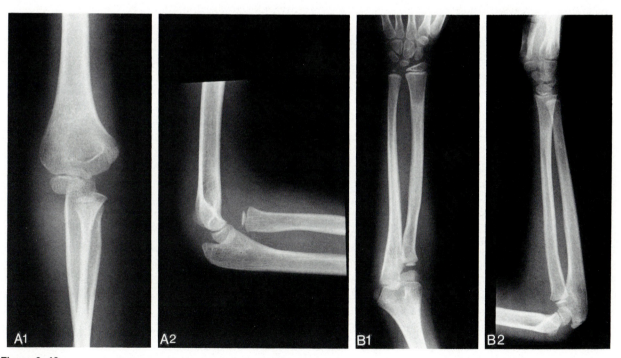

Figure 6–48
Anterior dislocation of the radial head without fracture or plastic deformation of the ulna. *A*, A 5-year-old girl fell from a height of 4 feet. *B*, There was no evidence of fracture in the forearm on initial or subsequent films.

and rotational forces are likely to be involved. The final position of the displaced radial head may be either anterolateral or posterolateral, depending on the rotational position of the forearm at the time of the primary adduction injury.[57] The metaphyseal fracture of the ulna usually occurs just below the coronoid process. An associated radial nerve injury can occur, which generally resolves spontaneously within 6 to 8 weeks.

Type IV. The type IV lesion is due to forced pronation.[73]

Monteggia Equivalents. These will be discussed in more detail under the management of the specific injuries. Generally, Monteggia equivalents are the result of a fall creating a hyperpronation force on the extended outstretched arm. They account for 5% of all injuries to the elbow and forearm in children,[67] with the highest incidence between the ages of 5 and 10 years.

In children, the ulnar fracture is often a greenstick fracture. The angulation of the fracture may have been greater at the instant of injury than when the radiographs are made. In children the radial head may pull out of the intact annular ligament, whereas in adults the injury tears the ligament. In less severe injuries with minimum angulation of the ulnar fracture, the dislocation may be missed, with late recognition of the dislocation of the radial head more than a month after the injury.[35]

Diagnosis

It is essential in all injuries of the forearm to obtain both anteroposterior and lateral x-rays of the elbow and wrist. When one bone of the forearm is fractured, the presence of any shortening of that bone means that there is a dislocation of the proximal or distal radioulnar joint.[72, 73] Clinical signs and symptoms include pain, inability to move the elbow, and deformity, with fixed pronation of the forearm and hand.

The reduction of the radial head is best assessed on the true lateral x-ray view. A line drawn through the center of the radial head should pass through the center of the capitellum.[45] On the anteroposterior view, with the forearm in supination, a line is drawn tangentially to the bicipital tuberosity and head of the radius; another line is drawn tangentially to the other border of the radial head. These lines should encompass the entire capitellum. Prior to age 10 years the bicipital tuberosity is not sufficiently ossified to utilize this technique. In younger children, a line drawn through the center of the radial neck and head should pass through the center of the capitellum.[73] If an open wound is associated with a type I lesion, it is usually located anteriorly over the ulna. In type II lesions the dislocated radial head frequently perforates the skin in the posterolateral aspect of the elbow joint.[4]

Management of the Acute Injury

Approximately 90% of children with this injury have good to excellent results. In patients less than 13 years of age who are treated by initial closed reduction, the long-term results are excellent.[45] Open reduction is required if an adequate closed reduction cannot be achieved. This occurs more frequently in older children or when there has been a delay in diagnosis or treatment.

Type I Fractures

Traction is applied with the forearm extended and supinated. The ulnar angulation is reduced, which frequently allows spontaneous reduction of the radial head. If this does not occur, the elbow is gently flexed while pressure is applied anteriorly over the head of the radius. Once the reduction is obtained, the elbow is immobilized in a long arm cast in full supination and flexion to 100 degrees, or as much flexion as the swollen elbow will tolerate.

In children, most of these injuries can be reduced with closed manipulation. If there is an oblique fracture of the ulna (especially in any obliquity that is from distal posterior to proximal anterior), the reduction may be difficult to maintain. Often these fractures will redisplace, causing late redislocation of the radial head. In this situation, fixation of the ulnar fracture is recommended. We have found that intramedullary fixation of the ulna is a very satisfactory method of fixation, decreasing the need for later extensive hardware removal and decreasing the risk for refracture after hardware removal (Fig. 6–49). If the fracture can be reduced by closed manipulation, a K-wire or Rush rod can be inserted percutaneously through the tip of the olecranon and across the fracture site. If the fracture cannot be reduced by closed manipulation, the ulnar fracture is exposed and then the fragments are pinned, using a retrograde pinning technique.[88] Once the ulnar fracture is reduced, the radial head reduction will usually be stable. This technique has been described in the section on diaphyseal fractures of the radius and ulna.

Occasionally the radial head does not reduce after anatomic reduction of the ulnar fracture owing to interposition of the annular ligament. Ogden states that the interposition is of three types: (1) partial;

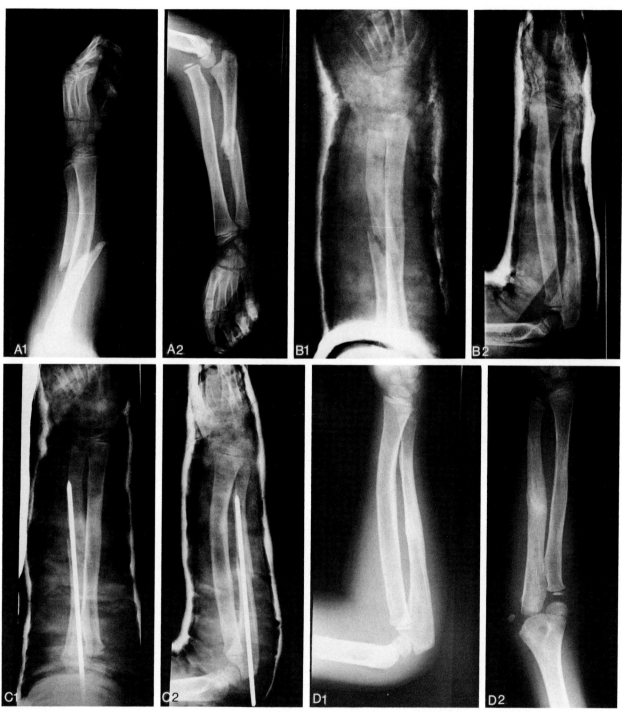

Figure 6–49

Compound Monteggia type I fracture that required intramedullary ulnar pinning. *A,* A 7-year-old boy fell in the park and sustained this injury with an open wound on the volar aspect of the forearm, caused by protrusion of the proximal ulnar fragment. A deformity of the distal radius and ulna seen on x-ray showed evidence of a previous fracture. A formal debridement was done by extending the anterior wound, and the fracture was reduced under direct vision. *B,* The fracture had displaced when reexamined at the time of secondary wound closure. *C,* Retrograde pinning of the ulna was therefore performed. This was difficult owing to the bowing in the ulna from the previous fracture. *D,* Follow-up x-rays at 2 months (the patient fractured his medial epicondyle after another fall).

(2) complete, in which the radial head pulls out of the intact ligament (most frequent); and (3) secondary to the presence of osteocartilaginous fragments.[64]

In this instance an open reduction of the radial head is performed using the posterior approach to the elbow or the Boyd approach.[10] The advantage of the Boyd approach is that both components of the Monteggia lesion can be approached via one incision. However, this approach has been criticized for increasing the chance of cross union. Another alternative is the use of two separate incisions. The portion of capsule and adjacent annular ligament is removed, and the annular ligament is repaired. If it cannot be repaired, it is reconstructed using the Bell-Tawse procedure. This will be described later under the management of complications.

Once the reduction has been obtained it is usually stable, and internal fixation is not necessary. Some authors have recommended a transcapitellar pin into the radial head to maintain the reduction.[9] We strongly advise against this technique because of the risk of pin breakage.[45, 96] Alternatively, the radius may be held in position by a K-wire passed through the radius into the ulna.[45] However, the potential for cross union exists with this technique.

Careful follow-up is essential, ensuring that adequate x-rays of the elbow and forearm are taken in both lateral and anteroposterior views. The arm is maintained in the long arm cast for 6 weeks or, alternatively, at 4 weeks changed to a cast brace for a further 2 weeks. The intramedullary pin is removed after the cast is removed; this usually can be done on an outpatient basis with local anesthetic. Range-of-motion exercises are then initiated. The child is cautioned not to participate in contact sports for 1 month following cast removal to avoid the possibility of refracture (Fig. 6–50).

Type II Fractures

Closed reduction under general anesthesia is usually successful. This is performed by extending the child's elbow with the forearm in supination, correcting the angulation of the ulna, and pushing with the thumb over the posterior aspect of the radial head. Alternatively, Bado suggests placing the elbow in 90 degrees of flexion and applying gentle traction and pronation.[4] The arm is then immobilized for 4 weeks in a long arm cast with the elbow in sufficient extension to obtain stability. The cast is changed to a long arm cast with elbow flexed for a further 2 weeks. Careful follow-up is essential. As for type I fractures, if the reduction of the ulna cannot be maintained, internal fixation may be necessary.

Type III Fractures

Closed reduction is performed by applying traction and putting abduction strain on the fully extended elbow, supinating the forearm while a direct ulnarward pressure is applied over the dislocated radial head. Once the lateral angulation is corrected, the supination of the forearm will tend to reduce the dislocation of the radial head because of the tightening of the interosseous ligament between the radius and the ulna.[57] The arm is then immobilized in flexion for 6 weeks. If the reduction is unsuccessful or cannot be maintained, open reduction of the ulnar fracture is performed.

Type IV Fractures

These fractures are extremely rare; as such, little has been written on the management of these injuries. Closed manipulation should consist of restoring the alignment of the ulnar fracture and strong supination to attempt to reduce both the radial head dislocation and the radial fracture.[37] Needless to say, these fractures are difficult to reduce by closed manipulation. As with other Monteggia fractures, the first step is accurate reduction of the ulna and fixation with the techniques described previously. If the ulnar fracture is unstable, plate fixation should be utilized instead of intramedullary pinning.

Following this, if closed manipulation of the radius fails, the radial shaft fracture should be exposed carefully. The posterior or Boyd approach to the radius should be used, with care to avoid injury to the posterior interosseous nerve. Generally, the radial head dislocation can be reduced easily at the same time that the radius is reduced, but annular ligament interposition may interfere with the reduction. For this reason, an extensile approach is recommended so that both the radial head and the radial shaft can be exposed if necessary. Ideally, separate incisions should be used for exposure to the radial and ulnar fractures to reduce the risk of cross union, but this is not always possible. The radial fracture should be fixed using a plate of the appropriate size. Intramedullary rod techniques that were described under management of radial shaft fractures can be used in younger children if the fracture is not too far proximal.

Monteggia Equivalents

These rare Monteggia variants will be discussed separately. In general, these fractures are more

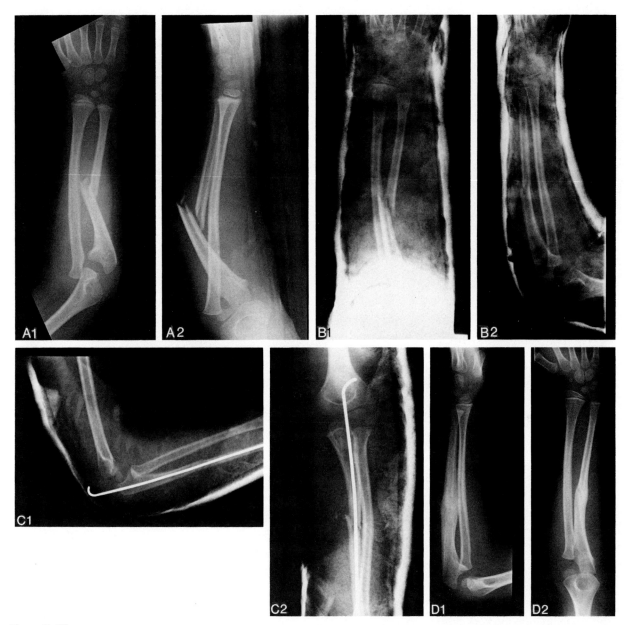

Figure 6–50

Monteggia type I fracture. *A,* A 5-year-old boy fell from a bicycle onto his left arm. He was treated with closed reduction under general anesthesia. *B,* In 2 weeks the fracture had redisplaced. Note the obliquity of the ulnar fracture, predisposing to recurrent deformity. *C–D,* Closed reduction and percutaneous pinning of the ulna were therefore undertaken, and the fracture subsequently healed in good position.

Illustration continued on following page

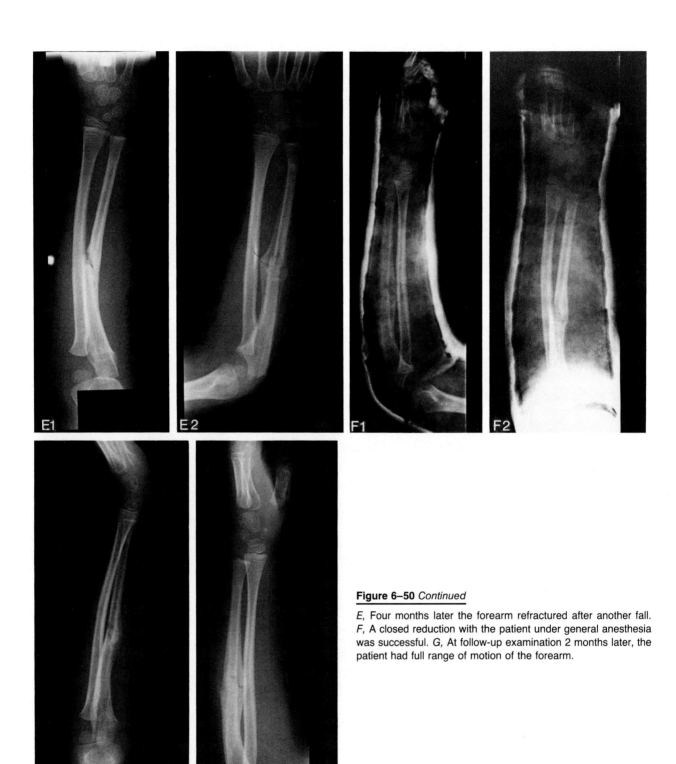

Figure 6–50 *Continued*
E, Four months later the forearm refractured after another fall. *F,* A closed reduction with the patient under general anesthesia was successful. *G,* At follow-up examination 2 months later, the patient had full range of motion of the forearm.

difficult to reduce by closed manipulation than are type I fracture-dislocations.

Anterior Dislocation of the Radial Head With Plastic Deformation of the Ulna. As discussed earlier, a significant number of missed anterior dislocations are associated with plastic deformation of the ulna. If the deformity in the ulna is not adequately corrected, this may lead to recurrent dislocation. In fact, the high recurrence rate in isolated anterior dislocations of the radial head in children is probably the result of unrecognized deformity in the ulna.[49]

The technique of reduction of the ulna has been discussed earlier. With the patient under general anesthesia, the ulna is reduced, the forearm is supinated, and pressure is applied over the anterior aspect of the radial head. A long arm cast is applied with the forearm supinated for 4 weeks. If there is recurrence of the dislocation, an osteotomy of the ulna may be necessary. Because of the possibility of recurrence,[67] follow-up should be extended to 1 year after the injury.

Fracture of the Shaft of the Ulna With a Fracture of the Radial Neck (Fig. 6–51). The most common mechanism of injury is a fall onto the outstretched hand with the forearm in any position of rotation and with a valgus strain on the extended elbow. The radial head is firmly secured against the radial notch of the ulna and the capitellum during valgus stress. The compression force fractures the radius at a relatively weak site at the neck or near the epiphyseal line, creating a Salter-Harris type II fracture. The pull of the biceps tendon displaces the distal radial fragment anteriorly and can cause the radial head to dislocate or subluxate posteriorly.[20]

There are three basic types of proximal radial fractures: (1) fractures of the neck with the head and shaft of the radius remaining in contact; (2) fractures through the radial neck or proximal epiphyseal plate with complete dislocation of the radial head; and (3) fractures through the radial neck or epiphyseal plate with the radial head remaining intact.[65]

A closed reduction may be performed using traction and varus stress. While rotating the forearm in alternating pronation-supination movements, the

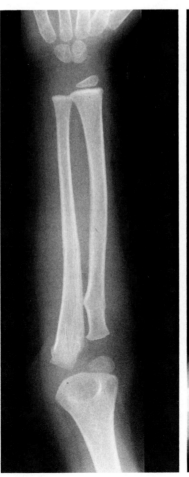
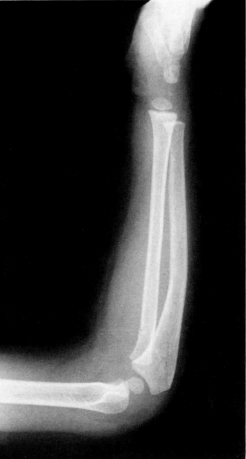

Figure 6–51

Monteggia type I variant. A 3-year-old boy fell off the bed and sustained a greenstick fracture of the ulnar shaft and a buckle fracture of the proximal third of the radius.

displaced radial fragment is reduced by applying direct pressure with the thumb. Reduction and internal fixation of the ulna will often allow an adequate closed reduction of the radial neck fracture. Up to 30 degrees of angulation in the radial neck is acceptable in younger children because of the bone's potential for remodeling. Although a closed reduction may be achieved, it is frequently difficult to maintain, and open reduction is then indicated. Of the children with fractures of the radial neck and head, 71% require operative treatment.[65] Open reduction of the radial neck fracture usually results in long-term elbow stiffness and should be avoided except for specific indications (Fig. 6–52).

If the radial neck fracture cannot be reduced satisfactorily and there is loss of pronation and supination of the forearm, open reduction is performed using a posterior approach to the radial head. Two separate incisions should be used in the open reduction of this fracture-dislocation, rather than a single large one, in order to avoid communication between the hematomas, which may increase the risk of cross union and permanent stiffness.[20] The stability of the reduction determines the necessity for fixation of the radial neck fracture, and this should be determined at the time of surgery. If necessary, K-wires should transfix the radial neck and head but should not enter the joint space. Because of the high risk of elbow stiffness, the elbow should be immobilized no longer than 3 weeks; a cast brace is applied for a further 2 weeks to allow early controlled motion. Unfortunately, even with open treatment, the results for this fracture are frequently poor owing to significant loss of motion or to cross union.[20]

Fracture of the Shaft of the Ulna With a Fracture of the Proximal Radius. This fracture pattern, the most common of the Monteggia variants, is not always differentiated from other shaft fractures of the radius and ulna. These can usually be reduced by closed manipulation, but the reduction can be difficult to maintain.[67] The fracture is manipulated using traction, with the elbow flexed in a right angle and the forearm in full supination. Over 50% of these injuries may require a second reduction.[67] Intramedullary fixation or plate fixation of the ulnar fracture can be used to maintain the ulnar reduction. If a satisfactory alignment of the radius cannot then be achieved, open reduction and fixation of the radial fracture should be undertaken, using a separate incision from the ulnar incision. The posterior interosseous nerve must be protected in this surgical approach.

Papavasiliou reported that in all cases in which there was 15 degrees of residual angulation of the ulna, there was a loss of 20 degrees of pronation.[67] Residual angulation should therefore be less than 15 degrees to produce an acceptable result.

Fracture of the Proximal Ulna in Association With Anterior Dislocation of the Radial Head. In this injury, the fracture of the olecranon is the result of a hyperextension injury to the elbow, and the forward dislocation of the radial head is produced by a concomitant pronation of the forearm.[33] Alternatively, there may be a sideways fall onto the outstretched hand,[87] or a fall onto the outstretched hand with the forearm supinated. The direction of angulation of the ulna is likely to be determined by the direction of the fall, which may produce varus, valgus, or hyperextension strain on the forearm.[100] Wright has reported the association of a fracture of the medial epicondyle in association with this variant.[100] These fractures are frequently comminuted or oblique and are consequently very unstable. Often difficult to reduce closed, they are equally difficult to stabilize with open reduction.

Some fractures can be managed by placing an intramedullary pin in the ulna, using the K-wire as a "joystick" to manipulate the fracture. Unfortunately, most of these fractures are located very proximally in the metaphyseal bone of the ulna so that the pin cannot securely control the proximal fragment, and this technique of reduction fails. If the fracture is oblique and there is little comminution, small-fragment lag screws can be used to secure the reduction. Otherwise a combination of screws, plates, and K-wires may be necessary. The radial head dislocation is usually easily reduced once the ulnar fracture is reduced. The arm should be immobilized postoperatively with the forearm in supination and the elbow flexed to maximize stability. Four weeks in the long arm cast plus an additional 2 weeks in an elbow cast brace is recommended.

Fracture of the Ulnar Diaphysis With Anterior Dislocation of the Radial Head and Fracture of the Olecranon. The basic principles of treatment are the same as for other type I Monteggia fracture-dislocations; i.e., once adequate reduction of the ulnar fractures has been obtained, the radial head dislocation can be reduced. The management of this variant is similar to that described for fracture of the ulnar metaphysis with fracture of the neck of the radius.

The most probable mechanism is a fall onto the outstretched hand with the forearm supinated, along with varus, valgus, or hyperextension strain on the forearm. From case reports in the literature it appears that with closed or open treatment there is a

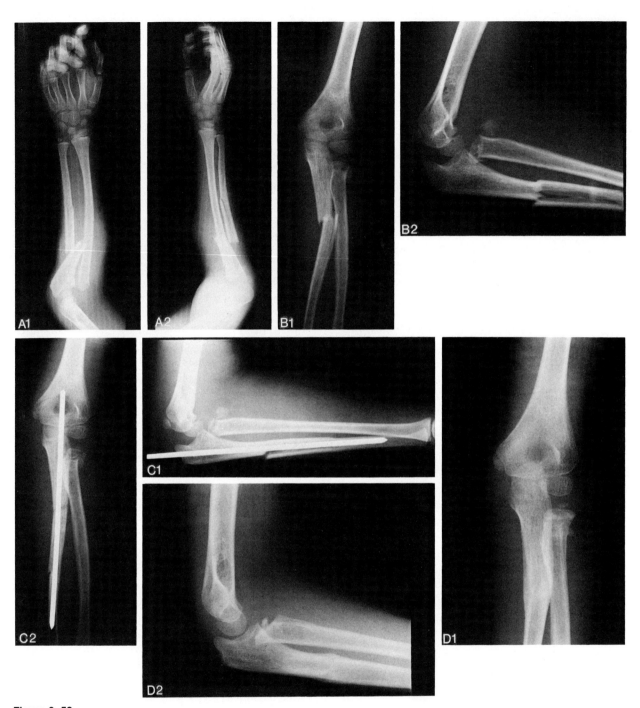

Figure 6-52

Monteggia-equivalent fracture A, An 8-year-old girl fell from a tree and sustained a displaced segmental fracture of the ulna and a displaced fracture of the radial neck. An anterior interosseous nerve palsy was noted. B, With the patient under general anesthesia a closed reduction was attempted, but the alignment could not be maintained. Fixation of the ulna by intramedullary pinning was performed. Examination with the patient under anesthesia using the image intensifier indicated that the radial head was stable and that the radial neck fracture ends were in an acceptable position. C, The early postoperative course was complicated by a compartment syndrome requiring fasciotomies. At the time of secondary wound closure under anesthesia, the radial head was inspected and the forearm put through a range of motion. The cortical fragment noted anteriorly was thought to be metaphyseal in origin, and it did not appear to contribute to the stability of the radial head and neck. At 4 weeks the above-elbow cast was replaced by a short arm cast, which was worn for an additional 2 weeks. The patient was then referred to physiotherapy for range of motion exercises. D, At radiologic follow-up 1 year later, the anterior deformity indicates that the previously noted fragment was, in fact, a portion of the radial head, indicating a Salter-Harris type IV fracture that had been misdiagnosed. However, the forearm remained stable, and the patient had nearly full range of motion. The anterior interosseous nerve injury was completely resolved. Further follow-up is indicated.

significant risk for loss of pronation and supination with this injury.[100] The management of the ulnar fracture is similar to that outlined for fractures of the ulnar metaphysis. A closed reduction of the radial neck fracture may be attempted, and if an adequate reduction cannot be achieved, open reduction is indicated.

Posterior Dislocation of the Elbow and Fracture of the Ulnar Diaphysis, With or Without Fracture of the Proximal Radius. The posterior dislocation of the elbow is reduced first, using traction and applying direct pressure posteriorly over the olecranon, flexing the elbow. Then the forearm is gently supinated.[4] The arm is immobilized in a long arm cast with the forearm in supination for 6 weeks. Alternatively, a cast brace may be applied at 4 weeks so that controlled range-of-motion exercises can be started earlier.

It has been suggested by Ravessoud that a displaced ulnar shaft fracture in association with a displaced lateral condylar fracture and intact radiohumeral articulation is a type III Monteggia equivalent.[71] He recommends open reduction and internal fixation of the lateral condylar fracture as well as open reduction and internal fixation of the ulnar shaft fracture to permit earlier mobilization of the elbow.[71] We recommend that the lateral condylar fracture be treated with open reduction and internal fixation with smooth K-wires. Depending on the location and degree of displacement of the ulnar fracture, the ulna is internally stabilized with an intramedullary pin or plate and screws. The elbow is immobilized for 3 weeks, after which time the smooth K-wires in the elbow are removed. The child is then allowed to move the elbow, either with or without a cast brace, depending on his or her age and the stage of the healing process in the ulna. The cast is removed at approximately 6 weeks, to be followed by further range-of-motion exercises.

Follow-up and Rehabilitation

Careful follow-up with adequate radiologic evaluation of the reduction of the radial head is essential. Comparison views of the opposite elbow can be helpful, since in the anteroposterior view, lateral subluxation of the radial head can be difficult to evaluate. Displacement of the radial head can frequently recur, with loss of reduction of the ulna. If open reduction of the radial head has been necessary, aggressive physiotherapy should be undertaken after cast removal because of the high risk of elbow stiffness.

Complications

Factors leading to poor results include failure to obtain anatomic reduction of the ulna; persistence or recurrence of dislocation of the radial head; heterotopic ossification, including synostosis of the proximal parts of the radius and ulna; nerve injury; and compartment syndrome.[65, 72]

Late Diagnosis or Redislocation

The neglected or unrecognized redisplaced Monteggia fracture-dislocation can cause pain, decrease in range of motion of the elbow, decrease in forearm rotation, and unstable cubitus valgus.[34, 48] Persistent dislocation in a child is rarely painful, and while it may limit pronation, it does not usually interfere with the motion of the elbow.[35] However, because of continued growth of the radius in the dislocated position the cubitus valgus may increase and the radial head may enlarge, distorting the supinator muscle and causing pressure on the posterior interosseous or radial nerve with possible late development of a progressive radial nerve palsy.[34, 48] For this reason, it is recommended that all such lesions in children be reduced.

The classic treatment was to leave the radial head dislocated and excise it at skeletal maturity, if necessary. However, it is generally agreed that the radial head should never be excised in children.[9] The resultant loss of growth in the radius inevitably would produce progressive radial deviation at the wrist joint and progressive valgus deformity at the elbow.[77]

Old Monteggia fracture-dislocations should be treated with open reduction of the persistently dislocated radial head with reconstruction of the annular ligament. Recurrence of radial head subluxation after reduction has been linked to insufficient correction of the ulnar deformity.[35] Therefore, in order to achieve reduction of the radial head, a corrective ulnar osteotomy is usually necessary. When there is marked limitation of flexion due to severe long-standing anterior dislocation of the radial head, an osteotomy of the radius with angular correction or shortening may also be required.[34]

The annular ligament, in most instances, has become a mass of fibrous tissue and scar that must be excised to allow reduction of the radial head. Reconstruction of the annular ligament using a fascial graft is then necessary (Fig. 6–53). If the annular ligament is found to be intact, transection and repair may be sufficient to restore stability without resorting to fascial graft reconstruction. The

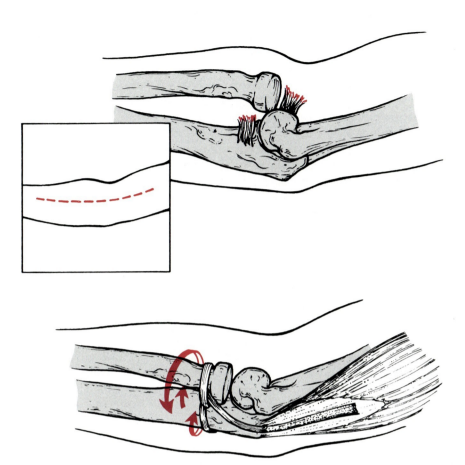

Figure 6–53

Annular reconstruction of the proximal radioulnar joint. (From Bell-Tawse, A.J.S. The treatment of malunited anterior Monteggia fractures in children. J Bone Joint Surg 47-B:720, 1965.)

likelihood of postoperative stiffness may be decreased with the simpler procedure.[35]

This procedure can be recommended only for children who have no major intraarticular injury, no damage to the epiphyseal centers, and only mild adaptive changes of the radial head. If there is significant overgrowth of the radius as well as secondary changes in the proximal and distal radioulnar joints, anatomic reduction of the radial head will not provide good articulation of those joints and is contraindicated.[35] In this situation, the classic treatment of late excision after skeletal maturity or interposition arthroplasty may be considered only if there are clinical indications for intervention.

Procedure (Bell-Tawse Annular Ligament Reconstruction With Lloyd-Roberts Modification). The patient should be positioned prone on the operating table with the upper extremity resting on a hand table. A Boyd approach is recommended. The elbow joint is entered through a lateral capsular incision. The interposed soft tissues, which may include joint capsule and annular ligament, are carefully removed, avoiding injury to the articular cartilage. Usually the radial head can be reduced with anterior pressure and supination of the forearm. If the reduction cannot be obtained in this manner, osteotomy of the ulna should be considered and performed at this stage. The radial head, once reduced, is usually stable. A 1×7 cm strip of fascia is then dissected from the lateral portion of the triceps tendon, preserving its distal attachment on the olecranon. A subperiosteal tunnel is fashioned so that the strip can be passed medial to the olecranon at a point opposite the origin of the annular ligament. The strip is then passed around the neck of the radius and sutured to itself or secured through a drill hole in the ulna.[34] If the triceps tendon is unsuitable, a free tendon graft as recommended by Watson-Jones should be used.[7]

Lloyd-Roberts recommended passing a K-wire percutaneously through the capitellum and into the proximal radius to stabilize the reduction.[49] As discussed previously, we do not recommend this procedure because of the frequency of complications, including pin breakage and irreversible joint stiffness.[96] The arm should be immobilized in a long arm cast with the forearm in supination and the elbow flexed to 80 degrees. We feel that immobilizing the elbow in a position less than 90 degrees may allow room inside the cast for some swelling and decrease the possibility of development of a compartment syndrome. Once the swelling has subsided, a new snug long arm cast is applied. Six weeks after the surgery, range-of-motion exercises are begun. The complication of cross union of the proximal radius and ulna has been encountered using this technique,[91] and therefore early motion with continuous passive motion and subsequently cast bracing is recommended if the radial head is sufficiently stable intraoperatively.

Malunion

Varus angulation of the ulna is the most common residual deformity; unlike posterior angulation, it is not associated with redislocation of the radial head. In the study by Olney and Menelaus, up to 25 degrees of angulation was still consistent with full range of motion of the elbow and forearm.[65]

Nerve Injuries

Nerve palsies secondary to the Monteggia fracture-dislocation occur in 11 to 20% of cases.[4, 65] The posterior interosseous nerve is most frequently injured in type III lesions, with lateral dislocation of the radial head; but this injury can also occur in type I injuries (Fig. 6–54).[65] The injury may be caused by direct pressure from the radial head, compression at the proximal edge of the arcade of Frohse, or entrapment between the radial head and the ulna, or it may be due to traction.[56, 82] Surgical exploration of the nerve is not indicated, since the radial nerve usually undergoes spontaneous recovery within 6 months of the injury.[11, 65] If early recovery of the nerve is not apparent with electromyographic (EMG) evaluation within 3 months of the injury, surgical exploration is warranted.

Ulnar nerve injury can also occur from compression within the cubital tunnel. If recovery does not take place spontaneously, surgical decompression is frequently successful.[84] Injuries to the radial nerve and median nerve have also been reported in association with the Monteggia lesion. Recovery occurred in all cases within 6 months of the injury.[65]

GALEAZZI FRACTURES

Although first described by Sir Astley Cooper in 1822, this fracture pattern has been named after Riccardo Galeazzi, who in 1934 described his experience with the fracture of the distal radius accompanied by a disruption of the distal radioulnar joint. This is a rare injury in children, with the peak incidence between 9 and 12 years of age.[53, 94]

Classification

No formal classification has been described for this fracture. The classic type is a fracture of the shaft of the radius in association with a dislocation of the distal radioulnar joint. The fracture occurs most frequently at the junction of the middle and distal thirds of the radius but may occur within the distal third of the radius.[94] Another variation of this lesion includes fractures of both radius and ulna, or double fractures of the radius in association with a dislocation of the distal radioulnar joint.[53] The configuration of the fracture is usually transverse, and less frequently oblique or spiral. It can be displaced anteriorly or posteriorly.[94]

In children, the Galeazzi equivalent is a fracture of the radius associated with a separation of the distal ulnar epiphysis or a fracture of the distal 2 cm of the ulna (Fig. 6–55).[72, 94] In this case the distal radioulnar joint is not disrupted because the ulnar epiphysis remains attached to the distal end of the radius. Reckling noted that the Galeazzi equivalent fracture is more likely to occur in children because the epiphyseal plate is weaker than the articular disk (Fig. 6–56).[72]

The Essex-Lopresti fracture, which is a fracture of the radial neck or head associated with a dislocation of the distal radioulnar joint, is not generally considered to be a Galeazzi fracture.[53] The mechanism of injury is a longitudinal force on the outstretched hand that creates a compressive force through the radial head into the capitellum. This has not been reported in children. However, we have encountered a variant of this fracture in a 12-year-old girl (Fig. 6–57).

Mechanism of Injury

The usual mechanism of injury is a fall on the outstretched hand combined with extreme pronation of the forearm. The articular disk tears or becomes detached at the extremes of pronation and extension of the wrist, with dislocation occurring secondary to the rotational forces. A direct blow may be responsible in a minority of cases.[53] Distal fractures tend to be associated with more severe trauma than do proximal injuries and frequently are the result of a fall from a height.[94]

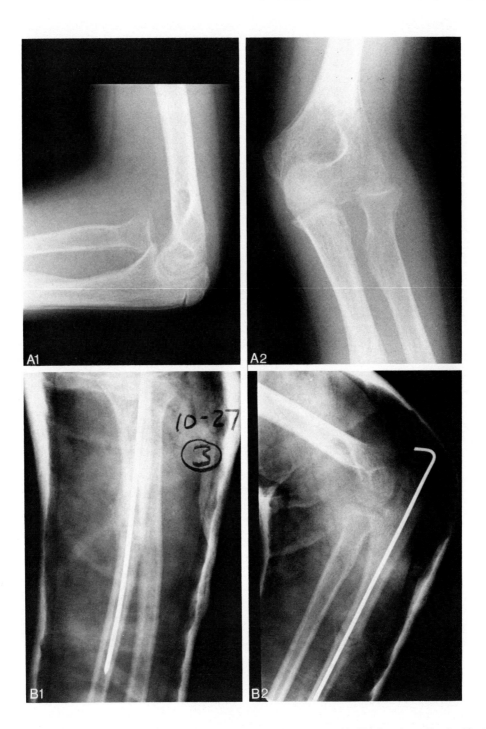

Figure 6-54

Recurrent radial head dislocation after a Monteggia fracture-dislocation. *A,* An 11-year-old girl fell and sustained a Monteggia fracture-dislocation. She was treated by closed manipulation and casting in hyperflexion. After 5 weeks the cast was removed, and she was found to have redislocation of the radial head. *B,* With the patient under general anesthesia, an osteoclasis of the ulna and intramedullary fixation were performed. Initial x-rays showed that the radial head seemed to be reduced. There was full range of motion of the forearm in the operating room. The patient was immobilized in a long arm cast. Postoperatively she had a posterior interosseous palsy.

Illustration continued on following page

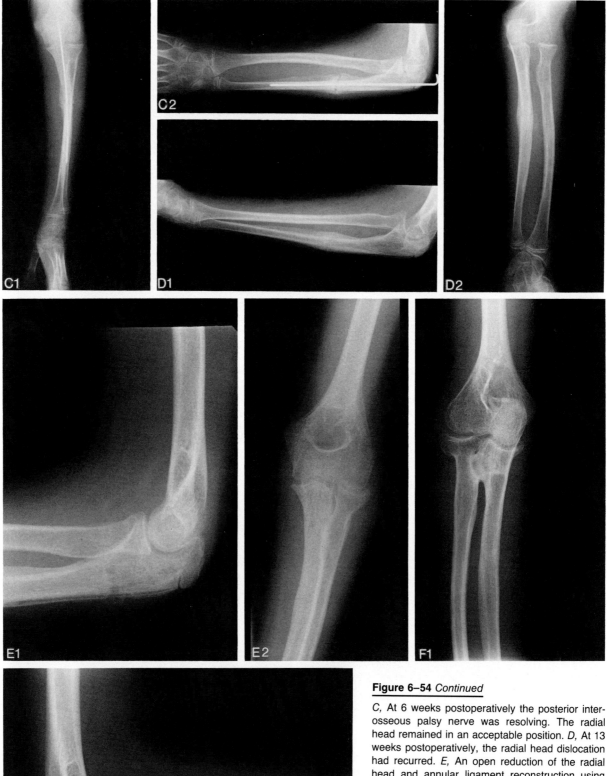

Figure 6–54 *Continued*

C, At 6 weeks postoperatively the posterior interosseous palsy nerve was resolving. The radial head remained in an acceptable position. *D,* At 13 weeks postoperatively, the radial head dislocation had recurred. *E,* An open reduction of the radial head and annular ligament reconstruction using the Lloyd-Roberts modification of the Bell-Tawse procedure were done. Postoperatively the child was treated in a continuous passive motion machine. *F,* At 3 months after the operative procedure, she had developed a proximal radioulnar synostosis. Her forearm is fixed in slight supination, and she may ultimately require a repositioning osteotomy.

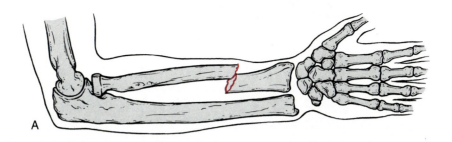

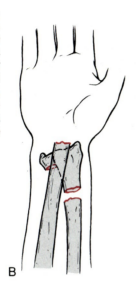

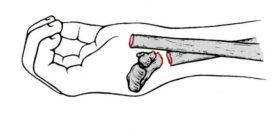

Figure 6–55

A, Galeazzi fracture-dislocation. *B,* Galeazzi-equivalent lesion, which consists of a fracture of the distal radius in association with a separation of the distal ulnar epiphysis or a fracture of the distal 2 cm of the ulna. (From Reckling, F.W. Unstable fracture-dislocations of the forearm [Monteggia and Galeazzi lesions]. J Bone Joint Surg 64-A:857, 1982.)

A complete dislocation of the distal radioulnar joint always involves rupture of the articular disk and of the associated dorsal and volar distal radioulnar ligaments. The Galeazzi fracture-dislocation is unstable owing to (1) disruption of the triangular fibrocartilage complex and (2) mechanical factors acting on the distal fragment of the radius. The most important stabilizing force is provided by the triangular fibrocartilage.[53, 73] The question of whether the triangular fibrocartilage is ruptured is the crucial one in determining the presence of a Galeazzi lesion. Some authors feel that avulsion of the ulnar styloid process is an indication of disruption of the triangular fibrocartilage.[53]

The mechanical factors acting on the distal fragment of the radius contribute to the instability of this fracture. The brachioradialis tends to shorten the radius via its insertion into the radial styloid; the pronator quadratus rotates the distal radial fragment toward the ulna; and the force of the thumb abductors and extensors tends to relax the radial collateral ligament and shorten the radial side of the wrist. The weight of the hand also acts as a strong volar displacing force.[53, 73]

Diagnosis

The clinical appearance is an angular concave deformity on the radial side of the forearm, which seems shortened. The distal radioulnar joint may be deformed, swollen, and painful. The ulnar head may seem to protrude and may be slightly more mobile than usual. An apparently solitary fracture of the radius should raise clinical suspicion of disruption of the distal radioulnar joint. Adequate anteroposterior and lateral x-rays are important in making the correct diagnosis. Walsh and co-workers found that the diagnosis had been missed in 41% of cases.[94]

Management

Most of these fractures in children can be managed with closed treatment.[53, 72, 94] If the radial fracture is very accurately reduced and the forearm is immobilized in full supination, the torn articular disk and associated ligaments will be approximated and will heal in an appropriate position.[72, 73, 94] The arm should be immobilized in an above-elbow plaster cast with the forearm in supination for about 6

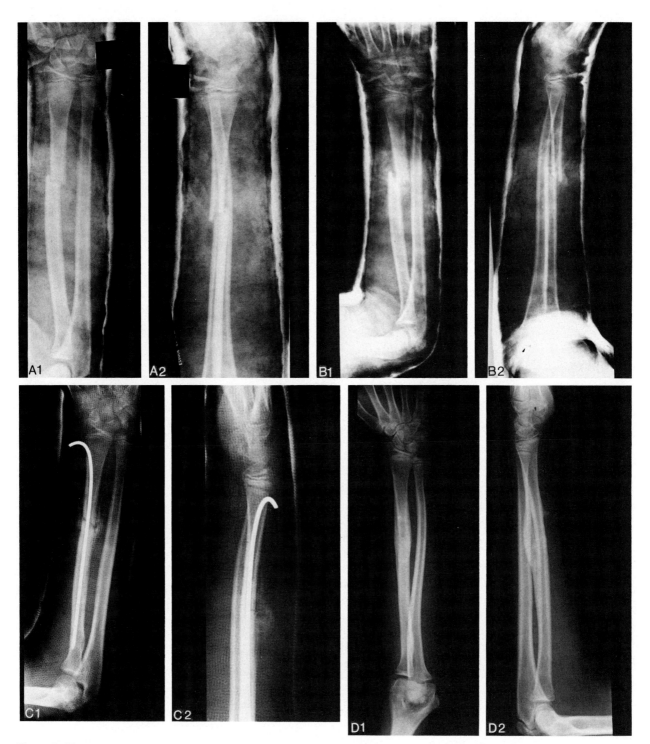

Figure 6–56

Galeazzi-equivalent fracture. *A,* An 11-year-old boy with a fracture of the radius associated with plastic deformation of the distal ulna. *B,* Although initially in good position, the fracture displaced. The plastic deformity was not corrected. *C,* A closed intramedullary pinning of the radius was performed. The pin was removed at 6 weeks. *D,* Follow-up study shows excellent alignment of both radius and ulna.

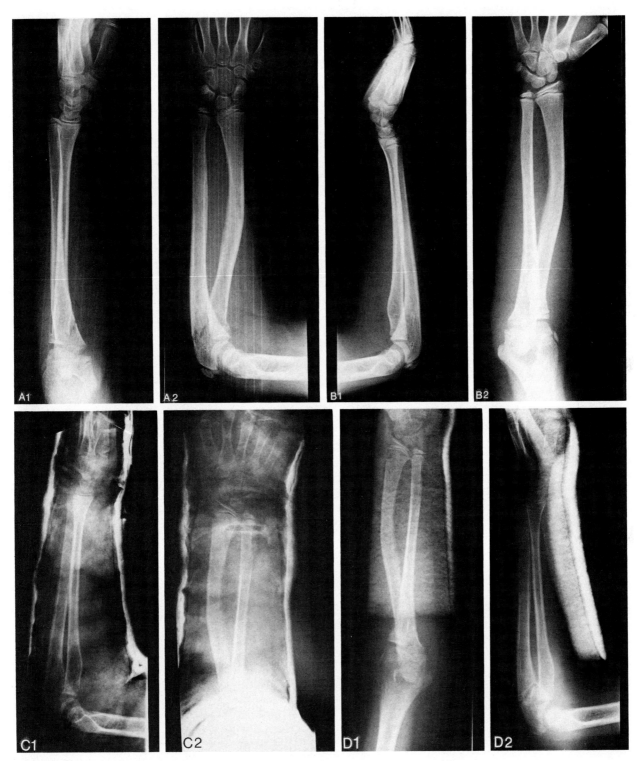

Figure 6–57

Essex-Lopresti variant. *A,* A 12-year-old girl tripped and fell onto her outstretched arm. She complained of pain in the elbow and wrist. Undisplaced fractures of the radial neck and olecranon are visible. Note the soft tissue swelling over the dorsal wrist, the widening of the distal radioulnar joint, and the dorsal dislocation of the distal ulna. *B,* X-rays of the opposite forearm, taken for comparison, confirmed that the distal radioulnar joint in the injured forearm was abnormal. The anatomic configuration of the radius was identical to that of the injured forearm, ruling out previous injury as a cause of the apparently excessive bowing of the radius. *C,* The patient was treated in a long arm cast with the forearm in supination. The distal radioulnar joint was reduced in this position. The cast was maintained for 4 weeks. *D,* It was replaced by a short arm splint for 2 additional weeks. At follow-up examination the patient remained asymptomatic, with full range of motion of the forearm.

weeks. This holds true for both anterior and posterior displacements of the radial fracture.[94] Follow-up should be on a weekly basis until the fracture healing is apparent on x-ray (Fig. 6-58).

An oblique fracture pattern in the radius is relatively unstable. If the fracture of the distal radius cannot be maintained in less than 10 degrees of angulation and without shortening of greater than 4 mm, open reduction of the distal radius should be considered.

Complications

Malunion with recurrent radioulnar subluxation can occur. This complication is very rare in the pediatric age group. Poorer results are seen if the diagnosis is delayed and if the forearm has been immobilized in an incorrect position or in a below-elbow cast.[94] If recurrent subluxation becomes a clinical problem, surgical reconstruction of the distal radioulnar joint should be considered. Rarely, nerve injuries have been described in association with the Galeazzi fracture and include injuries to the ulnar nerve at the distal ulna and an interosseous nerve palsy.[53, 74]

Wrist Injuries

DISLOCATION OF THE DISTAL RADIOULNAR JOINT

Isolated dislocations of the distal radioulnar joint are uncommon. They are more likely to occur in older children who are approaching maturity. This injury is in reality a dislocation of the radiocarpal complex from the ulna, although commonly it is described as a dorsal or volar dislocation of the distal ulna.[16, 27, 31, 61] With this injury, damage is to the triangular fibrocartilage complex in association with the dorsal or volar radioulnar ligaments.

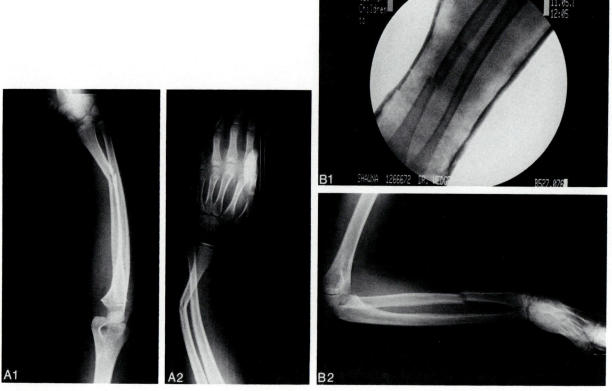

Figure 6-58

Fracture of the distal third of the radius. *A,* A 7-year-old girl fell, suffering a fracture of the distal radius and a greenstick fracture of the ulna. The pronation deformity in the forearm is well visualized on these films, since an anteroposterior view of the radius and ulna is seen in conjunction with a lateral view of the wrist. The distal radioulnar joint does not appear to be disrupted. *B,* The fracture was reduced with the patient under general anesthesia and the forearm placed in supination. A 50% end-on apposition of the radius was obtained, and this was accepted.

Illustration continued on facing page

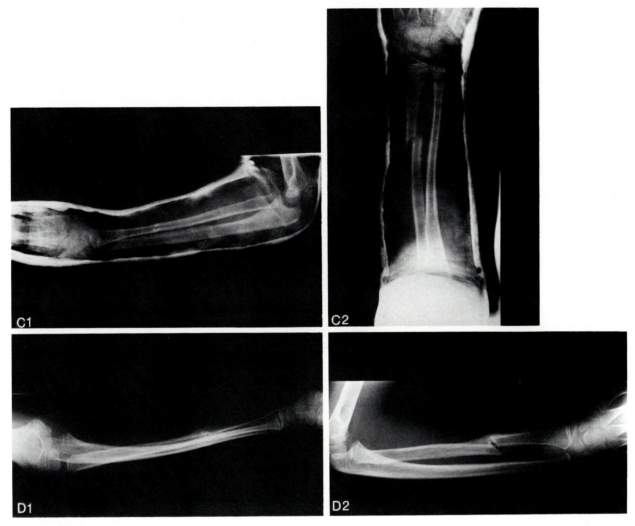

Figure 6–58 Continued

C, The interosseous distance is narrowed proximally, and the fracture has displaced slightly. This was accepted. *D,* The injury continued to heal uneventfully, and follow-up examination confirmed full range of motion of the forearm.

Mechanism of Injury

The mechanism of injury is usually a fall on the outstretched hand. Hypersupination injuries can result in a tear of the volar radioulnar ligament, causing volar displacement of the distal ulna. Injury to the dorsal radioulnar ligament occurs with hyperpronation injuries, resulting in dorsal dislocation of the distal ulna (Fig. 6–59).[61, 76]

Diagnosis

The distal ulna is usually tender, and pain can be elicited with compression of the distal radius and ulna. Any attempt to pronate or supinate the forearm will be painful. With dorsal dislocation of the ulna, as for Galeazzi fractures, careful physical examination will reveal a dorsal prominence of the distal ulna along with fixed pronation of the forearm.

If the dislocation is volar, the normal dorsal prominence of the distal ulna may disappear, and there may be a slight prominence on the anterior aspect of the wrist. Frequently there is a marked furrow on the medial side of the distal extensor aspect of the forearm. The distal forearm has a narrowed appearance and is fixed in supination.[76] Adequate anteroposterior and lateral views of the wrist are important to make the correct diagnosis. Comparison views of the opposite forearm are frequently necessary. Volar displacement of the ulna in relation to the radius is best seen on the lateral radiograph, and commonly the ulnar styloid process is broken at its base.[76] The ulna and radius may appear to be overlapping on the anteroposterior view.

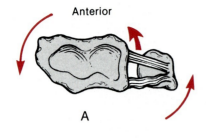
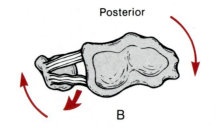
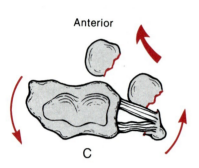
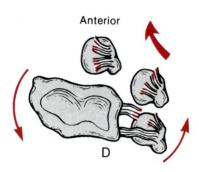

Figure 6–59

End-on views of the radioulnar joint in supination *(A)* and in pronation *(B)*, showing the suggested mechanism of injury in distal radioulnar dislocations. *C–D,* Possible variations of the injury. (From Rose-Innes, A.P. Anterior dislocation of the ulna at the interior radioulnar joint. J Bone Joint Surg 42-B:515, 1960.)

Management

The dislocation is reduced by reversing the mechanism of injury and applying direct pressure over the distal ulna. The arm is immobilized in a long arm cast for 6 weeks with the forearm in supination for dorsal dislocations and in pronation for volar dislocations.

If the dislocation has been missed, symptomatic injuries can be treated by soft tissue reconstructive procedures, including rerouting of the tendon of extensor carpi ulnaris or use of a fascial sling.[76] Unfortunately, the results of this surgery are not always effective. The Darrach procedure, i.e., excision of the distal ulna, should be avoided in growing children to prevent the late complication of dislocation of the radial head. At the end of growth, chronic symptoms can be relieved by distal ulnar excision.[61]

CARPAL DISLOCATIONS

Carpal dislocations are rare in children. They are more likely to occur in those who are approaching skeletal maturity and hence can be treated as adult fractures. The mechanism of these injuries is usually a crush that may or may not be associated with a fall.[61]

Management

Undisplaced fractures can be treated in a short arm cast for 6 weeks. Closed reduction of displaced fractures can be difficult. Traction is best applied using finger traps, and with the aid of the image intensifier to check the reduction, the wrist is manipulated into radial or ulnar deviation, dorsiflexion, and palmar flexion (Fig. 6–60). Usually these fractures are unstable, and percutaneous pinning using one to three K-wires must be performed. A short arm cast is maintained for 6 weeks, at which time the pins are removed. These fractures are likely to redisplace, and weekly x-ray follow-up is recommended (Fig. 6–61). If an adequate closed reduction cannot be obtained, an open reduction is performed through a dorsal or volar approach.

FRACTURES OF THE CARPAL BONES

The lunate, scaphoid, and pisiform frequently have more than one center of ossification, which may be mistaken for a fracture. The developing carpus is mostly cartilage, and because of its cushioning effect, this makes fracture or dislocation of the carpus in children extremely rare.[61] The scaphoid is the most commonly injured carpal bone, with most fractures occurring in children between the ages of 10 and 15 years. Although fractures of the lunate, capitate, and pisiform have been reported, these are rare.[61]

Mechanism of Injury

Fractures of the scaphoid constitute 0.45% of children's upper limb fractures. Like most pediatric

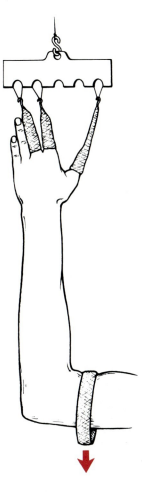

Figure 6–60

Application of traction using finger traps. (From King, R.E. Fractures of the shafts of the radius and ulna. In: Rockwood, C.A.J.; Wilkins, K.E.; King, R.E., eds. Fractures in Children. Vol 3. Philadelphia, J.B. Lippincott, 1984, pp. 301–362.)

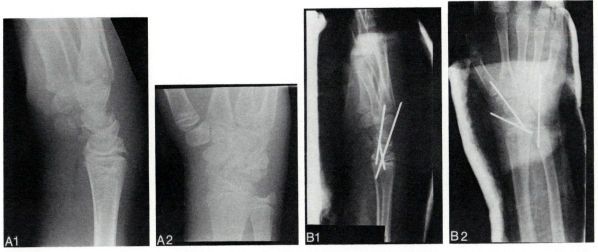

Figure 6–61

Greater arc fracture of the wrist A, A 12½-year-old girl suffered a fracture when a metal railing fell on her right wrist. B, A closed reduction was performed with the patient under general anesthesia using pronation and radial deviation of the wrist to reduce the scaphoid and radial styloid fractures. The fractures were pinned percutaneously, and a short arm thumb spica cast was applied. The fracture was carefully followed with weekly x-rays to ensure that the reduction was maintained.

forearm injuries, they usually result from a fall on the outstretched hand (Fig. 6–62). The fractures occur most frequently in the distal pole (59%) and mainly at the scaphoid tuberosity, presumably the result of an avulsion injury. Fractures of the waist of the scaphoid are less common (33%).[14]

Diagnosis

Similar to adult scaphoid fractures, there is swelling over the dorsal aspect of the radiocarpal joint and especially over the anatomic snuffbox. Wrist motion is limited by pain. There is tenderness over the anatomic snuffbox and scaphoid tuberosity. These fractures are best visualized radiographically on the oblique or pronated view. Fracture displacement is rare. Incomplete or single cortex fractures occur in 23% of pediatric cases.[14]

Management

Initial x-rays may be normal in 12% of cases.[14] If there is a clinical suspicion of a scaphoid fracture, the wrist should be immobilized in a thumb spica cast for 2 weeks, at which time the x-rays are repeated. If there is no evidence of a fracture at that time, the cast can be safely removed. If a scaphoid fracture is detected, the cast is reapplied for another 4 weeks.

Most scaphoid fractures in children heal within 6 weeks of injury, and nonunion is rare. The prime cause of delayed union or nonunion is a delay in diagnosis or displacement of the fracture. Continued immobilization will usually result in fracture union. If union is not obtained by 6 months after the injury, autogenous bone grafting, using an anterior approach to the scaphoid, is indicated.[14, 80]

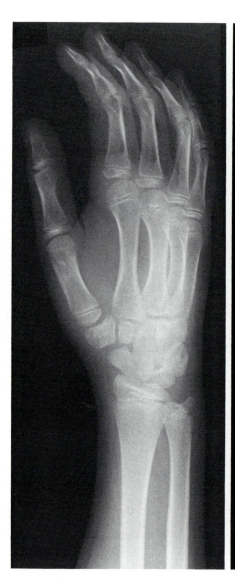
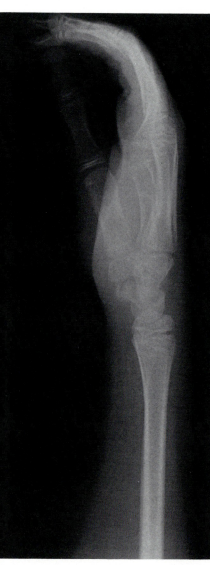

Figure 6–62

Fracture of the scaphoid tuberosity. A 12-year-old boy slipped in the schoolyard and landed on the extended right hand. He was treated in a thumb spica cast for 6 weeks, and the fracture healed uneventfully.

CARPOMETACARPAL DISLOCATIONS

These injuries are rare in children and are usually the result of violent trauma. They most frequently occur in combination with fractures of the adjoining metacarpal. Carpometacarpal dislocation of the thumb is especially uncommon because the stress causes a growth plate injury to the adjacent physis.

Management

After closed reduction, pin fixation to the adjacent metacarpals and carpus is recommended because these fracture-dislocations tend to be unstable. If an adequate closed reduction cannot be accomplished, open reduction through a dorsal approach should be undertaken.[30, 38, 78, 97] The hand and wrist are immobilized in a short arm cast with the hand in the "position of safety" (i.e., with the metacarpophalangeal joints immobilized at 90 degrees and the interphalangeal joints extended) for 4 weeks. The child is then started on exercises to recover range of motion in the hand. The pins are removed at 6 weeks from the time of injury.

Fractures and Dislocations of the Hand

INCIDENCE

Hand trauma is certainly very common in childhood, both early as toddlers begin to explore the world around them and later as young teenagers assert their independence. The epidemiology of these injuries reflects the changing patterns of activity throughout the growing years. Hastings and Simmons have undertaken a retrospective review of 354 pediatric hand fractures with a minimum 2-year follow-up.[106] All patients were under 18 years of age. The peak incidence of fractures was in the early teenage years, possibly related to contact sports. A smaller peak was seen in infancy, related mostly to crush injuries in doors. The etiology varies with age, but overall Hastings and Simmons found that the mechanisms included torque and angulation (34%), crush (21%), direct blow (10%), axial compression (9.5%), unknown (24%), and in one case, a pathologic fracture.[106] The little finger is involved most commonly (30%); the thumb is involved in 20% and the other fingers in near-equal distributions (index, 16%; middle, 16%; and ring fingers, 18%). Fractures of the proximal phalanx account for nearly half the injuries seen (43%), while fractures of the metacarpals and remaining phalanges are evenly distributed.

PRINCIPLES OF TREATMENT

Anesthesia

Anesthesia both for closed reduction of phalangeal fractures and for the treatment of open injuries of the fingertip is best accomplished with a digital nerve block at the base of the affected digit. Infants and small children are bundled in a sheet or secured in a papoose-like wrap before the part is prepared. A 1% solution of lidocaine without epinephrine is instilled using a 3 ml syringe and a 27 or 30 gauge needle. A small bead of anesthetic is placed under the dorsal skin on the radial side of the digit, and through this the needle is advanced almost to the palmar skin along the shaft of the proximal phalanx. After the plunger is withdrawn to ensure that a vessel has not been punctured, the anesthetic is instilled while the needle is slowly withdrawn. A line of solution is then deposited along the dorsal surface of the digit, and, finally, the ulnar side is injected. No more than 1 ml of anesthetic should be required for one finger, since a greater amount risks vascular compromise by compression. Median nerve blocks at the wrist or ulnar nerve blocks at the cubital tunnel can be used for metacarpal fractures, but we prefer hematoma blocks to reduce the risk of direct injection into the nerve. General anesthesia is rarely required for closed fractures in children but is frequently necessary in dislocations and open fractures with soft tissue injuries.

Manipulation

The manipulation of fractures and dislocations can prove quite difficult in children, given their small size. Adequate anesthesia is the key. An assistant who can both comfort and control the child is invaluable. Flexion of the metacarpophalangeal (MP) or interphalangeal (IP) joints of the finger usually aids in securing sufficient purchase as well as in improving control of the reduction. Occasionally it is necessary to use a fulcrum in manipulating fractures at the base of the proximal phalanx. A pencil or smooth pen barrel, being a familiar, non-threatening object, is effective.

Immobilization

Since most hand fractures in children can be satisfactorily treated with immobilization alone,[108] an understanding of the attendant principles is warranted. If the adult position of hand immobilization with the wrist and IP joints in extension and the MP joints flexed is used in small children, they can often pull their fingers into a fist and escape the bandage. In order to reduce the risk of the child's shedding the plaster, the wrist and MP joints are extended; this makes the effective lever arm for control of the metacarpal bones and phalanges together, reducing the chance of the child's flexing the fingers in the splint.

Immobilization of the small child's hand requires a more thorough effort than may be necessary in the adult. Plasters for children under 6 years of age should routinely extend above the flexed elbow, even to splint fingers or metacarpals. Skin glue can be used to enhance the security of the bandage. In older children a forearm plaster slab is sufficient. Our preference is to use a volar or dorsal slab, or both, as necessary in the first few days following injury. On follow-up examination the bandage is removed, repeat radiographs are taken, and, if the reduction is satisfactorily maintained, a circumferential plaster is applied. If the fracture is not sufficiently stable to remain reduced during the period required for films, it probably requires at least pin fixation, if not open reduction.

While plates and screws have become a standard method of fixation in adult hand fractures, such fixation is possible only occasionally in children's hand fractures.[114] The extensive dissection and periosteal stripping required for internal fixation increase the risk of devascularizing the epiphyses of small bones. In addition, the bulk of the hardware often precludes its use. In contrast to adults, the thick periosteum of children's bones can be used to advantage in providing a strong hinge against which to reduce a fracture. K-wires in sizes of 0.028, 0.035, and 0.045 inch are easily used to provide secure fixation. K-wires can be allowed to protrude through the skin with no untoward effects,[108] and, if they are left in place less than 4 weeks, pin tract infection is rare.

Many methods are available to facilitate elevation of a child's hand following reduction. We prefer a stockingette bandage with the proximal end split and tied around the chest and the opposite end suspended from an intravenous pole. Alternatively, the bandage can be secured to an overhead line of twill tape running from one end of the crib to the other.[116]

FRACTURES

In the majority of cases, fractures of the child's hand can be treated successfully by closed means.

Leonard and Dubravcik reviewed a large series of 263 hand fractures in children under 17 years of age.[108] Treatment consisted of splinting alone in 75% of cases, manipulation and splinting in 15%, and open reduction in 10%. Their particular indications for open reduction included open wounds and fractures of the phalangeal neck.

Fracture healing in a child is very rapid, occurring in about half the time required for an adult. Nonunion is extremely rare.[118] For these reasons, immobilization can often be limited to 3 weeks, particularly when the metaphysis or epiphysis is involved. Overtreatment may be a major source of complications.[118]

Malalignment may be corrected by remodeling with growth.[104] In general, fractures displaced within the plane of joint motion remodel quite satisfactorily, whereas those deviating laterally from the joint plane do less well. Rotational deformity does not correct with further growth and may not be acceptable. Therefore, limited indications exist for the operative treatment of fractures of the hand in a child (see below). When surgery is undertaken, however, particular care is required to manage delicate tissues and small bones.

Epiphyseal injury is a common finding in fractures in the child's hand. Hastings and Simmons found that 34% of their cases involved the epiphysis in the injury, with fractures through closing or recently closed epiphyses seen up to age 17 years.[106] The Salter-Harris classification of epiphyseal fractures[113] is described elsewhere (see Chapter 2). Salter-Harris type II injuries predominate (78.7%), with Salter-Harris types III (13.1%) and I (7.4%) being less common and Salter-Harris types IV (1.8%) and V being rare. Salter-Harris II injuries peak in the early teenage years. These fractures occurred in the proximal phalanx in 69% with the border digits predominating, injury in the little finger being the most common single fracture[106] and usually resulting from an abduction injury. Growth disturbance arising from injury to the epiphyseal plate is rare but is always a concern.

In general, Salter-Harris I and II injuries are treatable by closed reduction and immobilization and carry a favorable prognosis. Salter-Harris III and IV fractures are, by definition, intraarticular and should be opened and reduced anatomically to lessen the resulting joint incongruity and subsequent risk of late osteoarthritis. Clearly, it is necessary to assess the size of the intraarticular fragment and the feasibility of securing adequate fixation before proceeding. Types III and IV injuries have a worse prognosis. Treatment in the rare type V injury is dictated by the usually open nature of the wound and must be individualized to the case. The prognosis for normal growth in type V injuries is very guarded.

Distal Phalanx

Salter-Harris I and II fractures are the childhood equivalent of the mallet finger.[104] The flexor remains attached to the distal fragment, angulating it volarward, while the extensor is attached to the epiphysis, holding it in extension. The nail bed stays with the distal fragment. In the adolescent the mallet finger usually presents as a Salter-Harris III with a small intraarticular fragment. Usually this can be treated with splinting in extension, which should produce good or excellent results in 80% of patients.[111] This treatment can be used in open injuries as well, in which even the skin need not be closed.[111]

Recommendations for the operative treatment of displaced fragments vary widely. Campbell[104] favors anatomic reduction. McFarlane and Hampole[111] feel that operation is justified in an avulsion fracture of more than one third of the articular surface of the distal phalanx. One K-wire is placed to hold the fragment and another to hold the distal interphalangeal (DIP) joint in extension for 3 weeks. Splinting is maintained for 6 weeks. Niechajev[112] suggests that operation be reserved for those with subluxation of the distal phalanx or with fragments displaced more than 3 mm. He uses a pull-out wire to hold the already reduced fragment in place.

In fractures of the volar aspect of the DIP joint, an avulsion injury of the profundus tendon must always be considered. These injuries are seen in teenagers and involve the ring finger in 75% of cases.[107] Although in the majority of these injuries either no fracture or a small flake fracture will be seen, in unusual cases a large bony fragment may represent an intraarticular component sufficient to require K-wire fixation.[107] In small children, a 25 or 27 gauge hypodermic needle may be a suitable substitute for achieving fixation. Avulsions of the profundus tendon occur without fracture as well; in these cases surgery for the tendon injury is required, with either a direct tendon repair or fixation with a pull-out wire.

Open fractures of the distal phalanx are often accompanied by injury to the nail bed. Although a full discussion of these injuries is beyond the scope of this chapter, some points bear emphasis. Zook and co-workers[120] studied 290 consecutive nail bed injuries over a 5½ year period. After reviewing their results they concluded that nail bed lacerations should be repaired under tourniquet control and loupe magnification after removing the nail plate.

For the nail bed, 7-0 chromic sutures were used, and 5-0 or 6-0 nylon sutures for the skin component of the lacerations. If a fracture of the distal phalanx is associated with a nail bed injury, it is important to reduce the fracture as accurately as possible in order to achieve a flat nail bed.[119] A K-wire may sometimes be necessary to maintain the reduction. In multiply comminuted fractures the fragments should be reduced as much as possible and the nail plate used as a splint.[119] These authors prefer the use of the original nail for splinting open the eponychial fold rather than a piece of gauze, as postoperative discomfort is reduced.[120] Wood[118] prefers to leave the nail plate attached in fractures of the distal phalanx, levering it back into position under the eponychial fold, to further splint the fracture.

Middle Phalanx

Fractures of the middle phalanx usually result from forces applied directly to the bone, whereas loads applied to the whole digit commonly injure the base of the proximal phalanx. Transverse fractures of the shaft of the middle phalanx can be treated in a fashion comparable to that for the proximal phalanx (see below), with unstable fractures requiring pinning. Longitudinal crush injuries are often stable and minimally displaced and, if not intraarticular, can be treated with protective immobilization alone.

Oblique fractures of the distal middle or proximal phalanx should be very carefully assessed radiologically, since they are often intraarticular, with the fracture splitting the two articular condyles (Fig. 6-63). Treatment of this injury, once diagnosed, is controversial. Campbell[104] recommends following undisplaced fractures radiologically for evidence of slippage and intervening if necessary. Our preference is to pin these fractures with a single oblique K-wire to obviate the later displacement that can occur. Mobilization is undertaken after 3 weeks.

Epiphyseal injuries in the middle phalanx are uncommon. Most laterally directed forces cause injury to the epiphyseal plate of the proximal phalanx. Closed reduction and appropriate immobilization should prove adequate.

Proximal Phalanx

Salter-Harris II fractures of the base of the proximal phalanx are extremely common injuries and can almost all be treated by closed reduction and splinting (Fig. 6-64).[104] A digital nerve block is used. The MP joint is flexed, and a finger or pencil is placed in the appropriate web to allow a fulcrum on which the fracture can be reduced. Postreduction radio-

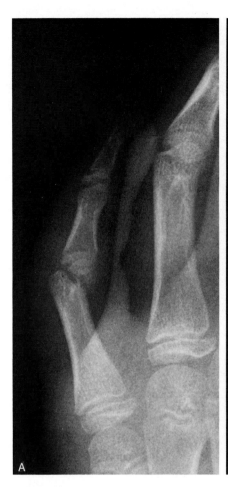
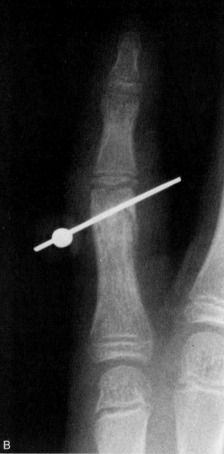

Figure 6–63

After falling from his bicycle, this 13-year-old was found to have an oblique fracture of the distal proximal phalanx. *A*, The fracture splits the two condyles. *B*, Closed reduction was successful with a single oblique K-wire being used to hold the fracture. The pin was left in place for 16 days before mobilization.

graphs are taken to confirm the reduction, and the finger is loosely "buddy-taped" to its neighbor. Plaster immobilization for 3 weeks with radiologic review after 3 to 7 days is undertaken.

In older children, however, Salter-Harris III or IV fractures may be seen, often as the epiphysis is beginning to close. These are intraarticular injuries which, given a fracture fragment of sufficient size to allow purchase with a K-wire, should be reduced anatomically (Fig. 6–65). Open reduction is usually required to provide adequate mobilization of the fracture, but care must be taken not to strip the periosteum, and hence the blood supply, to the epiphysis. The patient or family should be warned that these injuries may result in premature closure of the epiphysis with subsequent growth disturbance.

Hyperextension injuries to the MP joint can cause tears of the volar plate that present radiographically as small avulsion fractures of the volar base of the proximal phalanx. These injuries usually occur after the epiphyseal plates are closed. Tenderness and swelling are noted over the volar aspect of the joint but without ligament instability. Treatment consists of immobilization with the MP joint in flexion for 10 days followed by gradual mobilization.

Transverse phalangeal shaft fractures are usually stable and can be treated by immobilization alone.[108] If the fracture is unstable (meaning failure to obtain or maintain an adequate reduction), percutaneous pinning is used.[104] In particular, pinning or open reduction may be required in spiral fractures of the proximal phalanx, which are often very unstable (Fig. 6–66).[118] The use of plates for fixation may be considered in teenagers of adult size with closed epiphyses.

Fractures of the head or neck of the proximal phalanx must be examined very carefully. Truly undisplaced fractures of the neck of the proximal phalanx (supracondylar fractures) can be treated with splinting.[104] Rotation of the fragment in distal fractures of the proximal phalanx in children can easily be missed, however, particularly if true lateral radiographs are not obtained.[105] The distal fragment, which is small, may be rotated dorsally by as much as 180 degrees, with the intact collateral ligaments

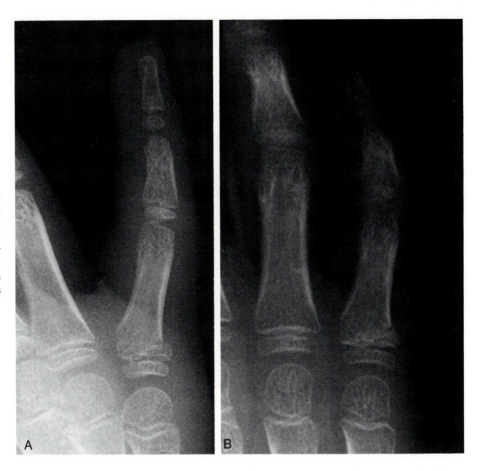

Figure 6–64

This 9-year-old boy fell down the stairs at home. *A,* He sustained a Salter-Harris II injury to the proximal phalanx of his little finger. Reduction was undertaken under digital block. *B,* Good maintenance of the reduction was seen at 3 weeks, when the finger was mobilized.

acting as the pivot point. On casual inspection, the radiograph appears to reveal a minimally displaced fracture, but the articular surface of the proximal phalanx may be facing directly into the fracture site. Open reduction is mandatory.[105] In those cases in which the dorsal angulation of distal fractures of the proximal phalanx has been missed or ignored, little remodeling is likely to occur, as there is no physis. A volar surgical approach with removal of the bone causing the block to flexion is described as a late reconstruction.[115]

Metacarpals

The degree of acceptable volar angulation in a fracture of the fifth metacarpal neck is controversial. Authors vary in their opinions, with some stating that 35 degrees of volar angulation of a boxer's fracture is acceptable,[102] and others recommending reduction of fractures at the neck of the metacarpal only if angulated more than 40 degrees into the palm or if unstable.[114] Our recommendation is to first attempt closed reduction under local anesthesia followed by plaster fixation. If on subsequent views taken 3 to 7 days later angulation greater than 30 degrees is seen, the patient is taken to the operating room, where a single longitudinal K-wire is placed after further closed reduction. This conclusion is based on the observation that most of these injuries occur in teenagers nearing the end of growth and that power grip may be affected if the fifth ray is angulated. In addition, inadequately treated or reduced fractures may present late with a tender lump in the palm. Reduction is achieved by holding the MP joint in 90 degrees of flexion, applying longitudinal traction, and pushing firmly over the dorsal convexity of the fracture. A K-wire is passed retrograde through the metacarpal head. Long-term follow-up of these injuries often reveals loss of the normal prominence of the fifth metacarpal head, and the patient and family should be made aware of this possible outcome.

Epiphyseal injuries of the metacarpal head are uncommon. Four were seen in a series of 103 fractures in 100 patients of all ages.[110] All were Salter-Harris III injuries that were treated with

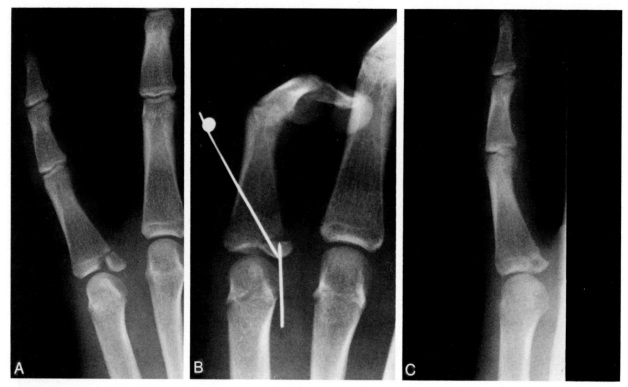

Figure 6–65

While playing lacrosse, this 17-year-old sustained a hyperextension injury of the little finger. *A*, This produced a Salter-Harris III fracture of his almost-closed epiphysis. Open reduction was undertaken by splitting the extensor tendon and rotating the small fragment through 90 degrees. *B*, Two K-wires were used for fixation. *C*, Two months later, consolidation of the fracture is seen with little articular deformity.

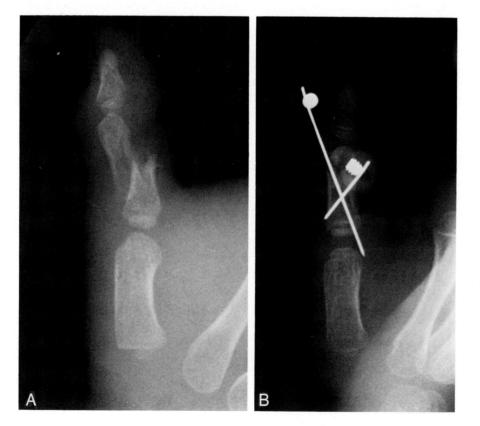

Figure 6–66

This 4-year-old fell on his outstretched hand. *A*, A spiral fracture of the proximal phalanx of the thumb is seen; closed reduction was not possible. At open reduction the extensor tendon was found to be torn away from the bone, with the ragged periosteum at the fracture site preventing reduction. *B*, Two K-wires were used to secure the reduced fracture fragments.

splinting and careful mobilization at 3 weeks, and all did well.

Avascular necrosis of the metacarpal head has been seen following blunt trauma. This is a difficult lesion to diagnose, since in the early stages the radiographs may be normal. This injury should be considered if there is a traumatic effusion of the MP joint.[110] The joint should be aspirated and the hand splinted. Late follow-up reveals stiffness and pain and radiologic evidence of collapse of the metacarpal head.

Fractures of the bases of the second through fifth metacarpals are frequently stable, and, if so, reduction is not required. Splinting in a forearm plaster is sufficient treatment.[114] If significantly malaligned, these fractures can be fixed with percutaneous K-wires.

Thumb

Most fractures of the thumb metacarpal occur at its base. Unlike in the adult thumb, the ligaments and capsule at the base of the thumb are extremely strong, with the weakest point at the physis and the proximal metaphysis. Salter-Harris II fractures are seen, but commonly the shaft of the metacarpal is fractured just distal to the epiphysis. The intraarticular fractures seen so often in adult practice are extremely uncommon in children.

Wood[118] accepts 30 degrees of angulation in fractures of the base of the thumb metacarpal that are angulated in a radial direction. In ulnar angulation, open reduction is often required, and redisplacement may be seen if closed treatment is used.[118] The translocation of the fragments relative to each other is often more of a concern than the angular deviation. Of particular note, the distal fragment can become lodged into the cleft between the bases of the first and second metacarpals. Such fractures require careful reduction to remove the potential bony block that might reduce the mobility of the carpometacarpal (CMC) joint of the thumb (Fig. 6–67).

Closed reduction of proximal shaft fractures of the thumb is made difficult by the inability to obtain sufficient control of the metacarpal fragment through the swollen thenar mass. In some cases, it may be of benefit to attempt reduction after several days have elapsed to allow resolution of the swelling. Open reduction, when indicated, is best approached through an incision between the glabrous and nonglabrous skin along the radial aspect of the thumb. Unlike in the adult fracture-dislocation, exposure of the CMC joint is not required.

DISLOCATIONS

Interphalangeal Joints

Dorsal dislocation of the DIP joint is rare in childhood[104] and is usually produced by a direct blow to the end of the finger (Fig. 6–68). Initial treatment is by closed reduction under local or, if necessary, general anesthesia. The finger is then immobilized for 10 days before gentle range of motion is encouraged. Failure of closed reduction requires an open dorsal approach with possible division of the collateral ligament.[104]

Dislocations of the proximal interphalangeal (PIP) joint in children are also rare. When they occur, the displacement is usually dorsal (Fig. 6–69). Closed manipulation should be sufficient treatment, with immobilization as described earlier. Irreducible injuries with an interposed volar plate or those that are unstable after reduction owing to collateral ligament injury[104] should be opened and repaired directly. Irreducible volar dislocations of the PIP joint, in contrast, have not been reported in the child.[104]

Metacarpophalangeal Joint

Dislocations of MP joints of digits other than the thumb and index finger are uncommon but have been reported[103] and can be treated using the principles described below.

Index Finger

Dislocation of the MP joint of the index finger may be either reducible or not. These injuries are characteristically caused by a hyperextension injury of the joint. With sufficient force the volar plate is torn and becomes interposed in the joint, and the lumbrical and flexor tendons cinch the neck of the metacarpal on its radial and ulnar sides, respectively. This combination renders the dislocation irreducible and is sometimes seen as the result of force applied to an otherwise reducible dislocation during attempted reduction. If gentle closed reduction fails, a volar zigzag surgical approach is recommended (Fig. 6–70).[109] Division of the A1 pulley may be sufficient to release the flexor noose; however, the volar plate usually requires axial incision to achieve adequate release. The joint is immobilized in 60 degrees of flexion for 10 days before gradual movement is begun.

Dislocation of the MP joint of the index metacarpal in the child may be complicated by vascular compromise of the physis of the metacarpal head or

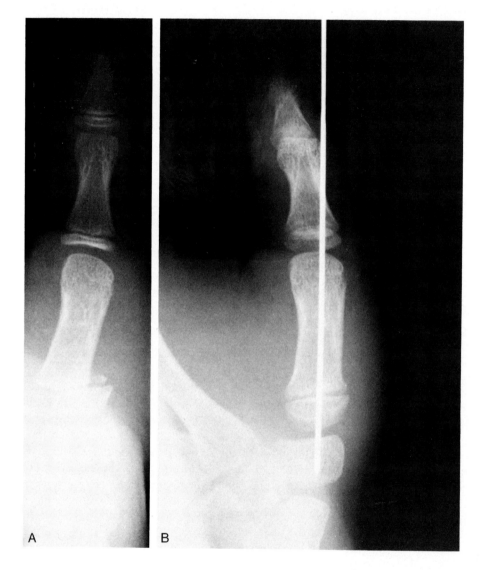

Figure 6–67

This 12-year-old fell from his bicycle, producing a Salter-Harris II fracture of the thumb metacarpal. *A,* Of note, the proximal end of the distal fragment is displaced toward the base of the second metacarpal, giving a potential bony block to unimpeded movement of the thumb CMC joint. *B,* Closed reduction was not possible immediately, but 5 days later, the swelling having subsided, manipulation achieved an excellent position that was fixed with a single axial K-wire.

Figure 6–68

A, A hyperextension injury dislocated the DIP joint of this 7-year-old's little finger. *B,* Reduction was undertaken with use of a digital block and was followed by splinting for 10 days.

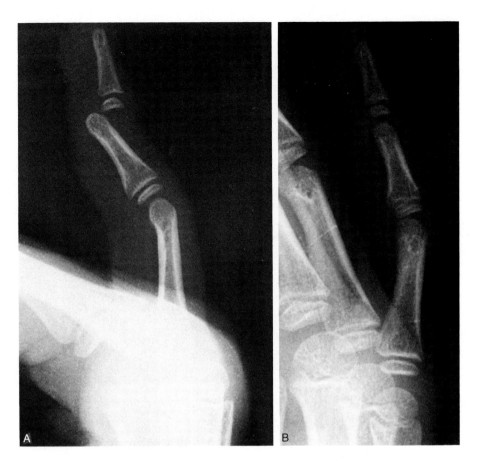

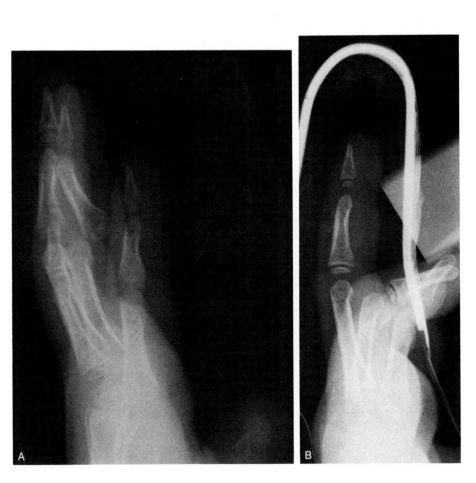

Figure 6–69

A window fell on the hand of this 3-year-old. *A,* A dorsal dislocation of the PIP joint is seen. *B,* Reduction was accomplished with use of local anesthesia. Immobilization was used for 3 weeks in this young child, with normal range of motion returning thereafter.

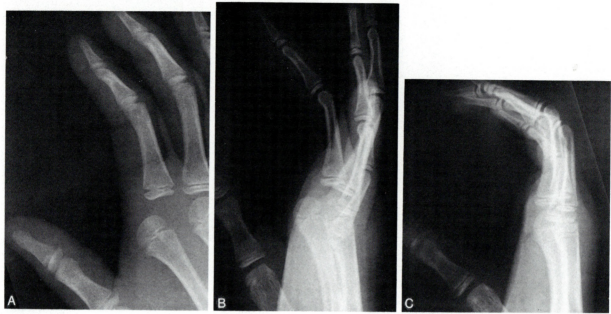

Figure 6–70

This 11-year-old dislocated the MP joint of the index finger. *A*, The oblique radiograph shows the widened joint space produced by the interposition of the volar plate. *B*, On the lateral view, the dorsal dislocation can be seen, with the second metacarpal head appearing unsatisfied in the palm. *C*, An open approach with division of the A1 pulley was required to achieve reduction in this case.

by osteochondral fracture, with either leading to subsequent deformity with growth. In addition, the vascular supply may be compromised by the operative exposure.[109]

Thumb

Irreducible dislocations of MP joints other than the index are rare.[104] In the thumb, ligament injury or fracture is much more commonly seen. Mild cases of forcible abduction and extension of the thumb usually yield a sprain of the ulnar collateral ligament of the MP joint. Stronger force produces a Salter-Harris III fracture of the base of the proximal phalanx or a proximal metacarpal shaft fracture. Ulnar collateral ligament avulsion without fracture is rare,[104] but if it should occur, Stener[117] observed that the proximal end of the ulnar collateral ligament of the MP joint of the thumb can fold back past the proximal edge of the adductor expansion. Displacement occurs during the extreme of forced abduction of the thumb when the proximal edge of the aponeurosis slides over the head of the metacarpal. This displacement renders nonoperative treatment of the lesion impossible.

Accurate descriptions of the pathologic anatomy of dislocation of the MP joint of the thumb are not new. Barnard[103] felt that the rent in the capsule supporting the volar plate entraps the head of the metacarpal. He goes on to describe in some detail a comparable dislocation of the MP joint of the little finger. When seen, dislocation of the MP joint of the thumb often requires open reduction. The head of the metacarpal is usually found protruding through the joint capsule and the flexor pollicis brevis,[118] which must be repaired.

SUMMARY

Trauma to the child's hand is common, with large numbers of fractures and some dislocations being seen in the emergency room. Most injuries can be treated in the emergency room setting except for those with associated injuries to nerve or tendon, which require general anesthesia for adequate management.

Early and frequent follow-up is the key in the closed management of fractures to confirm the adequacy of both the reduction and the splint. Immobilization can be maintained in infants and children for 3 weeks without risking development of significant residual stiffness. Injuries to the epiphyseal plate are common, since the ligaments and periosteum are strong and the epiphyses relatively weak. These injuries heal rapidly and without growth disturbance if appropriately treated.

REFERENCES

Forearm and Wrist

1. Abram, L. J.; Thompson, G. H. Deformity after premature closure of the distal radial physis following a torus fracture with a physeal, compression injury. Report of a case. J Bone Joint Surg 69-A:1450–1453, 1987.
2. Aitken, A. P. The end results of the fractured distal radial epiphysis. J Bone Joint Surg 17:302–308, 1935.
3. Amit, Y.; Salai, M.; Chechik, A.; et al. Closing intramedullary nailing for the treatment of diaphyseal forearm fractures in adolescence: a preliminary report. J Pediatr Orthop 5:143–146, 1985.
4. Bado, J. L. The Monteggia lesion. Clin Orthop 50:71–86, 1967.
5. Bailey, D. A.; Wedge, J. H.; McCulloch, R. G.; et al. Epidemiology of fractures of the distal end of the radius in children as associated with growth. J Bone Joint Surg 71-A:1225–1231, 1989.
6. Bell, M. F.; Hill, R. J.; McMurtry, R. Y. Ulnar impingement syndrome. J Bone Joint Surg 67-B:126–129, 1985.
7. Bell Tawse, A. J. S. The treatment of malunited anterior Monteggia fractures in children. J Bone Joint Surg 47-B:718–723, 1965.
8. Blount, W.; Shaefer, A.; Johnson, J. Fractures of the forearm in children. JAMA 120:111, 1942.
9. Blount, W. P. Forearm fractures in children. Clin Orthop 51:93–107, 1967.
10. Boyd, H. B. Surgical exposure of the ulna and proximal third of the radius through one incision. Surg Gynecol Obstet 71:87–88, 1940.
11. Boyd, H. B.; Boals, J. C. The Monteggia lesion. Clin Orthop 66:94–100, 1969.
12. Canale, S. T.; Puhl, J.; Watson, F. M.; Gillespie, R. Acute osteomyelitis following closed fractures. J Bone Joint Surg 57-A:415–418, 1975.
13. Christensen, J. B. A study of the interosseous distance between the radius and ulna during rotation of the forearm. J Bone Joint Surg 46-B:778–779, 1964.
14. Christodoulou, A. G.; Colton, C. L. Scaphoid fractures in children. J Pediatr Orthop 6:37–39, 1986.
15. Creasman, C.; Zaleske, D. J.; Ehrlich, M. G. Analyzing forearm fractures in children. The more subtle signs of impending problems. Clin Orthop 188:40–53, 1984.
16. Dameron, T. B. Traumatic dislocation of the distal radioulnar joint. Clin Orthop 83:55–63, 1972.
17. Daruwalla, J. S. A study of radioulnar movements following fractures of the forearm in children. Clin Orthop 139:114–120, 1979.
18. Evans, E. M. Fractures of the radius and ulna. J Bone Joint Surg 33-B:548–561, 1951.
19. Evans, E. M. Rotational deformity in the treatment of fractures of both bones of the forearm. J Bone Joint Surg 27:373–379, 1945.
20. Fahmy, N. R. M. Unusual Monteggia lesions in children. Injury 12(5):399–404, 1980.
21. Friberg, K. S. I. Remodelling after distal forearm fractures in children. I. The effect of residual angulation on the spatial orientation of the epiphyseal plates. Acta Orthop Scand 50:537–546, 1979.
22. Friberg, K. S. I. Remodelling after distal forearm fractures. II. The final orientation of the distal and proximal epiphyseal plates of the radius. Acta Orthop Scand 50:731–739, 1979.
23. Friberg, K. S. I. Remodelling after distal forearm fractures in children. III. Correction of residual angulation in fractures of the radius. Acta Orthop Scand 50:741–749, 1979.
24. Fuller, D. J.; McCullough, C. J. Malunited fractures of the forearm in children. J Bone Joint Surg 64-B:364–367, 1982.
25. Gainor, B. J.; Olson, S. Combined entrapment of the median and anterior interosseous nerves in a pediatric both-bone forearm fracture. J Orthop Trauma 4(2):197–199, 1990.
26. Gandhi, R. K.; Wilson, P.; Mason Brown, J. J.; Macleod, W. Spontaneous correction of deformity following fractures of the forearm in children. Br J Surg 50:5–10, 1962.
27. Gibson, A. Uncomplicated dislocation of the inferior radio-ulnar joint. J Bone Joint Surg 7:180–188, 1925.
28. Greulich, W. W.; Pyle, S. I. Radiographic Atlas of Skeletal Development of the Hand and Wrist, 2nd ed. Stanford, CA, Stanford University Press, 1964.
29. Gupta, R. P.; Danielsson, L. G. Dorsally angulated solitary metaphyseal greenstick fractures in the distal radius: results after immobilization in pronated, neutral, and supinated position. J Pediatr Orthop 10(1):90–92, 1990.
30. Hazlett, J. W. Carpometacarpal dislocations other than the thumb: A report of 11 cases. Can J Surg 11:315–322, 1968.
31. Heiple, K. G.; Freehafer, A. A. Isolated traumatic dislocation of the distal end of the ulna or distal radio-ulnar joint. J Bone Joint Surg 44-A:1387–1394, 1962.
32. Hogstrom, H.; Nilsson, B. E.; Willner, S. Correction with growth following diaphyseal forearm fracture. Acta Orthop Scand 47:299–303, 1976.
33. Hume, A. C. Anterior dislocation of the head of the radius associated with undisplaced fracture of the olecranon in children. J Bone Joint Surg 39-B:508–512, 1957.
34. Hurst, L. C.; Dubrow, E. N. Surgical treatment of symptomatic chronic radial head dislocation: a neglected Monteggia fracture. J Pediatr Orthop 3(2):227–230, 1983.
35. Kalamchi, A. Monteggia fracture-dislocation in children. Late treatment in two cases. J Bone Joint Surg 68-A:615–619, 1986.
36. Kay, S.; Smith, C.; Oppenheim, W. L. Both-bone midshaft forearm fractures in children. J Pediatr Orthop 6(3):306–310, 1986.
37. King, R. E. Fractures of the shafts of the radius and ulna. In: Rockwood, C. A. J.; Wilkins, K. E.; King, R. E., eds. Fractures in Children, Vol. 3. Philadelphia, J.B. Lippincott, 1984, pp. 301–362.
38. Kleinman, W. B.; Grantham, S. A. Multiple volar carpometacarpal dislocation. J Hand Surg 3:377–382, 1978.
39. Knight, R. A.; Purvis, G. D. Fractures of the forearm in adults. J Bone Joint Surg 31-A:755–764, 1949.
40. Kramhoft, M.; Solgaard, S. Displaced diaphyseal forearm fractures in children: classification and evaluation of the early radiographic prognosis. J Pediatr Orthop 9(5):586–589, 1989.
41. Langkamer, V. G.; Ackroyd, C. E. Removal of forearm plates (a review of the complications). J Bone Joint Surg 72-B(4):601–604, 1990.
42. Lascombes, P.; Prevot, J.; Ligier, J. N.; et al. Elastic stable intramedullary nailing in forearm shaft fractures in children: 85 cases. J Pediatr Orthop 10(2):167–171, 1990.
43. Lee, B. S.; Esterhai, J. L.; Das, M. Fracture of the distal radial epiphysis. Clin Orthop 185:90–96, 1984.
44. Lesko, P. D.; Georgis, T.; Slabaugh, P. Irreducible Salter-Harris type II fracture of the distal radial epiphysis. J Pediatr Orthop 7(6):719–721, 1987.

45. Letts, M.; Locht, R.; Weins, J. Monteggia fracture-dislocations in children. J Bone Joint Surg 67-B:724–727, 1985.
46. Levinthal, D. H. Fractures in the lower one-third of both bones of the forearm in children. Surg Gynecol Obstet 790–799, 1933.
47. Lewallen, R. P.; Peterson, H. A. Nonunion of long bone fractures in children: a review of 30 cases. J Pediatr Orthop 5(2):135–142, 1985.
48. Lichter, R. L.; Jacobsen, T. Tardy palsy of the posterior interosseous nerve with a Monteggia fracture. J Bone Joint Surg 57-A:124–125, 1975.
49. Lloyd-Roberts, G. C.; Bucknill, T. M. Anterior dislocation of the radial head in children. J Bone Joint Surg 59-B:402–407, 1977.
50. Mabrey, J. D.; Fitch, R. D. Plastic deformation in pediatric fractures: mechanism and treatment. J Pediatr Orthop 9(3):310–314, 1989.
51. Manoli, A. Irreducible fracture-separation of the distal radial epiphysis. J Bone Joint Surg 64-A:1095–1096, 1982.
52. Matthews, L. S.; Kaufer, H.; Garver, D. F.; Sonstegard, D. A. The effect on supination-pronation of angular malalignment of fractures of both bones of the forearm. J Bone Joint Surg 64-A:14–17, 1982.
53. Mikic, Z. D. Galeazzi fracture-dislocations. J Bone Joint Surg 57-A:1071–1080, 1975.
54. Moore, T. M.; Lester, D. K.; Sarmiento, A. The stabilizing effect of soft-tissue constraints in artificial Galeazzi fractures. Clin Orthop 194:189–194, 1985.
55. Morrey, B. F.; Askew, L. J.; An, K.; Chao, E. Y. A biomechanical study of normal functional elbow motion. J Bone Joint Surg 63-A:872–877, 1981.
56. Morris, A. H. Irreducible Monteggia lesion with radial-nerve entrapment. J Bone Joint Surg 56-A:1744–1746, 1974.
57. Mullick, S. The lateral Monteggia fracture. J Bone Joint Surg 59-A:543–545, 1977.
58. Nelson, O. A.; Buchanan, J. R.; Harrison, C. S. Distal ulnar growth arrest. J Hand Surg 9A(2):164–171, 1984.
59. Nielsen, A. B.; Simonsen, O. Displaced forearm fractures in children treated with AO plates. Injury 15(6):393–395, 1984.
60. Nilsson, B. E.; Obrant, K. The range of motion following fracture of the shaft of the forearm in children. Acta Orthop Scand 48:600–602, 1977.
61. O'Brien, E. T. Fractures of the hand and wrist region. In: Rockwood, C. A.; Wilkins, K. E.; Kin, R. E., eds. Fractures in Children, Vol. 3. Philadelphia, J. B. Lippincott, 1984, pp. 229–299.
62. Ogden, J. A. Complications. In: Ogden, J. A., ed. Skeletal Injury in the Child. Philadelphia, W. B. Saunders, 1990, pp. 247–248.
63. Ogden, J. A. Injury to the growth mechanisms. In: Ogden, J. A., ed. Skeletal Injury in the Child. Philadelphia, W. B. Saunders, 1990, pp. 97–174.
64. Ogden, J. A. Radius and ulna. In: Ogden, J. A., ed. Skeletal Injury in the Child. Philadelphia, W. B. Saunders, 1990, pp. 451–526.
65. Olney, B. W.; Menelaus, M. B. Monteggia and equivalent lesions in childhood. J Pediatr Orthop 9(2):219–223, 1989.
66. Papavasiliou, V.; Nenopoulos, S. Ipsilateral injuries of the elbow and forearm in children. J Pediatr Orthop 6(1):58–60, 1986.
67. Papavasiliou, V. A.; Nenopoulos, S. P. Monteggia-type elbow fractures in childhood. Clin Orthop 233:230–233, 1988.
68. Posman, C. L.; Little, R. E. Radioulnar synostosis following an isolated fracture of the ulnar shaft. Clin Orthop 213:207–210, 1986.
69. Ranawat, C. S.; Defiore, J.; Straub, L. R. Madelung's deformity. An end-result study of surgical treatment. J Bone Joint Surg 57-A:772–775, 1975.
70. Rang, M. Children's Fractures, 2nd ed. Philadelphia, J. B. Lippincott, 1982, p. 197 ff.
71. Ravessoud, F. A. Lateral condylar fracture and ipsilateral ulnar shaft fracture: Monteggia equivalent lesions? J Pediatr Orthop 5(3):364–366, 1985.
72. Reckling, F. W. Unstable fracture-dislocations of the forearm (Monteggia and Galeazzi lesions). J Bone Joint Surg 64-A:857–863, 1982.
73. Reckling, F. W.; Cordell, L. D. Unstable fracture-dislocations of the forearm. Arch Surg 96:999–1007, 1968.
74. Reckling, F. W.; Peltier, L. F. Riccardo Galeazzi and Galeazzi's fracture. Surgery 58:2453–2459, 1965.
75. Roberts, J. A. Angulation of the radius in children's fractures. J Bone Joint Surg 68-B:751–754, 1986.
76. Rose-Innes, A. P. Anterior dislocation of the ulna at the inferior radio-ulnar joint. J Bone Joint Surg 42-B:515–521, 1960.
77. Salter, R. B.; Harris, W. R. Injuries involving the epiphyseal plate. J Bone Joint Surg 45-A:587–622, 1963.
78. Sandzen, S. C. Fracture of the fifth metacarpal resembling Bennett's fracture. Hand 5:49–51, 1973.
79. Seriat-Gautier, B.; Jouve, J. L. Les décollements—fractures de l'extrémité inférieure du radius à déplacement antérieur chez l'enfant. Chir Pediatr 29:265–268, 1988.
80. Southcott, R.; Rosman, M. A. Non-union of carpal scaphoid fractures in children. J Bone Joint Surg 59-B:20–23, 1977.
81. Spinner, M.; Kaplan, E. B. The quadrate ligament of the elbow—Its relationship to the stability of the proximal radio-ulnar joint. Acta Orthop Scand 41:632–647, 1970.
82. Spinner, M.; Freundlich, B. D.; Teicher, J. Posterior interosseous nerve palsy as a complication of Monteggia fractures in children. Clin Orthop 58:141–145, 1968.
83. Stanitski, C. L.; Micheli, L. J. Simultaneous ipsilateral fractures of the arm and forearm in children. Clin Orthop 153:218–222, 1980.
84. Stein, F.; Grabias, S. L.; Deffer, P. A. Nerve injuries complicating Monteggia lesions. J Bone Joint Surg 53-A:1432–1436, 1971.
85. Sullivan, C. M.; Mubarak, S. J. Diagnosis and treatment of upper extremity compartment syndrome. Techniques Orthop 4(3):30–37, 1989.
86. Tarr, R. R.; Garfinkel, A. I.; Sarmiento, A. The effects of angular and rotational deformities of both bones of the forearm. J Bone Joint Surg 66-A:65–70, 1984.
87. Theodorou, S. D. Dislocation of the head of the radius associated with fracture of the upper end of the ulna in children. J Bone Joint Surg 51-B:700–706, 1969.
88. Thompson, H. A.; Hamilton, A. T. Monteggia fracture. Internal fixation of the fractured ulna with intramedullary Steinmann pin. Am J Surg 79:579–584, 1950.
89. Vainionpaa, S.; Bostman, O.; Batiala, H.; Rokkanen, P. Internal fixation of forearm fractures in children. Acta Orthop Scand 58:121–123, 1987.
90. Vender, M. I.; Watson, H. K. Acquired Madelung-like deformity in a gymnast. J Hand Surg 13A(1):19–21, 1988.
91. Vince, K. G.; Miller, J. E. Cross-union complicating fracture of the forearm. Part II: Children. J Bone Joint Surg 69-A:654–661, 1987.

92. Voto, S. J.; Weiner, D. S.; Leighley, B. Redisplacement after closed reduction of forearm fractures in children. J Pediatr Orthop 10(1):79–84, 1990.
93. Voto, S. J.; Weiner, D. S.; Leighley, B. Use of pins and plaster in the treatment of unstable pediatric forearm fractures. J Pediatr Orthop 10(1):85–89, 1990.
94. Walsh, H. P. J.; McLaren, C. A. N.; Owen, R. Galeazzi fractures in children. J Bone Joint Surg 69-B:730–733, 1987.
95. Warren, J. D. Anterior interosseous nerve palsy as a complication of forearm fractures. J Bone Joint Surg 45-B:511–512, 1963.
96. Wedge, J. H.; Robertson, D. E. Displaced fractures of the neck of the radius. J Bone Joint Surg 64-B:256, 1982.
97. Whitson, R. O. Carpometacarpal dislocation. A case report. Clin Orthop 6:189–195, 1955.
98. Wolfe, J. S.; Eyring, E. J. Median-nerve entrapment within a greenstick fracture. J Bone Joint Surg 56-A:1270–1272, 1974.
99. Worlock, P.; Stower, M. Fracture patterns in Nottingham children. J Pediatr Orthop 6(6):656–660, 1986.
100. Wright, P. R. Greenstick fracture of the upper end of the ulna with dislocation of the radio-humeral joint or displacement of the superior radial epiphysis. J Bone Joint Surg 45-B:727–731, 1963.
101. Zehntner, M. K.; Jakob, R. P.; McGanity, P. L. Growth disturbance of the distal radial epiphysis after trauma: operative treatment by corrective radial osteotomy. J Pediatr Orthop 10(3):411–415, 1990.

Hand

102. Almquist, E. E. Hand injuries in children. Pediatr Clin North Am 33(6):1511–1522, 1986.
103. Barnard, H. L. Dorsal dislocation of the first phalanx of the little finger: Reduction by Farabœuf's dorsal incision. Lancet 1:88–90, 1901.
104. Campbell, R. M., Jr. Operative treatment of fractures and dislocations of the hand and wrist region in children. Orthop Clin North Am 21:217–243, 1990.
105. Dixon, G. L.; Moon, N. F. Rotational supracondylar fractures of the proximal phalanx in children. Clin Orthop (83):151–156, 1972.
106. Hastings, H., 2nd; Simmons, B. P. Hand fractures in children. A statistical analysis. Clin Orthop 188:120–130, 1984.
107. Leddy, J. P.; Packer, J. W. Avulsion of the profundus tendon insertion in athletes. J Hand Surg 2(1):66–69, 1977.
108. Leonard, M. H.; Dubravcik, P. Management of fractured fingers in the child. Clin Orthop Rel Res 73:160–168, 1970.
109. Light, T. R.; Ogden, J. A. Complex dislocation of the index metacarpophalangeal joint in children. J Pediatr Orthop 8(3):300–305, 1988.
110. McElfresh, E. C.; Dobyns, J. D. Intra-articular metacarpal head fractures. J Hand Surg [Am] 8(4):383–393, 1983.
111. McFarlane, R. M.; Hampole, M. K. Treatment of extensor tendon injuries of the hand. Can J Surg 16:366–375, 1973.
112. Niechajev, I. A. Conservative and operative treatment of mallet finger. Plast Reconstr Surg 76(4):580–585, 1985.
113. Salter, R. B.; Harris, W. R. Injuries involving the epiphyseal plate. J Bone Joint Surg 45-A:587–622, 1963.
114. Segmuller, G.; Schonenberger, F. Fractures of the hand. In: Weber, B. G.; Bruner, C.; Freuler, F., eds. Treatment of Fractures in Children and Adolescents. New York, Springer-Verlag, 1980, pp. 218–225.
115. Simmons, B. P.; Peters, T. T. Subcondylar fossa reconstruction for malunion of fractures of the proximal phalanx in children. J Hand Surg [Am] 12(6):1079–1082, 1987.
116. Stalter, K.; Smoot, E. C.; Osler, T. Method for elevating the pediatric hand. Plast Reconstr Surg 81(5):788, 1988.
117. Stener, B. Displacement of the ruptured ulnar collateral ligament of the metacarpo-phalangeal joint of the thumb. A clinical and anatomical study. J Bone Joint Surg 44-B:869–879, 1962.
118. Wood, V. E. Fractures of the hand in children. Orthop Clin North Am 7(3):527–542, 1976.
119. Zook, E. G. Nail bed injuries. Hand Clin 1(4):701–716, 1985.
120. Zook, E. G.; Guy, R. J.; Russell, R. C. A study of nail bed injuries: Causes, treatment, and prognosis. J Hand Surg [Am] 9(2):247–252, 1984.

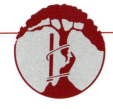

Neil E. Green, M.D.

7

Fractures and Dislocations About the Elbow

Fractures about the elbow are extremely common. Hanlon and Estes estimated that upper extremity injuries account for 65% of all fractures and dislocations in children. Lichtenberg claimed that fractures about the distal forearm are the most common injuries and that fractures and dislocations about the elbow are next in frequency. Elbow injuries occur more often among the skeletally immature than they do in the adult.[17, 107]

Fractures of the Distal Humerus

ANATOMY

Ossification

The ossification of the distal humerus progresses with age. At birth the metaphysis of the distal humerus is ossified; however, none of the structures that constitute the epiphysis is ossified. The capitellum is the first structure to ossify and may be seen radiographically as early as 6 months of age, according to Silberstein and co-workers.[121] Haraldsson, in his classic article in 1959,[51] stated that the capitellum may ossify as early as 1 month of age; however, 6 months is probably the youngest age at which this ossification center is seen (Fig. 7–1). Although ossification of the capitellum may not take place until as late as 2 years of age, Silberstein states that it is invariably present by that time.[121]

The medial epicondyle is the next ossification center to appear. It may be seen radiographically as early as 5 years of age in some but may not appear until 9 years in others. The medial epicondyle forms its own ossification center of the distal humerus, whereas the capitellum, the trochlea, and the lateral epicondyle fuse to form a single ossification center. The trochlea, which appears next, may become ossified as early as age 7 years but more commonly begins to ossify between 9 and 10 years of age. The lateral epicondyle is the last portion of the epiphysis

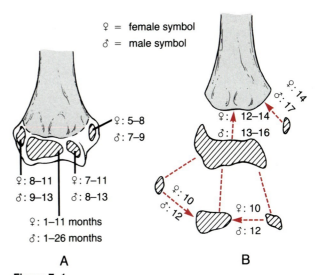

Figure 7–1

Ossification and fusion of the growth centers of the distal end of the humerus. *A*, Appearance of the ossification centers of the distal end of the humerus in the early years. If the wear of the ossification center begins before the age of 1 year, the designation is noted with the letter "m," for "months." *B*, Fusion of the ossification centers of the distal humerus. (Adapted from Haraldsson, S. On osteochondrosis deformans juvenilis capituli humeri including investigation of intra-osseous vasculature in distal humerus. Acta Orthop Scand [Suppl] 38, 1959.)

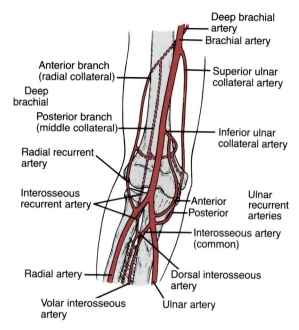

Figure 7–2

The vascular supply about the elbow is rich, with excellent collateral circulation. The collateral circulation is usually sufficient to maintain viability of the extremity in the event of occlusion of the brachial artery.

condyles are both extraarticular. The elbow capsule attaches to the ulna distal to the olecranon and coronoid process, leaving these as intraarticular structures. In addition, the entire radial head is located within the capsule, making it intraarticular. There are two elbow fat pads between the capsule and the distal humerus—one anterior and the other posterior. The radiographic appearance of these fat pads may aid in diagnosing injuries about the elbow; with an elbow effusion, one or both may become elevated from the surface of the distal humerus as seen on the lateral radiograph.[90]

Radiographic Anatomy

Different radiographic lines have been described to help in the radiographic diagnosis of fractures of the distal humerus. Bauman's angle may be helpful in determining the adequacy of reduction of a supracondylar fracture of the distal humerus.[6] This angle is defined as the angle created by the intersection of the distal humerus to ossify. It may be identified radiographically as early as 8 to 9 years of age.

The capitellum and trochlea may fuse as early as age 10 years, but this usually begins by age 12 years. This combined ossification center fuses to the lateral epicondyle at the same time, forming the main body of the epiphysis of the distal humerus. The epiphysis fuses to the metaphysis of the distal humerus as early as age 12 to 13 years, which signals the end of longitudinal growth of the distal humeral physis. Finally, the medial epicondyle fuses to the distal humerus between 14 and 17 years of age.

Vascular Anatomy

The collateral circulation about the elbow is rich and usually sufficient to maintain adequate circulation to the forearm and hand even if there is interruption of the main blood supply from the brachial artery (Fig. 7–2). Although interruption of the brachial artery may not result in loss of the limb, it will usually produce some signs of ischemia, such as claudication and cold intolerance.[67, 68, 73, 77, 144]

Joint Anatomy

The entire articular surface of the distal humerus is intraarticular; however, the medial and lateral epi-

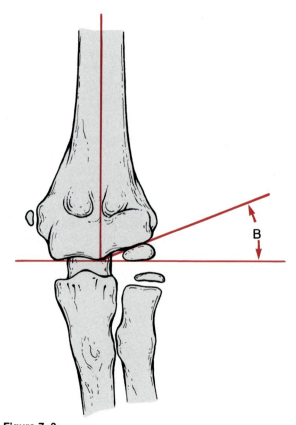

Figure 7–3

Bauman's angle is the angle formed between a line that follows the metaphysis of the lateral side of the distal humerus, i.e., the physis of the capitellum, and a line perpendicular to the axis of the humerus.

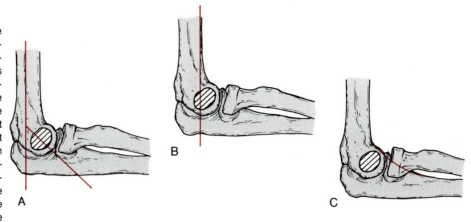

Figure 7–4

Radiographic lines that may be demonstrated on a lateral radiograph of the elbow. *A*, The capitellum of the distal humerus is angulated anteriorly approximately 30 degrees. This may be demonstrated by drawing a line parallel to the midpoint of the shaft of the distal humerus; where that line intersects with a line drawn through the midpoint of the capitellum indicates the anterior inclination of the capitellum. *B*, The anterior humeral line is a line drawn down the outer edge of the anterior cortex of the distal humerus. As the line is drawn distally through the capitellum the line should pass through the middle of the capitellum. *C*, The anterior coronoid line is a line drawn along the coronoid fossa of the proximal ulna, which is then continued proximally. It should just touch the capitellum anteriorly. The line will lie posterior to the most anterior portion of the capitellum if the capitellum is angulated anteriorly. If the capitellum is angulated posteriorly, the line will no longer touch the capitellum.

of a line drawn along the physis of the capitellum and a line perpendicular to the longitudinal axis of the humerus as seen on the anteroposterior radiographs (Fig. 7–3).

Silberstein and colleagues[121] have defined other lines to facilitate the diagnosis of fractures of the distal humerus as viewed on the lateral radiograph. The anterior coronoid line is drawn along the coronoid and continued proximally. It should just touch the capitellum anteriorly in the normal elbow. If the capitellum is angled or displaced anteriorly, this line will intersect or lie posterior to the capitellum.

The anterior humeral line is drawn along the anterior cortex of the humerus.[111] It should pass through the middle of the ossified capitellum as seen on a lateral radiograph. If this line passes anterior to the middle of the capitellum, the capitellum or the distal humerus has been displaced posteriorly. Conversely, if it passes posterior to the middle of the capitellum, the distal humerus has been displaced anteriorly (Fig. 7–4).

Silberstein has noted that the physis of the capitellum is wider posteriorly than anteriorly when viewed on a lateral radiograph. This may be mistaken for an injury to the physis if one is not familiar with the normal radiographic anatomy (Fig. 7–5).

Carrying Angle of the Elbow

The carrying angle of the elbow is the clinical measurement of varus-valgus angulation of the arm with the elbow fully extended and the forearm fully supinated. The intersection of the line along the midaxis of the upper arm with the line along the midaxis of the forearm defines this angle. Beals has shown that the carrying angle varies widely among

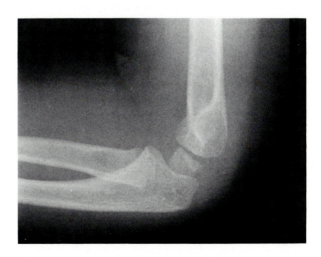

Figure 7–5

Lateral radiograph of the normal elbow. The physis of the capitellum is slightly wider posteriorly than it is anteriorly. This is seen on normal radiographs and should not be confused with an injury to the physis.

individuals. The angle increases with age, and there is no consistent difference between males and females. The carrying angle of a given elbow is best evaluated by comparing that angle with the carrying angle of the contralateral elbow.

Supracondylar Fractures

ANATOMY

The distal humerus is unique in design. Although the medial and lateral columns are strong, they are connected by a very thin wafer of bone that is only 1 mm thick in the central portion.[6, 27] This central thin area of the distal humerus is produced by the olecranon fossa posteriorly and the coronoid fossa anteriorly (Fig. 7–6). It is because of this distinct anatomy of the distal humerus that the supracondylar fracture is so unstable. If the distal fragment rotates even slightly, the medial column of the distal fragment does not line up with the medial column of the proximal fragment, and only the very thin bone between the two columns abuts. Dameron[27] compared this circumstance to attempting to balance the blades of two knives on one another. Since this is impossible, the two fragments invariably rotate and then tilt, producing an angular deformity of the elbow.

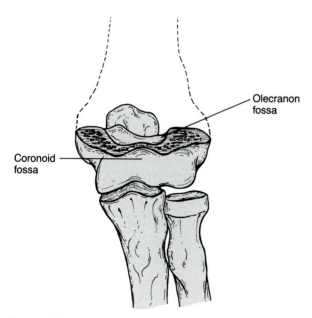

Figure 7–6

Cross section of the distal humerus through the region of the coronoid fossa. Note that the midportion of the humerus is extremely thin at this level, whereas the medial and lateral sides (columns) are thicker.

INCIDENCE

This fracture occurs most often in the immature skeleton and is usually seen in the first decade of life.[33, 55, 146] This is the most common fracture about the elbow in children, accounting for about 60% of the total.[34, 83] Two types of supracondylar fractures may result depending upon the mechanism of injury. The extension type occurs in over 96% of supracondylar fractures, whereas the flexion type constitutes less than 4% of these injuries.

MECHANISM OF INJURY

Supracondylar fractures of the distal humerus may be produced by either a hyperextension or a flexion injury. An injury that results from a fall on the outstretched hand with the elbow hyperextended causes the more common extension type of fracture. If the injury occurs from a fall on the olecranon with the elbow flexed, the less common flexion type of supracondylar fracture results.

Various investigators have been able to produce the flexion type of supracondylar fracture in both immature cadavers and monkeys.[1, 7, 107] Henrikson[55] studied children who had sustained a supracondylar fracture of the humerus and found that their uninjured opposite elbow was capable of more than the average amount of hyperextension. The ability to hyperextend the elbow is believed to direct the force from the fall on the outstretched hand to the anatomically weak olecranon fossa, resulting in a fracture. Because ligamentous laxity is greatest in the young, the peak incidence of this fracture is in the first decade of life.

CONSEQUENCES OF INJURY

The hyperextension force produces the fracture, which begins as a crack in the anterior cortex of the supracondylar area of the humerus. As the hyperextension moment progresses the anterior periosteum stretches over the fracture of the anterior cortex. This has been termed a stage I fracture by Abraham and co-workers.[1] If at this point the hyperextension force ceases, a nondisplaced or minimally angulated fracture occurs. Radiographically one may see a decrease in the normal anterior inclination of the capitellum on the lateral view.

A stage II fracture is the result of continued hyperextension of the elbow. Hence the distal fragment continues to angle posteriorly but does not displace. In a stage III injury the anterior periosteum is completely torn, and the distal fragment is displaced posteriorly. Although the anterior periosteum is completely torn in a stage III fracture, the posterior periosteum is usually intact and is used as a hinge to assist in closed reduction of the fracture. If the fracture is displaced posteromedially, which is usually the case, a medial periosteal hinge usually exists in addition to the posterior periosteum.

ASSOCIATED INJURIES

Nerve Injuries

There is a relatively high risk of nerve injury associated with supracondylar fracture of the distal humerus in children—between 7% and 15.5%, according to published reports.[10, 24, 39, 41, 65, 73, 75, 86, 127] Forty-five percent of the nerve injuries involve the radial nerve and 32% the median nerve. The ulnar nerve is less commonly involved, being injured about 23% of the time.[143] Ulnar nerve injury is more often associated with the flexion type of supracondylar fracture of the humerus. Although the radial nerve is most frequently injured according to the literature, we have found the anterior interosseous to be the most commonly injured nerve. As the proximal fragment displaces anteriorly, the median nerve with its associated anterior interosseous nerve is stretched anteriorly. This especially risks the anterior interosseous branch because it is tethered under the fibrous arch that arises from the deep head of the pronator teres.[65, 127]

Vascular Injuries

Although the consequences of vascular injury associated with supracondylar fracture of the distal humerus may be significant, the incidence of permanent vascular compromise of the extremity is very low. It occurs in less than 1% of all supracondylar fractures of the distal humerus.[101, 144] The brachial artery is usually protected by the brachialis muscle. If the displacement of the fracture is great, the brachialis muscle may be torn and the protection it provides to the brachial artery lost.

The proximal fragment of the supracondylar fracture is usually displaced anteriorly. If the brachialis muscle is torn, the anterior spike of the proximal fragment is displaced significantly. The brachial artery may become tethered and occluded by this spike of bone because the artery is tethered to the distal fragment by the supratrochlear artery.[115] This occlusion is usually relieved by reducing the fracture. The artery may also become entrapped within the substance of the fracture.[130] In this instance the circulation is usually satisfactory until one attempts reduction of the fracture with manipulation or traction. The reduction of the fracture with an entrapped brachial artery will result in loss of the radial pulse and possibly compromise of the circulation of the extremity.

CLASSIFICATION

Supracondylar fractures of the distal humerus may be classified by the direction of displacement of the proximal fragment. If the child falls on the outstretched hand with the elbow extended, an extension type of supracondylar fracture will result. In this type, by far the most commonly seen, the proximal fragment of the humerus is displaced anteriorly. The flexion type of supracondylar fracture of the distal humerus occurs from a fall on the olecranon with the elbow flexed. This injury is much less common, constituting less than 4% of all supracondylar fractures.[144]

Extension type supracondylar fractures are usually classified according to the amount of displacement of the two fragments. This classification was originally proposed by Gartland and is still the most useful.[42] Type I is a nondisplaced fracture. The fracture line may be easily visible or very indistinct. Good lateral views and observation of fat pad elevation help identify this fracture radiographically.

A type II fracture is an angulated fracture with an intact posterior cortex. On the lateral radiograph one can identify the posterior angulation of the distal fragment by the position of the capitellum. Normally the capitellum is angulated anteriorly about 30 degrees. This may also be documented radiographically by observation of the anterior humeral line, which normally crosses the middle of the capitellum on the lateral radiograph of the elbow. If this line runs anterior to the middle of the capitellum, one must suspect a type II supracondylar fracture of the distal humerus (see Fig. 7–4). Abraham and colleagues[1] have shown that the anterior periosteum is torn in the type II fracture; however, it is not completely torn and maintains some continuity anteriorly.

A type III supracondylar fracture is completely displaced, having lost all continuity of the two fragments of the distal humerus. The fracture is most often displaced posteromedially, although infrequently it may displace posterolaterally. Much has been written about the displacement of the distal fragment. It has been thought that posteromedial displacement is best held reduced with pronation of the forearm, because the soft tissues help close the lateral side of the fracture with the forearm in pronation. Conversely, if the fracture is displaced posterolaterally, supination is the position of choice for immobilization of the reduced fracture.

Extension Type Supracondylar Fracture

HISTORY

Children who are old enough to provide an adequate history will complain of pain in the elbow region with inability to move the elbow. They will have fallen on the outstretched hand with the elbow extended. This will be the rule for the type II and type III fractures; children who sustain type I injuries, however, may not have the total restriction of movement that is seen in the more displaced type of fractures.

PHYSICAL EXAMINATION

The physical examination of the patient with a supracondylar fracture of the distal humerus will depend upon the type of fracture sustained. If the fracture is nondisplaced, the swelling may not be great; however, there will be point tenderness in the supracondylar region of the distal humerus.

Children who sustain a type II fracture will have pain with attempted movement of the elbow but may be able to initiate a small amount of elbow motion because of the stability of the fracture.

Those who have sustained a type III fracture will have the most pain and swelling. These children are unable to initiate any movement of the elbow because of pain. When such a child is seen in an emergency department, the elbow is usually splinted in extension, which is the position of the elbow at the time of injury. Generally, there is significant swelling about the elbow, mostly about the distal humerus. With significant displacement of the fracture, there will be ecchymosis of the skin in the antecubital region of the elbow. When the proximal fragment of the humerus has penetrated the brachialis muscle, there may be puckering of the skin in the front of the elbow, indicating the severity of the fracture displacement. Little else can be discerned about the fracture itself because of the amount of pain and swelling with this injury. The forearm is generally pronated, because the distal fragment is usually internally rotated. This internal rotation must be corrected at the time of closed reduction.

A complete neurovascular evaluation of the arm is essential, because this fracture is notorious for producing some form of neurovascular damage. It is not uncommon for the radial pulse to be absent at the time of initial evaluation. This may be secondary to the tethering of the artery over the anterior surface of the proximal fragment of the distal humerus. If the pulse is absent, one should attempt a gentle reduction to relieve the pressure on the artery, if possible. Although absence of the radial pulse causes concern, the pulse usually returns, and rarely is the artery torn. Arterial spasm may be differentiated from arterial rupture or occlusion with the use of a Doppler probe. The collateral circulation around the elbow is extensive, which allows for sufficient circulation to the arm to maintain viability, in most instances, even if the artery is damaged. This is different from the circulation around the knee, where the popliteal artery is crucial, since the collateral circulation in this area is insufficient to maintain viability of the lower leg.[46]

The examination of the forearm is critical to determine the status of the circulation to the forearm and hand. If the pulse is absent, the limb will be viable if the collateral circulation is adequate; however, signs of ischemia are common. This is determined by examination of perfusion and function of the forearm and hand and by the presence of a pulse on Doppler examination. Volkmann's ischemia has been associated with this fracture. One must carefully look for the signs of impending ischemia, which are pain, compartment tightness, and decreasing motor and sensory function. The classic finding is pain out of proportion to the injury and especially pain with passive extension of the fingers. If there is any question of compartment ischemia, measurement of the compartment pressures of the forearm should be undertaken.

The neurologic examination should include a motor and sensory check of the the median, ulnar, and radial nerves. In addition, one should look carefully for injury to the anterior interosseous nerve. This branch of the median nerve is a pure motor nerve. It supplies motor function to the flexor pollicis longus and the flexor digitorum profundus to the index finger. Inability to flex the distal joints of the thumb and index finger indicates injury to this nerve.

RADIOGRAPHIC EVALUATION

An accurate radiographic diagnosis of a type III fracture of the supracondylar region of the distal humerus is usually not difficult. The accurate diagnosis of a type I or even a type II fracture may pose more difficulty. As previously mentioned, the use of the fat pad signs on the lateral radiographs will be helpful in localizing the trauma to the region of the elbow joint. In addition, on the lateral radiograph one should look for any alteration in the intersection of the capitellum with the anterior humeral line, for if this line crosses anterior to the middle of the capitellum, a type I or II supracondylar fracture is likely to be present.

MANAGEMENT

Type I Fracture

Although this fracture is nondisplaced, the distal fragment may be angulated posteriorly as seen on the lateral radiograph. Treatment will depend upon the extent of posterior angulation of the distal fragment. Rang states that reduction is not required if the posterior angulation is 20 degrees or less. Normally the capitellum is angulated anteriorly about 30 degrees. Even if the capitellum is in a straight line with the longitudinal axis of the humerus, remodeling of the injury should be able to correct this amount of angulation if the growth potential is sufficient. For some time, however, there will be more than normal elbow extension and less than normal elbow flexion because of the extension angulation of the distal fragment.

One pitfall in treating this fracture lies in not recognizing associated medial angulation of the fracture; if left uncorrected, this will produce a cubitus varus deformity that will not correct with growth. Although rare in a type I fracture, one may nevertheless identify medial compression of a type I fracture (Fig. 7–7). Compression of the medial side of this fracture may be identified clinically by inspecting the arm with full elbow extension to compare the carrying angle with that of the normal uninjured elbow. The use of Bauman's angle on an anteroposterior radiograph may also be helpful.

In general, this fracture requires immobilization for comfort and protection. The immobilization should not be circular even though this injury does not generally swell as much as the displaced supracondylar fracture. It is usually better to apply a long posterior splint with medial and lateral side splints to immobilize the elbow. The elbow should be placed in about 90 degrees of flexion unless there is enough swelling to suggest possible compromise of the circulation. In that instance the elbow should be extended until comfort and circulation are optimal. Three weeks of immobilization is usually sufficient for healing. At that time the splints are removed,

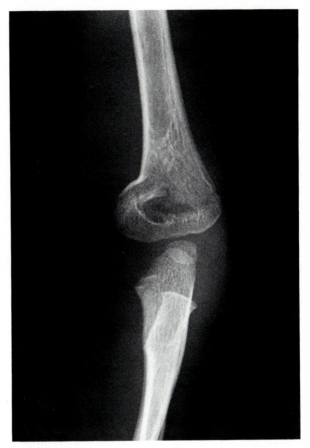

Figure 7–7

This anteroposterior radiograph of the distal humerus and elbow shows a nondisplaced supracondylar fracture. Note the compression of the metaphysis on the medial side. The lateral side is straight and has not been compressed. This has produced a cubitus varus deformity that should be corrected.

and if healing is judged to be adequate radiographically, the child is allowed unrestricted motion of the elbow.

Type II Fracture

Type II fractures are similar to type I fractures, although the severity of the angulation of the distal fragment is greater. In type II fractures the anterior cortex is broken, but the posterior cortex remains intact. In addition to posterior angulation, there may be some rotation of the distal fragment.

There is disagreement about the need for reduction of these fractures. Gartland[42] feels that even if the distal fragment has lost all its anterior angulation, as seen on the lateral radiograph, reduction of the fracture is not necessary because the deformity will remodel. Mann[78] is even more optimistic about the remodeling of these fractures in children. He stated that remodeling should be expected to be complete even if the fracture was angulated posteriorly 10 degrees. A significant amount of remodeling is possible about the distal humerus because of the proximity to the elbow joint. In addition, the younger the child at the time of injury, the greater the amount of remodeling potential. One must remember, however, that remodeling is possible only in the plane of motion of the elbow joint. In other words, only anterior or posterior angulation may remodel, whereas varus or valgus angulation will not correct with growth. Varus compression of the medial side of the fracture is more likely in a type II than in a type I fracture. Varus angulation of the elbow may be assessed in the same way as for a type I fracture, i.e., with full elbow extension, although this may not be possible because of pain. Bauman's angle on the injured side should be compared with its counterpart on the opposite uninjured side. If there is still a question of varus deformity, the patient should be anesthetized so that the arm can be thoroughly examined.

If there is medial compression of the fracture, it should be corrected with a valgus force (see Fig. 7–7). The elbow should be immobilized with the elbow in 90 degrees of flexion if swelling allows, and the forearm should be pronated. If correction of the posterior angulation of the distal fragment is not necessary but correction of medial compression is required, one may wish to immobilize the elbow in full extension to better stabilize the elbow after correction of the varus deformity. Usually these fractures are stable and do not require internal fixation, but some that have a rotational deformity as well as posterior angulation may require percutaneous fixation (Fig. 7–8).

Type III Fracture

The type III fracture is defined as a completely displaced supracondylar fracture, in which both the anterior and the posterior cortices have lost contact with each other. In most instances there is no bone contact of the proximal fragment with the distal fragment. This fracture carries the greatest risk of neurovascular injury. Much has been written about its treatment, which has evolved so that at present closed reduction with percutaneous pinning is accepted as the best method. The same treatment is also preferred for the fracture that is not reducible and for the one in which the neural or vascular status changes during fracture reduction.

TREATMENT

Skin Traction

Because of the risk of vascular compression resulting in Volkmann's ischemia of the forearm, traction

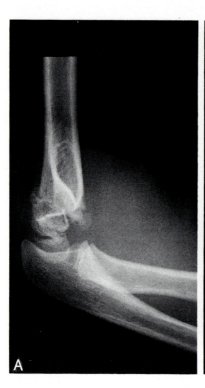
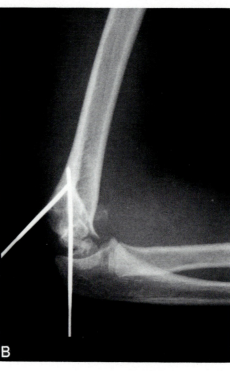

Figure 7–8

Type II supracondylar fracture of the distal humerus. *A,* Lateral radiograph of the distal humerus demonstrating posterior angulation of the distal fragment of the distal humerus. Note that if one drew the anterior humeral line, it would no longer intersect the capitellum; neither would the coronoid line lie on the anterior aspect of the capitellum. In addition, the capitellum has lost its normal 30 degrees of angulation. *B,* Postreduction radiograph of the distal humerus.

became a popular mode of treatment of this fracture. Both skin and skeletal traction have been used.

Dunlop's traction is skin traction applied to the arm with the child supine.[30, 32] Traction straps are applied to the forearm with the arm supinated. A counterweight is hung from the upper arm to help with pulling the proximal fragment of the humerus posterior to approximate the distal fragment. Longitudinal traction is then applied to the supinated forearm with the elbow flexed about 45 degrees. There have been several modifications of this technique. Ingebrightsen's method involved skin traction that was applied as overhead traction.[30, 144] Traction was applied to the upper arm, which pulled vertically. Traction applied to the forearm pulled horizontally with the elbow flexed close to a right angle. Graham described extension skin traction that was applied to the arm with the elbow in full extension.

Regardless of the type of skin traction used, the results seemed to be about the same, even though there were isolated reports of excellent outcomes. While the problem of compartment ischemia seemed to be lessened with the use of skin traction, the incidence of cubitus varus was unacceptably high in most series. For example, Piggot reported good results with extension skin traction, as did Dodge with Dunlop's traction.[30, 102] On the other hand, D'Ambrosia and Zink found an unacceptably high incidence of cubitus varus as did Prietto with skin traction.[26, 104] Because of the risk of cubitus varus, the use of skin traction for the treatment of this fracture has essentially been abandoned in the United States.

Skeletal Traction

Skeletal traction has been the most popular contemporary traction treatment of this fracture. In general, traction is applied to the fracture through the proximal ulna with the elbow in flexion. Initially traction was accomplished through the use of a Kirschner wire (K-wire) placed transversely through the proximal ulna. The wire is inserted with the child sedated. An axillary block may be used, although some prefer general anesthesia for fracture reduction and application of traction because it allows continuous monitoring of compartment function.[71] The pin must be inserted under sterile conditions. The point of insertion is important because of the proximity of the ulnar nerve. Therefore, the pin is inserted from the medial side of the arm at about the level of the coronoid process of the ulna, which is about 2.5 cm distal to the tip of the olecranon.[46, 123–125] For placement of the pin the elbow should be flexed to allow the nerve to move anteriorly and to be better able to feel the landmarks. A smooth pin is used because nerve injury is less likely than with a threaded pin if the pin is placed too close to the nerve. Once the pin has been inserted in the ulna, the arm is placed in traction.

Because of the risk of injury to the ulnar nerve a winged screw has been preferred by some authors.[34, 87, 96, 100] The screw is inserted into the proximal ulna at the same distance from the tip of the olecranon that is the site for the insertion of the traction wire. Instead of being inserted transversely it is inserted into the ulnar cortex in line with the longitudinal axis of the humerus. Another advantage of the screw is the fact that it has multiple holes in its wing so that the direction of pull of the traction may be altered to adjust for varus or valgus deformity.

Although some have advocated sidearm traction, most authors have preferred overhead traction because it elevates the elbow, thereby helping to reduce swelling.[26, 50, 72] In addition, D'Ambrosia and Zink pointed out that with the arm overhead the forearm rotates into pronation, which is the preferred position of the forearm in fractures that are displaced posteromedially.[26] Pronation is believed to close the lateral side of the fracture, which decreases the risk of cubitus varus.

For the application of sidearm traction, after the pin or screw is inserted, the child is placed supine on the edge of the bed with the fractured arm overhanging the side of the bed. The elbow is flexed to a right angle with the hand pointing to the ceiling. Skin traction straps are placed on the forearm and connected to a pulley and weights sufficient to support the arm. The skeletal traction is also connected to weights through a separate pulley. Additional weights may be suspended from the upper arm to help pull the proximal fragment of the humerus posteriorly.

For the application of overhead skeletal traction the direction of the traction is vertical through a series of pulleys. The forearm is suspended in a sling. Because there is usually an internal rotation deformity of this fracture, the hand is directed to the opposite upper corner of the bed (for example, if the right humerus is fractured, the hand is pointed toward the left upper corner).

Radiographs of the distal humerus are important to assess the efficacy of the traction; however, the anteroposterior view is difficult to obtain. One must extend the elbow enough to enable an adequate anteroposterior radiograph to be obtained, and this motion in itself may alter the position of the reduction of the fracture.

Kramhoft and associates[71] have reduced the fracture under general anesthesia and placed the extremity in traction with the patient still in the operating room. Frequently the fracture was remanipulated under anesthesia one or more times during the traction treatment. Other authors have placed the arm in skeletal traction, expecting the traction itself to reduce the fracture acceptably.[26, 34] Traction is usually maintained for 2 to 3 weeks. Hammond recommended 2 weeks of traction, after which the arm was placed in a cast.[50] Others, such as Fahey,[34] left the patient in traction for 2-1/2 to 3 weeks and then placed the arm in a sling.

Use of skeletal traction for the treatment of this fracture has generally had better results than has the use of skin traction.[26, 36, 71, 99] Nevertheless, the use of any kind of traction poses problems. The long hospital stay required for completion of traction care is generally not acceptable as long as alternative methods, providing equivalent or improved treatment, are available.

Closed Reduction and Cast Treatment

Closed reduction and cast treatment of this fracture is the preferred means of management in many centers. Reduction of the fracture is generally accomplished with the patient under general anesthesia. With the elbow extended, gentle longitudinal traction is applied to the supinated forearm with countertraction applied to the upper arm by an assistant. The medial or lateral displacement is then corrected with finger pressure over the medial or lateral epicondyle. Most of these fractures are displaced posteromedially, and they are also internally rotated. To bring the medial column of the distal fragment anterior to meet the medial column of the proximal fragment, the distal fragment should be externally rotated.[26] At this point the fracture is reduced by flexing the elbow while maintaining the longitudinal traction. In addition, the thumb of the surgeon should push the olecranon forward to eliminate the posterior displacement of the distal fragment. The elbow must be flexed maximally to hold the fracture reduced while radiographs are obtained to assess the quality of the reduction.

The lateral radiograph is relatively easy to obtain, but the arm should not be rotated to obtain this view. Instead the placement of the arm should be maintained and the machine moved to the crosstable position. The anteroposterior view is not possible, so that one must obtain the so-called Jones view, which is a transcondylar one. This is achieved by placing the subject's upper arm on the radiographic cassette. The elbow is maximally flexed with the forearm pronated. The radiographic tube is placed over the distal humerus and directed perpendicular to the distal humerus. In essence, one is obtaining an anteroposterior radiograph of the distal humerus through the overlying forearm. This radiograph is understandably difficult to interpret because of the overlying bone and soft tissue.

The position of the elbow is critical for maintaining the reduction of the fracture. To control the reduction, acute flexion of the elbow is necessary. This position tightens the posterior periosteum of the distal humerus and also tightens the triceps muscle, which tends to lock the reduction in place. Many authors have recommended pronation of the forearm for those fractures that are posteromedially displaced; this also prevents cubitus varus. Salter felt that there is an intact medial periosteal hinge that becomes taut with the forearm in pronation and with the fracture reduced. Griffin[47] and Rang also endorse this concept. They all agree that the fracture must be reduced first. Acute elbow flexion is required to tighten the posterior periosteal hinge. Once the posterior periosteal hinge is tight, with maximum elbow flexion the pronation of the elbow will tighten the medial periosteum; this will close the lateral fracture surfaces, reducing the degree of varus. Arnold and co-workers[5] recommended pronation as the position of stability of this fracture after reduction. They felt that the brachioradialis and the wrist extensors become tight with pronation of the forearm, which tends to close the fracture on the lateral side and thereby reduce the amount of varus deformity.

Thus, regardless of the rationale, all authors agree that acute flexion of the elbow with pronation of the forearm is required to stabilize a displaced fracture of the supracondylar region of the distal humerus. The problem with this position of the elbow is that acute flexion increases the tension in the already swollen elbow, increasing the risk of vascular compromise by reducing the arterial flow to the forearm and the venous outflow from the forearm. Less than acute flexion is frequently required to maintain adequate circulation to the distal arm in patients with displaced supracondylar fractures. Unfortunately, anything less than acute flexion risks loss of fracture reduction, because with even minor degrees of extension of the elbow the posterior periosteum becomes lax, allowing fracture displacement.

This dilemma led to the currently accepted methods of treatment of this fracture. It became obvious that since acute flexion was necessary to maintain reduction, another means of maintenance of the reduction was necessary to reduce the risk of vascular compromise. This led to the development of internal fixation of these fractures, an approach that is accepted as the standard today.

CURRENT METHOD OF TREATMENT
Closed Reduction and Percutaneous Pinning

One of the major problems with this fracture is the risk of development of cubitus varus. This deformity is not the result of a growth disturbance but rather is the direct result of malreduction of the fracture or loss of reduction. When one looks at the distal humerus, where this fracture occurs, it becomes evident that the width of the humerus is only 2 to 3 mm, at most, across the olecranon fossa. Therefore, if a supracondylar fracture is not anatomically reduced, the medial column of the proximal and distal fragments will not line up. The medial column of the distal fragment is posterior to the proximal portion of the medial column because of malrotation of the fracture fragments. Thus the proximal fragment is balancing on a fragment of bone 2 mm thick. As one can imagine, it is impossible to maintain varus-valgus alignment unless the medial columns of the two fragments are opposing. Hence, not only must the reduction be accurate, but also the reduction must be maintained, for any rotation of the distal fragment displaces the medial column of the distal fragment posterior to the medial column of the proximal fragment. This leads to tilting of the distal fragment into varus, with the development of cubitus varus.

The modern era of treatment of this fracture began in 1948 with a description by Swenson of percutaneous pinning of fractures of the distal humerus in adults.[132] In 1961 Casiano reported the use of this technique in children.[18] Since this description there have been multiple reports of the use of percutaneous pinning for the maintenance of reduction of the displaced supracondylar fracture.[34, 36, 37, 47] Some authors recommend the use of two lateral pins in order to avoid the ulnar nerve. Others advise using a very small incision on the medial side to be able to palpate the medial condyle so as to avoid the nerve. This may be helpful in the very swollen elbow. The drawback to the use of two lateral pins is that the fixation provided is less secure biomechanically than that provided by crossed pins. Two lateral pins may still allow rotation of the fracture, enabling the medial column to rotate posteriorly, unless the starting points of the two pins are widely separated—this is very difficult because of the small size of the distal fragment. Once the medial column support is lost, the fracture may tilt into varus.[145]

The reduction must be good before the fracture is stabilized with pins. Some authors have felt that malrotation of the fracture is not significant because this can be compensated for by the shoulder, which has such wide rotational motion. While this is true, the problem with a malrotated supracondylar fracture is that the fracture surfaces that oppose each other if the fracture is not adequately reduced are the very thin proximal and distal portions of the olecranon fossa. As mentioned, trying to maintain this fracture reduced in this circumstance is difficult at best; it is easy for the fracture to tilt medially without medial column support, resulting in cubitus varus. If the pin fixation is very secure, maintenance of the reduction is possible; however, most authors who reported their results of closed pinning of this fracture also recorded a variable incidence of cubitus varus.

Aronson and Prager[6] have used Bauman's angle to determine the adequacy of the reduction of this fracture intraoperatively. They recommend the use of two lateral pins to stabilize the fracture. If Bauman's angle is within 4 degrees of that of the opposite uninjured elbow, the reduction is accepted. If, on the other hand, the angle is greater, a repeat reduction is performed and a radiograph of the distal humerus obtained. This is repeated until Bauman's angle lies within a satisfactory range. With this attention to the reduction these authors reported no instances of cubitus varus. This points out the need for an excellent reduction of this fracture to reduce the incidence of a cubitus varus deformity.

Although Aronson and Prager[6] supported the use of Bauman's angle for determination of the adequacy of reduction, others have not found the use of this angle to be of benefit. Nacht and colleagues[91] found that the precise margin of the lateral condyle was not distinct, making the measurement of Bauman's angle difficult. They stated further that this angle was not helpful in children under the age of 3 years, because it is impossible to define bony landmarks in the elbow at this age.

Technique. The elbow should be reduced as soon as the child is brought to the operating room, in order to be able to work with an elbow that is not too swollen. Even if the child presents to the hospital with a grossly swollen elbow, it is better to reduce the fracture at that time rather than wait for the swelling to decrease, which will take days. The child is placed on a radiolucent operating table and anesthetized with general anesthesia. He or she is positioned supine with the involved extremity completely free. The shoulder of the involved extremity should be positioned at the edge of the table so that the remainder of the arm can hang free over the edge. This allows free access to the C-arm. Flynn has used a special bracket over which the elbow is flexed to help with the stabilization of the elbow during the pinning procedure.

The arm is sterilely prepared, and the fracture is reduced by first extending the elbow with longitudinal traction applied to the forearm. An assistant places countertraction on the upper arm. Medial or lateral displacement is corrected, and the forearm is externally rotated to correct the internal rotation deformity. The elbow is then flexed maximally, maintaining the traction. The surgeon's thumb is used to push the olecranon forward, which assists in the reduction. Maximum elbow flexion is maintained.

The reduction is assessed with the fluoroscope. The lateral projection is easy to obtain; however, it is important to move the radiographic machine rather than the elbow, because rotation, especially internal rotation, of the arm may cause loss of reduction of the fracture. The anteroposterior projection is more difficult to obtain because extension of the elbow before pinning will result in loss of the reduction, and one may use the Jones (transcondylar) view. If, however, the reduction appears to be satisfactory as seen on the lateral projection, the fracture should be pinned. Once stabilized, the elbow may be extended to view the fracture on the anteroposterior projection. The carrying angle is also observed with the elbow extended.

Smooth pins are used to lessen the risk of injury to the physis and the ulnar nerve. They should be inserted with the assistance of a power drill. The lateral pin is inserted through the lateral epicondyle, angling cephalad at about 35 to 45 degrees and slightly posterior. One may use the C-arm image to assist in pin placement. The medial pin is then inserted through the medial epicondyle. Care must be taken to avoid injury to the ulnar nerve, which usually can be palpated in its groove behind the epicondyle. If significant swelling obscures the landmarks, manual pressure may help locally decrease the swelling. If this is unsuccessful, a small incision may be made over the medial epicondyle to assist in pin placement. This pin is placed at the same angle as the lateral pin. To increase stability the far cortex of the humerus must be just engaged by the pins (Fig. 7–9).

Once the fracture is stabilized the elbow may be extended, enabling one to view the carrying angle and to obtain a true anteroposterior radiograph. The pins are bent outside the skin, and the arm is splinted with the elbow in flexion. To prevent compression the plaster should not be circular. The exact amount of elbow flexion is dictated by the amount of swelling and by the radial pulse.

The child should be hospitalized until it is certain that the risk of circulatory compromise is past. The arm is placed in a sling. Follow-up requires repeat radiographs in a about a week to be certain that the reduction is not lost. Three weeks of immobilization is all that is usually required. At that time the splint and pins are removed if radiographs demonstrate sufficient healing. Unprotected motion, but with activities restricted, is allowed so as to encourage use of the arm and movement in the elbow.

Open Reduction and Internal Fixation

Open reduction and internal fixation of this fracture were once thought to be not indicated except in rare circumstances. Later reports, however, showed excellent results with the use of open reduction.[11, 120, 141] We have lowered our indications for open reduction of supracondylar fractures, concluding that open reduction is indicated for open fractures; when there is circulatory compromise or neurologic loss during or after closed reduction; and when an adequate closed reduction cannot be obtained. The last case is the least defined, but almost all reports of closed reduction and pinning cite a risk of development of cubitus varus with this technique.[4, 34, 39, 90, 145] To decrease this risk, a near-perfect reduction of the fracture should be sought, because this prevents the medial tilt of the medial column, which causes the cubitus varus deformity. We therefore proceed to open reduction if an excellent closed reduction cannot be achieved.

Technique. A medial incision is made over the medial side of the distal humerus and elbow. The ulnar nerve is protected. The periosteum over the proximal fragment will have been stripped by the injury. The fracture is explored to be certain that no neural or vascular structure is trapped. Less than 1 mm of periosteum is elevated from the distal fragment to prevent circulatory embarrassment of the distal fragment. The fracture is then reduced and cross-pinned. If an anatomic reduction is not possible, a lateral approach is made to assure a perfect reduction. The pins are left protruding from the skin and are bent.

One is always amazed at the minimal discomfort that these children experience because of the de-

Figure 7-9

Displaced extension type supracondylar fracture. *A*, Anteroposterior radiograph of a supracondylar fracture of the distal humerus. *B*, Intraoperative post-reduction anteroposterior radiograph demonstrating good reduction of the fracture. The lateral pin was withdrawn several millimeters. *C*, Intraoperative lateral radiograph of the fracture showing the correction of the posterior displacement and restoration of architecture of the distal humerus. The pins are bent outside the skin. *D*, Lateral radiograph of the elbow taken 6 months after the injury demonstrates normal anatomy of the distal humerus.

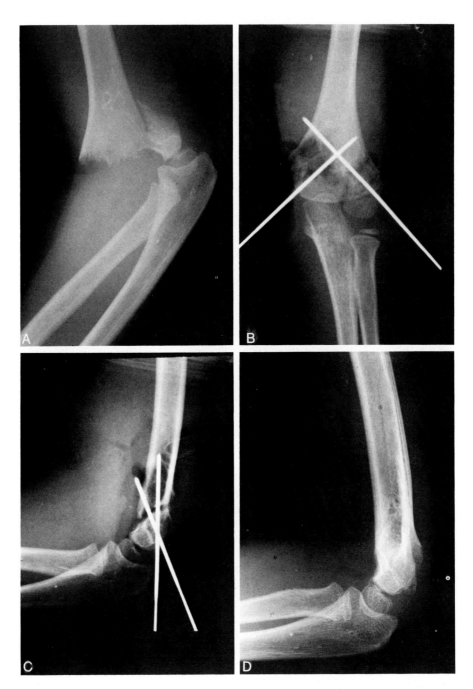

compression of the hematoma. They can usually be discharged from the hospital the day following surgery. Their follow-up is the same as that for closed pinning. The pins are usually removed and motion begun 3 weeks after surgery. The risk of myositis ossificans, which has discouraged operation on these fractures in the past, has not been a problem in our experience; nor has it been reported as a complication in the published series.[11, 105, 120, 141]

COMPLICATIONS

Vascular Compromise

Vascular problems may be grouped into two types: namely, acute, from interruption of the blood supply to the arm, and subacute, or Volkmann's ischemia. Acute vascular insufficiency is fortunately uncommon. There is excellent collateral circulation about the elbow, which usually provides sufficient blood flow to the arm even if the brachial artery is damaged.[67, 73, 75, 114, 145] The mere absence of the radial pulse on palpation is not an indication of vascular insufficiency. In fact, the radial pulse may be absent because of spasm, only to return after reduction of the fracture. On the other hand, loss of the pulse during reduction may indicate obstruction from too much elbow flexion or entrapment of the artery in the fracture.

The vascular status to the extremity is judged by the skin color, temperature of the extremity, functioning of the arm, amount of pain, and radial pulse. The first step in management of supracondylar fractures of the humerus with vascular compromise should be closed reduction under general anesthesia. If the circulation improves, immobilization of the fracture may be carried out. However, if ischemia persists, the brachial artery should be explored. The absence of a pulse as detected by a Doppler probe can help confirm the vascular insufficiency.[145] An arteriogram may be performed in the operating room before repair of the artery is undertaken. Ligation of the artery to eliminate spasm, although once popular, is not indicated. An open reduction and pin fixation of the fracture are also performed.

Some have recommended the use of traction in the face of vascular insufficiency.[46, 97] If the circulation improves, they advise continuing the entire treatment of the fracture with the use of traction. If the circulation does not improve within 1 hour of initiation of traction, however, arterial exploration is recommended.

Volkmann's ischemia is most common in those fractures treated with the elbow flexed acutely. Fortunately, it is much less frequent with the use of traction, percutaneous pinning, or open reduction and pinning. For that reason, closed reduction and flexion treatment of this fracture are not recommended. Pinning of the fracture allows the elbow to be extended sufficiently to decrease the risk of ischemia.

The signs and symptoms of forearm ischemia are well known. Suffice it to say that pain should alert one to its presence. In addition, pain with passive finger extension is an early sign.[46] Measurement of compartment pressure and early fasciotomy if the pressure is high will help reduce the risk of permanent damage.

Neurologic Injury

The incidence of neurologic injury varies greatly in published reports, with some authors reporting few if any, and others reporting an incidence as high as 15%.[10, 24, 38, 40, 65, 75, 86, 127] Most series report that radial nerve injury is the most common, with median nerve injury next and ulnar nerve injury the least common. Spinner and Schreiber[127] reported a high incidence of injury to the anterior interosseous nerve with supracondylar fracture of the distal humerus. We have also found that injury to this nerve is the most common with supracondylar fracture. Because it is purely a motor nerve and may be detected only if the flexion of the distal joints of the thumb and index fingers is tested, it is possible to miss its presence. Spinner and Schreiber[127] found that the nerve passes through a fibrous arch 2 to 3 cm below the joint. This fibrous arch, which arises from the deep head of the pronator teres, may tether the nerve, causing it to stretch with anterior displacement of the proximal fragment of the distal humerus.

Regardless of the nerve injured, almost all reports found that these nerves recover spontaneously.[21, 24, 40, 58, 65] Routine nerve exploration was not recommended by these authors unless there was no nerve recovery at all within 3 months. However, Jones and Louis[65] reported recovery beginning as late as 4 to 5 months after injury. It is, however, recommended that nerve exploration be performed if nerve function deteriorates during or following closed reduction of the fracture.[40, 74]

Cubitus Varus

This is the most common persistent deformity resulting from malreduction or loss of reduction of supracondylar fractures. The exact incidence of this deformity varies widely according to the series from a low of 0% to a high of 60%.[4, 6, 25, 29, 46, 78, 87] This deformity is not the result of a growth arrest of the distal humeral physis, although some modern authors have clung to this belief.[55, 59] Some have felt that lateral growth stimulation resulting from the fracture produces the varus deformity.[9, 16, 59, 99] Medial tilt of the distal fragment producing varus deformity is almost universally accepted as the cause.[30, 39, 42, 72, 122, 124] Because of the anatomy of the distal humerus, with the very thin metaphysis, a near-anatomic reduction is necessary to allow the proximal and distal medial columns of the humerus to abut, providing fracture stability. Lack of contact of the two medial columns, which results from persistent posterior rotation of the medial side of the distal fragment, allows the fracture to tilt into varus.

Detection of this deformity requires full elbow extension, which may help explain the impression that this deformity occurs after the fracture has healed. If the fracture is immobilized for a prolonged period, loss of elbow extension may persist. The deformity may not be recognized until full elbow extension is finally achieved.

Although the cubitus varus or gunstock deformity may be unsightly, it does not limit function,[5, 30] and because it is the result of malunion it will not progress. Correction of the deformity is easiest when the child is approaching skeletal maturity, because one is able to achieve solid fixation without concern for the physis of the distal humerus. Ippolito and co-workers[60] found that correction deteriorated with continued growth in those patients who underwent osteotomy to correct cubitus varus. Most patients and their families desire correction when the deformity is noticed. Several methods of correction have been proposed. King and Secor[70] proposed a medial opening wedge osteotomy that is fixed with Steinmann pins and a Riedel clamp. Coventry and Henderson[24] prefer a lateral closing wedge osteotomy for correction. Other authors have been concerned about both loss of correction and undercorrection with this approach.[109, 134] If this type of osteotomy is stabilized with K-wires, the arm should be immobilized in extension to better control the correction. Oppenheim and associates[96] felt that there is a critical angle for the insertion of the lateral pin, because if the angle is too acute the pin will slide off the opposite cortex of the humerus. On the other hand, if the angle is too obtuse the pin will not cross the osteotomy site.

Because of the risk of loss of correction with pin fixation, French[40] described fixation of the lateral closing wedge osteotomy with the use of two screws linked with a wire. The screws are placed on either side of the osteotomy. To help correct the rotational deformity the two screws may be offset. With the elbow extended, the osteotomy is closed and a wire is placed around the two screws and then tightened. The correction of the carrying angle may then be checked with the elbow extended and the forearm supinated. Bellemore also used this technique and obtained better results than with pin fixation.

DeRosa and Graziano[29] described an osteotomy that they attribute to Lloyd-Roberts in which the inferior cut of the osteotomy does not reach the lateral cortex; instead it stops 0.5 cm short and then is connected to the proximal cut with a vertical cut. This leaves a lateral spike of bone attached to the distal fragment. Once the osteotomy is closed it may be stabilized with a single screw placed from the lateral spike across the osteotomy (Fig. 7–10).

Flexion Type Supracondylar Fracture

These fractures are much less common than the extension type. Wilkins[144] estimated the incidence to be about 2.5% of all supracondylar fractures; Fowles and Kassab[39] found the incidence to be slightly higher. This fracture is the result of a fall on the point of the flexed elbow. When these children are seen in an emergency department the elbow is held flexed, in contrast to the extended elbow seen with the extension type of supracondylar fracture. These fractures are more stable in extension than in flexion because the anterior periosteum is intact. However, a long arm cast with the elbow extended is cumbersome. Rang found that this type of cast would not stay on, and he attached a pelvic band to help keep the cast in place.

The treatment of this fracture should be similar to the treatment for the extension type. If the fracture is nondisplaced, simple immobilization is all that is necessary. If the distal fragment is simply angulated anteriorly, reduction and immobilization with the elbow in extension are usually successful (Fig. 7–11). If the fracture is displaced, closed reduction and pinning should be performed. Fowles and Kassab[39] had better results with open reduction and pin fixation. They found that the distal fragment had become buttonholed through the triceps in those fractures that were not reducible.

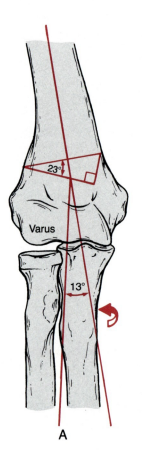
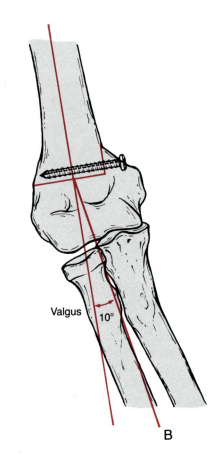

Figure 7–10

Closing wedge osteotomy of the distal humerus. *A*, The osteotomy is designed to correct the varus deformity of the distal humerus, leaving a small buttress of metaphysis that will allow for screw fixation of the osteotomy. *B*, The appearance of the osteotomy after the wedge of bone has been removed and the osteotomy has been stabilized with a screw.

Figure 7–11

Lateral radiograph of the flexion type supracondylar fracture of the distal humerus. *A*, Lateral radiograph demonstrating the anterior angulation of the distal fragment. *B*, Lateral radiograph of the elbow taken 6 months after fracture reduction shows correction of the anterior angulation. The fracture was reduced with extension of the elbow and maintained in an extension long arm cast.

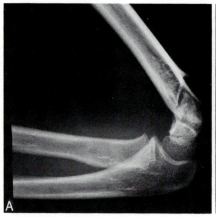
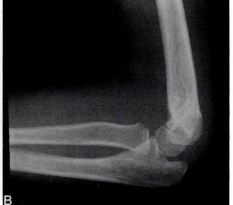

Fracture-Separation of the Distal Humeral Physis

INCIDENCE

The exact incidence of this fracture is not known because it has been underdiagnosed.[27] DeLee and colleagues[28] reviewed three cases of infantile supracondylar fractures that had been reported by MacAfee and concluded that these were actually fracture-separations of the distal humeral physis. At one time this injury was thought to be very rare; however, it is now seen and recognized more frequently.

MECHANISM OF INJURY

Two clear mechanisms of injury seem to be the cause of this fracture. It may be the result of birth trauma. One must be able to differentiate this injury from a brachial plexus palsy, because neonates will frequently not move a painful extremity, thereby mimicking paralysis. Holda and colleagues[56] reported that after the neonatal period, a fall from a height was the cause of the fractures in their series. However, three of their seven patients were under the age of 1 1/2 years, making child abuse more likely. DeLee and associates reported that child abuse was proven or suspected in 6 of their 16 patients.[28] One must therefore strongly suspect the possibility of child abuse when one sees this fracture in a young child.

CLASSIFICATION

DeLee and co-workers[28] classified this injury based on the age of the child and the presence or absence of ossification of the capitellum. Type A occurs in infants from birth to 9 months of age. There is no ossification center present in the capitellum at this age, and there is no metaphyseal bony fragment attached to the distal fragment. Type B occurs in children 7 months to 3 years of age. The ossification center of the capitellum is present radiographically, and there may or may not be a fragment of the metaphysis (Thurston-Holland sign) displaced with the epiphysis. Type C occurs in children 3 to 7 years of age. The capitellum is well ossified, and there is a large Thurston-Holland metaphyseal fragment seen on the radiograph.

DIAGNOSIS

These children present with marked swelling about the elbow; the physical appearance of the joint resembles that of an elbow dislocation. Gentle manipulation of the elbow will reveal a muffled crepitus that is thought to be diagnostic of epiphyseal separation. It is the result of two cartilaginous surfaces rubbing together and should be distinguished from bony crepitus.

On the anteroposterior radiograph the radius and ulna are displaced in relation to the humerus. However, the radius and ulna are in their normal relationship to each other. This injury must be distinguished radiographically from an elbow dislocation, from a displaced fracture of the lateral condyle of the distal humerus, and from a supracondylar fracture of the distal humerus.

On an anteroposterior radiograph of a normal elbow a line drawn along the longitudinal axis of the radius passes through the capitellum regardless of the position of the elbow. If this line does not pass through the capitellum, there is a dislocation of the radius, an elbow dislocation, or a displaced fracture of the lateral condyle of the distal humerus. In a fracture-separation of the distal humeral physis, the relationship of the radius to the capitellum remains intact; however, the radius and ulna lose their normal relationship with the distal humerus. In addition, the capitellum is displaced medially. The fracture-separation of the distal humeral physis is usually displaced medially, whereas the elbow dislocation is usually displaced laterally (Fig. 7–12).

A displaced fracture of the lateral condyle of the distal humerus may be distinguished by the fact that the radius and ulna retain their normal relationship with the humerus; however, because the capitellum is displaced the radius does not retain its normal relationship with it. A supracondylar fracture is uncommon in the very young. In addition, a fracture line should be seen above the epiphysis.

In the very young (before the capitellum has ossified) the fracture-separation is most easily confused with an elbow dislocation. Elbow dislocation is very uncommon in this age group, however. In addition, the forearm is displaced laterally with dislocation of the elbow. The radius and ulna are displaced medially with the epiphysis of the distal humerus with a fracture-separation of the distal humeral physis. Arthrography of the elbow joint may be useful in assisting with the diagnosis, especially when the capitellum has not yet ossified (Fig. 7–13).

TREATMENT

Unlike the supracondylar fracture, this fracture is usually stable because it occurs through the thicker distal end of the humerus below the thin supracon-

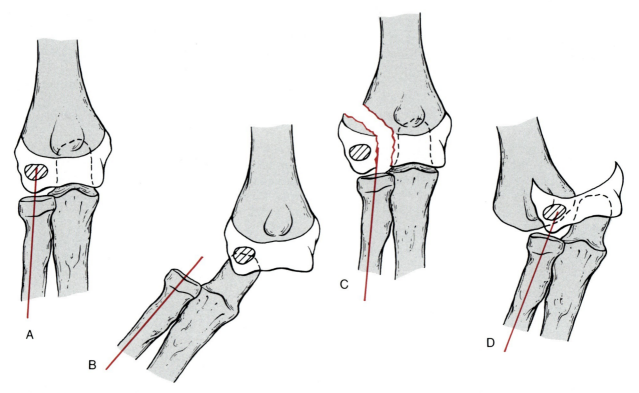

Figure 7–12

Comparison of injuries about the distal humerus. *A*, The normal relationships about the distal humerus. *B*, Dislocation of the elbow. The line drawn along the longitudinal axis of the radius no longer intersects the capitellum. The capitellum, however, remains in its normal relationship to the distal humerus. *C*, Displaced fracture of the lateral condyle. The longitudinal axis of the proximal radius does not intersect the capitellum, and the capitellum is displaced from its normal position on the distal metaphysis of the humerus. *D*, Fracture-separation of the distal humeral physis. Note that the capitellum is displaced from its normal position on the lateral side of the metaphysis of the distal humerus but that it maintains its normal relationship with the radial head. (Adapted from DeLee, J.C.; Wilkins, K.E.; Rogers, L.F.; Rockwood, C.A. Fracture-separation of the distal humerus epiphysis. J Bone Joint Surg 62-A:46, 1980.)

dylar region. Therefore, cubitus varus deformity is less likely to develop than it is after supracondylar fracture.[27] Nevertheless, Holda and co-workers[56] found that five of their seven patients developed a cubitus varus deformity.

DeLee and colleagues[28] recommend closed reduction if the fracture is fresh; however, if the fracture is old they recommend splinting the arm until the fracture is solid without attempts at reduction. The findings of Holda and associates[56] tend to corroborate this because their results with more aggressive treatment were poor. Mizuno and co-workers[89] obtained good results with open reduction through a posterior approach.

With this injury our preference for treatment is to first investigate the possibility of child abuse. If necessary, the child may be admitted to the hospital to facilitate this inquiry. Admission may also be warranted to observe for circulatory change. If reduction is required, closed reduction is performed by placing gentle traction on the forearm. The medial displacement of the distal fragment is then corrected. Any malrotation is corrected, and the elbow is flexed to 90 degrees with the forearm pronated, because the medial displacement recurs if the forearm is supinated.[27] The arm is splinted for 3 weeks, after which unrestricted motion is allowed (Fig. 7–14).

Fracture of the Lateral Condyle of the Distal Humerus

INCIDENCE

This fracture is relatively common, occurring in 12 to 16.8 % of fractures about the elbow in children.[37, 88, 148]

MECHANISM OF INJURY

There are two theories as to the cause of this fracture. Avulsion of the lateral condyle of the

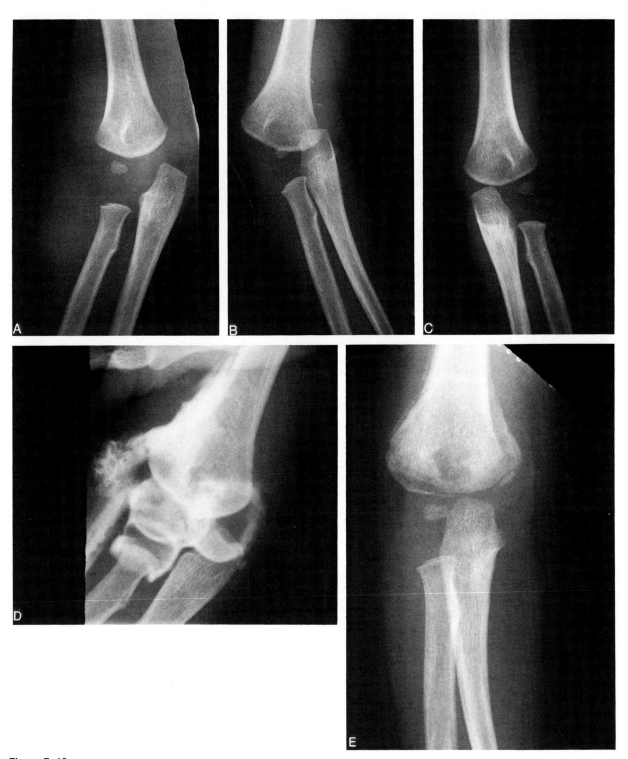

Figure 7-13

Fracture-separation of the distal humeral physis. *A*, Anteroposterior radiograph of the injured extremity. The capitellum is displaced medially. *B*, Anteroposterior stress view of the same elbow demonstrating the marked instability and further displacement of the capitellum medially. *C*, Anteroposterior view of the opposite normal extremity showing the normal relationship between the capitellum and the distal humeral metaphysis. *D*, Arthrogram of the elbow showing that the capitellum and proximal radius are well aligned and that the capitellum is displaced medially. *E*, Anteroposterior radiograph of the same elbow 3 weeks after injury that shows healing of the fracture. The capitellum remains slightly displaced medially.

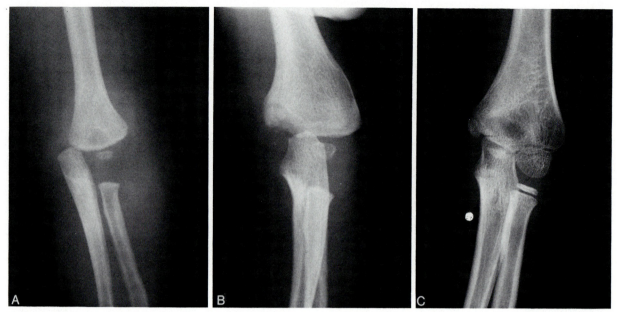

Figure 7-14

Displaced fracture of the distal humeral physis. *A,* Anteroposterior radiograph of the distal humerus taken at the time of injury demonstrates medial displacement of the capitellum. Note that the longitudinal axis of the radius intersects the capitellum. *B,* Anteroposterior radiograph of the elbow taken 3 months after injury. The displacement was not corrected at the time of immobilization. *C,* Follow-up radiograph 5 years post injury demonstrating remodeling of the distal humerus. The patient clinically had full mobility in the elbow.

humerus may result from a fall on the outstretched hand with the forearm supinated. A varus force on the arm transmits the force through the forearm extensor musculature to its attachment on the lateral condyle of the humerus, resulting in avulsion of the condyle.[61, 106, 112] Using a similar mechanism, Jakob and colleagues were able to reproduce this injury in young cadavers, confirming this as a possible etiology (Fig. 7-15).[61]

Both Stimson[129] and Fahey,[34] however, believed that this fracture was the result of a compression injury. Stimson[129] produced this fracture in cadavers with a force directed to the outstretched hand with the elbow flexed. Undoubtedly, both mechanisms of injury are possible.

CLASSIFICATION

Milch[88] has classified this fracture according to the location of the fracture line through the distal humerus. If the fracture line is lateral to the trochlear groove, the fracture may or may not displace; however, the elbow joint does not dislocate (Fig. 7-16). As long as some or all of the trochlea remains unfractured, it serves as a lateral buttress for the coronoid-olecranon ridge of the ulna, preventing lateral displacement of the ulna. This fracture, termed a type I by Milch, may cross through the ossification center of the capitellum, or it may go through a portion of the trochlea, leaving the capitellum intact (Figs. 7-17 and 7-18). The fracture line in a type II fracture lies at or medial to the trochlear groove. As a consequence of the loss of the trochlear abutment, the ulna and radius are displaced laterally (Fig. 7-19).

Salter and Harris[116] have classified these fractures as type IV fractures, because the fracture line begins in the metaphysis, crosses the physis, and enters into the epiphysis. Some have felt that because the trochlea is not ossified at the age when this fracture usually occurs, this does not actually cross the physis and therefore should be called a type II fracture in the Salter and Harris classification.[15] While this is technically correct, and the risk of growth arrest of the physis is probably less when the trochlea is not ossified, the fracture does indeed fulfill the Salter-Harris criteria for a type IV fracture.

Jakob and co-workers[61] also classified this fracture according to the amount of displacement of the capitellum seen radiographically (Fig. 7-20). A type I fracture is actually a partial fracture that is nondisplaced. The fracture line does not go through the entire cartilaginous epiphysis, and therefore the joint surface is intact. This fracture may be able to

Figure 7–15

Displaced fracture of the lateral condyle of the distal humerus with a nondisplaced fracture of the olecranon. *A*, Anteroposterior radiograph demonstrates the fracture of the olecranon and the medial displacement of the capitellum. From this radiograph one can appreciate that the injury occurred with a varus force with the elbow in extension. The capitellum was therefore avulsed. *B*, Lateral radiograph showing the fracture to be one of the lateral condyle, including the entire capitellum and a portion of the metaphysis of the distal humerus. *C*, Postreduction intraoperative radiograph of the distal humerus that shows reduction and pinning of the fracture.

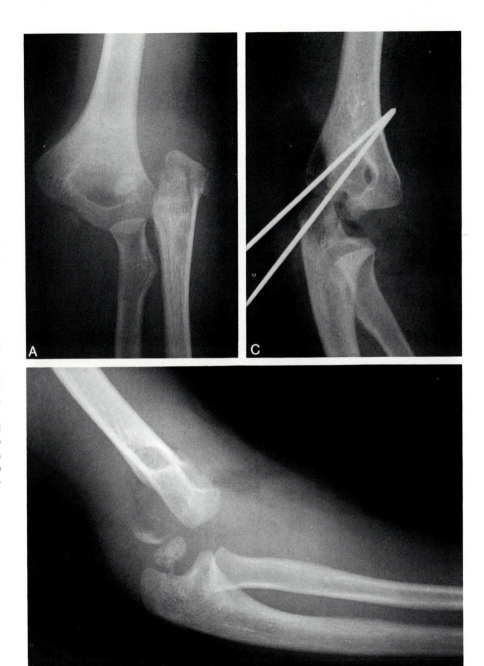

Figure 7–16

A, Drawing of the distal humerus showing the trochlear groove and the capitellotrochlear sulcus. *B*, A type I fracture of the lateral condyle. The fracture line is lateral to the trochlear groove. The relationship between the proximal forearm and distal humerus remains intact. The capitellum may be displaced partially or totally. *C*, The fracture line goes through the trochlear groove, making the elbow joint unstable. The radius and ulna may therefore become displaced laterally.

233

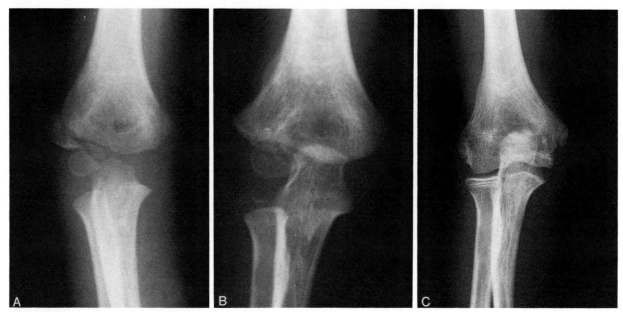

Figure 7–17

A, Milch type I fracture of the lateral condyle. The fracture line crosses through the midportion of the ossification center of the capitellum. This fracture was originally treated with cast immobilization; when the patient was referred at 6 weeks post injury, the fracture was still displaced. Open reduction and internal fixation of the fracture were performed. B, Four months post reduction the fracture is healed. C, Seven years post open reduction of the fracture the distal humerus appears normal.

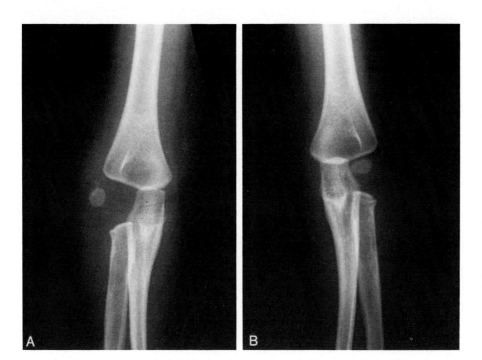

Figure 7–18

A, Anteroposterior radiograph of the distal humerus of a child who sustained a displaced type I fracture of the lateral condyle of the distal humerus. Note that the capitellum is displaced laterally but that the radius and ulna have maintained their normal relationship with the distal humerus. B, Lateral radiograph of the opposite normal extremity taken for comparison. Note the normal lateral angulation of the proximal humerus.

Figure 7–19

Displaced Milch type II fracture of the lateral condyle. *A*, Anteroposterior radiograph demonstrating the fracture of the lateral condyle with lateral displacement of the fracture along with lateral displacement of the proximal radius and ulna. The fracture line travels through the trochlear groove or medial to it. Because of the loss of elbow stability, there is displacement of the radius and ulna laterally. *B*, Lateral radiograph of the distal humerus demonstrating the large fragments of the lateral condyle. *C*, Postreduction anteroposterior radiograph that shows the fracture to be reduced and pinned. *D*, Follow-up radiograph 1 year later shows healing of the fracture.

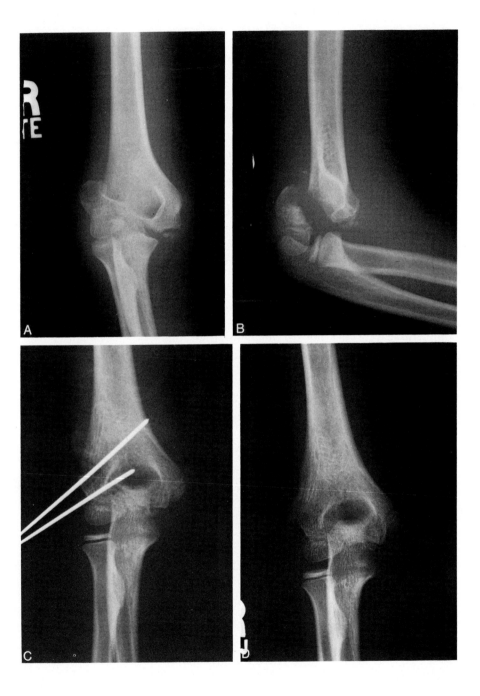

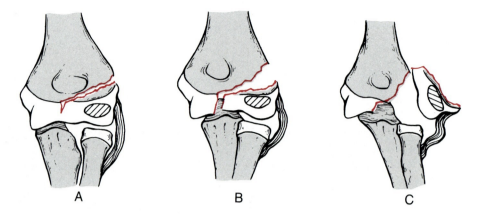

Figure 7–20

Classification of lateral condylar fractures according to the amount of displacement. *A*, Type I fracture. Note that the fracture line enters the cartilaginous surface of the distal humerus between the capitellum and trochlea but that the fracture is not complete into the articular surface in the fractures and therefore is nondisplaced. *B*, Complete fracture (type II). The fracture is complete through the articular surface but is not displaced out of the elbow joint. *C*, Complete fracture with complete displacement of the lateral condyle (type III).

be treated without surgical reduction. A type II fracture is a complete fracture that extends completely through the articular surface. The capitellum may be laterally displaced, but it is not rotated. A type III fracture is completely displaced, and the capitellum is rotated out of the joint. There is complete loss of the normal relationship of the proximal radius to the capitellum (Fig. 7–21).

DIAGNOSIS

Clinically there is swelling of the elbow that is most marked laterally. Most of the tenderness is localized here also. The fracture is usually easily identified radiographically if the capitellum is well ossified and if it is displaced. Oblique radiographs of the elbow may assist in the diagnosis of a nondisplaced or

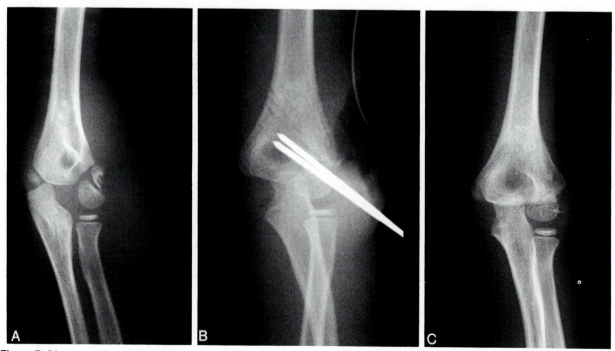

Figure 7–21

Totally displaced fracture of the lateral condyle of the distal humerus. *A*, Anteroposterior radiograph of the distal humerus showing the displaced and rotated fracture of the lateral condyle of the distal humerus. *B*, Intraoperative anteroposterior radiograph of the fracture of the distal humerus. *C*, Anteroposterior radiograph taken 7 months post fracture.

minimally displaced fracture. There may be difficulty in differentiating this fracture from a type I fracture of the distal humeral physis or from a dislocation of the elbow if the fracture is lateral to the trochlear groove and if the capitellum is not ossified. While arthrography will be helpful, it should be borne in mind that fracture of the lateral condyle is very rare in this age group, whereas fracture-separation of the entire physis is more common.

TREATMENT

Nondisplaced type I fractures may be treated with immobilization only. It has been our experience that the nondisplaced fracture is less common than the displaced fracture. One must be absolutely certain that the fracture is truly nondisplaced before electing to treat it nonoperatively. Frequent radiographs out of plaster must be obtained to ensure that displacement does not occur during the 3 weeks of immobilization. To assure that the fracture does not displace, closed pinning of the fracture may be performed, followed by 3 weeks of cast immobilization. The pins are then removed, and motion is begun. This should probably be performed if one is not certain that the fracture is truly nondisplaced.

Type II fractures may occasionally be reduced closed and then secured by percutaneous pins. One must be certain, however, that an anatomic reduction has been obtained; otherwise a poor result will ensue.[51, 146] Because the fracture is intraarticular the joint surface must be reconstituted perfectly to prevent the development of an irregular articular surface. Nonunion is another problem seen with this fracture and is common in those displaced fractures treated nonoperatively (Fig. 7–22). The third reason for obtaining a perfect reduction is that this is a Salter-Harris type IV fracture, which will usually result in a growth arrest if not reduced perfectly. In this fracture, however, because the epiphyseal portion of the fracture usually goes through the cartilaginous portion of the epiphysis, growth arrest is less likely.[51] In general, displaced type II and all type III fractures must be reduced perfectly, which usually requires an open reduction with pin fixation.[33, 34, 36, 37, 51, 61, 63, 87, 115, 125, 140]

A Kocher approach to the lateral side of the distal humerus is used. Once the fracture is exposed the periosteum of the distal humerus is elevated a few millimeters to visualize it. The periosteum on the distal fragment must be elevated no more than 1 to 2 mm from the fracture surface to protect the blood supply to this fragment. However, it is imperative that the entire fracture be visible. One must see the anterior joint surface to be certain that an anatomic reduction has been obtained. The fracture is secured with two smooth Kirschner pins. Intraoperative radiographs are obtained to ascertain the quality of the reduction (see Fig. 7–21). The elbow is immobilized for 3 weeks, after which the pins are removed and motion is begun. Some authors have recommended suture fixation; however, this is not secure enough and nonunion may result.[25, 146]

Delayed Open Reduction

Some authors have felt that if this fracture is seen late, open reduction should not be performed.[51, 61, 87, 106] They reported a high incidence of avascular necrosis, probably because of the extensive soft tissue stripping necessary to mobilize the fracture. Jakob and co-workers[61] recommend no treatment if the fracture is seen after 3 weeks. This has not been our experience in three patients seen between 6 and 8 weeks post injury. They all underwent open reduction with pin fixation. One was a Milch type I fracture in which the fracture line went directly through the ossification center of the capitellum and would have resulted in a growth arrest if not reduced (see Fig. 7–17). All these fractures united without avascular necrosis or growth arrest, and all patients regained and maintained full elbow motion.

COMPLICATIONS

Nonunion and Cubitus Valgus

Nonunion is usually the result of inadequate internal fixation or failure to perform it. Suture fixation of this fracture was popular for a time.[25] However, the incidence of nonunion has led most authors to abandon this technique in favor of pin fixation. Nonunion may also result from misdiagnosis of this fracture. If there is minimal displacement and the metaphyseal fragment is small, there is a chance that the fracture may not be correctly identified. Because this is an intraarticular fracture, nonunion is believed to be the result of synovial fluid bathing the fracture and preventing union.[51]

The treatment of an established nonunion is controversial. Some have recommended no treatment or a delay in treatment until the child is close to skeletal maturity.[51, 61] Flynn and associates[37] recommended grafting to obtain union in order to prevent valgus and a tardy ulnar nerve palsy. Some patients with a nonunion will have pain, especially if the dominant extremity is involved, which is usually

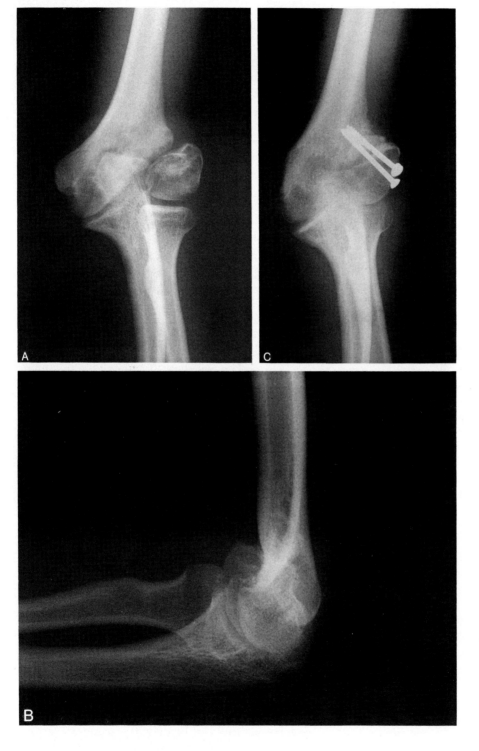

Figure 7–22

Nonunion fracture of the lateral condyle of the distal humerus. *A*, Anteroposterior radiograph demonstrating the nonunion of the lateral condyle of the distal humerus. *B*, Lateral radiograph of the elbow. The lateral condyle is freely mobile and moves proximally with elbow flexion, and distally and posteriorly with elbow extension. *C*, Anteroposterior radiograph taken after open reduction and internal fixation with bone grafting of the nonunion.

secondary to the elbow instability. The lateral condylar fragment most often is completely mobile, which allows increased valgus stress to the elbow.

Internal fixation and grafting of these mobile nonunions generally results in loss of some elbow motion; however, the tradeoff may be beneficial if the pain can be relieved.[81] The metaphyseal fragment should be stabilized to the main portion of the metaphysis with compression screws, and a bone graft should be added (see Fig. 7–22).

Fracture of the Medial Condyle of the Humerus

This fracture is very uncommon, accounting for less than 2% of all elbow fractures in children.[14, 144] Two mechanisms of injury have been proposed, as is the case for the lateral condylar fracture.[19, 38, 69, 139] The fracture may occur from a fall on the outstretched hand with the elbow extended and result in avulsion of the medial condyle.[19, 39] Varma and Srivastava[139] stated that their two patients sustained their injuries by a fall on the olecranon, the olecranon having been driven into the trochlea to fracture the medial condyle.

CLASSIFICATION

Kilfoyle[69] devised a classification identical to the one used for the lateral condyle fracture. The type I fracture is nondisplaced, and the fracture line does not go into the articular surface. The fracture line in a type II fracture goes through the articular surface, but the fracture is essentially nondisplaced. The type III fracture is totally displaced and rotated. Bensahel and co-workers,[14] using a similar classification, claimed that these different injuries occur in different age groups. The type I injury occurs in children less than 5 years of age. The type II fracture may be seen in any age group, and the type III fracture occurs in a somewhat older child. In their series this fracture was seen in children with an average age of 7 years.

DIAGNOSIS

This fracture may be difficult to diagnose because it is frequently seen before the ossification of the trochlea begins. Clinically the child will have a swollen, painful elbow with the majority of the pain and swelling on the medial side. This injury is most commonly mistaken for a fracture of the medial epicondyle. Clinically the examination of the two injuries will be different. The avulsion of the medial epicondyle in the young child usually is accompanied by an elbow dislocation. The elbow is likely to be unstable with a valgus force. On the other hand, because the medial side of the elbow joint is fractured, there will be varus instability with a fracture of the medial condyle of the distal humerus (Fig. 7–23).

Radiographically a fracture is suggested if the medial condyle is markedly displaced. One should also look for a fleck of bone avulsed from the metaphysis. An arthrogram of the elbow may be necessary to confirm the diagnosis.

TREATMENT

Type I fractures will heal with simple immobilization; however, type II fractures should be stabilized with percutaneous pinning if the reduction is anatomic. If there is a question of the adequacy of the reduction, open reduction and pinning of the fracture should be performed. A type III fracture must undergo open reduction and pin fixation. The elbow should be immobilized for 3 weeks, followed by pin removal and mobilization.

Fracture of the Medial Epicondyle

INCIDENCE

This is a relatively common injury, occurring in about 10% of children's elbow fractures,[87, 144] and typically in an older age group. The majority are seen in adolescents (between 10 and 14 years of age)[12, 69, 125, 146] in males (more than 75%).[122]

MECHANISM OF INJURY

This injury is the result of an avulsion of the medial epicondyle. A valgus force combined with contraction of the forearm flexor muscles (Smith, Kilfoyle, Wilson). If the valgus force is great enough, an elbow dislocation will result, in addition to the avulsion of the medial epicondyle. In many series of medial epicondyle fractures, most occur along with elbow dislocation.[69, 87, 146]

CLASSIFICATION

Most systems of classification of this fracture are similar and are based on the amount of displacement of the fragment and whether or not it is entrapped

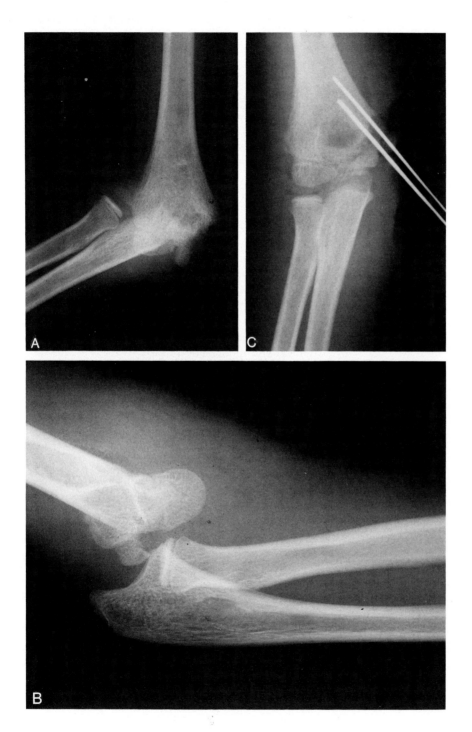

Figure 7–23

Displaced fracture of medial condyle of the distal humerus. *A,* Anteroposterior radiograph of the elbow. Note the displacement of the medial epicondyle. Note also that the trochlea has been displaced but is positioned behind the distal metaphysis of the distal humerus and therefore is difficult to visualize. *B,* The lateral radiograph of the elbow shows that the injury includes both the epicondyle and the trochlea. This is therefore a fracture of the entire lateral condyle. *C,* Anteroposterior radiograph taken intraoperatively demonstrates reduction and internal fixation with smooth pins.

Table 7–1

Classification of Fractures of the Medial Epicondyle

I. Undisplaced
II. Minimally displaced (<5 mm)
III. Displaced (>5 mm)
    Elbow not dislocated or reduced
    Epicondyle not in joint
    Epicondyle in joint
    Elbow dislocated

in the elbow joint (Table 7–1).[12, 122, 144] Woods and Tullos[146] have also classified this injury; however, their classification pertains to the teenager, who is very near the age of closure of the apophysis of the medial epicondyle.

DIAGNOSIS

The diagnosis of this fracture is generally easy. There will be a history of a valgus injury to the arm. The child will have pain and swelling localized to the medial side of the elbow. In the case of an elbow that also dislocated but spontaneously reduced, there will be generalized pain and swelling; however, the point tenderness will be greatest medially. Radiographically the apophysis of the medial epicondyle may appear wider than normal in the nondisplaced fracture. Frequently a comparison radiograph of the opposite elbow will be of benefit.

Woods and Tullos[146] have recommended that a stress radiograph be performed to determine the amount of instability. They perform the stress test with the patient supine and the elbow flexed to a right angle. The shoulder is externally rotated with the upper arm resting on the table; the elbow and forearm are suspended over the edge of the table. If the elbow is unstable, the medial side of the elbow will widen, which can be demonstrated with an anteroposterior radiograph of the elbow taken in this position.

TREATMENT

The treatment of this fracture depends upon the amount of displacement of the epicondyle. For nondisplaced and minimally displaced (<5 mm) fractures, most recommend immobilization of the elbow in 90 degrees of flexion for 5 to 7 days for comfort.[15] Elbow motion is then begun to prevent stiffness of the elbow. Treatment of fractures that are displaced more than 5 mm remains controversial. In 1950 Smith[123] stated that even displaced fractures healed, although with a fibrous union, and also that no disability resulted from this fibrous union. He said that the loss of motion seen as a result of this fracture could be prevented with early motion. Bernstein and colleagues[15] have also recommended closed treatment for displaced fractures of the medial epicondyle.

Others have felt that valgus instability of the elbow is an indication for open reduction and pin fixation, especially in the dominant arm of an athlete.[107, 108, 146] Woods and Tullos[146] have shown that medial elbow stability depends upon the medial collateral ligament of the elbow and the forearm flexor muscles. They demonstrated the three bands of the medial collateral ligament. The eccentric position of the epicondyle assures that one of the bands of the ligament will remain taut throughout the range of elbow motion. However, when the medial epicondyle is displaced, the entire collateral ligament displaces with it. The ligament loses its tightness, leading to medial instability of the elbow (Fig. 7–24). It therefore seems reasonable to openly reduce and internally fix a displaced fracture with valgus instability (Fig. 7–25).

Ulnar nerve symptoms were once felt to be an indication for exploration of the fracture.[20, 69, 135] On the other hand, Bernstein and associates[15] found no permanent ulnar nerve injuries as a result of this fracture and recommended observation. Patric and Sneddon also found no permanent ulnar nerve injuries in a review of published material. Median nerve injury, while very uncommon, is an indication

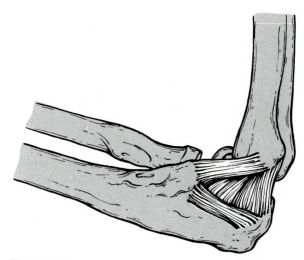

Figure 7–24

Drawing of the ulnar collateral ligament of the elbow. Note the anterior band, posterior band, and oblique band.

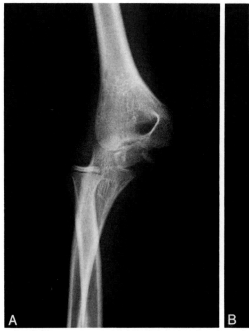
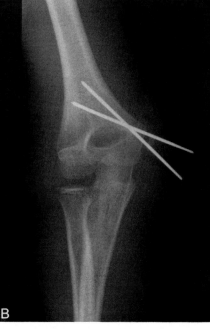

Figure 7–25

Elbow dislocation with fracture of the medial epicondyle. *A*, Anteroposterior radiograph of the elbow. The relationship between the radius and ulna and the humerus is lost because of the elbow dislocation. The medial epicondyle has been displaced. *B*, The elbow dislocation is reduced, and the medial epicondyle has been stabilized with smooth pins.

for nerve exploration. This nerve may rarely become entrapped in the elbow joint as a result of an elbow dislocation with an associated fracture of the medial epicondyle (Fig. 7–26).[43, 82, 105, 110]

The displaced medial epicondyle may become entrapped in the elbow joint when reduction of the dislocation is done. This fragment must be removed from the joint. Roberts[111] recommended using a

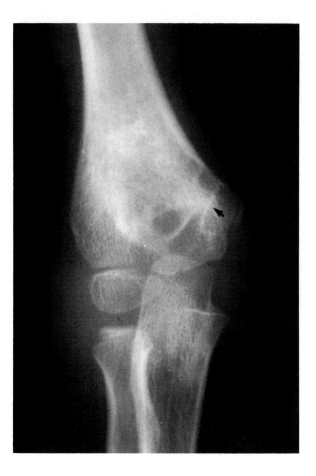

Figure 7–26

Anteroposterior radiograph taken 4 months after dislocation of the elbow. Note the cortical depression in the distal humerus just proximal to the medial epicondyle (*arrow*). This marks the location of the median nerve that became entrapped in the elbow joint after the dislocation.

closed maneuver. He placed a valgus stress on the elbow joint with the forearm supinated to try to dislodge the epicondyle. This seems reasonable if one plans to treat this fracture closed. However, if one plans to openly reduce and pin the unstable medial epicondyle, open removal of the epicondyle at the time of pin fixation should be performed.

Fracture of the Lateral Epicondyle

This is an extremely uncommon injury. It is probably the result of an avulsion of the epicondyle along with the attachment of the forearm extensor muscles. The treatment is immobilization for comfort, with early mobilization.

T-CONDYLAR FRACTURES

Incidence and Classification

Although rare in the pediatric age group, these fractures are seen in the teenager. Usually the physis of the distal humerus is closed or very near the end of growth. Jarvis and D'Astous[62] reported on 16 patients with this injury; the average age of their patients was 12 years, 9 months. These authors also classified the fractures into three groups. Type I is a nondisplaced fracture (however, they found no type I fractures in their series). Type II fractures are displaced. These authors define displacement as greater than 1 mm of separation or step-off of the articular surface. A type III fracture is a fracture-dislocation; it occurred only once in their series.

Treatment

T-condylar fractures must be treated just as one would treat any intraarticular fracture. If the joint surface is displaced, open reduction and internal fixation should be performed. Most recommend a posterior approach through the triceps, which provides the best visualization of the fracture. An olecranon osteotomy may be performed in the skeletally mature patient. The internal fixation devices used will depend upon the type of fracture and the degree of instability. In some relatively stable fractures, lag screws will provide excellent fracture stability (Fig. 7–27).

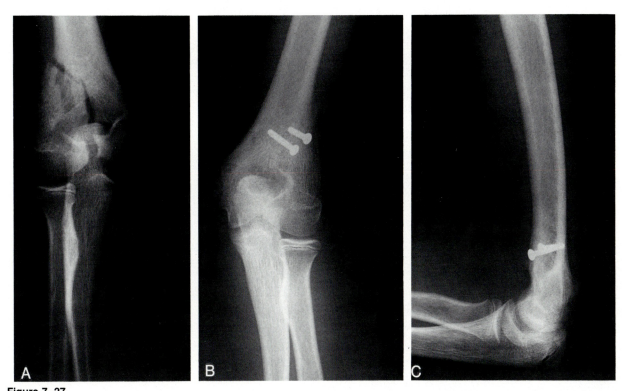

Figure 7–27

T-condylar fracture of the distal humerus. *A*, Anteroposterior radiograph demonstrates the displaced T-condylar fracture of the distal humerus. *B*, Anteroposterior radiograph after open reduction and internal fixation with two lag screws. *C*, Lateral radiograph after open reduction of the fracture.

Fracture of the Proximal Radius

INCIDENCE

Fractures about the proximal radius occur in about 8% of all elbow fractures in children.[34, 144] These fractures are different from those seen in adults because in children most involve the neck of the radius and the physis rather than the head.[55] Most occur in children between the ages of 9 and 12 years.[55, 94, 109, 137, 139]

ANATOMY

The normal proximal radius angulates close to the head of the radius. This may be mistaken for a fracture if one is not aware of this normal angulation. There is a normal lateral angulation of up to 15 degrees as seen on the anteroposterior radiograph (Fig. 7–28). On the lateral radiograph the normal angulation is about 5 degrees.[138]

MECHANISM OF INJURY

Fractures of the proximal radius in the mature patient frequently involve an injury of the head of the radius. In the skeletally immature patient, however, the head of the radius is mostly cartilage, and the force is directed to the physis and the metaphysis. A fracture of the neck of the radius in children may occur in one of two ways. A fall on the outstretched hand with the elbow extended transmits a valgus force to the neck of the radius, resulting in a fracture. If the fracture involves the physis of the proximal radius, any of the four types of fractures of the physis described by Salter and Harris may occur.[116] In addition, the fracture line may involve the metaphysis of the radius only without injury to the physis.

The proximal radius may also be fractured in association with a posterior dislocation of the elbow. The injury that results is usually a fracture through the physis. Jeffrey[63] described displacement of the epiphysis of the radius posteriorly. This fracture occurs when the elbow dislocation spontaneously reduces after posterior dislocation. The capitellum fractures the radial epiphysis as the elbow reduces, pushing the epiphysis posteriorly. Newman[94] later showed that the radial epiphysis may also be fractured through the physis at the time of the posterior elbow dislocation. Since the injury occurs at the time of the dislocation rather than during the reduction, the radial epiphysis is displaced anteriorly.[63, 94]

CLASSIFICATION

Authors have classified fractures of the proximal radius in children in different manners.[62, 94, 95, 144] Wilkins combined these groupings, relying heavily on the those of Jeffrey[63] and Newman,[94] to produce his own classification.[144] He divided valgus injuries into three types according to location of the fracture line. The injuries resulting from posterior elbow dislocation are divided into two groups according to

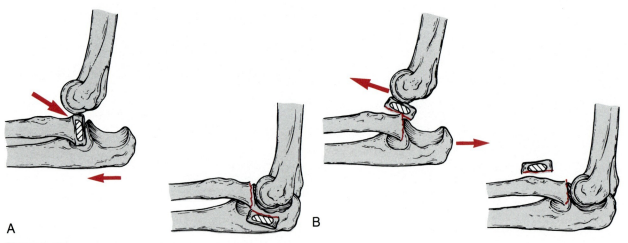

Figure 7–28

Displaced fracture of the radial neck. *A*, The neck is fractured as an elbow dislocation reduces, pushing the radial head posteriorly. *B*, Displacement of the radial head and neck anteriorly. At the time of elbow dislocation the radial head and neck remain anterior to the radius through the metaphysis of the radius. *A* from Jeffrey, C.C. Nonunion of epiphysis of the lateral condyle of the humerus. J Bone Joint Surg 40:396, 1958. *B* from Newman, J.J. Displaced radial neck fractures in children. Injury 9:114, 1977.)

> **Table 7–2**
> **Classification of Fractures of the Proximal Radius**
>
> I. Valgus fractures
>   Type A: Salter-Harris types I and II
>   Type B: Salter-Harris type IV
>   Type C: Fracture of the radial metaphysis only
> II. Fractures secondary to posterior elbow dislocation
>   Type D: Reduction injuries
>   Type E: Dislocation injuries

From Wilkins, K. E. Fractures and dislocations of the elbow region. In: Rockwood, C. H.; Wilkins, K. E.; King, R. E., eds. Fractures in Children. Philadelphia, J. B. Lippincott, 1984.

whether the radial head is displaced anteriorly or posteriorly (Table 7–2).

DIAGNOSIS

The diagnosis of displaced fracture of the neck of the radius is usually easily made radiographically. Some nondisplaced fractures may be difficult to visualize radiographically, however, and rotational views of the proximal radius may be helpful. The clinical examination of the patient should alert one to the diagnosis. The child will have tenderness over the radial head. Rotation of the forearm will produce pain in the lateral elbow that may radiate distally in the forearm.

MANAGEMENT

There is disagreement about the need for reduction of angulated fractures of the radial neck in children. It is known that these fractures will remodel and that this remodeling may be considerable, because of the degree of movement of the radiohumeral and radioulnar joints. Nevertheless, the literature is replete with articles recommending treatment for angulated radial neck fractures. Some, such as Salter and Harris[116] and Jones and Esah,[66] have favored anatomic position and have recommended accepting no more than 15 degrees of angulation. Fahey[34] accepted 25 degrees of angulation, while Rang[107] and Jeffrey[63] accepted 30 degrees of angulation as did Tibone and Stolz.[136] Henrikson[55] felt that 35 degrees of angulation was acceptable as did McBride and Monnet.[84] However, Vahvanen[138] believed that only 10 degrees of angulation of the proximal radius will correct spontaneously with growth.

There is therefore no clearly documented indication for the need of reduction of these fractures. Most currently feel, however, that up to 30 degrees of angulation may be accepted if there is sufficient growth remaining to expect remodeling. If the angulation is greater, a closed reduction of the fracture should be attempted. Patterson[101] described a maneuver used for reduction of this fracture. With an assistant providing countertraction on the upper arm, the surgeon supinates the forearm and applies longitudinal traction. At the same time the elbow is forced into varus by the assistant. Before reduction the forearm should be rotated until the position of maximum tilt of the radial head is directed laterally.[63] The thumb of the surgeon then pushes the radial head back into place.

In 1981 Angelov[3] described a method of percutaneous reduction of the angulated radial neck. A double-pronged instrument is inserted percutaneously and is used to push the head of the radius into the correct position. Recently Bernstein also reported on the successful use of this technique (Fig. 7–29).

Open reduction is indicated if the fracture cannot be reduced satisfactorily by either closed or percutaneous means. The radial head and neck should be approached through a lateral Kocher approach to the elbow. Care is taken to avoid injury to the radial nerve, which may be exposed to protect it.[66] Rang[107] advocates pronation of the forearm to avoid injury to the nerve. Some authors have preferred to use no means of internal fixation after reduction of this fracture, feeling that the fracture is inherently stable.[95, 108, 110] Most authors, however, recommend the use of pin fixation to ensure maintenance of the reduction.[66, 107] The pin should be inserted into the edge of the radial head and cross the fracture obliquely (Fig. 7–30). A pin through the capitellum that crosses the elbow joint and then enters the radial head should not be used, because the pin is likely to break.[94]

The length of immobilization of the elbow will depend upon the nature of the fracture and upon the type of reduction used. If the fracture is minimally angulated and no reduction is necessary, the elbow should be immobilized for comfort for 5 to 7 days only. Elbow motion is begun to avoid loss of motion. If the fracture has been reduced, immobilization for 3 weeks is sufficient. The elbow should be immobilized in 90 degrees of flexion, because if significant elbow motion is lost as a result of the injury, function of the elbow will be best if the motion that remains is about at the neutral or functional position.

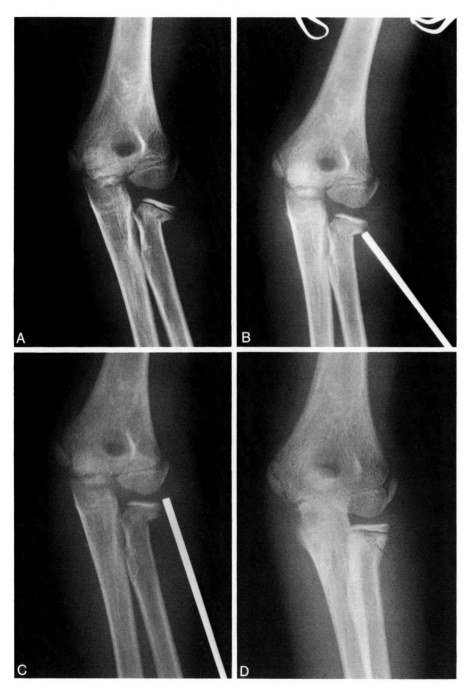

Figure 7–29

Angulated fracture of the radial neck. *A*, Anteroposterior radiograph of the elbow. There is a fracture of the radial neck that is angulated 45 degrees. *B*, Anteroposterior radiograph with a percutaneously inserted Steinmann pin. The blunt end of the Steinmann pin has been inserted against the head and neck of the radius proximal to the fracture. *C*, The fracture has been reduced by general pressure with the blunt end of the Steinmann pin against the radial head. *D*, Anteroposterior radiograph. There has been complete correction of the angulation of the fracture.

Figure 7–30

Displaced fracture of the radial neck. *A*, Lateral radiograph of the elbow. The radial neck is displaced posteriorly. *B*, Anteroposterior radiograph. Radial head and neck are displaced posteriorly and angulated laterally. *C*, Anteroposterior radiograph of the elbow after open reduction and internal fixation with two smooth Steinmann pins. The pins have been placed along the edge of the radial head and neck across the metaphysis and across the physis.

Illustration continued on following page

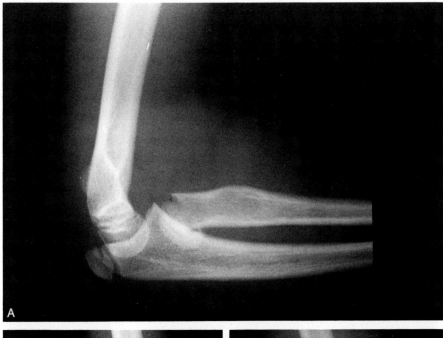
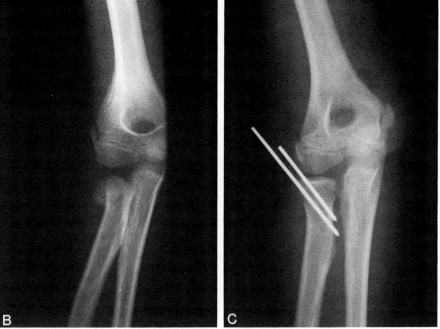

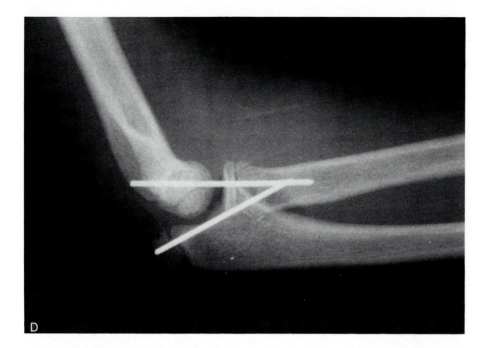

Figure 7-30 Continued
D, Lateral radiograph taken postoperatively.

Olecranon Fractures

INCIDENCE

These fractures are relatively uncommon, constituting 5% of all fractures about the elbow.[34, 83, 144] Newell[93] reported on 40 cases seen over a 40-year period, most of which were minimally displaced. Wilkins[144] stated that less than 20% require surgical treatment.

MECHANISM OF INJURY

Fracture of the olecranon may be the result of a fall on the olecranon with the elbow flexed. An intra-articular fracture is the usual result. It may be nondisplaced, or it may displace enough to require reduction. Olecranon fractures in children may also result from a fall on the outstretched hand with the elbow extended. If the elbow does not hyperextend, but the fall is accompanied by a varus or valgus force, a fracture of the olecranon may result. These injuries are usually greenstick fractures. Bado[8] has classified them as Monteggia fractures because a valgus force that produces a fracture of the olecranon will usually fracture the neck of the radius. On the other hand, a varus-directed force may result in dislocation of the head of the radius.

CLASSIFICATION

The most commonly used classification is that of Matthews, although others have described these fractures as a variant of the Monteggia fracture-dislocation (Table 7-3) (see Chapter 6).

TREATMENT

Most of these fractures are nondisplaced and therefore require no reduction. Extension injuries associated with a dislocation of the head of the radius require treatment (see Chapter 6). Occasionally, flexion injuries of the olecranon are displaced and require open reduction. The type of fixation that is used will depend upon the type of fracture sustained (Fig. 7-31).

Dislocation of the Elbow Joint

INCIDENCE

Dislocation of the elbow is a rare injury in children. Henrikson found 45 elbow dislocations in children

---

Table 7-3
Classification of Fractures of the Olecranon

- Type I—Undisplaced; no associated injury
- Type II—Undisplaced with fracture of proximal radius or supracondylar fracture
- Type III—Undisplaced but with soft tissue damage, e.g., neurovascular damage
- Type IV—Displaced fracture

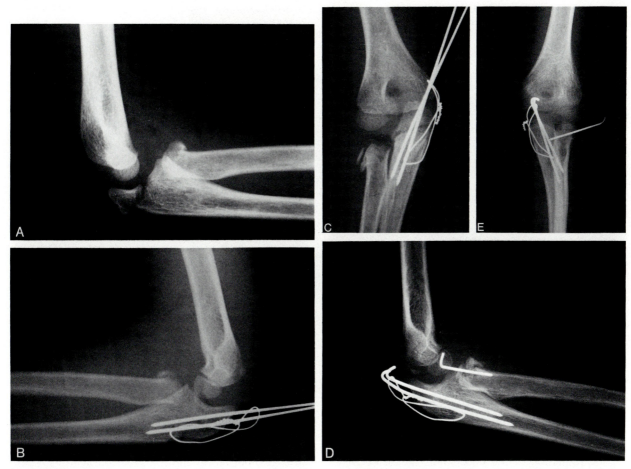

Figure 7–31

Fracture of the olecranon and radial neck. *A*, Lateral radiograph of the elbow showing the displaced fracture of the olecranon with anterior displacement of the distal ulna and radius. Note the displaced fracture of the radial neck. *B*, Intraoperative lateral radiograph of the elbow after open reduction and internal fixation of the olecranon with two smooth pins and a tension band wire. *C*, Anteroposterior radiograph of the elbow after reduction of the olecranon. The radial head and neck are still displaced out of the elbow joint. *D*, Lateral radiograph after open reduction of the radial head. *E*, Anteroposterior radiograph after open reduction of the radial head. The radial head is fixed with a smooth pin that enters the edge of the radial head and crosses the metaphysis and physis.

among 1579 elbow injuries, an incidence of about 3%.[55] While these injuries may occur at almost any age, the peak incidence is during the second decade of life.[75, 92, 144]

MECHANISM OF INJURY

Two likely mechanisms may be responsible for dislocation of the elbow joint. Both probably require a posteriorly directed force. If this force is directed in a posterior direction only, a straight posterior dislocation of the elbow will occur (Fig. 7–32). There is disagreement as to whether the elbow is in flexion or hyperextension at the time of injury.[63, 98] If there is first a valgus force combined with a posteriorly directed force, avulsion of the medial epicondyle in the skeletally immature patient will occur (see Fig. 7–25).

CLASSIFICATION

Elbow dislocations in adults have been classified by Stimson.[129] This classification is dependent upon the direction of displacement of the ulna; for example, if the ulna is displaced posteriorly, this is classified as a posterior dislocation. The two main groups are based upon the proximal radioulnar joint. If that joint is intact, a pure dislocation of the elbow joint is present. That dislocation may be posterior, which is by far the most common; it may also be in a medial or lateral direction. Stimson also described an anterior dislocation, which is extremely rare.[74, 92, 111]

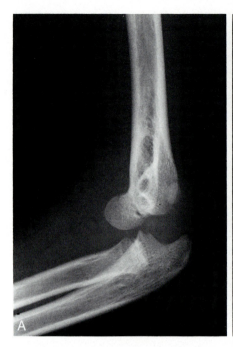
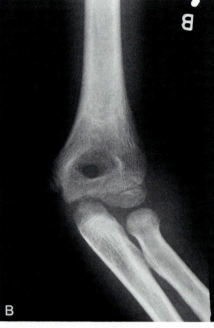

Figure 7–32

Posterior dislocation of the elbow. *A*, Lateral radiograph of the elbow. The ulna and radius are displaced posteriorly. *B*, Anteroposterior radiograph of the posterior dislocation of the elbow.

His second main group includes those elbow dislocations in which the proximal radioulnar joint is also disrupted.

TREATMENT

Closed reduction of the dislocation should be performed as soon as possible. Prior to any treatment a complete evaluation of the neurovascular status of the extremity must be made, because injury to the brachial artery and the median and, less commonly, the ulnar nerve may occur at the time of dislocation. Anesthesia, to reduce the discomfort and to relax the musculature about the elbow, will greatly facilitate the reduction. Although one may choose general anesthesia, an axillary block will usually provide both pain control and muscle relaxation. Self-administered nitrous oxide may also be used.

Regardless of the method of anesthesia, reduction of the dislocation requires traction to dislodge the coronoid process and the radial head from their posterior position. Before applying traction one must first correct any lateral displacement to try to prevent entrapment of the median nerve within the elbow joint.[43] Once the medial or lateral displacement has been corrected, the forearm should be supinated. Then distal and longitudinal traction is applied, with the patient's elbow flexed, while an assistant holds the upper arm to provide countertraction. The assistant stabilizes the upper arm, and the traction with the elbow in flexion may effect the reduction. The surgeon may also use the thumb and fingers to push the olecranon forward while continuing the traction.

The stability of the elbow should be checked. Usually the elbow will be stable, and 2 to 3 weeks of immobilization is all that is required. At the end of that time, elbow motion is encouraged to regain function. If the elbow is unstable at the time of reduction, it should be immobilized in the position of stability for a minimum of 3 weeks and possibly longer. Following that time a removable splint should be worn. While motion is encouraged, full extension is not attempted until 6 weeks after the injury.

Instability of the dislocation may also result from entrapment of the medial epicondyle within the elbow joint. Careful inspection of the radiographs will reveal the position of the medial epicondyle. If it is within the elbow joint after reduction, it must be removed either by manipulation or, more commonly, by open reduction, after which it is internally fixed with pins.

COMPLICATIONS

Vascular Compromise

Disruption of the brachial artery in association with elbow dislocation has been reported, but fortunately it is rare.[53, 68, 77] Brachial artery injury is more common with open elbow dislocation.[53, 68, 77] Louis and co-workers[77] stated that with brachial artery laceration in association with elbow dislocation there is disruption of the collateral circulation about the elbow, resulting in severe ischemia of the forearm. This requires immediate arterial exploration and vascular repair.

Neurologic Injury

Both ulnar and median nerve injuries have been reported to occur with dislocation of the elbow. Injuries to the ulnar nerve have been associated with valgus dislocations, with avulsion of the medial epicondyle. These nerve lesions have been transient.[40]

Median nerve lesions, on the other hand, have been uncommon; when they occur, however, they may produce profound nerve damage because the nerve may become entrapped within the elbow joint as a result of the elbow dislocation.[43, 48, 79, 82, 105, 107, 110]

Hallett[49] described three mechanisms by which the median nerve may become entrapped within the elbow joint. In the first type the nerve becomes entrapped within the joint after a valgus dislocation. The medial epicondyle is avulsed, or the forearm flexor muscles are detached along with tearing of the ulnar collateral ligaments. The nerve slips behind the humerus during the dislocation and becomes entrapped within the joint after the reduction. In the second type the nerve is caught in the healing fracture of the medial epicondyle. In type III the nerve becomes looped anteriorly in the joint.

Hallett considered the diagnosis of this injury to be difficult because of absence of pain. Our experience has been otherwise.[45] We encountered a 7-year-old girl who had dislocated her elbow 4 months previously. After the dislocation she complained of pain in her arm, and because of her refusal to extend the elbow she was referred for physical therapy. In spite of this the patient never regained elbow extension and continued to complain of elbow pain. By the time she was seen by us she had a complete median nerve lesion. The nerve was found to be looped around the posterior humerus, entering the elbow joint posteriorly. Radiographically there was a cortical depression in the ulnar side of the distal humerus caused by the nerve, as described by Matev[82] (see Fig. 7–27). The nerve required resection and anastomosis because the portion within the joint was found to be nothing but scar. The patient regained near-total normal motor function and almost normal sensation in the median nerve distribution.

RECURRENT DISLOCATION

Because recurrent dislocation of the elbow is uncommon, there have been few reports of this complication. Osborne and Cotterill[98] believed that recurrence was the result of failure of reattachment of the posterolateral capsule and ligaments of the elbow joint. If an elbow dislocation is produced by a valgus injury to the elbow, the medial epicondyle and medial collateral ligaments are avulsed. In the cases of recurrent dislocation described, the instability has been on the lateral rather than the medial side.[137] These dislocations, therefore, most likely result from a posteriorly directed force rather than a valgus injury. We have observed, as have others, that there is an avulsion of the capsule and lateral collateral ligaments along with a small piece of bone and cartilage from the lateral side of the elbow.[97, 137]

The treatment of recurrent dislocation of the elbow requires repair of the lax posterolateral structures of the elbow. Osborne and Cotterill[98] described a method of reattachment of the capsule and lateral collateral ligaments to restore elbow stability. These structures are incised in line with their fibers beginning at the humeral epicondylar ridge. The incision is continued distal to the annular ligament. The bone of the lateral epicondyle is roughened, and the capsule and collateral ligament are reattached to the bone with sutures.

DIVERGENT ELBOW DISLOCATION

This is an uncommon type of elbow dislocation.[28, 53, 57] The probable mechanism is an axial load on the elbow with the forearm pronated, resulting in both an elbow dislocation and disruption of the proximal radioulnar articulation (Fig. 7–33).[57] The elbow joint is reduced first; the divergence of the radius and ulna is then reduced by pronation of the forearm.

Radial Head Dislocation

INCIDENCE

Isolated traumatic dislocation of the head of the radius is extremely rare. This injury is most frequently associated with fracture of the ulna, thus being a type of Monteggia fracture-dislocation.[87] Hamilton and Parkes stated that suspected isolated radial head dislocations in children were most likely associated with bending of the ulna. If the ulna did not appear bent on the radiographs, they concluded that it had regained its normal shape.

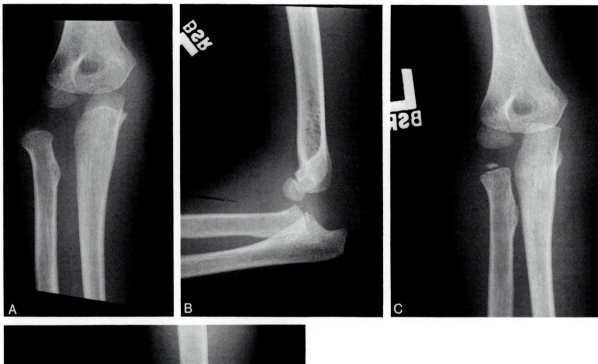

Figure 7–33

Divergent dislocation of the elbow. A, Anteroposterior radiograph of the elbow demonstrating the separation between the radius and the ulna. B, Lateral radiograph of the elbow. There is a posterior dislocation of the radius and ulna. C, Anteroposterior radiograph after closed reduction demonstrating restoration of the normal anatomy of the elbow. D, Lateral radiograph of the elbow following reduction. (From Holbrook, J.L.; Green, N.E. Divergent pediatric elbow dislocation. Clin Orthop 234: 72, 1988.)

The annular ligament stabilizes the head of the radius and prevents dislocation. The annular ligament may be torn with the forearm in pronation.[142, 143]

DIFFERENTIATION FROM CONGENITAL DISLOCATION OF THE RADIUS

Frequently, congenital radial head dislocation is not noticed by the patient or the family because the arm function is normal. Usually, when the child sustains a relatively minor injury to the elbow, the radial head dislocation is observed. The differentiation from the true acute injury may be made by careful examination of the extremity. Although the child with a congenital dislocation and recent trauma may have pain, it is usually less severe than one would expect with a traumatic dislocation. The elbow motion, especially in rotation, will most likely be greater than expected.

The radiographs will demonstrate dysplasia of the radiohumeral joint (Fig. 7–34). The capitellum may be hypoplastic. The radial head is usually dome-shaped without the central depression that is normally present and that one would see with a traumatic dislocation of a normal radial head.[2, 80, 85]

MANAGEMENT

Surgical treatment of true congenital dislocation of the head of the radius is not warranted in the child, because attempts at reduction have not been rewarding. The child with essentially normal elbow function will probably lose elbow motion and func-

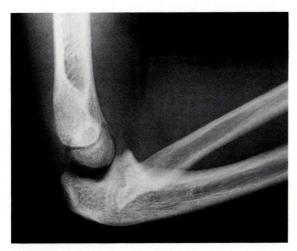

Figure 7–34
Congenital dislocation of the radial head. On the lateral radiograph the radial head is displaced posteriorly and has migrated proximally. The radial neck is narrow and dysplastic, which indicates a long-standing dislocation.

tion after surgical reduction. Neglected traumatic dislocation, on the other hand, has been treated with open reduction with good results, even when the interval between the trauma and the surgical reduction has been more than 3 years.[13, 76] Use of a strip of the triceps tendon to reconstruct the annular ligament has been advocated.[13, 76]

Subluxation of the Radial Head

INCIDENCE

While subluxation of the radial head is the most accurate description of this injury, it is also known by the terms "pulled elbow" and "nursemaid's elbow." It is probably the most common traumatic elbow injury in children. It has been estimated to occur in 15 to 27% of all elbow injuries in children less than 10 years of age.[22, 126] Although the average age of incidence is between 2 and 4 years, we have encountered this injury in children up to age 8 years.

MECHANISM

This injury is produced with the forearm in pronation. With longitudinal traction and the forearm in pronation, the annular ligament tears at its attachment to the radius. The head of the radius moves distally, and as the traction is released the annular ligament becomes caught between the radial head and the capitellum.[117, 132] The tear in the annular ligament may be small, and only a small portion of the annular ligament is caught between the radial head and the capitellum. With a large tear, more of the annular ligament will become entrapped, and reduction of the subluxation will be more difficult.

This injury is not seen in older children; Salter and Zaltz claimed that this injury is rare after the age of 5 years because the ligament becomes thicker with age and resists tearing.[117] The shape of the radial head is oval rather than circular. The sagittal diameter in supination is greater than the coronal diameter of the radial head; therefore the subluxation is able to be reduced with the forearm in supination.

The radial head subluxation results from a pull on the child's extended arm. Typically, the arm is pulled by a parent, or a person walking with the child, who assists the child to step up onto a sidewalk. However, the injury may occur whenever someone pulls on the child's extended and pronated forearm. Children may even produce the injury themselves. If the child grabs something to break a fall, radial head subluxation may result.

MANAGEMENT

The child with radial head subluxation holds the arm flexed at the elbow with the forearm pronated. The initial pain quickly subsides, and the child may return to play but will not use the injured extremity. The infant may hold the arm limp. This pseudoparalysis may cause concern that brachial plexus stretch may have occurred.

A careful examination of the arm will reveal pain in the elbow only. Radiographs should be obtained to rule out another injury. The subluxation is then reduced by forcefully supinating the forearm with the elbow in 60 to 90 degrees of flexion. With the forearm forcefully supinated, the elbow is fully flexed maximally.[126] The surgeon's thumb is placed over the radial head. As the radial head reduces one is able to palpate and hear the click of reduction. The greater the tear in the annular ligament the more forceful the supination that will be required. Although a palpable or audible reduction is usually observed, this is not always the case. Nevertheless, the child will begin to use the arm quickly after the subluxation is reduced. The child should be observed until the arm is used. Immobilization of the arm is not necessary and should not be used. It is important for the family to be able to observe the child's use of the arm. If use of the arm is not normal, the family should be instructed to bring the child back for reevaluation.

REFERENCES

1. Abraham, E.; Powers, T.; Witt, P.; et al. Experimental hyperextension supracondylar fractures in monkeys. Clin Orthop 171:309–318, 1982.
2. Almquist, E.E.; Gordon, L.H.; Blue, A.I. Congenital dislocation of the head of the radius. J Bone Joint Surg 51-A:1118–1127, 1969.
3. Angelov, A. A new method for treatment of the dislocated radial neck fracture in children. In: Chapchal, G., ed. Fractures in Children. New York, Georg Thieme, 1981, pp. 192–194.
4. Arino, V.L.; Lluch, E.E.; Ramirez, A.M.; et al. Percutaneous fixation of supracondylar fractures of the humerus in children. J Bone Joint Surg 59-A:914–916, 1977.
5. Arnold, J.A.; Nasca, R.J.; Nelson, C.L.: Supracondylar fractures of the humerus. J Bone Joint Surg 59-A:589–595, 1977.
6. Aronson, D.D.; Prager, B.I. Supracondylar fractures of the humerus in children. A modified technique for closed pinning. Clin Orthop (219):174–184, 1987.
7. Ashhurst, A.P.C. An Anatomical and Surgical Study of Fractures of the Lower End of the Humerus. Philadelphia, Lea & Febiger, 1910.
8. Bado, J.L. The Monteggia lesion. Clin Orthop 50:71–86, 1967.
9. Bakalim, G.; Wilppula, E. Supracondylar humeral fractures in children. Acta Orthop Scand 43:366–374, 1972.
10. Banskota, A.; Volz, R.G. Traumatic laceration of the radial nerve following supracondylar fracture of the elbow. A case report. Clin Orthop (184):150–155, 1984.
11. Basom, W.C. Supracondylar and transcondylar fractures in children. Clin Orthop 1:43–48, 1953.
12. Bede, W.B.; Lefebure, A.R.; Rostman, M.A. Fractures of the medial humeral epicondyle in children. Can J Surg 18:137–142, 1975.
13. Bell Tawse, A.J. The treatment of malunited anterior Monteggia fractures in children. J Bone Joint Surg 47-B:718–723, 1965.
14. Bensahel, H.; Csukonyi, Z.; Badelon, O.; Badaoui, S. Fractures of the medial condyle of the humerus in children. J Pediatr Orthop 6:430–433, 1986.
15. Bernstein, S.M.; King, J.D.; Sanderson, R.A. Fractures of the medial epicondyle of the humerus. Contemp Orthop 12:637–641, 1981.
16. Brewster, A.H.; Karp, M. Fractures in the region of the elbow in children. An end-result study. Surg Gynecol Obstet 71:643–649, 1940.
17. Buhr, A.J.; Cooke, A.M. Fracture patterns. Lancet 1:531–536, 1959.
18. Casiano, E. Reduction and fixation by pinning "banderillero." Milit Med 125:262–264, 1961.
19. Chacha, P.B. Fracture of medial condyle of humerus with rotational displacement. J Bone Joint Surg 52-A:1453–1458, 1970.
20. Collins, R.; Lavine, S.A. Fracture of the medial epicondyle. Clin Proc Child Hosp (Wash) 20:274–277, 1964.
21. Corkery, P.H. The management of supracondylar fractures in the humerus in children. Br J Clin Pract 18:583–591, 1964.
22. Corrigan, A.B. The pulled elbow. Med J Aust 2:187–189, 1965.
23. Costigan, P.G. Subluxation of the annular ligament at the proximal radio-ulnar joint. Alberta Med Bull 17:7–9, 1952.
24. Coventry, M.B.; Henderson, C.C. Supracondylar fractures of the humerus: 49 cases in children. Rocky Mt Med J 53:458–465, 1956.
25. Crabbe, W.A. Treatment of fracture separation of the capitular epiphysis. J Bone Joint Surg 45-B:722–726, 1963.
26. D'Ambrosia, R.; Zink, W. Fractures of the elbow in children. Pediatr Ann 11:541–548, 550–553, 1982.
27. Dameron, T.B. Transverse fractures of distal humerus in children. Instr Course Lect 30:224–235, 1981.
28. DeLee, J.C.; Wilkins, K.E.; Rogers, L.F.; Rockwood, C.A. Fracture-separation of the distal humerus epiphysis. J Bone Joint Surg 62-A:46–51, 1980.
29. DeRosa, G.P.; Graziano, G.P. A new osteotomy for cubitus varus. Clin Orthop 236:160–165, 1988.
30. Dodge, H.S. Displaced supracondylar fractures of the humerus in children: Treatment by Dunlop's traction. J Bone Joint Surg 54-A:1408–1418, 1972.
31. Dowd, G.S.; Hopcroft, P.W. Varus deformity in supracondylar fractures of the humerus in children. Injury 10:297–303, 1979.
32. Dunlop, J. Transcondylar fractures of the humerus in childhood. J Bone Joint Surg 21-A:59–73, 1939.
33. Eliason, E.L. Dressing for supracondylar fractures of the humerus. JAMA 82:1934–1935, 1924.
34. Fahey, J.J. Fractures of the elbow in children. Instr Course Lect 17:13–46, 1960.
35. Flynn, J.C.; Richards, J.R., Jr. Non-union of minimally displaced fractures of the lateral condyle of the humerus in children. J Bone Joint Surg 53-A:1096–1101, 1971.
36. Flynn, J.C.; Matthews, J.G.; Benoit, R.L. Blind pinning of displaced supracondylar fractures of the humerus in children. J Bone Joint Surg 56-A:263–273, 1974.
37. Flynn, J.C.; Richards, J.F., Jr.; Saltzman, R.I. Prevention and treatment of non-union of slightly displaced fractures of the lateral humeral condyle in children. An end-result study. J Bone Joint Surg 57-A:1087–1092, 1975.
38. Fowles, J.V.; Kassab, M.T. Displaced fractures of the medial humeral condyle in children. J Bone Joint Surg 62-A:1159–1163, 1980.
39. Fowles, J.V.; Kassab, M.T. Displaced supracondylar fractures of the elbow in children. A report on the fixation of extension and flexion fractures by two lateral percutaneous pins. J Bone Joint Surg 56-B:490–500, 1974.
40. French, P.R. Varus deformity of elbow following supracondylar fractures of the humerus in children. Lancet 2:439–441, 1959.
41. Galbraith, K.A.; McCullough, C.J. Acute nerve injury as a complication of closed fractures or dislocations of the elbow. Injury 11:159–164, 1979.
42. Gartland, J.J. Management of supracondylar fractures of the humerus in children. Surg Gynecol Obstet 109:145–154, 1959.
43. Graham, H.A. Supracondylar fractures of the elbow in children. 1. Clin Orthop 54:85–91, 1967.
44. Graham H.A. Supracondylar fractures of the elbow in children. 2. Clin Orthop 54:93–102, 1967.
45. Green, N.E. Entrapment of the median nerve following elbow dislocation. J Pediatr Orthop 3:384–386, 1983.
46. Green, N.E.; Allen, B.A. Vascular injuries associated with dislocation of the knee. J Bone Joint Surg 59-A:236–239, 1977.
47. Griffin, P.P. Supracondylar fractures of the humerus. Pediatr Clin North Am 22:477–486, 1975.

48. Haddad, R.J., Jr.; Saer, J.K.; Riordan, D.C. Percutaneous pinning of displaced supracondylar fractures of the elbow in children. Clin Orthop 71:112–117, 1970.
49. Hallett, J. Entrapment of the median nerve after dislocation of the elbow. J Bone Joint Surg 63-B:408–412, 1981.
50. Hammond, G. The management of supracondylar fractures of the humerus in children. Surg Clin North Am 22:747–762, 1952.
51. Haraldsson, S. On osteochondrosis deformans juvenilis capituli humeri including investigation of intra-osseous vasculature in distal humerus. Acta Orthop Scand (Suppl) 38, 1959.
52. Hardacre, J.A.; Nahigian, S.H.; Froimson, A.I.; Brown, J.E. Fractures of the lateral condyle of the humerus in children. J Bone Joint Surg 53-A:1083–1095, 1971.
53. Harvey, S.; Tchelebi, H. Proximal radio-ulnar translocation. J Bone Joint Surg 61:447–449, 1979.
54. Henderson, R.S.; Robertson, I.M. Open dislocation of the elbow with rupture of the brachial artery. J Bone Joint Surg 34-B:636–637, 1952.
55. Henrikson, B. Supracondylar fracture of the humerus in children. Acta Chir Scand (Suppl):369, 1966.
56. Holda, M.E.; Manolia, A.; LaMont, R.L. Epiphyseal separation of the distal end of the humerus with medial displacement. J Bone Joint Surg 62-A:52–57, 1980.
57. Holbrook, J.L.; Green, N.E. Divergent pediatric elbow dislocation. Clin Orthop 234:72–74, 1988.
58. Holmberg, L. Fractures in the distal end of the humerus in children. Acta Chir Scand (Suppl):103, 1945.
59. Hoyer A. Treatment of supracondylar fracture of the humerus by skeletal traction in an abduction splint. J Bone Joint Surg 34-A:623–637, 1952.
60. Ippolito, E.; Moneta, M.R.; D'Arrigo, C. Post-traumatic cubitus varus: Long-term follow-up of corrective humeral osteotomy in children. J Bone Joint Surg 72-A:757–765, 1990.
61. Jakob, R.; Fowles, J.V.; Rang, M.; Kassab, M.T. Observations concerning fractures of the lateral humeral condyles in children. J Bone Joint Surg 57-B:430–436, 1975.
62. Jarvis, J.G.; D'Astous, J.L. The pediatric T-supracondylar fracture. J Pediatr Orthop 4:697–699, 1984.
63. Jeffrey, C.C. Nonunion of epiphysis of the lateral condyle of the humerus. J Bone Joint Surg 40:396–405, 1958.
64. Johansson, O. Capsular and ligament injuries of the elbow joint. Acta Chir Scand (Suppl) 287, 1962.
65. Jones, E.T.; Louis, D.S. Median nerve injuries associated with supracondylar fractures of the humerus in children. Clin Orthop 150:181–186, 1980.
66. Jones, T.R.W.; Esah, M. Displaced fracture of the neck of the radius in children. J Bone Joint Surg 53-B:429–439, 1971.
67. Kamal, A.S.; Austin, R.T. Dislocation of the median nerve and brachial artery in supracondylar fractures of the humerus. Injury 12:161–164, 1980.
68. Kilburn, P.; Sweeney, J.G.; Silk, F.F. Three cases of compound posterior dislocation of the elbow with rupture of the brachial artery. J Bone Joint Surg 44-B:119–121, 1982.
69. Kilfoyle, R.M. Fractures of the medial condyle and epicondyle of the elbow in children. Clin Orthop 41:43–50, 1965.
70. King, D.; Secor, C. Bow elbow (cubitus varus). J Bone Joint Surg 33-A:572–576, 1951.
71. Kramhoft, M.; Keller, I.L.; Solgaard, S. Displaced supracondylar fractures of the humerus in children. Clin Orthop (221):215–220, 1987.
72. Lagenskiold, A.; Kivilaakso, R. Varus and valgus deformity of the elbow following supracondylar fracture of the humerus. Acta Orthop Scand 38:313–320, 1967.
73. Liddell, W.A. Neurovascular complications in widely displaced supracondylar fractures of the humerus. J Bone Joint Surg 49-B:806, 1967.
74. Linscheid, R.L.; Wheeler, D.K. Elbow dislocations. JAMA 194:113–118, 1965.
75. Lipscomb, P.R.; Burselson, R.J. Vascular and neural complications in supracondylar fractures of the humerus in children. J Bone Joint Surg 37-A:487–492, 1955.
76. Lloyd-Roberts, G.C.; Bucknill, T.M. Anterior dislocation of the radial head in children. J Bone Joint Surg 59-B:402–407, 1979.
77. Louis, D.S.; Ricciardi, J.E.; Spengler, D.M. Arterial injury: A complication of posterior elbow dislocation. J Bone Joint Surg 56-A:1631–1636, 1974.
78. Mann, T.S. Prognosis in supracondylar fractures. J Bone Joint Surg 45-B:516–522, 1963.
79. Mannerfelt, L. Median nerve entrapment after dislocation of the elbow. J Bone Joint Surg 50-B:152–155, 1968.
80. Mardam-Bey, T.; Ger, E. Congenital radial head dislocation. J Hand Surg 4:316–320, 1979.
81. Masada, K.; Kawai, H.; Kawabata, H.; et al. Osteosynthesis for old established non-union of the lateral condyle of the humerus. J Bone Joint Surg 72-A:32–40, 1990.
82. Matev, I. A radiological sign of entrapment of the median nerve in the elbow joint after posterior dislocation. J Bone Joint Surg 58-B:353–355, 1976.
83. Maylahn, D.J.; Fahey, J.J. Fractures of the elbow in children. JAMA 166:220–228, 1958.
84. McBride, E.D.; Monnet, J.C. Epiphyseal fracture of the head of the radius in children. Clin Orthop 16:264–271, 1960.
85. McFarland, B. Congenital dislocation of the head of the radius. Br J Surg 24: 41–49, 1936.
86. McGraw, J.J.; Akbarnia, B.A.; Hanel, D.P.; et al. Neurological complications resulting from supracondylar fractures of the humerus in children. J Pediatr Orthop 6:647–650, 1986.
87. McKeever, P.; Bernstein, S.; King, J.D.; et al. Percutaneous reduction of angulated radial neck fractures in children: A report of 15 cases. Presented at AAOS Annual Meeting, New Orleans, February 1990, p. 209.
88. Milch H. Fractures and fracture-dislocations of humeral condyles. J Trauma 4:592–607, 1964.
89. Mizuno, K.; Hirohata, K.; Kashiwagi, D. Fracture-separation of the distal humeral epiphysis in young children. J Bone Joint Surg 61-A:570–573, 1979.
90. Murphy, W.A.; Siegel, M.J. Elbow fat pad with new signs and extended differential diagnosis. Radiology 124:659–665, 1977.
91. Nacht, J.L.; Ecker, M.L.; Chung, S.M.; et al. Supracondylar fractures of the humerus in children treated by closed reduction and percutaneous pinning. Clin Orthop (177):203–209, 1983.
92. Neviaser, J.S.; Wickstrom, J.K. Dislocation of the elbow: A retrospective study of 115 patients. South Med J 70:172–173, 1977.
93. Newell, R.L. Olecranon fractures in children. Injury 7:33–36, 1975.
94. Newman, J.H. Displaced radial neck fractures in children. Injury 9:114–121, 1977.
95. O'Brien, P.I. Injuries involving the radial epiphysis. Clin Orthop 41:51–58, 1965.
96. Oppenheim, W.; Davlin, L.B.; Leipzig, J.M.; Johnson,

E.E. Concomitant fractures of the capitellum and trochlea. J Orthop Trauma 3:260–262, 1989.
97. Ormandy, L. Olecranon screw for skeletal traction of the humerus. Am J Surg 127:615–616, 1974.
98. Osborne, G.; Cotterill, P. Recurrent dislocation of the elbow. J Bone Joint Surg 48-B:340–346, 1966.
99. Ottolenghi, C.E. Acute ischemic syndrome: Its treatment; prophylaxis of Volkmann's syndrome. Am J Orthop 2:312–316, 1960.
100. Palmer, E.E.; Niemann, K.M.W.; Vesely, D.; et al. Supracondylar fracture of the humerus in children. J Bone Joint Surg 60-A:653–656, 1978.
101. Patterson, R.F. Treatment of displaced transverse fractures of the neck of the radius in children. J Bone Joint Surg 16:695–698, 1934.
102. Piggot, J. Supracondylar fractures of the humerus in children. Analysis at maturity of fifty-three patients treated conservatively. Letter. J Bone Joint Surg 68-A:1304, 1986.
103. Piggot, J.; Graham, H.K.; McCoy, G.F. Supracondylar fractures of the humerus in children. Treatment by straight lateral traction. J Bone Joint Surg 68-B:577–583, 1986.
104. Prietto, C.A. Supracondylar fractures of the humerus. J Bone Joint Surg 61-A:425–428, 1979.
105. Pritchard, D.; Linscheid, R.L.; Svien, H.J. Intra-articular median nerve entrapment with dislocation of the elbow. Clin Orthop 90:100–103, 1973.
106. Ramsey, R.H.; Griz, J. Immediate open reduction and internal fixation of severely displaced supracondylar fractures of the humerus in children. Clin Orthop 90:130–132, 1973.
107. Rang, M. Children's Fractures. Philadelphia, J.B. Lippincott, 1983.
108. Rang, M.; Moseley, C.F.; Roberts, J.M.; et al. Symposium: Management of displaced supracondylar fractures of the humerus. Contemp Orthop 18:497–535, 1989.
109. Reidy, J.A.; Van Gorden, G.W. Treatment of displacement of the proximal radial epiphysis. J Bone Joint Surg 45-A:1355, 1963.
110. Roaf, R. Foramen in the humerus caused by the median nerve. J Bone Joint Surg 39-B:748–749, 1957.
111. Roberts, P.H. Dislocation of the elbow. Br J Surg 56:806–815, 1969.
112. Rogers, L.F.; Malave, S., Jr.; White, H.; Tachdjian, M.O. Plastic bowing, torus and greenstick supracondylar fractures of the humerus: Radiographic clues to obscure fractures of the elbow in children. Radiology 128:145–150, 1978.
113. Rohl, L. On fractures through the radial condyle of the humerus in children. Acta Chir Scand 104:74–80, 1953.
114. Rowell, P.J.W. Arterial occlusion in juvenile humeral supracondylar fracture. Injury 6:254–256, 1974.
115. Rutherford, A. Fractures of the lateral humeral condyle in children. J Bone Joint Surg 67-A:851–856, 1985.
116. Salter, R.B.; Harris, W.R. Injuries involving the epiphyseal plate. J Bone Joint Surg 45:587–592, 1963.
117. Salter, R.B.; Zaltz, C. Anatomic investigations of the mechanism of injury and pathologic anatomy of "pulled elbow" in young children. Clin Orthop 77:134–143, 1971.
118. Schwab, G.H.; Bennett, J.B.; Woods, G.W.; Tullos, H.G. Biomechanics of elbow instability: The role of the medial collateral ligament. Clin Orthop 146:42–52, 1980.
119. Sharp, I.K. Fractures of the lateral humeral condyle in children. Acta Orthop Belg 31:811–816, 1965.
120. Shifrin, P.G.; Gehring, H.W.; Iglesias, L.J. Open reduction and internal fixation of displaced supracondylar fractures of the humerus in children. Orthop Clin North Am 7:573–581, 1976.
121. Silberstein, J.J.; Brodeur, A.E.; Graviss, E.R.; Atchawee, L. Some vagaries of the medial epicondyle. J Bone Joint Surg 63:524–528, 1981.
122. Smith, F.M. Children's elbow injuries: Fractures and dislocations. Clin Orthop 50:7–30, 1967.
123. Smith, F.M. Medial epicondyle injuries. JAMA 142:396–402, 1950.
124. Smith, F.M. Displacement of the medial epicondyle of the humerus into the elbow joint. Ann Surg 124:410–425, 1946.
125. Smith, F.M.; Joyce, J.J. Fractures of lateral condyle of humerus in children. Am J Surg 7:324–239, 1954.
126. Snellman, O. Subluxation of the head of the radius in children. Acta Orthop Scand 28:311–315, 1959.
127. Spinner, M.; Schreiber, S.N. Anterior interosseous nerve paralysis as a complication of supracondylar fractures of the humerus in children. J Bone Joint Surg 51-A:1584–1590, 1969.
128. Staples, O.S. Dislocation of the brachial artery. J Bone Joint Surg 47-A:1525–1532, 1965.
129. Stimson, L.A. A Practical Treatise on Fractures and Dislocations. Philadelphia, Lea Brothers and Co., 1900.
130. Stone, J.S. Fractures of the elbow in children. J Orthop Surg 3:395–400, 1921.
131. Sweeney, J.G. Osteotomy of the humerus for malunion of supracondylar fractures. J Bone Joint Surg 57-B:117, 1975.
132. Swenson, A.L. The treatment of supracondylar fractures of the humerus by Kirschner wire transfixion. J Bone Joint Surg 30-A:993–997, 1948.
133. Tayob, A.A.; Shively, R.A. Bilateral elbow dislocations with intra-articular displacement of medial epicondyles. J Trauma 20:332–335, 1980.
134. Theodorou, S.D. Dislocation of the head of the radius associated with fracture of the upper end of the ulna in children. J Bone Joint Surg 51-B:700–706, 1969.
135. Theodorou, S.D.; Ierodiaconou, M.N.; Roussis, N. Fracture of the upper end of the ulna associated with dislocation of the head of the radius in children. Clin Orthop (228):240–249, 1988.
136. Tibone, J.E.; Stoltz, M. Fracture of the radial head and neck in children. J Bone Joint Surg 63-A:100–106, 1981.
137. Trias, A.; Comeau, Y. Recurrent dislocation of the elbow in children. Clin Orthop 100:74–77, 1974.
138. Vahvanen, V. Fracture of the radial neck in children. Acta Orthop Scand 49:32–38, 1978.
139. Varma, B.P.; Srivastava, T.P. Fracture of the medial condyle of the humerus in children: A report of 4 cases including the late sequelae. Injury 4:171–174, 1972.
140. Wadsworth, T.G. Premature epiphyseal fusion after injury of the capitulum. J Bone Joint Surg 46-B:46–49, 1964.
141. Weiland, A.J.; Meyer, S.; Tolo, V.T.; et al. Surgical treatment of displaced supracondylar fractures of the humerus in children. J Bone Joint Surg 60-A:657–661, 1978.
142. Wiley, J.J.; Galey, J.P. Monteggia injuries in children. J Bone Joint Surg 67-B:728–731, 1985.
143. Wiley, J.J.; Pegington, J.; Horwich, J.P. Traumatic dislocation of the radius at the elbow. J Bone Joint Surg 56-B:501–507, 1974.
144. Wilkins, K.E. Fractures and dislocations of the elbow region. In: Rockwood, C.H.; Wilkins, K.E.; King, R.E., eds. Fractures in Children. Philadelphia, J.B. Lippincott, 1984, p. 363.
145. Wilson, P.D. Fractures and dislocations in the region of the elbow. Surg Gynecol Obstet 56:335–359, 1933.
146. Woods, G.M.; Tullos, H.G. Elbow instability and medial epicondyle fracture. Am J Sports Med 5:23–30, 1977.

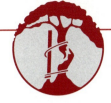

Lawrence X. Webb, M.D.

8

Fractures and Dislocations About the Shoulder

Clavicle

Relevant Anatomy

The clavicle, or collar bone, is an S-shaped bone at the anterior root of the neck. By articulating with the sternum medially and with the scapula at the acromion process laterally, it serves as an osseous connection between the axial skeleton and the upper extremity. In cross section, the medial two thirds of the clavicle is rounded or prismatic, and the lateral one third is flattened. The anterosuperior aspect of the clavicle is subcutaneous.

The clavicle provides an attachment for the pectoralis major on the medial two thirds of its anterior surface and for the deltoid on the lateral one third of its anterior surface. Inferiorly, through its middle two fourths, it affords an attachment for the subclavius muscle and its enveloping clavipectoral fascia, while providing an attachment for both portions of the coracoclavicular ligament laterally and for the costoclavicular ligament medially. On its posterior aspect, the clavicle provides an attachment in its lateral one third for the trapezius and for the clavicular head of the sternocleidomastoid muscle medially. The subclavian vessels and brachial plexus lie posterior to the junction of the medial two thirds and the lateral one third of the bone.[39]

Developmental Anatomy

The clavicle is the first bone to begin to ossify, which it does from two primary ossification centers that appear during the fifth or sixth week of fetal life.[34, 78] In contradistinction, it is one of the last to completely ossify, with its medial physis not closing until age 24 to 26 years.[55]

FRACTURES OF THE MEDIAL END OF THE CLAVICLE AND PSEUDOSTERNOCLAVICULAR JOINT DISLOCATIONS

Incidence

Fracture of the medial end of the clavicle in a child occurs infrequently, accounting for only about 5% of all clavicular fractures.[98] Medial physeal fractures are more common than medial shaft fractures, and the former can mimic sternoclavicular joint dislocations in the adult.[87]

Mechanism

Because the medial physeal plate does not close until about age 24 or 25 years,[39, 55] medial injuring forces usually produce an epiphyseal fracture rather than a dislocation of the sternoclavicular joint.[87] The most common mechanism of injury is thought to be compression of the shoulder toward the midline. Whether displacement occurs retrosternally or prosternally is determined by the secondary force vectors on this intershoulder compression.[27] A direct force can also fracture the end of the clavicle; in this case, displacement is always posterior.

Diagnosis

The patient will have a history of either a blow to the medial end of the clavicle or sternal area or an indirect mechanism, as when the shoulder is used to butt another player in a contact sport. Physical examination will reveal local swelling and tenderness about the medial end of the clavicle (Fig. 8–1). When the displacement is posterior, there may be symptoms of respiratory embarrassment, dysphagia, dysphonia, or distended neck veins from compression on the neighboring trachea, esophagus, recurrent laryngeal nerve, or great vessels, respectively. X-rays angled so as to minimize the effect of obscuring overlying tissues, e.g., the "serendipity" view of Rockwood[27] (Fig. 8–2) or the Hobbs view[48] with the medial end of the clavicles and the sternoclavicular joints visualized bilaterally for comparison, usually confirm the diagnosis. Computed tomography is helpful in delineating more clearly the direction and extent of displacement and the relation of the displaced fracture to neighboring structures.

Treatment

Nondisplaced fractures of the medial end of the clavicle can be managed symptomatically and have a good prognosis. A "bump" should be expected and will remodel to some extent with time, especially in the younger child. A life threat exists when hypoxia or hypercapnia is present secondary to a posteriorly displaced medial portion of the clavicle, and an adequate airway should be secured as part of the patient's primary treatment.[1] An anteriorly displaced medial clavicular fracture can sometimes be reduced by drawing the patient's shoulders backward and apart; this maneuver is sometimes easier when the patient is supine and a folded towel is placed between the shoulder blades.

Posterior displacements can sometimes be reduced percutaneously and directly; i.e., following a suitable anesthetic and skin preparation, a sterile towel clip is used to grab the medial end of the clavicle and manipulate it to its reduced position. Maintenance of the reduction is usual if the displacement is posterior, but reduced anterior dislocations are notoriously less stable. Sometimes the displacing forces can be negated successfully by a figure-of-eight plaster wrap and an arm sling. This reduction should be maintained for a month. The medial clavicular physis in a child has a great remodeling capacity, and late pain and deformity following an anteriorly displaced medial clavicular fracture are seldom seen.

Open reduction should be reserved for open injuries requiring debridement, for posterior displacements that are adversely affecting neighboring vital structures, and for displacements that cannot be reduced (and that reduction maintained) by closed techniques.[8, 32, 87] Internal fixation with metal implants is inadvisable and has been reported to be associated with potentially grave complications.[19] Alternatively, a suture or two placed strategically through drill holes in the outer portion of the neighboring sternum or sternoclavicular ligament and the medial end of the clavicle should suffice to "fix" the reduction until it heals.[87]

One additional, albeit rare, indication for an open reduction is in cases of a scapulothoracic dissociation. In this instance, an anatomic reduction helps "set" the scapula in the correct position on the thoracic wall and facilitates the repair of the torn scapular suspensory musculature close to its correct resting length.

FRACTURED CLAVICULAR SHAFT AT BIRTH

Incidence

The clavicle is the most commonly fractured bone in the newborn.[102] The incidence of clavicular birth fractures ranges from 2.8 to 7.2 per 1000 term deliveries, and clavicular fractures represent from 84 to 92% of all obstetric fractures.[20, 33, 79, 102]

Mechanism and Diagnosis

Clavicular injury at birth has been shown to correlate with birth weight, inexperience of the delivering physician, and midforceps delivery.[20] The mechanism of fracture production is indirect, i.e., an axial compression at the time of passage through a narrow birth canal. The most common fracture site is at the junction of the lateral one third and the middle one third of the bone. The fracture is almost always nondisplaced or is only minimally displaced; often it is unappreciated initially, being discovered as a lump over the clavicle at about 10 days after birth. This lump is the most definitive sign of the fracture; earlier than 10 days, an asymmetric Moro reflex has been reported to be fairly specific for a clavicular fracture in the newborn.[108] Occasionally, the fracture is manifest by "pseudoparalysis" of the arm (Fig. 8–3).[20, 68] In this instance, the differential diagnosis should include fracture of the proximal humerus; sepsis of the shoulder joint; clavicular, scapular, or proximal humeral osteomyelitis; and brachial plexus palsy.[68, 102, 108] It should be borne in mind that two of these diagnoses can coexist, e.g., fracture with brachial plexus palsy or fracture with infection.[18, 125]

Figure 8–1

Fracture of medial end of clavicle. *A*, This patient sustained multiple injuries; the prominence of the right medial clavicle is obvious. *B*, A chest x-ray shows the asymmetry consistent with a medial physeal injury (the epiphysis is unossified). Incidental note is made of the contralateral first rib fracture.

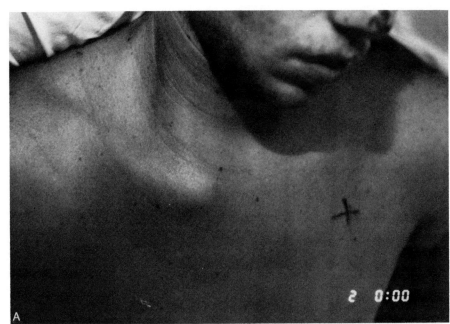

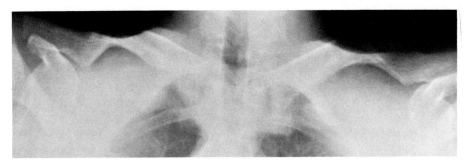

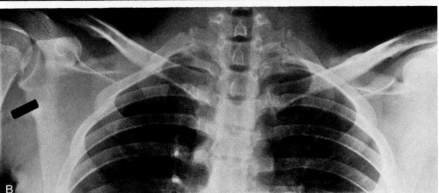

Figure 8–2

A "serendipity" or cephalic tilt roentgenogram of a 14-year-old child. No fractures or dislocations are noted. The film is obtained by placing a non-grid cassette behind the supine patient's head and neck and angling the beam cephalad 40 degrees from a distance of 45 to 60 inches.

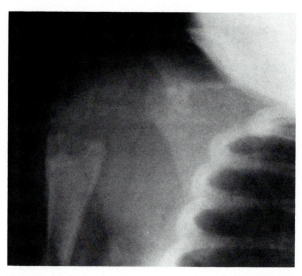

Figure 8–3

Pseudoparalysis of the shoulder. This 4-week-old infant with pseudoparalysis following injury was treated for a clavicle fracture. The child was seen again in follow-up at 2½ weeks, at which time a "sucked candy" appearance of the proximal humeral metaphysis was apparent. Aspiration confirmed an osteomyelitis. The differential diagnosis of pseudoparalysis in such a case is clavicular, proximal humeral, or scapular trauma; brachial plexus palsy; or sepsis of joint and/or neighboring bone.

Treatment

In the rare case in which upper extremity movements elicit tenderness or in cases of pseudoparalysis, splinting the upper extremity to the chest wall with a stockinette stretch bandage or a similar soft, expandable bandage for approximately 10 days is appropriate.[14, 27, 57]

FRACTURED CLAVICULAR SHAFT IN CHILDHOOD

Incidence

Fracture of the clavicle is the most common childhood fracture.[114] The most common portion of the bone to fracture is the shaft, and such fractures account for approximately 85% of all childhood clavicular fractures.[76]

Mechanism

The most common mechanism of the clavicular shaft fracture is a fall onto the shoulder. This mechanism accounted for 87% of the 150 prospectively studied cases carefully documented in the report by Stanley and co-workers.[114] Often, the bone breaks where it changes shape (concave to convex and cross-sectionally from round to flat). Less commonly, the bone is fractured by a direct blow; this accounted for 7% of Stanley's cases, with the remaining 6% of the patients having fallen on their outstretched hand.[114]

Associated Injuries

High-energy trauma is associated with a larger number of fragments and greater fragment displacements, with a consequent higher likelihood for injury to surrounding nonosseous structures, such as the brachial plexus, the neighboring vessels, or the apex of the lung.[52, 76, 89, 121]

Diagnosis

Characteristically, the child will hold the elbow of the affected limb with the opposite hand and tilt the head toward the affected side so as to minimize the displacing pull by the sternocleidomastoid and trapezius muscles. X-rays are confirmatory, although for nondisplaced fractures they may be read initially as negative. Close attention paid to the periclavicular soft tissue shadow and use of a soft tissue technique may detect subtle injuries. Overlying structures may obscure a medial physeal injury, and a Rockwood "serendipity" view (40 degree cephalic tube angle)[27] or a Hobbs projection[48] may be helpful. Children with appropriate histories and point tenderness over the clavicle but negative primary x-rays usually demonstrate a confirmatory small puff of callus at the site of injury on follow-up x-rays obtained 3 or 4 weeks later.

Treatment

More than 200 methods for the nonoperative management of a clavicular shaft fracture have been described.[59] Most commonly these fractures are managed with an apparatus that draws the shoulder backward (e.g., a figure-of-eight plaster wrap, or a figure-of-eight bandage or strap). Patient comfort can be enhanced by placing the ipsilateral arm in a sling for the first couple of weeks.

A common residuum of the injury is a "bump" at the point where the fracture heals. The child and parents should be made aware of this on the initial visit. Characteristically, the bump becomes less distinct as the bone remodels over the next 6 to 9 months.[87] Long-term impairment as a consequence of a closed clavicular fracture managed in childhood using closed methods is a rarity.

Debridement followed by open reduction is indicated for the open clavicular shaft fracture. Internal

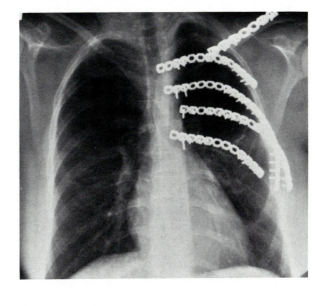

Figure 8–4
One infrequent indication for operative fixation of the clavicle is in an older adolescent with concomitant ipsilateral multiple rib fractures requiring stabilization. In this case an anatomic reposition of the clavicle fracture fragments permits an accurate "setting" of the scapula on the chest wall.

fixation is best avoided but may be necessary to prevent impingement of displaced sharp bone ends on neighboring vital structures or to prevent their protruding through the wound.[117] A 3.5 mm or 2.7 mm reconstruction plate is appropriate internal fixation; one should avoid using pins. A delayed wound closure and arm support in a figure-of-eight bandage or a sling is appropriate. Open reduction may also be indicated for significantly displaced nonreducible fractures, e.g., those that have buttonholed through the trapezius or the fascia, with secondary tenting of the skin.[66] We have also plated the clavicle in an older adolescent with a fracture associated with multiple rib fractures and a flail chest, which needed to be managed by a thoracotomy and rib stabilization (Fig. 8–4). In this patient, the stabilization of the clavicle contributed to the stabilization of the chest wall and set the scapulothoracic articulation at the correct point on the thoracic wall. This indication for clavicular osteosynthesis is seen infrequently, even at major trauma centers (personal communication, J.W. Meredith, Wake Forest University Medical Center; and B. Claudi, Technical University of Munich, 1992).

FRACTURE OF THE DISTAL END OF THE CLAVICLE

Relevant Anatomy

Two anatomic facts greatly enhance our understanding of trauma to the distal end of the clavicle in the child. The first is that the secondary ossification center at the distal end of the clavicle remains unossified until shortly before it unites with the diaphysis at approximately age 19 years.[120] The second is that the thick periosteal sleeve surrounding the distal clavicle and its epiphysis provides a strong attachment for the acromioclavicular and coracoclavicular ligaments.[93] These anatomic relationships make it easier to understand why fracture in this region is much more common than dislocation of the acromioclavicular joint. When the distal clavicle fractures in a child, it creates a rent in the periosteal sleeve, and with displacement the ossified lateral metaphysis herniates through the rent while the unossified epiphysis is retained in the sleeve. Because the epiphysis is cartilage and is radiolucent, it gives the x-ray appearance of what is, in an adult, an acromioclavicular joint dislocation.

Incidence

The outermost aspect of the clavicle, including the acromioclavicular joint, accounts for 10% of the fractures of the clavicle[2, 76, 98]; these occur with greater frequency than do fractures at the medial end of the bone.[27]

Mechanism of Injury

This injury is produced by a force on the point of the shoulder, i.e., a fall or a blow. The patient presents with pain and tenderness on the point of the shoulder. If the fracture is displaced, there may be deformity of the shoulder and upward tenting of the skin. X-rays of the shoulder demonstrate a high-riding lateral clavicular metaphysis in relation to the neighboring acromion. Occasionally, there is an associated fracture of the base of the coracoid process.[31, 130]

Classification

Distal clavicular fractures have been classified into three types by Dameron and Rockwood,[27] with type I being a fracture without displacement; type II, a displaced fracture, nonarticular; and type III, a fracture involving the acromioclavicular joint (Fig. 8–5).

Treatment

In view of the tremendous remodeling potential, i.e., the osteogenic capacity of the retained periosteal sleeve, these injuries should be managed nonoperatively. Treatment usually consists of a simple sling or shoulder Velpeau immobilization for 3 weeks, followed by gentle functional shoulder exercises. There have been several reports of Y-shaped distal clavicles or distal clavicular duplication ascribed to developmental causes[37, 122]; Ogden has suggested a traumatic etiology as well—with one limb of the Y being the original, now upwardly displaced, lateral clavicular metaphysis (Fig. 8–6).[87] The condition is asymptomatic and does not require treatment. As a rule, one should expect a normal-appearing and normally functioning shoulder following distal clavicular fracture in a child.

ACROMIOCLAVICULAR JOINT INJURY

A true injury to the acromioclavicular joint is rare in the child but is seen in the older adolescent.[27] The injury mechanism is the same as in the adult, i.e., a blow to or a fall on the point of the shoulder. Allman[2] has classified these injuries into three types: type I, a mild sprain of acromioclavicular ligaments without a subluxation of the joint; type II, a sprain of the ligament with subluxation of the joint but no alteration in the coracoid-clavicle distance; and type III, a dislocation of the joint with an increase in the coracoid-clavicle distance, which implies a disruption in the coracoclavicular ligament (Fig. 8–7).

Treatment for types I and II injuries should consist of a simple form of immobilization, such as a sling or shoulder Velpeau bandage for 3 or 4 weeks. This should be followed by functional shoulder exercises, with gradual progression of movement dictated by patient comfort. Type I injuries do well as a rule. Type II injuries are occasionally accompanied by late sequelae, i.e., weakness and pain with shoulder movement. Affected individuals may be candidates for a reconstruction procedure, such as a Weaver-Dunn reconstruction, in their early adult years.

There has been some discussion in the recent

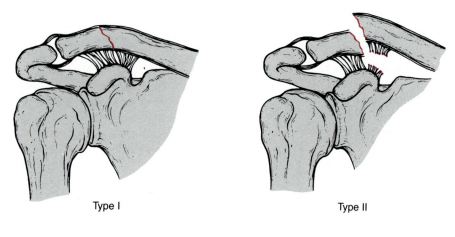

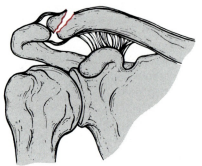

Figure 8–5

Distal clavicle fractures classified into three types by Dameron and Rockwood[27]: Type I is nondisplaced and nonarticular; type II is displaced and nonarticular; type III is intraarticular.

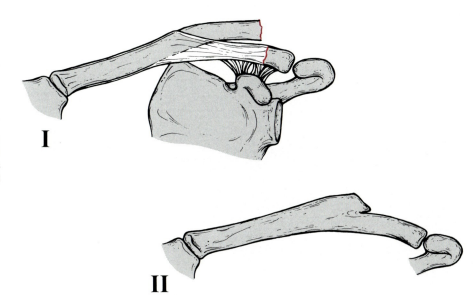

Figure 8–6

I, Distal clavicular fracture in an immature individual with upward displacement. *II*, Healing occurs within the retained periosteal sleeve.

literature on adult acromioclavicular fractures about the best method of managing the type III injury. Indications for open treatment include acromioclavicular joint injuries in conjunction with scapulothoracic dissociation,[3, 84] irreducible injuries wherein the clavicle is subcutaneous and buttonholed through the fibers of the trapezius,[91, 85] and open injuries requiring debridement and irrigation. These uncommon indications notwithstanding, nonoperative management[62, 118] is the treatment of choice for this injury in the adolescent and should be as outlined above.

Scapula

Developmental Anatomy

The scapula starts to ossify from a single center at the eighth week of fetal life.[128] The center for the middle of the coracoid process forms at 1 year of age and that for the base of the coracoid/upper portion of the glenoid at 10 years.[58] At puberty, two to five centers form in the acromion and fuse by age 22 years; failure of fusion of any of these centers gives rise to the variant "os acromiale" (Fig. 8–8).[65] A horseshoe-shaped secondary center at the inferior rim of the glenoid, a center for the medial border, and a center for the inferior angle form and later fuse with the remainder of the bone by age 22 years.[39, 72, 107]

Anatomy

The scapula is a flat bone applied to the posterosuperolateral chest wall; it is richly invested with muscle attachments (n = 17) on both its superficial and its deep aspects, with only the dorsal edge of its spine and acromion being subcutaneous. It artic-

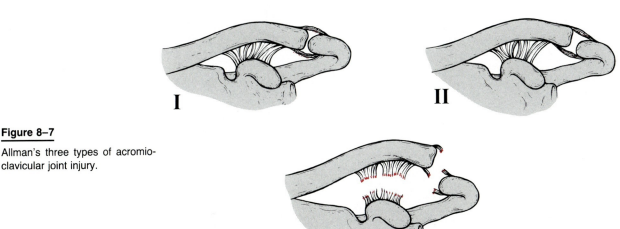

Figure 8–7

Allman's three types of acromioclavicular joint injury.

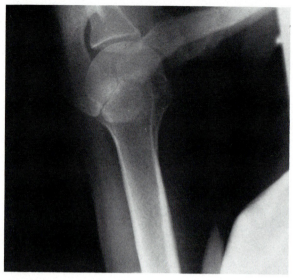

Figure 8–8

This is one of several possible patterns of "os acromiale," discovered incidentally on an axillary lateral projection of this patient's glenohumeral joint.

ulates with the clavicle at the acromioclavicular joint, with the humerus at the glenohumeral joint, and functionally with the chest wall at the scapulothoracic articulation (not a true joint). The muscles that house the scapula participate in shoulder movements by rotating as well as translating the scapula on the chest wall.[50, 53] The articular surface of the glenoid is pear-shaped; a fibrocartilaginous labrum on its rim helps center the humeral head in the glenoid during function. The bony projections, i.e., the acromion and coracoid process, are oriented at 120 degrees to each other and to the axillary border of the scapula when viewed from the true lateral aspect of the bone (the so-called "Y" view of the scapula; Fig. 8–9).[103]

Incidence and Classification

Fractures of the scapula are rare in children[4, 28] and are classified according to the portion of the bone that is fractured, i.e., the body, the glenoid, the acromion, or the coracoid.[25]

Body Fractures

Body fractures occur as the result of a direct, significant trauma. With the large amount of surrounding muscle, deformity is rarely evident. Clues on physical examination include abrasions, ecchymoses, neighboring wounds, swelling, and tenderness. True anteroposterior (AP) and lateral x-ray views are usually diagnostic, but opposite-side comparison views are often necessary to detect subtle injuries in the child.

A scapulothoracic dissociation can be diagnosed on an AP view of the chest (Fig. 8–10).[30] Associated injury to the brachial plexus,[97] vascular structures,[3] and chest wall[3] should be searched for. Scapulothoracic dissociation has not been reported in newborn or very young children but has been reported in two older children, aged 8 and 11 years.[3, 84] Both children underwent an operative repair of the detached sus-

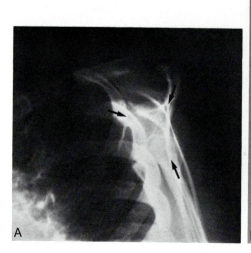
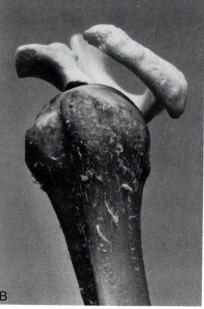

Figure 8–9

A "Y" view (A) of the glenohumeral joint with corresponding view of the dry bony scapula and overlying humerus (B).

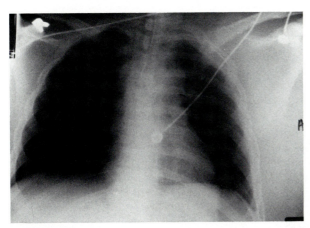

Figure 8–10

Scapulothoracic dissociation. The main radiographic findings are asymmetry of the shoulder girdle with the affected side (*left*) being laterally displaced.

pensory muscles and open restoration of the articulation with the clavicle.

In general, body fractures, like dissociations, imply a large amount of force and associated injury to the underlying chest, and injury to neighboring structures (subclavian and axillary vessels, brachial plexus) should be searched for. These fractures are managed by sling immobilization of the shoulder for 2 to 3 weeks, followed by gentle mobilization, e.g., pendulum exercises with progression over several weeks to full activity in accord with patient comfort and findings on physical and roentgenographic examinations.

GLENOID FRACTURES

Fractures of the glenoid are caused by forces transmitted to the shoulder by a fall on a flexed elbow.[66] Whether a dorsal or an anterior rim fragment results is determined by the position of the arm at the time of injury. Computed tomography is especially useful in assessing the size and significance of these fractures. If the fragment is large, the humeral head may be subluxed; with dislocation, there may be significant displacement of the associated glenoid rim fragment.[66]

For minimally displaced glenoid fragments not associated with humeral head subluxation or dislocation, the recommended treatment is sling immobilization for 3 weeks followed by gentle functional exercises. For the seldom encountered situation of a large fragment being associated with humeral head subluxation or dislocation, operative anatomic reduction with a lag screw (Fig. 8–11) or a small "hook"[131] or "spring"[71] plate and repair of associated capsular tears are indicated. Careful preoperative planning is strongly recommended, and the surgical approach is dictated by the location of the fragment to be fixed. Postoperatively, the patient's arm is immobilized in a sling for 3 weeks followed by gentle functional exercises. Screws or plates should be removed after 3 months.[66]

ACROMIAL FRACTURES

Fractures of the acromion are rare but can result from a direct force on the point of the shoulder.[73] A failure of one of the several acromial epiphyses to fuse, i.e., os acromiale (see Fig. 8–8),[65] should not be mistaken for a fracture. Opposite-side comparison x-rays may be helpful, as may reference to an appropriate skeletal roentgenographic atlas.[56, 58] The usual treatment consists of sling immobilization for 3 weeks, followed by early functional shoulder exercises.

CORACOID FRACTURES

A fracture of the coracoid process is uncommon in the child.[87] The two fracture patterns seen when the injury does occur represent an avulsion by the pull of the acromioclavicular ligaments or an avulsion from the conjoined tendon of the coracobrachialis and short head of the biceps brachii.[9] The first type of fracture occurs through the physis at the base of the coracoid and the upper quarter of the glenoid[46, 60, 130]; the second type occurs through the tip of the coracoid.[25] Coracoid fractures can accompany distal clavicular fractures, apparent acromioclavicular joint injuries, and shoulder dislocations.[12, 119, 129] The injury can be demonstrated by the Stryker notch view[43] or by an axillary lateral view when the gantry is widened to include the coracoid on the film (Fig. 8–12). Treatment usually consists of sling immobilization of the shoulder for 3 weeks followed by gentle functional shoulder exercises.

Glenohumeral Joint Dislocation

Developmental Anatomy

Between 4½ and 7 weeks after fertilization, the proximal upper limb bud blastema differentiates into the scapula, the humerus, and an interzone.[36] This interzone and its surrounding mesenchyme give rise to the capsule and intraarticular structures of the glenohumeral joint.[35] Differentiation of these struc-

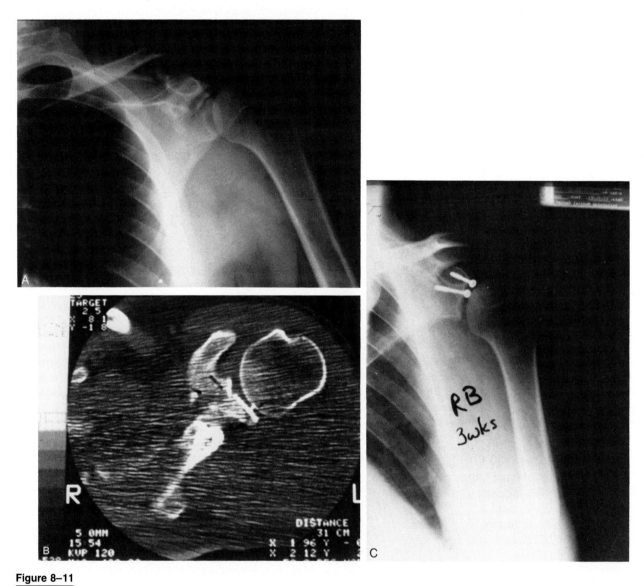

Figure 8–11

A, An intraarticular fracture of the glenoid; there was an associated acromioclavicular separation and acromial fracture. *B*, CT scan demonstrates the step-off displacement in the joint. *C*, The articular fragment was repositioned anatomically via an anterior approach. The fragment was held in place by means of two lag screws.

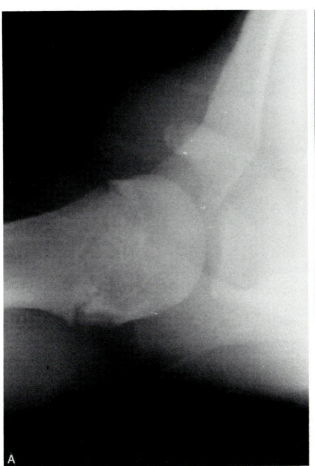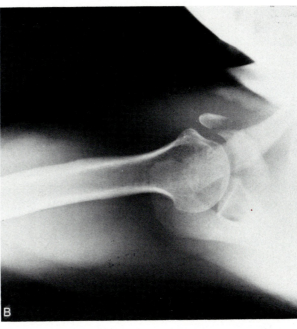

Figure 8–12

A, The coracoid is adequately visualized on the axillary lateral projection when the gantry is wide. *B*, The tip of the coracoid has been avulsed in this mature individual.

tures is complete by 7 to 8 weeks post fertilization; thereafter the joint cavity and its surrounding structures as well as the supporting elements, such as the rotator cuff muscles and tendons, increase in absolute size while maintaining relative size.[35]

Anatomy

The glenohumeral articulation is a true synovial joint of the ball-and-socket variety. The joint comprises the rather shallow, pear-shaped glenoid and the spherical head of the humerus. The closely related capsule, its associated glenohumeral ligaments, and its overlying rotator cuff tendons provide a mobile and dynamic extension of the shallow glenoid cavity, which centers the spherical humeral head within that cavity and enables it to pass through a greater arc of motion than any other joint in the body.[53] However, the major reliance of the glenohumeral joint on soft tissue support makes it the most prone to subluxate or dislocate.[86]

Incidence

During childhood, the open proximal humeral physis is the mechanically weak link in the glenohumeral articulation, and thus skeletal trauma to the region is most often manifest by a Salter-Harris type II[106] proximal humeral fracture. During adolescent years, as the proximal humeral growth plate begins to close, there is a rise in the incidence of glenohumeral dislocation. In the series reported by Rowe and colleagues of some 500 glenohumeral dislocations seen over a 20-year period, only 8 (1.2%) occurred in children under age 10 years, whereas 99 (19.8%) occurred in patients aged 10 through 20 years.[101] Approximately half the injuries in the 10- to 20-year group (48/99) were recurrent dislocations.[101] Recurrence rates have ranged from 20%[101] to 100%[4] in children under 10 years and from 48%[101] to 90%[4] in patients between ages 10 and 20 years. Dislocation of the shoulder during infancy is very rare but has been reported in association with brachial plexus palsy[63, 64] and sepsis[40] and as a congenital deformity.[23, 41]

Classification

Glenohumeral dislocation may be classified according to the direction of the dislocation, i.e., anterior, posterior, or inferior (the last two are rare). They may also be classified according to etiology, as shown in Figure 8–13.

Mechanism of Injury

The anterior glenohumeral dislocation is usually produced by a force on the outstretched hand with the shoulder in abduction, external rotation, and elevation, causing forward levering of the humeral head and secondary stretching of the anterior and inferior capsular tissues. Eighty-five percent have anterior and inferior capsular detachment from the glenoid neck—the so-called Bankart lesion.[7] Posterior dislocation can accompany epileptic seizures and convulsions due to electroshock and is explained by the powerful override of the internal rotators, which lever the humeral head in the opposite (posterior) direction.[107, 123]

Many patients with a history of atraumatic dislocation can voluntarily sublux or dislocate the shoulder. Those who perform this atraumatic voluntary type of dislocation are more likely to be children or adolescents than adults.[100] In the initial report by Rowe and co-workers on the subject,[100] 20 of 26 (80%) patients were 16 years or younger; psychiatric factors were found to play an important role in these voluntary dislocations. Whether this ability is spontaneous or is acquired after an initial traumatic injury is unclear. In Rowe's series,[100] 11 patients could recall no specific episode of initial trauma; the remaining 15 could recall a minor twist or a fall.

Diagnosis

A traumatic dislocation causes pain and swelling about the shoulder. The attitude of the arm will depend on the type of dislocation; i.e., with an anterior dislocation, it will be held abducted and slightly externally rotated; with a posterior dislocation, it will be fixed in adduction and internal rotation; and with an inferior dislocation, it will be held in abduction with the forearm lying on or behind the patient's head (the so-called luxatio erecta position). An atraumatic dislocation causes no or minimal pain and swelling.

A careful neurovascular examination should be performed routinely. Injury to the axillary nerve of the brachial plexus as well as the rotator cuff tendons is sometimes seen in association with glenohumeral dislocation and should be searched for. In their series of 226 anterior dislocations, Pasila and associates,[88] reported 11% brachial plexus injuries, 8% axillary nerve injuries, and 11% rotator cuff tears. The neighboring axillary artery and vein are also liable to injury, particularly in excessively forceful reductions.[15]

When chronic instability is suspected, the examiner can demonstrate glenohumeral laxity by manually stabilizing the scapula and exerting gentle anterior-to-posterior, posterior-to-anterior, or inferior-to-superior forces on the humeral head with the

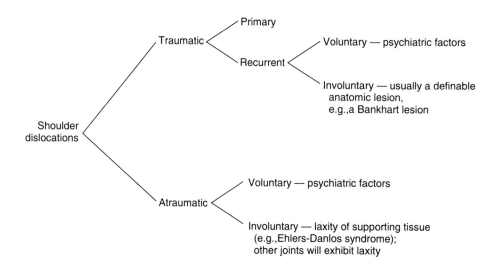

Figure 8–13

Etiologic classification of glenohumeral dislocations.

opposite hand and comparing the response with that of the opposite side. Alternatively, the examiner can elicit an apprehension sign by checking the limits of comfortable external rotation in varying degrees of abduction for both shoulders or by the Feagan test.[94] X-rays should include a "trauma series,"[95] i.e., an AP and lateral view in the plane of the scapula. Because the overlying humeral head and chest wall can obscure subtle rim fractures (as well as a fracture of the lesser humeral tuberosity), an axillary lateral view or a modified axillary lateral view[13] is also obtained.

Treatment

Reduction of an acute, traumatic dislocation can usually be accomplished safely using any of several classic methods. For immediate reduction of acute dislocation (as in those witnessed, preferably verified as a dislocation with a portable imaging device and treated on an athletic field), slight abduction and "derotation" of the affected arm with minimal traction, as described by O'Brien and associates,[86] can be attempted. The hippocratic method[47] consists of slow and gentle traction on the affected arm with gentle internal and external rotation to disengage the humeral head. The physician applies countertraction by placing his or her stockinged foot on the patient's chest wall across the anterior and posterior axillary folds (Fig. 8–14A). Alternatively, one can employ a modification of this technique using a twisted sheet across both axillary folds and around the chest with an assistant pulling on the sheet to provide countertraction (Fig. 8–14B).

The Stimson method[115] calls for positioning the patient prone and allowing the affected arm to hang from the edge of the table with a weight (5 to 10 lb) suspended from the end of the arm (Fig. 8–14C). Numerous other methods have been described by Milch,[75] Lacey,[61] Russell,[104] Janecki,[54] Mirick,[77] and White.[127]

After reduction, the neurovascular examination should be repeated and documented. A sling should be applied, followed by early motion with progression being dictated by patient comfort. A period of enforced shoulder immobilization has been shown in Hovelius' large prospective series of cases not to influence the recurrence rate.[51] Both the patient and

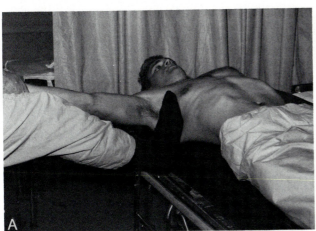
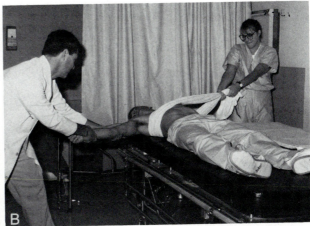
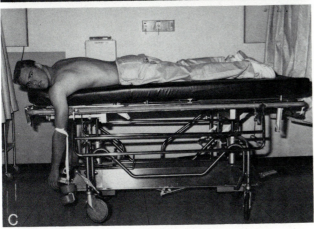

Figure 8–14

Glenohumeral reduction techniques. *A*, Hippocratic method. *B*, Modified hippocratic method. *C*, Stimson method.

the parents should be informed of the high likelihood for recurrence as well as of the maneuver that is likely to trigger it (for an anterior dislocation this would be elevation with external rotation), and of which sports are "dangerous" (for an anterior dislocation this might be tennis). Patients with recurring dislocations, especially if the dislocations are brought about by trivial activities of daily living that are hard to modify, are candidates for a repair directed toward the specifically implicated disorder, e.g., a Bankart repair[99] for a lax anterior capsule secondary to capsular avulsion from the anterior inferior glenoid neck.

Patients who are voluntary dislocators are best initially managed nonoperatively with a rehabilitation program aimed at strengthening the rotator cuff as well as the deltoid muscles[44, 80, 100] and perhaps with specific counseling directed toward modifying the underlying attention-seeking behavior pattern.[100] If this treatment is successful, any recurring dislocations will be of the involuntary variety and may be multidirectional. Surgical therapy with a capsular shift to correct this problem, as described by Neer and Foster,[81] would then be indicated.

Fractures of the Proximal Humerus

Developmental Anatomy

The primary ossification center for the humerus appears at about the sixth week of fetal life.[38] The ossification center for the humeral head appears at about the time of birth, that for the greater tuberosity between 7 months and 3 years, and that for the lesser tuberosity 2 years later. These proximal secondary ossification centers coalesce at about age 5 to 7 years.[39, 92, 96, 105] The proximal physis closes between ages 14 and 17 years in girls and between ages 16 and 18 years in boys.[39, 92, 96, 105]

Anatomy

The proximal physis is tent-shaped, its apex being located in the posteromedial portion of the proximal humerus on cross section (Fig. 8–15A).[87] A small portion of the posterior proximal and medial metaphysis is intracapsular and extracartilaginous. The capsular attachment provides a strong tether just distal to this.[39] This anatomic characteristic, in addition to the relative thickness of the posteromedial periosteum and thinness of the anterolateral periosteum,[26] may help explain the tendency for the metaphyseal fragment to buttonhole the periosteum anterolaterally when the proximal humerus is fractured and (in Salter-Harris type II injuries) for a small posteromedial piece of metaphysis to stay with the proximal fragment (Fig. 8–15B).

It should be noted that physeal fractures pass through the zone of hypertrophy adjacent to the zone of provisional calcification, sparing the zone of embryonal cartilage and thereby retaining the growth potential of the physis.[10, 26, 106] The proximal humeral physis contributes 80% of the longitudinal growth of the humerus, and thus fractures at that site have great remodeling potential.[10, 29, 82]

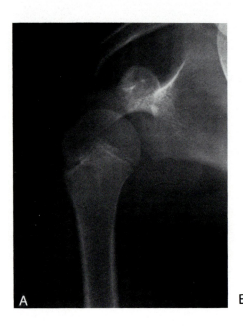
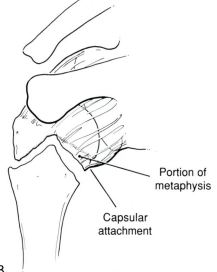

Figure 8–15

A, "Tent-shaped" proximal humeral physis. B, Glenohumeral capsular attachment site following a fracture.

Incidence

Fractures involving the proximal humeral growth plate represent approximately 0.45% of all childhood fractures[96] and approximately 3% of all epiphyseal fractures.[82] Salter-Harris type I injuries predominate in neonates and children under age 5 years[25]; metaphyseal fractures predominate in those between ages 5 and 11 years; and Salter-Harris type II injuries predominate in those over age 11 years.[25]

Mechanism of Injury

Injury in the newborn is usually attributable to the trauma of delivery. Hyperextension and excess rotation have been implicated.[24, 42, 109] The forces that bring about a fracture of the proximal humerus in children are most commonly indirect and result from a fall on the outstretched arm,[49, 69, 112] although a direct force, i.e., a blow on the posterolateral upper arm, was implicated as the most prevalent mechanism in one series.[82]

Diagnosis

Diagnosis can be difficult in the newborn. The findings can be subtle, such as irritability with arm movements, or can be more pronounced, such as pseudoparalysis, in which case they should be distinguished from entities such as septic arthritis (see Fig. 8–3), brachial plexus palsy, and distal clavicular injuries.[27, 38, 49] Plain films of the proximal humerus should be obtained with comparison views of the opposite limb; arthrography may help outline the position of the proximal (largely cartilaginous) fragment.[6, 16, 22, 27, 82]

In older children, pain, splinting, and arm dysfunction are present. Ecchymosis and swelling are variably present, and in displaced fractures the arm may be shortened and the proximal metaphysis bulging beneath the anterior aspect of the shoulder. Diagnostic plain x-rays at 90 degrees to each other should be obtained.

Classification

The Salter and Harris classification of epiphyseal injuries has been applied to physeal injuries of the proximal humerus.[106] As was pointed out earlier, most of the fractures of the proximal humerus in children under age 5 years are type I; 75% of the fractures in children over age 11 years are type II, with the remainder being type I. Metaphyseal fractures predominate between ages 5 and 11 years.[25]

Salter-Harris types III, IV, and V injuries are rarely seen.[25, 69] The single reported case of a Salter-Harris type III injury was associated with a dislocation in a 10-year-old child.[21]

Fracture stability (either before or after a closed reduction) is also a means of classifying these fractures (stable vs. unstable) and can be used to guide treatment.

Salter-Harris type II fractures were further subdivided into four grades by Neer and Horwitz, who used the extent of fracture displacement as the criterion for their grades (Table 8–1).[82]

It should be noted that grades III and IV are associated with varus angulation. In Neer and Horwitz's series,[82] shortening of from 1 to 3 cm was reported in 11% of group I and group II patients, versus 33% of group IV patients; no shortening resulted at the time of injury in any patient younger than 11 years. Thus, the remodeling potential (in years) may play more of a role in determining the final outcome than the extent of displacement.

Treatment

In general, fractures of the proximal humerus are managed by closed techniques. Nondisplaced fractures can be managed by sling-and-swathe immobilization followed by protected motion. Displaced fractures should be reduced and then managed as described above. When reduction cannot be achieved or when the reduction achieved is lost as the arm is brought to the chest wall, the decision must be made whether to accept this malposition (usually varus ± displacement), to make further attempts at reduction, or to employ more elaborate immobilization methods (which potentially entail greater morbidity). This decision should take into account the age of the patient (and thus the remodeling potential of the bone) as well as the fact that a functional shoulder can be expected regardless of

Table 8–1

Neer/Horwitz Classification of Proximal Humeral Fractures

Grade	Displacement
I	< 5 mm
II	< 1/3 shaft width
III	≤ 2/3 shaft width
IV	> 2/3 shaft width

From Neer, C. S., II; Horwitz, B. S. Fractures of the proximal lumeral epiphysial plate. Clin Orthop 41:24, 1965.

the method used.[10, 26, 112] With the more severely displaced varieties of growth plate injuries in the older child (>11 years), one can anticipate 1 to 3 cm of arm shortening and a loss of glenohumeral motion (abduction) of several degrees.[82]

Sherk and Probst[111] set up minimal guidelines for an acceptable reduction: an angulation of less than 20 degrees and a displacement of less than 50%. With these criteria met, an acceptable outcome can be expected.[17, 111]

The choices for treatment of displaced fractures are closed reduction with olecranon pin traction, a "salute" cast, closed reduction with percutaneous pinning,[11] or open reduction with internal fixation (usually percutaneous pinning). For the ventilator-dependent child or the child whose other injuries require an enforced recumbency, olecranon pin[92] or percutaneous winged screw[69] skeletal traction is well suited. For the child who is otherwise mobile, a "salute" cast is one alternative but can be associated with skin breakdown, abduction contracture, and brachial plexus injury.[11, 49, 92] Alternatively, and perhaps preferentially,[67] for the child with injuries requiring monitoring of the abdomen or chest, percutaneous Steinmann pin fixation can be performed coincident with reduction. Using an image intensifier with the child appropriately anesthetized,[11] two or three large Kirschner wires (K-wires) or small-diameter Steinmann pins are directed obliquely cephalad from the lateral metaphysis across the reduced physis and into the proximal epiphysis (Fig. 8-16). The pins are cut and "J"d at the ends outside or just under the skin, and a sterile dressing is applied. A simple sling-and-swathe or collar-and-cuff is then applied to support the limb until the fracture heals. The pins are usually removed at 2 to 3 weeks, at which time gentle pendulum exercises can be started.

Open reductions should be reserved for special circumstances, i.e., an open injury requiring a surgical debridement, associated glenohumeral dislocation (in which forceful attempts at closed reduction may be a hazard to neighboring soft tissue structures), vascular injuries, or in the rare circumstance when reduction is unsatisfactory in an adolescent owing to an interposed biceps tendon.[124] Vigorous attempts at reducing a glenohumeral dislocation associated with a fractured proximal humerus are potentially hazardous and place surrounding vessels and nerves at risk of serious injury. Skeletal stabilization (usually percutaneous pinning) is needed under these circumstances and enables one to control the position of the humeral head in the glenoid by positioning the arm against the chest wall. Reestablishing skeletal continuity also better enables one to assess the stability of the joint reduction.

If skeletal traction, a salute cast, or percutaneous pins are used, the immobilization can be switched at about 3 weeks, when the fracture is "sticky," to a simpler form, e.g., a collar-and-cuff or a sling-and-swathe (Fig. 8-17). Periods of gentle motion out of the sling can start at about that time also. The fracture is usually healed by 4 to 6 weeks, at which time light activities are permitted. Vigorous activities involving the shoulder can be resumed in a gradual stepwise fashion, with a series of intermediate goals along the way. The timetable depends on the individual and his or her healing capacity, the severity of the injury, and the type of stressful activity to be resumed (e.g., pole vaulting vs. kite flying).

Fractures of the Humeral Shaft

Developmental Anatomy

The humeral diaphysis begins to ossify at the sixth or seventh week of fetal life and is entirely ossified by birth.[38] On cross section, the shaft is cylindrical proximally and flattened distally in the coronal plane.[39] The posterior aspect of the bone provides the origin for the lateral head of the triceps (superolaterally) and for its medial head (inferomedially), with the "spiral groove" lying in between. The radial nerve and its accompanying artery have a close relation to the bone along this groove. Just proximal to its midpoint, the lateral aspect of the shaft provides the insertion for the deltoid muscle. Medially at this level is the attachment for the coracobrachialis. More proximally, the pectoralis major inserts into the lateral ridge of the intertubercular groove. The brachialis muscle has its origin from the distal half of the anterior aspect of the humeral shaft.[39] An appreciation of these muscle attachments is essential in understanding the deforming forces acting on the humeral fracture fragments (Fig. 8-18).

Incidence

The humeral shaft is less frequently fractured in children than in adults. Among the humeral shaft fractures of childhood, diaphyseal fractures are more common in children older than 12 years or younger than 3 years.[105] For children under age 10 years, the incidence of shaft fracture is approximately 26 per 100,000 per year.[96] Overall, shaft

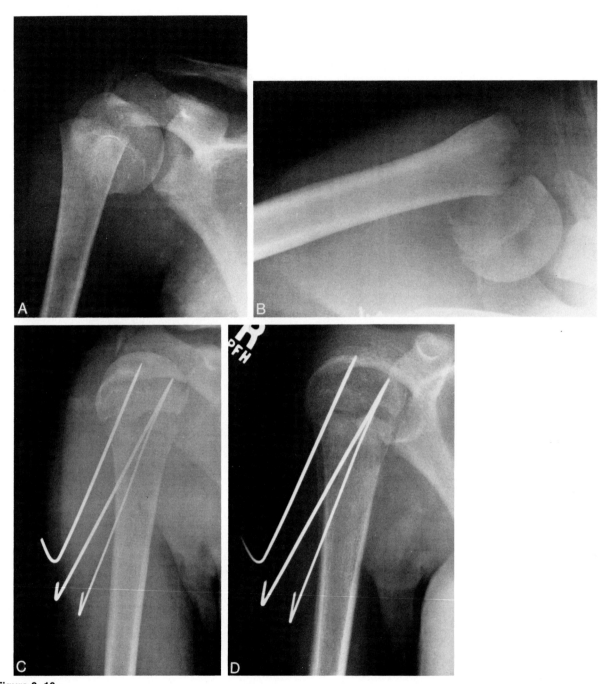

Figure 8–16

A–B, X-rays of the proximal humerus of a 14-year-old girl subsequent to a four-wheeler accident during which she sustained multiple trauma. *C*, Fracture was managed with a closed reduction and percutaneous pinning. *D*, At follow-up 4 weeks later the pins were removed; the patient quickly regained the normal use of her shoulder.

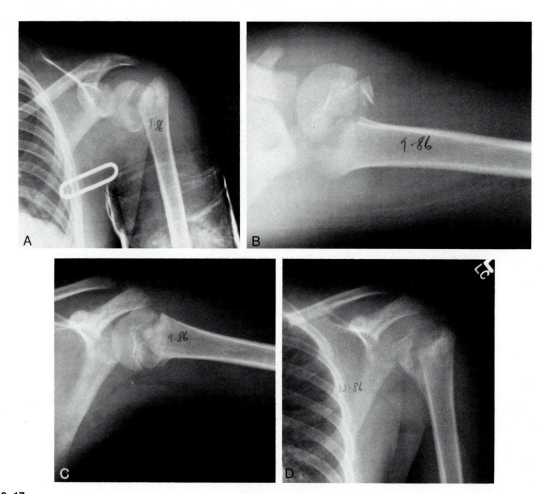

Figure 8–17

A–B, Type II proximal humerus fracture in a 12-year-old. C, Because abduction improved the alignment of the fracture, the patient was treated in abduction. D–E, One month later, early healing is evident. F–G, Three-month x-rays demonstrate more complete healing; the child had a normal shoulder by clinical examination.

fractures account for 2 to 5% of all fractures in children.[74]

Mechanism of Injury

Transverse or short oblique fracture patterns are the result of direct trauma to the arm, which is the most common mechanism of injury. Indirect trauma, e.g., a violent twisting, results in a spiral or long oblique fracture pattern; this is the pattern most commonly seen when child abuse is the cause.[92] Minor trauma may cause the humerus with an underlying unicameral bone cyst to fracture at the level of the cyst (Fig. 8–19)[83] and is the most common mode of presentation for this entity.[113]

Fracture at the junction of the middle and distal thirds of the shaft may be associated with injury to the closely related radial nerve,[92] and that injury should always be tested for by asking the patient to extend the ipsilateral metacarpophalangeal joints.

Diagnosis

Newborns may present with pseudoparalysis. Brachial plexus palsy, clavicular fracture, proximal humeral fracture, and infection should be differentiated.[109] The child with a greenstick fracture may present with minimal symptoms and tenderness. The older child with a displaced humeral shaft fracture will usually have a history of trauma to the arm. (The exception to this rule is the child whose unicameral bone cyst presents with a fracture brought about by an otherwise trivial use of the arm.[83]) There may be obvious deformity of the brachium if it has not already been splinted, and palpation will elicit tenderness over the arm. Plain x-rays in two views are confirmatory.

Treatment

Isolated closed injuries are best managed by closed methods. One takes advantage of the stout sur-

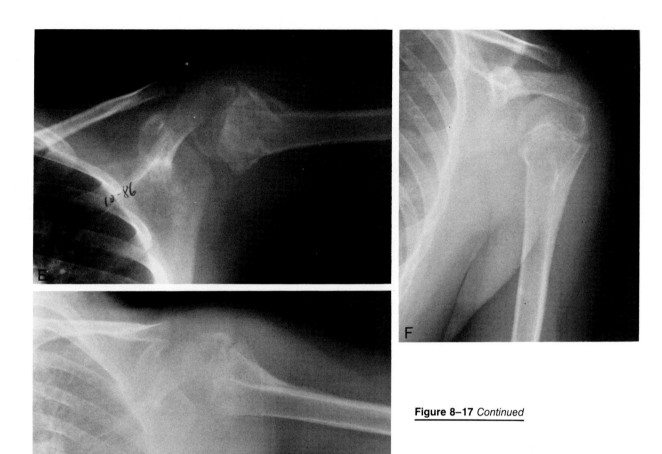

Figure 8–17 Continued

rounding periosteum by several methods, e.g., a hanging cast,[90] traction through an olecranon pin[70]/winged screw,[69] or the weight of the arm in a shoulder Velpeau[36]/collar-and-cuff type bandage.[126] Fracture in the newborn can be managed by splinting the arm to the chest wall.[5] Remodeling in newborns and very young children is robust. Maintenance of alignment is more important for fractures of the distal half of the humerus, because remodeling is less active there. As a guideline, one should strive to maintain this alignment within 15 degrees.[49] Bayonet apposition is not a problem; usually there is some overgrowth of the humerus.[45]

Most fractures are "sticky" by 3 to 4 weeks (2 to 3 weeks in newborns and very young children), and protected motion can be started then with brief periods out of the Velpeau or collar-and-cuff. By 6 to 8 weeks (3 to 6 weeks in newborns and very young children), most fractures have healed well enough to go without support. Subsequent rehabilitation of the upper extremity is tailored to the demands of the individual. For the young child, this can consist simply of the resumption of light play, with avoidance of activities that would risk a fall (e.g., skate boarding, climbing) until the humerus has remodeled sufficiently.

Associated radial nerve injuries should be observed for 16 to 20 weeks.[116] (The exception to this rule is the child who has radial nerve function at presentation but loses it during an attempt at reduction. Under these circumstances, the radial nerve should be explored.[110]) In those patients with no sign of return of function (the earliest returning motor function is the brachioradialis), the nerve should be explored, with neurolysis/neurorrhaphy if indicated.

Open fractures require a surgical debridement and irrigation. One should not primarily close the traumatic wound; coverage should be delayed until one is confident that the wound is clean (usually at

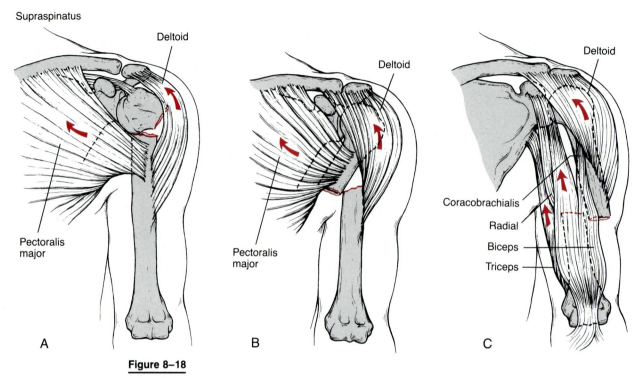

Figure 8–18

Muscle attachments (A–C) that direct deforming forces in proximal humeral fractures.

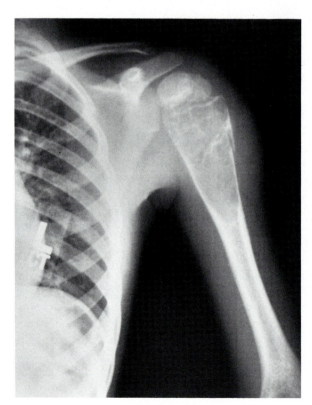

Figure 8–19

Proximal fracture of left humerus in a 5-year-old; the diagnosis of a unicameral bone cyst was made on the basis of the x-ray.

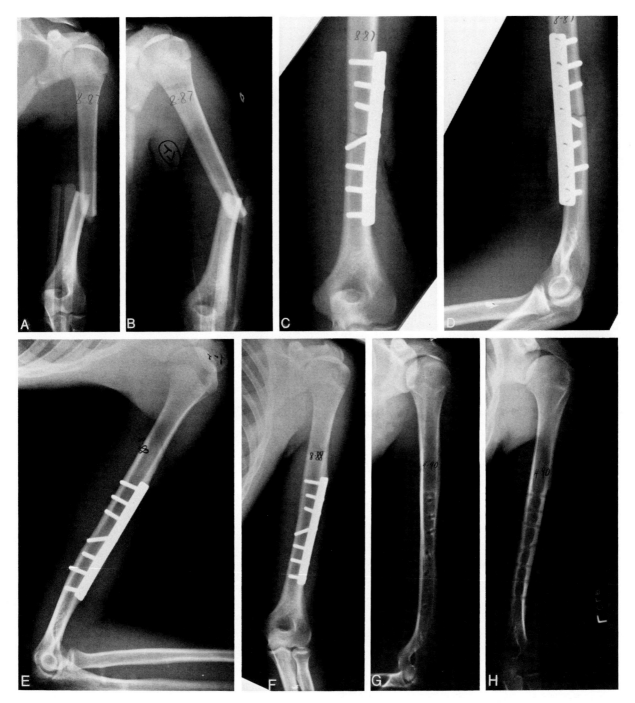

Figure 8-20

A-B, Fractured humerus in an older adolescent with multiple trauma, managed with an osteosynthesis. *C-H*, The osteosynthesis affords enhanced mobilization and pain-free limited upper extremity function. A disadvantage of the method is the need for a second operation to remove the implant after the bone has healed and remodeled.

day 5). Subsequent to the application of a sterile dressing, the fracture fragments can be stabilized using a shoulder Velpeau dressing or similar technique. Alternatively, an external fixator can be used if the wound is untidy and in need of frequent dressing changes. Internal fixation (Fig. 8–20), adroitly applied by a surgeon familiar with the method so as to minimize further local devascularization of wounded tissue, has a number of advantages in a polytraumatized child, especially one with associated chest or severe head trauma.[67] These advantages include early functional use of the extremity, easier nursing care of the patient, and greater ease in mobilizing the patient. These advantages must be weighed against the enhanced potential for local infection and the need for later implant removal.

Although seldom necessary in children, internal fixation can be considered in the aforementioned circumstances as well as when there is an associated vascular injury requiring repair or when there is nonunion of a shaft fracture. In the last instance, bone grafting and compression plating should be undertaken and elbow and shoulder motion recommenced.

Acknowledgments

The author wishes to thank Drs. Thomas Sumner and Robert Bechtold, Department of Radiology, The Bowman Gray School of Medicine of Wake Forest University, Winston-Salem, NC; Dr. Richard Lange, Department of Orthopaedic Surgery, University of Wisconsin Hospital, Madison, WI; John Faris, Forsyth Radiologic Associates, Winston-Salem, NC, and Dr. Paul Rush, Laurinburg, SC, for their help in the compilation of the figures for this chapter; and Barbara Crouse, Judith T. MacMillan, and Alma B. Doub for their help in the preparation of this manuscript.

REFERENCES

1. Advanced Trauma Life Support Program. 1988 Instructor Manual. Chicago, American College of Surgeons, 1989, pp. 31–56.
2. Allman, F.L., Jr. Fractures and ligamentous injuries of the clavicle and its articulation. J Bone Joint Surg 49-A:774–784, 1967.
3. An, H.S.; Vonderbrink, J.P.; Ebraheim, N.A.; et al. Open scapulothoracic dissociation with intact neurovascular status in a child. J Orthop Trauma 2:36–38, 1988.
4. Asher, M.A. Dislocations of the upper extremity in children. Orthop Clin North Am 7:583–591, 1976.
5. Åstedt, B. A method for the treatment of humerus fractures in the newborn using the S. von Rosen splint. Acta Orthop Scand 40:234–236, 1969.
6. Aufranc, O.E.; Jones, W.N.; Bierbaum, B.E. Epiphysial fracture of the proximal humerus. JAMA 207:727–729, 1969.
7. Bankart, A.S.B. Recurrent or habitual dislocation of the shoulder-joint. Br Med J 2:1132–1133, 1923.
8. Barth, E.; Hagen, R. Surgical treatment of dislocations of the sternoclavicular joint. Acta Orthop Scand 54:746–747, 1983.
9. Bateman, J.E. The Shoulder and Neck. Philadelphia, W.B. Saunders, 1972, pp. 436–438.
10. Baxter, M.P.; Wiley, J.J. Fractures of the proximal humeral epiphysis: Their influence on humeral growth. J Bone Joint Surg 68-B:570–573, 1986.
11. Beebe, A.C.; Bell, D.F. The management of severely displaced fractures of the proximal humerus in children. Techn Orthop 4:1–4, 1989.
12. Bernard, T.N., Jr.; Brunet, M.E.; Haddad, R.J., Jr. Fractured coracoid process in acromioclavicular dislocations. Report of four cases and review of the literature. Clin Orthop 175:227–232, 1983.
13. Bloom, M.H.; Obata, W.G. Diagnosis of posterior dislocation of the shoulder with use of Velpeau axillary and angle-up roentgenographic views. J Bone Joint Surg 49-A:943–949, 1967.
14. Blount, W.P. Fractures in Children. Baltimore, Williams & Wilkins, 1955.
15. Calvet, J.; LeRoy; LaCroix. Luxations de l'épaule et lésion vasulaires. J Chir 58:337–346, 1941–1942.
16. Campbell, J.; Almond, H.G.A. Fracture-separation of the proximal humeral epiphysis. A case report. J Bone Joint Surg 59-A:262–263, 1977.
17. Canale, S.T. Fractures and dislocations in children. In: Crenshaw, A.H., ed. Campbell's Operative Orthopaedics, Vol. 3, 7th ed. St. Louis, C.V. Mosby, 1987, pp. 1886–1889.
18. Canale, S.T.; Puhl, J.; Watson, F.M.; Gillespie, R. Acute osteomyelitis following closed fractures. Report of three cases. J Bone Joint Surg 57-A:415–418, 1975.
19. Clark, R.L.; Milgram, J.W.; Yawn, D.H. Fatal aortic perforation and cardiac tamponade due to a Kirschner wire migrating from the right sternoclavicular joint. South Med J 67:316–318, 1974.
20. Cohen, A.W.; Otto, S.R. Obstetric clavicular fractures. A three-year analysis. J Reprod Med 25:119–122, 1980.
21. Cohen, B.T.; Froimson, A.I. Salter III fracture dislocation of the glenohumeral joint in a 10-year-old. Orthop Rev 15:403–404, 1986.
22. Conwell, H.E. Fractures of the surgical neck and epiphyseal separations of upper end of humerus. J Bone Joint Surg 8:508–516, 1926.
23. Cozen, L. Congenital dislocation of the shoulder and other anomalies. Report of a case and review of the literature. Arch Surg 35:956–966, 1937.
24. Cumming, W.A. Neonatal skeletal fractures. Birth trauma or child abuse? J Can Assoc Radiol 30:30–33, 1979.
25. Curtis, R.J., Jr.; Rockwood, C.A., Jr. Fractures and dislocations of the shoulder in children. In:Rockwood, C.A. Jr.; Matsen, F.A., III, eds. The Shoulder, Vol. 2. Philadelphia, W.B. Saunders, 1990, pp. 991–1032.
26. Dameron, T.B.; Reibel, D.B. Fractures involving the proximal humeral epiphyseal plate. J Bone Joint Surg 51-A:289–297, 1969.

27. Dameron, T.B., Jr.; Rockwood, C.A., Jr. Fractures and dislocations of the shoulder. In: Rockwood, C.A., Jr.; Wilkins, K.E.; King, R.E., eds. Fractures in Children. Philadelphia, J.B. Lippincott, 1984, pp. 577–682.
28. DePalma, A.F. Surgery of the Shoulder, 2nd ed. Philadelphia, J.B. Lippincott, 1973, p. 28.
29. Digby, K.H. The measurement of diaphysial growth in proximal and distal directions. J Anat Physiol (Lond) 50:187–188, 1915–1916.
30. Ebraheim, N.A.; An, H.S.; Jackson, W.T.; et al. Scapulothoracic dissociation. J Bone Joint Surg 70-A:428–432, 1988.
31. Eidman, D.K.; Siff, S.J.; Tullos, H.S. Acromioclavicular lesions in children. Am J Sports Med 9:150–154, 1981.
32. Eskola, A. Sternoclavicular dislocation: A plea for open treatment. Acta Orthop Scand 57:227–228, 1986.
33. Farkas, R.; Levine, S. X-ray incidence of fractured clavicle in vertex presentation. Am J Obstet Gynecol 59:204–206, 1950.
34. Gardner, E. The embryology of the clavicle. Clin Orthop 58:9–16, 1968.
35. Gardner, E. The prenatal development of the human shoulder joint. Surg Clin North Am 43:1465–1470, 1963.
36. Gilchrist, D.K. A stockinette-Velpeau for immobilization of the shoulder girdle. J Bone Joint Surg 49-A:750–751, 1967.
37. Golthamer, C.R. Duplication of the clavicle ("os subclaviculare"). Radiology 68:576–578, 1957.
38. Gray, D. J.; Gardner, E. The prenatal development of the human humerus. Am J Anat 124:431–446, 1969.
39. Gray, H. Anatomy of the Human Body. [Edited by C. Clemente.] 30th American ed. Philadelphia, Lea & Febiger, 1985, pp. 226–236.
40. Green, N. E.; Wheelhouse, W.W. Anterior subglenoid dislocation of the shoulder in an infant following pneumococcal meningitis. Clin Orthop 135:125–127, 1978.
41. Greig, D.M. True congenital dislocation of the shoulder. Edin Med J 30:157–175, 1923.
42. Haliburton, R.A.; Barber, J.R.; Fraser, R.L. Pseudodislocation: An unusual birth injury. Can J Surg 10:455–462, 1967.
43. Hall, R.H.; Isaac, F.; Booth, C.R. Dislocations of the shoulder with special reference to accompanying small fractures. J Bone Joint Surg 41-A: 489–494, 1959.
44. Hawkins, R.J.; Koppert, G.; Johnston, G. Recurrent posterior instability (subluxation) of the shoulder. J Bone Joint Surg 66-A:169–174, 1984.
45. Hedström, O. Growth stimulation of long bones after fracture or similar trauma: A clinical and experimental study. Acta Orthop Scand (Suppl) 122:7–41, 55–62, 102–105, 1969.
46. Heyse-Moore, G.H.; Stoker, D.J. Avulsion fractures of the scapula. Skeletal Radiol 9:27–32, 1982.
47. Hippocrates. The Genuine Work of Hippocrates. [Translated by F. Adams.] Baltimore, Williams & Wilkins, 1939.
48. Hobbs, D. W. Sternoclavicular joint. A new axial radiographic view. Radiology 90:801, 1968.
49. Hohl, J.C. Fractures of the humerus in children. Orthop Clin North Am 7:557–571, 1976.
50. Hollinshead, W.H. The Back and Limbs, Vol. 5, 3rd ed. Philadelphia, Harper & Row, 1982, p. 319.
51. Hovelius, L. Anterior dislocation of the shoulder in teenagers and young adults. Five-year prognosis. J Bone Joint Surg 69-A:393–399, 1987.
52. Howard, F.M.; Shafer, S.J. Injuries to the clavicle with neurovascular complications. A study of fourteen cases. J Bone Joint Surg 47-A:1335–1346, 1965.
53. Inman, V. T.; Saunders, J.B.daC.M.; Abbott, L.C. Observations on the function of the shoulder joint. J Bone Joint Surg 26:1–30, 1944.
54. Janecki, C.J.; Shahcheragh, G.H. The forward elevation maneuver for reduction of anterior dislocations of the shoulder. Clin Orthop 164:177–180, 1982.
55. Jit, I.; Kulkarni, M. Times of appearance and fusion of epiphysis at the medial end of the clavicle. Indian J Med Res 64:773–782, 1976.
56. Keats, T.E. Atlas of Normal Roentgen Variants that May Simulate Disease, 4th ed. St. Louis, Mosby-Yearbook, 1988.
57. Key, J.A.; Conwell, H.E. Fractures of the clavicle. In: Key, J.A.; Conwell, H.E., eds. The Management of Fractures, Dislocations, and Sprains, 4th ed. St. Louis, C.V. Mosby, 1946, pp. 495–512.
58. Köhler, A. Borderlands of the Normal and Early Pathologic in Skeletal Roentgenology. [Edited by E.A. Zimmer. Translated and edited by J.P. Wilke.] 3rd American ed. New York, Grune & Stratton, 1968, pp. 156–159.
59. Kreisinger, V. Sur le traitement des fractures de la clavicule. Rev Chir 65:396–407, 1927.
60. Kuhns, L.R.; Sherman, M.P.; Poznanski, A.K.; Holt, J.F. Humeral-head and coracoid ossification in the newborn. Radiology 107:145–149, 1973.
61. Lacey, T., II; Crawford, H.B. Reduction of anterior dislocations of the shoulder by means of the Milch abduction technique. J Bone Joint Surg 34-A:108–109, 1952.
62. Larsen, E.; Bjerg-Nielsen, A.; Christensen, P. Conservative or surgical treatment of acromioclavicular dislocation: A prospective, controlled, randomized study. J Bone Joint Surg 68-A:552–555, 1986.
63. Laskin, R.S.; Sedlin, E.D. Luxatio erecta in infancy. Clin Orthop 80:126–129, 1971.
64. Lemperg, R.; Liliequist, B. Dislocation of the proximal epiphysis of the humerus in newborns. Report of two cases and discussion of diagnostic criteria. Acta Paediatr Scand 59:377–380, 1970.
65. Liberson, F. Os acromiale: a contested anomaly. J Bone Joint Surg 19:683–689, 1937.
66. Liechti, R. Fractures of the clavicle and scapula. In: Weber, B.G.; Brummer, C.; Freuler, F., eds. Treatment of Fractures in Children and Adolescents. New York, Springer-Verlag, 1980, pp. 87–95.
67. Loder, R.T. Pediatric polytrauma: Orthopaedic care and hospital course. J Orthop Trauma 1:48–54, 1987.
68. Madsen, E.T. Fractures of the extremities in the newborn. Acta Obstet Gynecol Scand 34:41–74, 1955.
69. Magerl, F. Fractures of the proximal humerus. In:Weber, B.G.; Brunner, C.; Freuler, F., eds. Treatment of Fractures in Children and Adolescents. New York, Springer-Verlag, 1980, pp. 88–117.
70. Magnuson, P.B. Fractures. Philadelphia, J.B. Lippincott, 1933, pp. 58–99.
71. Mast, J.W.; Jakob, R.; Ganz, R. Planning and Reduction Technique in Fracture Surgery. New York, Springer-Verlag, 1988, p. 244.
72. McClure, J.G.; Raney, R.B. Anomalies of the scapula. Clin Orthop 110:22–31, 1975.
73. McGahan, J.P.; Rab, G.T.; Dublin, A. Fractures of the scapula. J Trauma 20:880–883, 1980.
74. Mehmann, P. Fractures of the shaft of the humerus. In: Weber, B.G.; Brenner, C.; Freuler, F., eds. Treatment of

Fractures in Children and Adolescents. New York, Springer-Verlag, 1980, pp. 118–129.
75. Milch, H. Treatment of dislocation of the shoulder. Surgery 3:732–740, 1938.
76. Miller, D.S.; Boswick, J.A., Jr. Lesions of the brachial plexus associated with fractures of the clavicle. Clin Orthop 64:144–149, 1969.
77. Mirick, M.J.; Clinton, J.E.; Ruiz, E. External rotation method of shoulder dislocation reduction. J Am Coll Emerg Phys 8:528–531, 1979.
78. Moseley, H.F. The clavicle: Its anatomy and function. Clin Orthop 58:17–27, 1968.
79. Nasso, S.; Verga, A. La frattura della clavicola del neonato. Minerva Pediatr 6:593–597, 1954.
80. Neer, C.S., II. Involuntary inferior and multidirectional instability of the shoulder: Etiology, recognition, and treatment. Instr Course Lect 34:232–238, 1985.
81. Neer, C.S., II; Foster, C.R. Inferior capsular shift for involuntary inferior and multidirectional instability of the shoulder. A preliminary report. J Bone Joint Surg 62-A:897–908, 1980.
82. Neer, C.S., II; Horwitz, B.S. Fractures of the proximal humeral epiphysial plate. Clin Orthop 41:24–31, 1965.
83. Neer, C.S., II; Francis, K.C.; Marcove, R.C.; et al. Treatment of unicameral bone cyst. A follow-up study of 175 cases. J Bone Joint Surg 48-A:731–745, 1966.
84. Nettrour, L.F.; Krufky, E.L.; Mueller, R.E.; Raycroft, J.F. Locked scapula: Intrathoracic dislocation of the inferior angle. A case report. J Bone Joint Surg 54-A:413–416, 1972.
85. Neviaser, R.J. Injuries to the clavicle and acromioclavicular joint. Orthop Clin North Am 18:433–438, 1987.
86. O'Brien, S.J.; Warren, R.F.; Schwartz, E. Anterior shoulder instability. Orthop Clin North Am 18:395–408, 1987.
87. Ogden, J.A. Skeletal Injury in the Child, 2nd ed. Philadelphia, W.B. Saunders, 1990, pp. 327–338, 357.
88. Pasila, M.; Jaroma, H.; Kiviluoto, O.; Sundholm, A. Early complications of primary shoulder dislocations. Acta Orthop Scand 49:260–263, 1978.
89. Penn, I. The vascular complications of fractures of the clavicle. J Trauma 4:819–831, 1964.
90. Pollen, A.G. Fractures and Dislocations in Children. Baltimore, Williams & Wilkins, 1973, pp. 7–22.
91. Powers, J.A.; Bach, P.J. Acromioclavicular separations: Closed or open treatment? Clin Orthop 104:213–223, 1974.
92. Rang, M. Children's Fractures, 2nd ed. Philadelphia, J.B. Lippincott, 1983, pp. 143–156.
93. Rockwood, C.A., Jr. Fracture of the outer clavicle in children and adults. Abstract. J Bone Joint Surg 64-B:642, 1982.
94. Rockwood, C.A., Jr. Subluxations and dislocations about the shoulder. In: Rockwood, C.A., Jr.; Green, D.P., eds. Fractures in Adults, Vol. 1. Philadelphia, J.B. Lippincott, 1984, pp. 758–759.
95. Rockwood, C.A., Jr.; Szalay, E.A.; Curtis, R.J., Jr.; et al. X-ray evaluation of shoulder problems. In: Rockwood, C.A., Jr.; Matsen, F.A., III, eds: The Shoulder, Vol. 1. Philadelphia, W.B. Saunders, 1990, pp. 178–207.
96. Rose, S.; Melton, L.J., III; Morrey, B.F.; et al. Epidemiologic features of humeral fractures. Clin Orthop 168:24–30, 1982.
97. Rounds, R.C. Isolated fracture of the coracoid process. J Bone Joint Surg 31-A:662–663, 1949.
98. Rowe, C.R. An atlas of anatomy and treatment of midclavicular fractures. Clin Orthop 58: 29–42, 1968.
99. Rowe, C.R. Anterior dislocations of the shoulder: prognosis and treatment. Surg Clin North Am 43:1609–1614, 1963.
100. Rowe, C.R.; Pierce, D.S.; Clark, J.G. Voluntary dislocation of the shoulder. A preliminary report on a clinical, electromyographic, and psychiatric study of twenty-six patients. J Bone Joint Surg 55-A:445–460, 1973.
101. Rowe, C.R.; Zarins, B.; Ciullo, J.V. Recurrent anterior dislocation of the shoulder after surgical repair. Apparent causes of failure and treatment. J Bone Joint Surg 66-A:159–168, 1984.
102. Rubin, A. Birth injuries: Incidence, mechanisms, and end results. Obstet Gynecol 23:218–221, 1964.
103. Rubin, S.A.; Gray, R.L.; Green, W.R. The scapular "Y": A diagnostic aid in shoulder trauma. Radiology 110:725–726, 1974.
104. Russell, J.A.; Holmes, E.M., III; Keller, D.J.; Vargas, J.H., III. Reduction of acute anterior shoulder dislocations using the Milch technique: A study of ski injuries. J Trauma 21:802–804, 1981.
105. Salter, R.B. Textbook of Disorders and Injuries of the Musculoskeletal System. Baltimore, Williams & Wilkins, 1970, pp. 438–439.
106. Salter, R.B.; Harris, W.R. Injuries involving the epiphyseal plate. J Bone Joint Surg 45-A:587–622, 1963.
107. Samilson, R.L. Congenital and developmental anomalies of the shoulder girdle. Orthop Clin North Am 11:219–231, 1980.
108. Sanford, H.N. The Moro reflex as a diagnostic aid in fracture of the clavicle in the newborn infant. Am J Dis Child 41:1304–1306, 1931.
109. Scaglietti, O. The obstetrical shoulder trauma. Surg Gynecol Obstet 66:868–877, 1938.
110. Shaw, J.L.; Sakellarides, H. Radial-nerve paralysis associated with fractures of the humerus. A review of 45 cases. J Bone Joint Surg 49-A:899–902, 1967.
111. Sherk, H.H.; Probst, C. Fractures of the proximal humeral epiphysis. Orthop Clin North Am 6:401–413, 1975.
112. Smith, F.M. Fracture-separation of the proximal humeral epiphysis. Am J Surg 91:627–635, 1956.
113. Spjut, H.J.; Dorfman, H.D.; Fechner, R.E.; Ackerman, L.V. Tumors of Bone and Cartilage. Atlas of Tumor Pathology, 2d series, Fasc. 5. Washington, D.C., Armed Forces Institute of Pathology, 1971, pp. 347–390.
114. Stanley, D.; Trowbridge, E.A.; Norris, S.H. The mechanism of clavicular fracture. A clinical and biomechanical analysis. J Bone Joint Surg 70-B:461–464, 1988.
115. Stimson, L.A. An easy method of reducing dislocations of the shoulder and hip. Med Rec 57:356–357, 1900.
116. Szalay, E.A.; Rockwood, C.A., Jr. The Holstein-Lewis fracture revisited. Abstract. Orthop Trans 7:516, 1983.
117. Tachdjian, M.O. Pediatric Orthopedics, 2nd ed. Philadelphia, W.B. Saunders, 1990.
118. Taft, T.N.; Wilson, F.C.; Oglesby, J.W. Dislocation of the acromioclavicular joint: An end-result study. J Bone Joint Surg 69-A:1045–1051, 1987.
119. Taga, I.; Yoneda, M.; Ono, K. Epiphyseal separation of the coracoid process associated with acromioclavicular sprain. A case report and review of the literature. Clin Orthop 207:138–141, 1986.
120. Todd, T.W.; D'Errico, J., Jr. The clavicular epiphyses. Am J Anat 41:25–50, 1928.
121. Tse, D.H.W.; Slabaugh, P.B.; Carlson, P.A. Injury to the axillary artery by a closed fracture of the clavicle. A case report. J Bone Joint Surg 62-A:1372–1374, 1980.

122. Twigg, H.L.; Rosenbaum, R.C. Duplication of the clavicle. Skeletal Radiol 6:281, 1981.
123. Vastamäki, M.; Solonen, K.A. Posterior dislocation and fracture-dislocation of the shoulder. Acta Orthop Scand 51:479–484, 1980.
124. Visser, J.D.; Rietberg, M. Interposition of the tendon of the long head of biceps in fracture separation of the proximal humeral epiphysis. Neth J Surg 32:12–15, 1980.
125. Watson, F.M., Jr.; Whitesides, T.E., Jr. Acute hematogenous osteomyelitis complicating closed fractures. Clin Orthop 117:296–302, 1976.
126. Watson-Jones, R. Fractures and Joint Injuries, Vol. 2, 4th ed. Baltimore, Williams & Wilkins, 1955, pp. 503–507.
127. White, A.D.N. Dislocated shoulder—a simple method of reduction. Med J Aust 2:726–727, 1976.
128. Wilber, M.C.; Evans, E.B. Fractures of the scapula. An analysis of forty cases and a review of the literature. J Bone Joint Surg 59-A:358–362, 1977.
129. Wong-Pack, W.K.; Bobechko, P.E.; Becker, E.J. Fractured coracoid with anterior shoulder dislocation. J Can Assoc Radiol 31:278–279, 1980.
130. Zilberman, Z.; Rejovitzky, R. Fracture of the coracoid process of the scapula. Injury 13: 203–206, 1981–1982.
131. Zuelzer, W.A. Fixation of small but important bone fragments with a hook plate. J Bone Joint Surg 33-A:430–436, 1951.

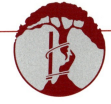

J. Andy Sullivan, M.D.

9

Fractures of the Spine in Children

Fractures of the spine in children are uncommon. Once recognized, most are easy to manage. Unrecognized or improperly managed, they may become catastrophic or fatal. Proper management depends upon knowledge of normal development of the spine and the normal radiographic variants that accompany this development.

Developmental Anatomy of the Spine

The first two cervical vertebrae vary in their development from the remaining cervical vertebrae and from the thoracic and lumbar vertebrae. The atlas (C1) usually develops from three ossification centers, one for the body and one for each of the neural arches (Fig. 9–1A).[1, 4, 54] Occasionally the body may be formed from two centers or may completely fail to appear, but the neural arches may extend forward and fuse.[4] The body also may fail to appear, resulting in failure of anterior fusion leaving a cleft. The ossification center for the anterior arch is present in approximately 20% of individuals at birth, appearing in the remainder during the first year of life. The anterior arch is occasionally bifid. Closure of the posterior arch of C1 is usually completed by the third year. Variations include an absent ring of C1 or failure to completely ossify. The ring of C1 reaches its normal adult size by age 4 years. The body joins the neural arches by a neurocentral synchondrosis that usually closes by the seventh year.

The axis (C2) develops from four separate centers (Fig. 9–1B). There is one for each of the neural arches, one for the center or body, and one for the odontoid. All the ossification centers are present at birth,[1, 4, 54] and fusion occurs by age 3 years. Before this time these synchondroses may be mistaken for fractures (Fig. 9–2). According to Freiberger and co-workers,[27] odontoid development occurs in the fifth fetal month by the ossification of two longitudinal primary centers that fuse at birth. The tip of the odontoid usually appears above the V-shaped shaft at around 6 to 7 years of age and fuses by the twelfth year. Failure to fuse may leave a small ossicle known as the ossiculum terminale. The dens, or odontoid process, sits on the centrum, or body, which is joined by the neural arches. It is separated from the centrum of the axis by a region of growth cartilage that disappears at age 5 to 7 years. In children, fractures can occur through this cartilaginous center. Fusion of the odontoid through the neural arches and the body of the axis occurs between the ages of 3 to 6 years.[1]

The facet joint changes in orientation with maturity. The angle of the C1–C2 facet is 55 degrees in the newborn and increases to 70 degrees at maturity.[51] In the lower cervical spine the angle of the facet joints is 30 degrees at birth and 60 to 70 degrees at maturity. These angles coupled with the greater ligamentous laxity in the young child explain the increased translational motion that is present.

Cervical vertebrae 3 to 7 and the thoracic and lumbar spine develop in a similar manner (see Fig. 9–1C).[1] Each is formed from three ossification centers, one for each neural arch and one for the vertebral centrum. A neurocentral synchondrosis joins these and disappears at around age 3 to 6 years. Ordinarily the arches fuse between age 2 to 4 years. In the cervical and thoracic vertebrae there are five secondary ossification centers. These include one each for the spinous processes, transverse proc-

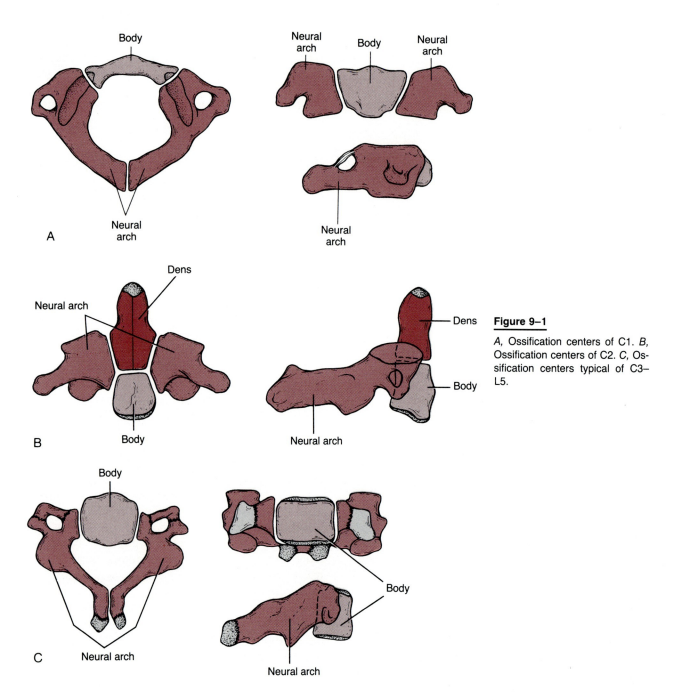

Figure 9–1

A, Ossification centers of C1. B, Ossification centers of C2. C, Ossification centers typical of C3–L5.

esses, and the vertebral end plate (the ring apophyses). In the lumbar spine there are two for the mamillary processes. These secondary ossification centers appear during puberty and fuse to the vertebrae by age 25 years. The child's spine usually has assumed adult characteristics and is near adult size by age 8 to 10 years, so radiologic studies of the spine except for the apophyses are comparable to those of the adult.

Each vertebra grows in height by enchondral ossification in each of the end plates. Increase in width occurs by perichondrial and periosteal appositional growth.

Relevant Anatomy

The skull articulates with the atlas through the two occipitoatlantal joints.[1] The predominant motion that occurs here is flexion and extension, with almost no rotation. There are four atlantoaxial joints, one anterior and one posterior to the odontoid and the

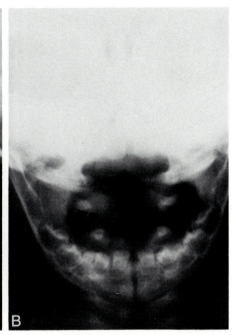

Figure 9–2

Axis ossification centers and synchondroses of C2. *A*, Lateral C-spine radiograph in an infant. The *arrowhead* points to an apparent cleft at the base of C2, which is the synchondrosis at the base of the odontoid. *B*, Anteroposterior radiograph of an infant. Note the bifid appearance and the cleft at the top of the odontoid.

remaining two between the atlas and axis articular processes. The transverse ligament is the first line of defense to prevent atlantoaxial dislocation.[25, 71] The stability of the articulation of the skull to the spine is enhanced by additional ligaments from the axis to the occiput. These include the alar ligaments (which serve as checkreins to limit rotation and to prevent the odontoid from impinging on the cord), the apical dental ligament, and the cruciate ligament. Once the odontoid has moved its transverse diameter, the alar, or check, ligaments are taut.

Steel[71] analyzed lateral flexion and extension cervical spine films of 50 normal adults and 50 normal children (ages 12 to 15 years). He also performed stress tests of the cervical spine. The first structure to fail in stress testing was the transverse ligament, followed by the accessory ligaments. Once the transverse ligament ruptures, the alar ligaments are insufficient to prevent catastrophic movement of the odontoid with further stress. When the transverse ligament fails, it ruptures near its attachment to the arch. The elasticity in the ligament causes it to shorten, and therefore it may fail to heal. Although the alar ligaments may heal after injury, they are not strong enough to prevent injury to the cord with additional stress.[25, 71]

In the review of radiographs, Steel found that the maximum translation of the odontoid in relation to the atlas was 3 mm in the adult (20% of the transverse diameter of the odontoid) and 4 mm in the child (30% of the transverse diameter of the odontoid).[71] Displacement of 3 to 5 mm is considered to be in the normal range in children. When this distance is exceeded, the transverse ligament is presumed to have ruptured. When the distance exceeds 10 to 12 mm, all ligaments have failed. Steel based the rule of thirds on the finding that at the level of the atlantoaxial articulation, one third of the space in the spinal canal is occupied by the odontoid and one third by the cord, leaving one third as the so-called space available for the cord (SAC) (Fig. 9–3).

The anatomy of C3 through C6 is similar. C7 has a very long, stout, nonbifid spinous process (vertebra prominens). The transverse processes of C7 are also very large, and the transverse process of the foramen is small. The vertebral artery passes anterior to the transverse process of C7, not through the foramina. Occasionally a cervical rib may occur in place of the transverse process of C7. The thoracic vertebrae are unique in that they have costal processes for articulation with the ribs. The lumbar vertebrae are the largest of all the vertebrae.

Anomalies of the Spine

CERVICAL

Cervical spine anomalies can include failure of formation or failure of segmentation. C1 can fail to segment from the skull, leading to narrowing of the foramen magnum and neurologic symptoms. Wedge-shaped vertebrae, bifid vertebrae, or a com-

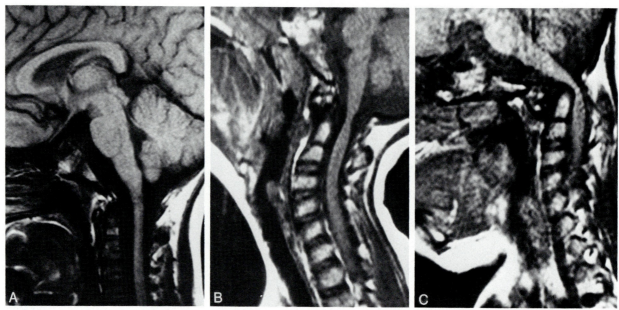

Figure 9–3

A, This MRI study shows a normal canal, the odontoid, the cord, and the remaining the space available to the cord. *B*, Extension MRI scan in a patient with Down syndrome demonstrating the odontoid, mild constriction of the cord at that level, and the space available to the cord. *C*, Flexion MRI scan demonstrating forward translation of C1 relative to the odontoid and tenting of the cord over the odontoid as the space available to the cord is compromised.

bination of these can also occur. Klippel and Feil[41] reported on a patient with a short neck, a low posterior hairline, and severe restriction of motion of the neck due to complete fusion of the cervical vertebrae. This is now known as the Klippel-Feil syndrome. Hensinger and colleagues[32] reviewed 50 patients with this classic triad of findings and added to these the constellation of associated anomalies that occur frequently in these patients. These include congenital scoliosis, renal anomalies, Sprengel's deformity, impaired hearing, synkinesia, and congenital heart disease.

Hensinger and associates[31] have reported on congenital anomalies of the odontoid process. These include aplasia (complete absence) with absence of the base; hypoplasia (partial absence), in which there is a stubby peg at the base of the odontoid located above the C1 articulation; and the most common anomaly, os odontoideum. The incidence of these anomalies is unknown, as they are frequently discovered incidentally.

THORACOLUMBAR

Thoracolumbar anomalies include failure of segmentation and failure of formation. These can lead to block vertebrae, wedge vertebrae, bifid vertebrae, and the most common, spina bifida occulta. The resultant spinal deformity depends on the severity, orientation, and location of the anomaly.

Radiology of the Spine

In children, the epiphyseal centers mentioned earlier and normal variants are often mistaken for fractures. The epiphyseal plates should be distinguished by their distinctive smooth appearance and their proper anatomic location. Normally, bifid structures are similarly distinguished from fractures, which have more irregular lines and develop sclerosis.

The articulation of the skull to the cervical spine can be difficult to evaluate radiographically. Anomalies of the odontoid can be confused with acute injury. In the cervical spine one must be aware of the phenomenon of pseudosubluxation and of the normal values for the soft tissue spaces.

Wholey and co-workers[81] also reviewed the relationship of the odontoid to the basion. The middle half of the odontoid lies directly beneath the basion (the midsagittal point of the anterior lip of the foramen magnum) and at an average distance of 5 mm from the basion (see Fig. 9–5). In infants and young children, this distance may be as much as 1 cm. These investigators stated that a variation greater than 1 to 2 cm in the relationship of the odontoid to the basion requires further evaluation. They felt that this relationship was much more reproducible than the drawing of McGregor's or Chamberlain's lines.

In another series of radiographs in children, an increased distance between the odontoid process and the anterior arch of the atlas was noted during flexion.[11] Movement of 3 mm or more was observed on the roentgenograms made with the neck in flexion in 14 children (20%) in this age group. With extension there was overriding of the anterior arch of the atlas on the odontoid in 14 of 70 patients (20%). In this study, overriding was present when more than two thirds of the viable anterior arch of the atlas lay above the superior margin of the odontoid process.

Dolan[17] has reviewed the many ways in which the cervicobasilar relationship can be evaluated. Cervicobasilar abnormalities can be caused by occipital hypoplasia, trauma, tumor, infection, abnormal cranial ossification, and generalized bone disease.

Radiographic findings for odontoid agenesis or hypoplasia are usually a slight depression between the superior articular facets of C1 and C2.[28, 31] Lateral laminagrams or computed tomography (CT) may be helpful. Regardless of the method used, views in flexion and extension must be obtained. In os odontoideum there is a wide radiolucent gap demonstrable between the fragments (see Fig. 9-13C).[23, 26] The os odontoideum moves anteriorly with the ring of C1. This motion, normally less than 3 mm, in most symptomatic patients is up to 1 cm. Mach bands are an optical phenomenon that can be mistaken for a fracture. These dark and light lines appear at the borders of structures of different radiodensities. They are known to occur across the base of the dens, where they may mistaken for a fracture (Fig. 9-4).[14]

Wholey and co-workers[81] reviewed 600 lateral C-spine radiographs in children, looking at the retropharyngeal and retrotracheal spaces and the cervical canal diameter. They concluded that a retropharyngeal space greater than 7 mm and a retrotracheal space greater than 14 mm were abnormal in a child. The cervical canal area is 22 mm at C1 and 18 mm at C7. Between the ages of 3 and 6 years the child's spine gradually approaches adult dimensions. Prevertebral soft tissues are rather uniform in the adult, but in the young child they vary in thickness and shape and are more difficult to evaluate. Crying, position changes in the uncooperative patient, and the amount of adenoid lymphoid tissue may lead to a false impression of a widened prevertebral soft tissue space.[7]

Pseudosubluxation is a condition in which there is apparent displacement of one cervical vertebra on another on the lateral cervical spine radiograph, especially with flexion (Fig. 9-5). Cattell and Filtzer[12] obtained lateral flexion and extension radiographs in 160 randomly selected children between the ages of 1 to 16 years (10 per year). They stated that anterior subluxation of C2 on C3 was difficult

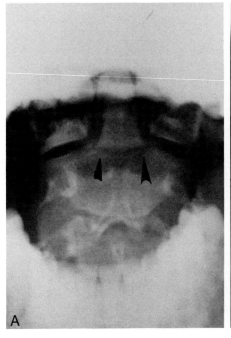
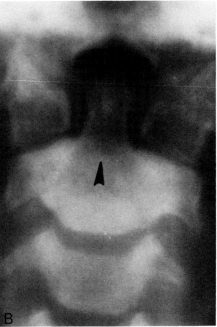

Figure 9-4

Mach bands. *A*, Note the apparent radiolucent line at the base of the odontoid *(arrowheads)*, which could be mistaken for a fracture. *B*, Tomogram demonstrating that there is no fracture.

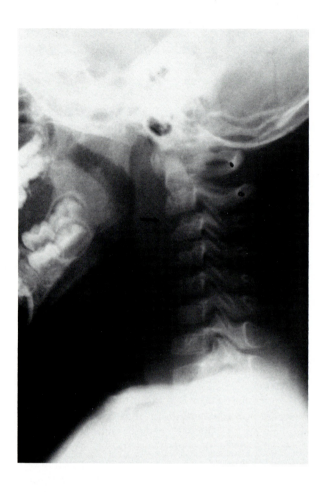

Figure 9–5

Pseudosubluxation. The arrow points to an apparent subluxation of C2 on C3, which in reality is within normal limits. This child was subsequently found to be normal. The arrow is in the retropharyngeal space, which also appears widened but is normal. The dots on the posterior spines are to draw Swischuk's line, which revealed that this spine was normal (see text). (Courtesy of Dr. Teresa Stacy.)

to measure in the young child because of poor bony landmarks or reference points. Using the posterior corners of C2 and C3, they were able to demonstrate striking anterior displacement as a result of combined forward shift and flexion of C2 on C3. This was described as marked in 9% (15 patients) and moderate in 15% (24 patients). Forty percent of patients less than age 8 years had anterior displacement. Based on this and other studies, pseudosubluxation of up to 4 mm is acceptable in the child.[4, 12, 58, 72, 77] The most common level is C2–C3, but displacement occurs at C3–C4 as well. Swischuk[73] has described a line that can be used to evaluate pseudosubluxation. It is drawn along the posterior arch of C1, C2, and C3. The line should pass within 1.5 mm of the posterior arch of C2 (Fig. 9–6); over 1.5 cm is considered nonphysiologic.

There are other radiographic variations that occur in children. In the very young child, reversal of a normal smooth anterior curve can be seen in the lateral projection. Cervical vertebrae are also noted to be wedge-shaped early in life, gradually achieving their adult shape on lateral view by age 8 years.[72] In the thoracic and lumbar spine of young children there are well-defined anterior and posterior indentations in the vertebral bodies that are seen on the lateral radiograph.[79] Posteriorly these result from the passage of vascular structures. Anteriorly they are created by a difference in density caused by the growth plates and vascular structures. The posterior notch is present at all ages but becomes less prominent with age. The anterior arch disappears with the normal development of the marrow space.

Incidence of Spinal Trauma in Children

Cervical spine injuries in children are relatively rare. Of 1299 cases of vertebral trauma seen at the Henry Ford Hospital, 631 were to the cervical spine.[30] Only 12 of these were seen in individuals less than 15 years of age (1.9%). An additional 6 patients were added to the series, so a total of 18 patients were reviewed. These injuries occurred more frequently in males than in females, and the incidence increased with age. Injuries in the age range 0 to 2 years were rare and were mainly the result of birth trauma. In

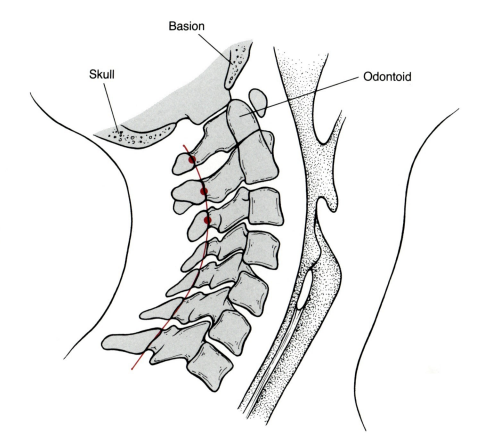

Figure 9–6

Line drawing of the cervical spine illustrating the basion, odontoid, and Swischuk's line.

the group 3 to 5 years, the most frequent mechanisms of injury were falls from a height, automobile accidents, and child abuse. In the age range 6 to 15 years, motor vehicle accidents and sport injuries accounted for most cases. Seven of 18 patients had a neurologic deficit. Only 5 of the 18 required surgery. Six of the 18 had associated major trauma to the head, chest, or abdomen. Swimming, diving, surfing, and motor vehicle accidents are among the major causes of spinal trauma in children.[3, 19, 33] Other studies have confirmed similar demographic data.[21, 37, 67] In this series,[30] there were four fractures of the odontoid, one dislocation of C1–C2, and six fracture-dislocations. Of the fracture-dislocation group, five developed neurologic complications, and three required surgery. Vertebral compression fractures were not seen.

Cervical spine injuries of all types may be more common than is currently recognized because of failure to diagnose these injuries. Aufdermaur[2] noted that fractures of the spine are rare in children, accounting for 2.5 to 3.3% of all spinal injuries. He was able to identify 12 spinal injuries at autopsy over an 8-year period. He also performed studies in three spines by stressing them in a vise to see where they would fracture. Roentgenograms of these spines revealed large gaping fissures and wide intervertebral joint spaces that perhaps suggested a lesion. The fracture was consistently through the end plate of the vertebral body. Of the spines seen at autopsy, seven of the injuries were in the cervical spine, four were in the thoracic spine, and one was in the lumbar spine. Ten of 12 injuries had been sustained during motor vehicle accidents, and 2 were from hyperextension at birth. Importantly, only 1 of the 12 subjects had been suspected of having a spine fracture before necropsy. These cases, then, represent a spinal injury incidence of 12% of 100 children coming to necropsy over that 8-year period. In three of the subjects it was felt that the fracture contributed directly to the death. These three had ligament injuries as well, indicating that the spine was unstable. A higher incidence of spine instability occurs in patients with Down syndrome, Morquio syndrome, and rheumatoid arthritis and in those with upper airway infection.

Spinal Injury in the Neonate

Spinal column and spinal cord injury can occur during delivery and are more common during breech delivery.[42, 52, 74] When associated with cephalic delivery, the injuries tend to occur in the upper cervical spine and are thought to result from rotation. Injuries associated with breech delivery are usually in the lower cervical spine and upper thoracic spine and are thought to result from traction (Fig. 9–7).[77] At necropsy, Shulman and co-workers[68] demonstrated transection of the cord with atlanto-occipital and atlantoaxial dislocations. In a series of 600 neonatal autopsies, Tawbin[74] found a 10% incidence of brain, brain stem, or spinal injuries.

Complete C6–C7 dislocation with locked facets has also been reported in an infant.[48] This child had sustained a difficult delivery owing to a large abdominal mass and was neurologically normal at birth. Complete C6–C7 dislocation with locked facets was discovered during a skeletal survey. The patient was successfully treated in traction but died at 6 months of other causes. Jones and Hensinger[38] have reported on C2–C3 dislocation in a child that occurred at birth and resulted in weakness and hypotonia.

The diagnosis was made at 2 years of age. Because of hypotonia and what was considered to be ligamentous laxity, a diagnosis of Larsen's syndrome had been made. The patient underwent spinal fusion at 20 months. One should include cervical spine injury in the differential diagnosis of a newborn with decreased tone, a nonprogressive neurologic deficit, and a negative history of familial neurologic disorders.[38, 52]

Spinal Cord Injury in Children

Spinal cord injury (SCI) in children is unique in several ways. Depending on the age at the time of injury and level of the lesion, children with SCI are almost certain to develop spinal deformity. They also have a high incidence of lower extremity problems. Unique to the pediatric patient is the syndrome of spinal cord injury without radiographic abnormality (SCIWORA).

SCIWORA

This syndrome is defined as spinal cord injury in a patient in whom there is no visible fracture on plain radiographs, linear tomograms, or CT. The patients can present with complete or incomplete SCI syndromes.

Various theories have been put forward to explain SCIWORA. The spinal column in the child is more elastic than the spinal cord and can undergo considerable deformation without being disrupted.[11] Leventhal[42] has shown that the spinal column can elongate up to 2 in without disruption, whereas the inelastic spinal cord will rupture with only ¼ in of elongation. A clinical example of this mechanism is the seat belt distraction injury pattern. Patients have been seen with SCIWORA and cerebrospinal fluid–mediastinal fistulas, demonstrating that the cord can be severely disrupted without demonstrable fracture or dislocation of the spinal column. This injury, then, would involve severe flexion and distraction.

Pang and co-workers[55, 56] have suggested hyperextension in the thoracic and lumbar spine as a probable mechanism. They have compared a series of SCIWORA patients who were run over by cars while lying prone or while lying supine.[55] Although both groups had a variety of visceral injuries that one would expect from such a crush, only those lying prone sustained a neurologic injury, suggesting that the SCIWORA was caused by hyperextending the spine.

Other factors in SCIWORA include the relatively

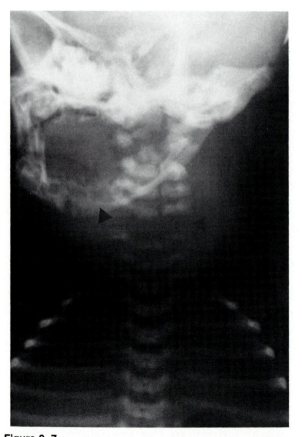

Figure 9–7

Dislocation of C4–C5 (*arrowheads*). This patient had abdominal dystocia, the result of a cephalic delivery with forceps. (Courtesy of Dr. Tim Tytle.)

large head to body size ratio in the child. Poor neck muscle development and head control may also be important. These speculations are supported by the fact that these injuries are more common in the younger child and in the upper cervical spine.[55, 57, 84] One must be particularly vigilant if the dire consequences of missing the diagnosis of SCIWORA syndrome are to be avoided. While motor and pedestrian accidents are the most frequent causes, the syndrome can occur with falls or in sports. It may also have a delayed onset.

The incidence of SCIWORA in patients with SCI has varied from 5 to 67%.[55, 56, 84] Yngve and colleagues[84] reviewed a series of 71 SCI patients from birth to age 1 year. Sixteen had SCIWORA, while 55 had SCI associated with osseous injury. In another series of 55 children with SCIWORA, 22 had complete or severe SCI and 33 had incomplete or mild SCI.[55] Ten lesions were in the upper cervical spine (C1–C4) and 33 in the lower (C5–C8); 12 were thoracic. The syndrome was more common and more likely to be severe in the younger child. All but 1 of the 22 patients with complete SCI were less than 8 years of age, and two thirds of the severely injured were less than 4 years of age. Younger children were also more likely to have upper cervical spine injuries. Fifteen of the patients in Pang's series[55] had a delayed onset of paralysis. Nine had transient warning signs, such as paresthesias or subjective paralysis. Eight patients sustained a second episode of SCIWORA after the initial event; the second event was always more severe than the initial injury. In all patients with a delayed onset of the syndrome, the spine had not been immobilized after the initial trauma, and all were neurologically normal before the second event. Four developed a complete SCI and were left with varying degrees of residual deficit. SCIWORA patients have a variety of associated injuries. In one series, 18 of the patients had a closed head injury.[56] Thoracic injuries were usually the result of severe trauma, and the crush injuries often had associated visceral injuries.

Pang[55] has stated that the prognosis depends on the results of the initial neurologic examination. To maximize the care of these patients he made the following recommendations: (1) Rule out occult fractures and dislocations that are unstable and require surgery. (2) Identify those patients who are likely to have late deterioration. (3) Prevent the recurrence of SCIWORA. After initial examination the patients should be evaluated by plain radiography, linear tomography, CT, and magnetic resonance imaging (MRI). None of these has proved reliable in detecting the osseous or ligamentous injury that must be present.[29] Myelography may be useful to localize the level of injury. In one series a displaced end plate was diagnosed by myelography.[84] Extravasation of myelographic dye from the spinal canal is a poor prognostic sign (Fig. 9–8). Pang and Pollack[55] found that somatosensory evoked potential (SSEP) studies were abnormal in 17 of 22 patients studied. The SSEP is particularly useful in patients with combined head trauma, in the young child, and as a baseline for recovery.

The indications for surgery in SCIWORA are the same as those for SCI and osseous injury. These patients usually have stable injuries and rarely require surgical stabilization. Laminectomy has not proved beneficial.[49, 55, 56, 84]

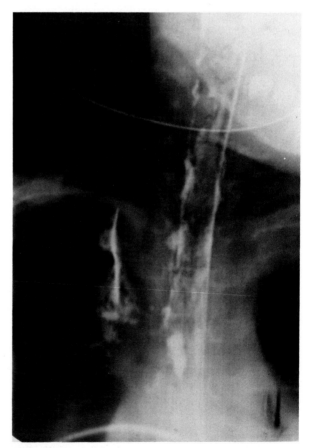

Figure 9–8

SCIWORA. This patient was struck by a car. In the emergency room he was noted to have a T4 level complete paraplegia. Plain radiography and CT studies were normal. The myelographic contrast medium extravasated into the chest at T4.

CHARACTERISTICS OF SPINAL CORD INJURY IN CHILDREN

Spinal cord injury in children is rare. Most occur as a result of motor vehicle accidents (38%), falls or jumps (16%), and gunshot wounds (13%).[33] Sports-related injuries are less frequent, diving being the most common (9%). All other sports account for 1% or less of the total. Spinal cord injury became a reportable condition in Oklahoma in 1987. From October 1987 to August 1989, 127 traumatic SCI patients were reported; none was less than 16 years old.

Spine fracture without spinal cord injury is more common than fracture with spinal cord injury.[29] Children make up a small percentage of all patients with acquired quadriplegia and paraplegia. Rang[64] reviewed the experience at Toronto Sick Children's Hospital over a 15-year period and found that paraplegia was three times more common than quadriplegia.

It is of utmost importance that all children with suspected spinal injury, even though it is relatively uncommon, be properly immobilized prior to extraction from a vehicle or prior to transport. Because of the large head size relative to body size, children under 10 years may need a recess in the spine board for the occiput or may need to be placed on double mattresses to protect the cervical spine. In one series of ten children less than 10 years of age with cervical spine injuries, lateral radiographs revealed that the spine was improperly positioned on a standard spine board.[34]

Upon arrival in the emergency room the patient should have the initial airway and cardiovascular status checked. A careful examination should be done to seek associated injuries. The child who is comatose or who has multiple organ system trauma or closed head trauma must be systematically evaluated for spinal injury. The neurologic examination must be complete and meticulous. The sensory level and motor function should be carefully documented. After routine radiography in two planes has been done, additional studies include supervised stress views, CT to demonstrate bony injury, and MRI to evaluate the spinal cord. A myelogram may be necessary.

Corticosteroids are often given in the hope that they will be beneficial. In a randomized, controlled study of methylprednisolone, placebo, and naloxone in the treatment of acute spinal cord injury, methylprednisolone produced improvement in motor and sensory recovery when evaluated at 6 weeks and 6 months.[9] The effect was limited to those treated within the first 8 hours of injury. Methylprednisolone was given as a bolus and for the first 23 hours after injury. The effect was observed in both complete and incomplete SCI. There was a higher incidence of wound infections, but the difference was not statistically significant. There was no increased risk of gastrointestinal bleeding. All the patients in the study were over 13 years of age, so that the effect on children is unknown. All patients with SCI should be given some type of antacid to protect against stress ulcers. Routine care includes a Foley catheter initially and then intermittent catheterization and a bowel program. Pressure sore prevention is of extreme importance and begins immediately.

Guidelines for management of spinal skeletal injury are the same as those discussed for SCIWORA. Children have a better chance than adults for some useful recovery from SCI. Hadley and co-workers[29] noted that 89% of pediatric patients with incomplete SCI improved; 20 patients with complete SCI had significant recovery as opposed to adults, who usually carry a worse prognosis. None of the patients sustained neurologic deterioration as a result of treatment. Children with both incomplete and complete SCI showed some recovery except in the thoracic area, where the prognosis was regarded as hopeless.[64] Laminectomy is not beneficial and can be harmful[49, 64, 67, 83] because it increases instability. In the cervical spine, swan neck deformity can occur after laminectomy.[69] Angular deformity at all levels is more likely after laminectomy in children.[47]

Children with acquired paraplegia require management by a variety of specialists, which is best delivered by a team approach. Specialists in orthopedics, pediatrics, urology, psychology, social services, physical and occupational therapy, orthotics, and education are crucial members of the team.

Several authors have looked at the risk of spinal deformity subsequent to SCI in children.[5, 6, 10, 40, 47] Mayfield and associates[47] reviewed 49 patients less than 18 years of age. In the 28 who developed SCI before the teenage growth spurt, all developed spinal deformities, 80% of which were progressive. Ninety-three percent developed scoliosis, 57% kyphosis, and 18% lordosis. Sixty-one percent of these patients required spinal fusion. In most patients orthotic management was unsuccessful, but in some it delayed the age at which fusion was necessary. These patients experienced a high complication rate after surgery, but 93% achieved a solid fusion. Thirteen had laminectomy without benefit. Pelvic obliquity was often a problem. In the patients who sustained their injury after the teenage growth spurt, two thirds developed acute angular deformity at the site of their fracture. Only 38% had a progressive deformity, which was usually not significant. Only one third of these patients required stabilization. Age, then, is very important because younger patients are at a higher risk for the development of deformity.

In other series the following additional factors were important in the development of deformity. The paralysis itself is the most important factor.[5] Children with simple fractures without SCI show good remodeling of the spine, and subsequent deformity is rare and not progressive.[35] In a series of paraplegias resulting from infections, tumors, and trauma, the cases caused by infection had the highest incidence of development of deformity, indicating that it is the paraplegia itself, rather than any injury to the bony column, that is most important.[5] The level of injury is important, with higher levels carrying a higher risk.[47] Spasticity and muscle imbalance are also contributory.[5] The development of pelvic obliquity can be catastrophic in the SCI patient with insensitive skin.[40] When pelvic obliquity develops, the pelvis follows the spine. Management of the deformity must balance the pelvis to produce a good sitting surface and a good result.[6, 40]

SPECIFIC CERVICAL SPINE INJURIES

Occiput–C1

Injuries at this level have been infrequently demonstrated in children.[22] It may well be that these injuries are so often associated with death that they are not diagnosed, as in the studies by Aufdermaur[2] (Fig. 9–9). In the study of Shulman and co-workers,[68] necropsy demonstrated transection of the cord with atlanto-occipital and atlantoaxial dislocation. Bohlman[8] has reported a case of a 14-year-old child with an occipit–C1 lesion that was not discovered until arteriography was performed.

A lesion is diagnosed by the demonstration of excessive mobility of the occiput on C1. There are no series available with specific treatment recommendations. Because of the potential for cord injury and death, these lesions should probably be reduced and an occiput–C1 or occiput–C2 fusion performed.

Subluxation of C1 on C2

There is minimal rotation between the occiput and C1.[1] Fifty percent of cervical spine rotation occurs between C1 and C2. There is, to a lesser extent, flexion, extension, and translation in this joint. Roughly one third of the canal is occupied by the odontoid, one third by the cord, and one third by the SAC.[71] When rotation exceeds normal, and particularly when the ligaments are disrupted, the odontoid can cause pressure on the spinal cord. In addition, the vertebral artery is immediately anterior to the transverse foramina of C1 and C2 and can be damaged with excessive displacement. This excessive mobility can be caused by rupture of the ligaments, fracture of the odontoid, or increased ligamentous laxity.

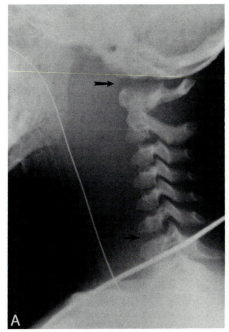
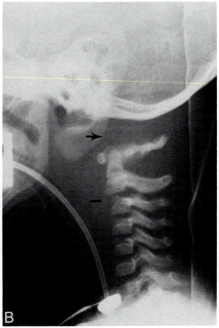

Figure 9–9

Atlanto-occipital dislocation. *A*, This 3-year-old female sustained multiple trauma and was placed on a respirator. Note the massive prevertebral swelling, dislocation of the atlanto-occipital joint, and dislocation of C6–C7. The patient died shortly after the study. *B*, This 3-year-old was struck by a car, resuscitated elsewhere, and transferred. Once again, note the hypopharyngeal soft tissue swelling and an additional injury at C2–C3. This patient also died. (Courtesy of Dr. Tim Tytle.)

Diagnosis of C1–C2 instability is suggested by a history of trauma to the cervical spine and confirmed by plain or tomographic views of the cervical spine and flexion-extension views showing excursion of greater than 5 mm between the anterior cortex of the dens and the posterior cortex of the anterior ring of C1. The neurologic condition of the patient must be meticulously documented. Although these injuries may fail to heal, a trial of conservative treatment in a halo vest or Minerva cast is indicated in the child. Additional pins may be required in the small infant or child to distribute the force of the halo pins.[50] If after a period of 2 to 3 months of this conservative care, the flexion-extension films indicate continued instability of greater than 5 mm, a C1–C2 fusion should be performed. My preferred technique is the same as that described and illustrated under os odontoideum.

There has been considerable interest in the incidence of C1–C2 instability in individuals with Down syndrome (DS).[13, 15, 61–63, 70, 78] In a series of 236 patients, 17% were found to have greater than 5 mm of instability.[61] Eighty-five percent were asymptomatic, while 15% had neurologic symptoms or findings.[62] In a more recent review of 404 patients,[62] 14.6% of patients had greater than 5 mm of displacement (59 of 404). Of these 59 patients, 53 were asymptomatic, and only 6 were symptomatic and required surgery. In follow-up there had not been significant changes clinically or radiographically.

After the early studies, the Committee on Sports Medicine of the American Academy of Pediatrics issued a policy statement.[13] The committee recommended that patients with DS having 5 to 6 mm of instability be restricted from participating in sports that carry a risk of stress to the head and neck. Those without instability were not restricted. Follow-up was not specified. The Special Olympics organization issued a bulletin that placed even greater restrictions on particular sports.[70] The bulletin led to the belief that all individuals with DS required examination and radiographic evaluation before participation in sports. In some instances this was interpreted as an annual requirement.

In a 1988 review, Davidson[15] found little support for the hypothesis that "instability" predisposes to neurologic compromise or dislocation. All cases of dislocation were preceded by several weeks of readily detectable physical signs; therefore, a carefully performed physical examination (including a neurologic examination) was more predictive. Davidson reached the following conclusions: (1) The incidence of atlantoaxial dislocation in DS is unknown. (2) There is no evidence that a radiograph is predictive.

One patient with a normal x-ray died of the condition. (3) There is no report of an atlantoaxial dislocation in a patient with DS during participation in sports.

Instability of the cervical spine in individuals with DS is a matter of concern to those individuals with the syndrome and to their caretakers. While instability occurs in a significant number of these individuals, the natural history of the condition is unknown. It is reasonable to obtain a baseline neurologic examination and flexion and extension films of the cervical spine. Repeat neurologic evaluation every 3 to 5 years is probably sufficient. These persons should not be unnecessarily restricted. If neurologic symptoms or signs develop, a more detailed work-up is necessary. If radiographic evaluation reveals an atlanto–dens interval of greater than 5 mm, the patient should refrain from sports that stress the cervical spine. Recognized treatment options exist for those with neurologic problems.[63] In one series, 7 of 236 patients had various neurologic deficits.[63] Early recognition and treatment led to good results. The patients with long-standing symptoms were minimally improved by surgery.

Atlantoaxial Rotary Fixation (AARF)

This condition, called by a variety of names, is a clinical condition in which there is usually pain, loss of cervical motion, and torticollis. In young patients with long-standing AARF, there may also be facial asymmetry. In the series of 17 cases of Fielding and Hawkins,[24] one of the striking features was the delay in diagnosis. The condition may be difficult to diagnosis with plain films, but plain tomography may be suggestive. Cineradiography or CT may be necessary to make the diagnosis.

In the series of Fielding and Hawkins,[24] there was an equal number of males and females, and the age range was from 7 to 68 years (average 20 years). Onset had been spontaneous in four, associated with minor trauma in three, and associated with upper respiratory infection (URI) in five; three had miscellaneous associated conditions. In another series of 16 children, 8 gave a history of minor trauma, 9 of recent URI, and 1 of juvenile rheumatoid arthritis.[60]

In Fielding's and Hawkins' series[24] the average delay to diagnosis was 11.6 months. Neck extension was usually decreased by as much as 50%. The characteristic position of the head was a 23 degree tilt to one side with a 20 degree rotation to the opposite side and slight flexion. Patients could actively make the deformity worse but were unable actively to correct it.

The diagnosis must be confirmed radiographically. On the open-mouth anteroposterior (AP) view, there is a lateral rotation of the mass of the atlas. The lateral mass that is forward appears wider and closer to the midline, and the other lateral mass appears smaller and farther away from the midline. This creates asymmetry between the odontoid process and the lateral mass. On the side on which the atlas is rotated posteriorly, the joint between the lateral masses is obscured. On the AP view, particularly with tilt and rotation, the spinous process appears markedly deviated from the midline and on the same side as the chin. Open-mouth views with rotation of 15 and 30 degrees to the right and left may be useful. On the lateral plain films, the lateral mass of the atlas is rotated forward to the position normally held by the oval anterior arch of the atlas. This can lead to constriction of the canal. With tilting of the atlas, the two halves of the posterior arch are not superimposed. Plain tomography shows that the lateral masses are in different planes. This can occur with positioning and is not diagnostic. Lateral cineradiography, when available, will show that the posterior arches of C1 and C2 move together rather than independently during neck rotation, confirming the diagnosis. Recently CT has been used for confirmation. The usual technique is to obtain 5 mm or 6 mm cuts from the occiput to C2. The lateral masses of C1 show rotary subluxation of 20 degrees (Fig. 9–10).[24] Dynamic CT, in which 3 mm cuts are first taken in routine fashion and then with right and left rotation, are reported to be of benefit in making the diagnosis.[60]

Fielding and Hawkins[24] divided this disorder into four grades depending upon the status of the atlantoaxial ligaments. Type I, the most common, is a rotary fixation without any anterior displacement of the atlas. In this type the transverse ligament is thought to be intact and the condition therefore more benign. Type II is potentially dangerous in that there is rotary fixation and anterior displacement of less than 3 to 5 mm, indicating a deficient transverse ligament that causes unilateral anterior displacement of one of the lateral masses. The last two types are more severe, since they are associated with rupture of all the ligaments. In type III the displacement is over 5 mm; this type is considered to be associated with deficiencies of transverse and secondary ligaments with both lateral masses displaced anteriorly. Type IV is an unusual type, in which there is posterior displacement of the atlas due to a deficient dens.

The origin of the condition is uncertain. Inflammation, ruptured ligaments, muscle contracture, and spasm have all been suggested. Trivial trauma and URI are probably among the most common causes.[14, 39, 60] Kawabe and co-workers[39] reviewed 17 cases and also performed autopsies on 6 infant cadavers. CT studies were done on 8 patients with AARF and compared with 95 normal studies. This article discusses a range of possible causes, noting that the facet angle of the axis is steeper in children than in adults. There is also a meniscus-like synovial fold found in the occipitoatlantal and atlantoaxial joints of children that is not present in adults. These investigators concluded that inflammation or effusion from trauma could cause infolding or rupture of these synovial folds that would result in AARF.

Figure 9–10

CT study of atlantoaxial rotary fixation. A, The view of C1. B, The view of C2 was obtained while the position of the head was maintained. Note the rotation of C2 relative to C1. (Courtesy of Dr. Tim Tytle.)

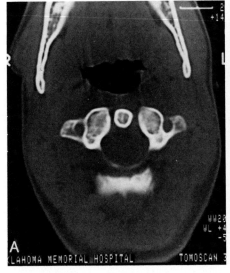
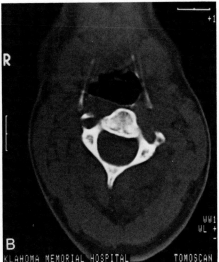

On the CT of patients with AARF the lateral mass of C1 showed rotary subluxation of 20 degrees anterolaterally.

The differential diagnosis of AARF includes congenital anomalies of the upper cervical spine, infection, anomalies of the dens, syringomyelia, tumor, ocular problems, and bulbar palsy. In AARF the sternocleidomastoid is elongated, whereas in most of the other conditions it is short.

With early detection the treatment is traction, usually with a halter, until the spasm is relieved and the deformity corrected. Maintenance of position in a collar is usually sufficient. In patients with long-standing deformity the condition is often irreducible or only incompletely reducible. In these patients the deformity may recur after conservative care unless fusion is carried out. In the series of Fielding and Hawkins,[24] which included adults and children, 11 of 13 patients were treated by skull traction followed by fusion with good results. In the four remaining patients, one died in traction, two declined surgery, and one had insufficient follow-up.

Marar and Balachandran[46] reviewed 12 children treated for AARF with traction and a Minerva jacket. Six of 12 had a good result with this treatment. Three of 12 did not undergo reduction but were symptom free. Likewise, 3 of 12 patients did not undergo reduction and had symptoms. One of them was treated by fusion and decompression of C1 and the foramen magnum. Phillips and Hensinger[60] reviewed 23 children (average age, 7 years to 6 months) treated for AARF. The key was early detection. Sixteen patients with symptoms of less than 1 month's duration responded to brief periods of halter traction (1.3 to 2.3 kg) and were then managed in some sort of cervical immobilization. Eleven of this group had their symptoms less than 1 week. The average hospital stay was 4 days. All seven patients who did not undergo reduction had had symptoms for longer than 1 month, and these patients were treated with fusion in situ. The specific type of fusion was not mentioned, but the point was made that no reduction was attempted.

Fractures of the Atlas

The atlas is a diminutive structure in the human. It is shielded from most forces. Most fractures of the atlas result from direct axial compression that drives the occipital condyles onto the atlas. The force is dissipated on the lateral masses (Fig. 9–11A). The usual fracture disrupts both the anterior and the posterior ring (Fig. 9–11B). The transverse ligament can be ruptured. SCI is rare. The fracture is hard to evaluate on the plain radiographs, but CT is an excellent means of demonstrating the injury (Fig. 9–11C). Most of these lesions will heal in a halo or Minerva cast or vest. Up to 6 months of immobilization may be necessary.

Fractures of the Axis

Fractures of the ring of C2, the so-called hangman's fracture, has been reported in an infant who struck his head and sustained a central cord syndrome in a motor vehicle accident.[80] The initial films were interpreted as being normal. Later films showed a fracture of C2 immediately behind the articular surface of the lateral mass. The neural arch of C2 remained with C3, while the head and C2 moved forward. This injury was treated by skull traction through burr holes. In 18 days there was return of neurologic function. By 22 days the spine was considered to be stable and was treated with a soft collar. At 14 months the child had residual weakness of the intrinsic muscles of the hand. This was believed to be a hyperextension injury. Many of these injuries are minimally displaced (Fig. 9–12). These injuries will heal with immobilization in a cast or halo.

Fractures of the odontoid and C1–C2 dislocations are the most common pediatric cervical spine injuries.[67] Fractures of the odontoid are usually associated with head trauma from motor vehicle accidents or falls from a height. The odontoid fracture is typically at the base, and the fragment moves with C1. The fracture can usually be reduced and held with halo traction or a halo vest or Minerva jacket for 6 to 8 weeks. Surgical reduction is rarely necessary. Results in the older child are similar to those in the adult. Fractures at the base and tip generally heal satisfactorily, whereas those at the level of the articular cartilage have a high failure rate when treated conservatively and usually require surgery. If unrecognized, these may fail to heal.

These acute injuries must be differentiated from os odontoideum, which typically has a remnant of the axis at the base and an apical segment separated by a wide gap (Fig. 9–13A, B). The apical segment is usually hypoplastic and may be seen with plain tomography or CT (Fig. 9–13C). Wollin[82] considered os odontoideum a developmental anomaly of the axis in which the odontoid was divided by a transverse gap and the apical segment was left reduced without the bony support of the base of the process. Fielding and Griffin,[23] however, believed that os odontoideum was an acquired lesion. They reported on three patients with radiographic evi-

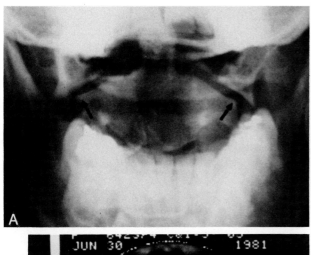
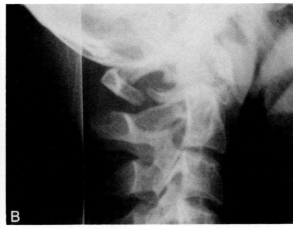
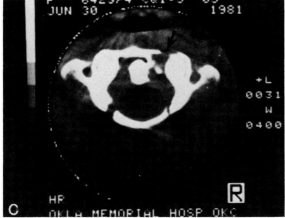

Figure 9–11

Fracture of C1 (Jefferson fracture). *A*, The AP view shows lateral displacement of the lateral mass and articulating facets of C1 on C2. *B*, The oblique view illustrates disruption of the posterior aspect of the ring of C1. *C*, The CT scan reveals the true extent of the injury. (Courtesy of Dr. Teresa Stacy.)

dence of a normal odontoid, all of whom developed an os odontoideum after trauma. One fell at 17 months, had a radiographically normal odontoid at 17 months, and gradually developed a lesion by age 6 years. Another had a normal x-ray at 18 months and an os odontoideum at age 8 years. These investigators concluded that this condition, rarely seen in young infants and rarely associated with congenital anomalies, is therefore probably not developmental.

Os odontoideum weakens the atlantoaxial joint, as it lacks a peg (Fig. 9–13*B*). In the cases described the retropharyngeal soft tissue space was wide, but there was no history of preceding URI to explain it; therefore it was thought to be swelling from the trauma. The proposed theory was that with trauma the blood supply was damaged and the development of the odontoid was compromised.

In Wollin's series of nine patients aged 10 to 68 years, two had severe symptoms.[82] Gwinn and Smith had seven patients aged 2 to 55 years, three of whom had severe symptoms.[28] These patients may be asymptomatic, have vague discomfort, or gradually develop partial or complete quadriparesis.

Instability is an indication for surgical stabilization, as additional trauma could be fatal. My preferred method of treatment is a C1–C2 fusion (Fig. 9–13*D–F*). The patient is positioned prone, Gardner-Wells tongs used to hold the head. Initial radiographs are obtained to be certain that the radiographic technique is sufficient and to confirm the position of C1 and C2. The exposure is facilitated if the cervical spine is in neutral flexion. One should be careful to avoid exposing any more than the area that is to be fused. An 18-gauge wire is passed under C1, and the free ends of the wire are passed back through the loop and tightened to grasp the ring of C1 (Fig. 9–13*D*). The head is then extended and the reduction confirmed by radiography (Fig. 9–13*E*). Overreduction must be avoided. A notch can be made in the inferior aspect of the spinous process of C2 to maintain the wire, or the wire can be passed through a hole in the spinous process if it is large enough. The wire is then twisted to maintain the

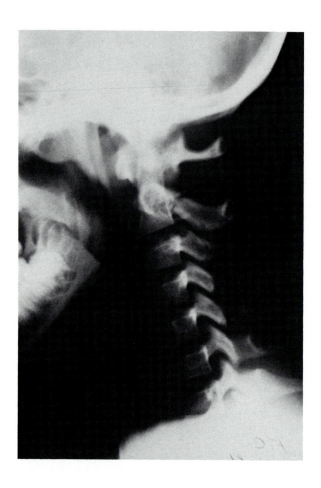

Figure 9–12

Fracture of C2 (Hangman's fracture).

position of the reduction (Fig. 9–13F). C1 and C2 are decorticated with rongeurs, and strips of iliac bone are packed around the area to be fused. Postoperatively the patient is placed in a SOMI orthosis for 3 months. Flexion-extension radiographs demonstrating stability are obtained before discontinuing the orthosis.

Fractures and Dislocations of C3–C7

Most of the fractures in the cervical spine in children occur at C1 and C2[37, 67]; fracture-dislocation in C3–C7, as seen in adults, is rare.[36, 59]

Evans and Bethem[21] reviewed 24 consecutive cases of cervical spine injuries in children, which represented 1.2 cases per year in their busy hospital. Their patients being somewhat older (average age 13 years), some were probably better considered as adults. One must consider the mechanism of injury when choosing a treatment mode. Evans and Bethem[21] believed that flexion injuries were the culprit in 42% and hyperextension dislocations in 12%. In contrast to other series of pediatric cervical spine fractures, 29% were upper cervical spine injuries and 71% involved C3 through C7.

No definite guidelines were given as to which patients could be treated closed and which ones required surgery. Treatment for most patients was nonoperative with tongs, Minerva casts, or halo or neck orthoses. In the three patients who were operated on, the anterior approach was contraindicated. In the flexion injuries that disrupt the anterior longitudinal ligament, this approach would increase the instability. Since most were flexion injuries, posterior spinal fusion with a wire and iliac graft was the treatment of choice. Nonoperative treatment was successful in 95% of patients. Evans and Bethem[21] concluded that surgery might be indicated for flexion injuries, which were associated with a high rate of late kyphosis. They further concluded that surgery might be indicated for burst fractures with neurologic injury in the hope that stabilization would enhance recovery. Most lower cervical spine fracture-dislocations will usually heal when treated closed. Laminectomy is not beneficial and has been shown to cause swan neck deformity and further instability.[69]

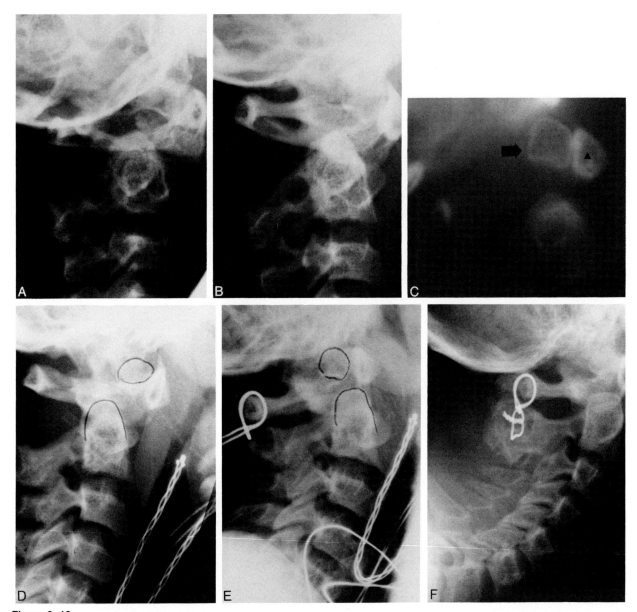

Figure 9-13

Os odontoideum. This patient fell from a tree, striking his neck on a branch. He was neurologically normal and had minimal findings for an acute cervical spine injury. *A,* His lateral C-spine x-ray was suggestive of instability at C1–C2. *B,* A lateral flexion view of C1–C2 showing displacement of C1 on C2. *C,* Tomograms revealed a rounded apical segment (*thick arrow*), a large gap above the remnant of the dens (*thin arrow*), and movement of the apical segment with the anterior aspect of C1. *D,* Operative radiograph prior to reduction. *E,* Radiograph with C1 reduced on C2 and the wire placed arond the ring of C1. *F,* Postoperative radiograph demonstrating the position of the wire.

Ligamentous instability can occur in children and adolescents, although it is less common than in adults. Pennecot and co-workers[59] described 16 cases of dislocation and ligamentous disruption, 5 at C1–C2 and 11 from C3 through C7. A constant feature was the loss of a normal lordosis and a stiff neck (Fig. 9–14). This was confirmed on lateral radiographs in neutral and active hyperflexion. On the roentgenogram there was widened interspinous space, loss of parallelism of the articular facets, kyphosis in the disk space, and posterior opening. Calcification in the interspinous ligament appeared at a delayed time, indicating disruption and healing in the ligament. A delay in diagnosis was common. Five of eight patients were treated with posterior spinal fusion after the injury. The indications for surgery were persistent pain and roentgenographic evidence of worsening of the condition. These investigators cautioned that the exposure must be carefully controlled to prevent extension of the fusion mass to levels beyond the intended fusion level.

THORACOLUMBAR SPINE FRACTURES

Thoracolumbar spine fractures in children are quite rare. As noted earlier, upper thoracic spine injuries can be incurred during birth. Thoracic and lumbar spine injuries in a young child can be the result of battering.[16] In the case shown in Figure 9–15 the child was noted to have a normal spine during the first year of life and a markedly deformed spine with paralysis at age 2 years. As in many of these cases, the history was vague. Initially a history of progressive neurologic deterioration was obtained, and a diagnosis of tuberculosis was suspected until the previous films were obtained. Child abuse was the final diagnosis.

Most thoracic and lumbar spine fractures in children result from motor vehicle accidents, pedestrian-vehicular accidents, or a fall from a height.[33] Adolescents engage in a wide variety of activities that can result in spinal fractures, including sports such as tobogganing and skiing, and can be victims of motorcycle and motor vehicle accidents.[34, 54]

Classification

No one has yet reviewed a series of pediatric or adolescent patients to apply the three-column classification system. These are frequently described as being a result of compression, distraction, or shear. Compression injuries occur when the spine is acutely flexed forward. In some situations, particularly sporting events, the spine may be partially flexed, causing preloading.

While it is unusual, pathologic fractures of the spine do occur. The patient in Figure 9–16 had been scheduled for a scoliosis evaluation. She was involved in a motor vehicle accident and sustained a fracture through T11. The final diagnosis was aneurysmal bone cyst. Pathologic fractures can occur in eosinophilic granuloma, in leukemia, and in other blood proliferative disorders. In a series from St. Jude's Hospital, 1.6% of children with acute lymphocytic leukemia (ALL) had vertebral compression fractures at the time of presentation.[65] The diagnosis of ALL was delayed in some because of the unusual presentation. Twenty-two had multiple-level involvement. The symptoms abated with treatment. One must also be aware of the vertebra plana seen

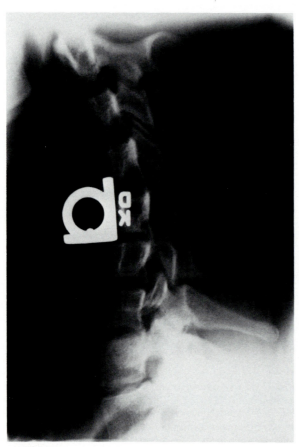

Figure 9–14
Unilateral facet dislocation. This skeletally mature patient gave a history of 3 months of pain following an automobile accident. She was neurologically normal. Note the reversal of the normal cervical lordosis and the anteriorly displaced inferior articulating facet of C6. While it is poorly reproduced, there is also increased interspinous distance. (Courtesy of Dr. Tim Tytle.)

Figure 9–15

Child abuse. *A,* This x-ray taken during the first year of life reveals multiple rib fractures and a normal spine. *B,* This subsequent film shows a healing fracture-dislocation at the thoracolumbar junction.

in eosinophilic granuloma that can be confused with a compression fracture.

Roaf[66] studied the mechanics of injury in fractures of the spine by subjecting cadaver spines of children and adults to load. With precompression and a normal disk, the annulus bulged but transmitted the load to the vertebral bodies. The blood was squeezed out of the body, and with continued pressure the bodies cracked. After the break the nuclear material extruded, and with further pressure the body disintegrated. With a dehydrated disk, prolapse occurred. Compression forces were mainly absorbed by the body. The healthy nucleus pulposus was incompressible. It was difficult to produce fractures with pure compression or pure flexion. A combination of rotation and compression could produce almost any of the commonly seen fracture patterns. Pure rotation was more likely to produce dislocation, whereas compression produced fractures.

Distraction injuries can be produced by wearing lap seat belts.[18, 75] American auto makers have

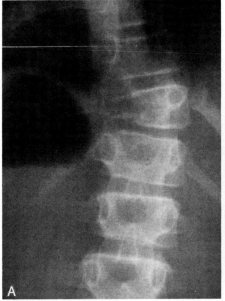
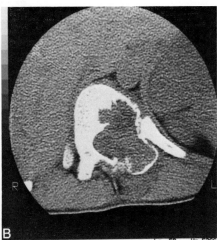

Figure 9–16

Pathologic fracture. *A,* A prior x-ray disclosed a 25 degree scoliosis with the apex at T11. This exposure was made after an automobile accident. Note the absent pedicle at T11, which could also be seen on the prior film. *B,* CT scan of T11 reveals destruction of the pedicle, erosion of the body, and extension into the soft tissues. Note the thin cortical shell over the soft tissue mass.

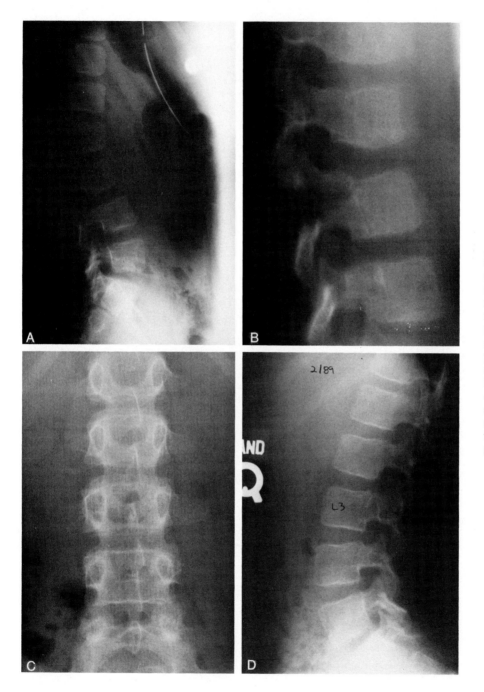

Figure 9–17

Distraction fracture-dislocation. *A*, Lateral spine film discloses loss of lumbar lordosis and increase in the interspinous distance between L2 and L3. *B*, Tomograms confirm a fracture through the spinous process and disruption of the disk space. An extension film over a bolster showed that the fracture could be reduced closed. AP (*C*) and lateral (*D*) spine x-rays 9 months later show healing of the fracture, which was treated in a plaster body jacket in extension.

lagged in providing shoulder type restraints for rear seat passengers. In addition, smaller children are not as effectively protected by existing shoulder harnesses. As the child is thrown forward, the lap belt, which is incorrectly positioned above the iliac crest, compresses the abdominal contents and forms a fulcrum. The more posteriorly located spine is distracted around this fulcrum, causing tension in the posterior aspect of the spine. If sufficient force is applied, this can cause tearing of the posterior ligaments or bony fracture and dislocation (Fig. 9–17). The classic Chance fracture is a bony injury through the vertebral body, the pedicles, and the spinous processes. Variations include pure facet dislocation with disruption of the disk space, and dislocation through the facet joints with fracture through the body (Fig. 9–18). One must examine carefully for intraabdominal injury, such as small bowel lacerations, renal damage, and rupture of the spleen.

A retrospective review of 365 CT studies for intraabdominal trauma revealed five pediatric cases of lap belt injury with lumbar spine injury.[75] These consisted of facet subluxation and anterior dislocation of L3 on L4. There were multiple compression fractures in one patient. In retrospect the fractures were visible on the AP radiograph, but the findings were quite subtle and best appreciated on the lateral view. Injuries of the lumbar spine occurred in less than 2% of injured children evaluated by CT. An absence of clinical symptoms may have led to failure to make the diagnosis. The child has a higher center of gravity, a large head, and an incompletely developed iliac crest, all of which may predispose to these injuries.

In another review of two cases of pediatric lumbar flexion distraction fractures associated with lap belts, the initial diagnosis was missed in both patients.[18] Retrospectively the injuries were visible on the AP radiographs, although they were best seen on the lateral lumbar spine view. One of these patients was treated conservatively, while the other was treated surgically. At follow-up, both had maintained their reduction and had remodeling of the vertebral body. A high index of suspicion is required to make the diagnosis of such injuries. Installation of adjustable shoulder restraints could perhaps prevent these seat belt injuries. Although the injury to the spine is

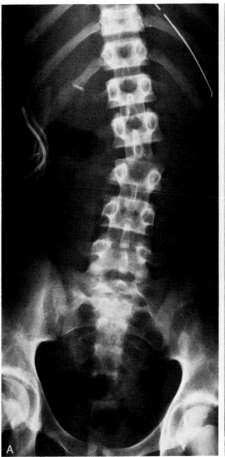
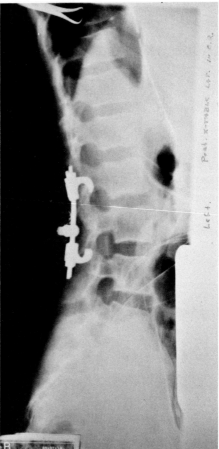

Figure 9–18

Facet dislocation. A, This patient sustained a distraction seat belt injury. She had an L2–L3 facet dislocation. She also sustained tears in the small bowel. B, The spine injury was treated by open reduction, internal fixation with Harrington compression rods, and limited fusion.

serious, without the seat belt many of these children would not have survived the accident or would have sustained other injuries, such as closed head trauma.

There have been 85 reported cases of fracture of the vertebral limbus (a fracture between the ring apophysis and the cartilaginous rim of the vertebral end plate).[20, 43, 76] Twenty-four of these were in patients aged 10 to 18 years. The injury most frequently is to the superior end plate of one of the midlumbar spines (Fig. 9–19). The mechanisms of injury have included weightlifting, shoveling, gymnastics, hyperextension, and trauma. The patients present with back and leg pain and spasm; often there is a paucity of neurologic signs. The diagnosis is rarely made on the plain radiographs. CT with or without contrast medium is useful, although the exact diagnosis may not be apparent. Often one is able only to make the diagnosis of a mass in the spinal canal. This must be differentiated from spinal stenosis or other causes, as decompression alone is of no benefit. The treatment of choice is excision of the loose fragment, which is more easily accomplished if the diagnosis is made early.

Intervertebral disk calcification occurs in children and can be confused with trauma or infection.[44, 45, 57] The patients present with pain, neurologic signs, and a radiograph that demonstrates calcification in the spinal canal. In most cases the course is benign, and the condition resolves with conservative care.

Diagnosis

One must approach pediatric patients who have multiple trauma with a high index of suspicion. Those who are comatose or poorly responsive are particularly at risk. A careful search should be made for sensory level and movement, ascertaining that movement is voluntary and not due to reflexes. Rectal examination for tone and cremasteric reflex is also important.

Radiographic evaluation in multiply traumatized patients routinely includes chest and abdominal AP and lateral radiographs and often CT studies. These must be carefully scrutinized, looking at the disk spaces, the posterior aspects of the spinous processes, and the shape of the vertebral body. Children may have compression fractures at multiple levels. Small areas of avulsion may be the only subtle findings, and often these can be confused with the normal ring apophysis. As noted by Aufdermaur,[2] rupture through the growth zone and disks may be minimally visible on an radiograph.

In the absence of spinal cord injury, progression of spinal deformity is rare. Children's vertebral bodies tend to remodel. In the review by Horal and co-workers,[35] 53% were normal at follow-up. The patients had no significant disability. Interbody fusion is usual.

Management

All children with fractures of the thoracic and lumbar spine, regardless of how minimal, should be admitted to the hospital. The risk of ileus and urinary retention is the same as in an adult. Pain must be managed, and the patient must be observed for the possibility of progressive neurologic deficit. The majority of children's fractures are stable and do not require operative intervention; unstable injuries, however, may require operation. One must determine the mechanism of injury in order to choose the type of instrumentation needed to restore stability. In general, the same indications exist for children as for adults. Fracture-dislocation with displacement should be reduced. The best decompres-

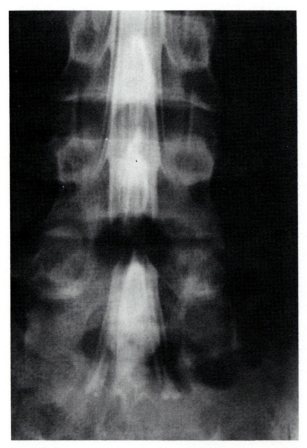

Figure 9–19

Fracture of the end plate. This myelogram reveals a near-complete block at L4–L5. At surgery the patient was found to have a fracture of the superior end plate of L5.

sion of the thoracic and lumbar spine is reduction. Laminectomy is not beneficial and can be detrimental. Instrumentation may be more difficult in children, owing to their smaller size. Until recently, Luque instrumentation was one of the only alternatives, but small hooks and other implants are now available for a variety of the spinal instrumentation systems.

With an incomplete neurologic injury, it is prudent to perform realignment as soon as the patient is stable. This is most often obtained by posterior spinal fusion with instrumentation and iliac grafting. These injuries are not surgical emergencies unless there is an open wound or progressive neurologic deficit.

Acknowledgment

I would like to thank Drs. Teresa Stacy and Tim Tytle for supplying some of the illustrations for this chapter. These are from the superb teaching files that they have developed for the Department of Radiology, University of Oklahoma, College of Medicine.

REFERENCES

1. Anson, B.J. Morris' Human Anatomy, 12th ed. New York, McGraw-Hill, 1953.
2. Aufdermaur, M. Spinal injuries in juveniles: Necropsy findings in twelve cases. J Bone Joint Surg 56-B:513–519, 1974.
3. Babcock, J.L. Spinal injuries in children. Pediatr Clin North Am 22:487–500, 1972.
4. Bailey, D.K. The normal cervical spine in infants and children. Radiology 59:712–719, 1952.
5. Banniza von Bazan, U.K.; Paeslack, V. Scoliotic growth in children with acquired paraplegia. Paraplegia 15:65–73, 1977–1978.
6. Bedbrook, G.M. Correction of scoliosis due to paraplegia sustained in paediatric age group. Paraplegia 15:90–96, 1977–1978.
7. Boger, D.C. Cervical prevertebral soft tissues in children: An unreliable soft tissue indicator of cervical spine trauma. Contemp Orthop 5:31–34, 1982.
8. Bohlman, H.H. Acute fractures and dislocations of the cervical spine. J Bone Joint Surg 61-A:1119–1142, 1979.
9. Bracken, M.B.; Shepard, M.J.; Collins, W.F.; et al. A randomized, controlled trial of methylprednisolone or naloxone in the treatment of acute spinal cord injury: Results of the Second National Spinal Cord Injury Study. N Engl J Med 322:1405–1411, 1990.
10. Burke, D.C. Traumatic spinal paralysis in children. Paraplegia 9:268–276, 1971.
11. Burke, D.C. Spinal cord trauma in children. Paraplegia 9:1–14, 1971.
12. Cattell, H.S.; Filtzer, D.L. Pseudosubluxation and other normal variations in the cervical spine in children. J Bone Joint Surg 47-A:1295–1309, 1965.
13. Committee on Sports Medicine. Atlantoaxial instability in Down syndrome. Pediatrics 74:152–154, 1984.
14. Daffner, R.H. Pseudofracture of the dens: Mach bands. Am J Roentgenol 128:607–612, 1977.
15. Davidson, R.G. Atlantoaxial instability in individuals with Down syndrome; A fresh look at the evidence. Pediatrics 81:857–865, 1988.
16. Dickson, R.A.; Leatherman, K.D. Spinal injuries in child abuse: A case report. J Trauma 18:811–812, 1978.
17. Dolan, K.D. Cervicobasilar relationships. Radiol Clin North Am 25:155–166, 1977.
18. Ebraheim, N.A.; Savolain, E.R.; Southworth, S.R.; et al. Pediatric lumbar seat belt injuries: Report of two cases. Orthopedics, in press.
19. Ehara, S.; El-Khoury, G.Y.; Sato, Y. Cervical spine injury in children. Radiologic manifestations. AJR 151:1175–1178, 1988.
20. Epstein, N.A.; Epstein, J.A.; Mauri, T. Treatment of fractures of the vertebral limbus and spinal stenosis in five adolescents and five adults. J Neurosurg 24:595–604, 1989.
21. Evans, D.L.; Bethem, D. Cervical spine injuries in children. J Pediatr Orthop 9:563–568, 1989.
22. Evarts, C.M. Traumatic occipital-atlantal dislocation. Report of a case with survival. J Bone Joint Surg 52-A:1653, 1970.
23. Fielding, J.W.; Griffin, P.P. Os odontoideum: An acquired lesion. J Bone Joint Surg 56-A:187–190, 1974.
24. Fielding, J.W.; Hawkins, R.J. Atlanto-axial rotary fixation (fixed rotary subluxation of the atlanto-axial joint). J Bone Joint Surg 59-A:37–44, 1977.
25. Fielding, J.W.; Cochran, G.B.B.; Lawsing, J.F., III; Hohl, M. Tears of the transverse ligament of the atlas: Clinical and biomechanical study. J Bone Joint Surg 56-A:1683–1691, 1974.
26. Fielding, J.W.; Hensinger, R.N.; Hawkins, R.J. Os odontoideum. J Bone Joint Surg 62-A:376–383, 1980.
27. Freiberger, R.H.; Wilson, P.H.; Nicolas, J.A. Acquired absence of the odontoid process. J Bone Joint Surg 47-A:1231, 1965.
28. Gwinn, J.L.; Smith, J.L. Acquired and congenital absence of the odontoid. Am J Roentgenol 88:424–431, 1962.
29. Hadley, M.N.; Zabramski, J.M.; Browner, C.M.; et al. Pediatric spinal trauma: Review of 122 cases of spinal cord and vertebral column injuries. J Neurosurg 68:18–24, 1988.
30. Henrys, P.; Lyne, E.D.; Lifton, C.; Salciccioli, G. Clinical review of cervical spine injuries in children. Clin Orthop 129:172–176, 1977.
31. Hensinger, R.N.; Fielding, J.W., Hawkins, R.J. Congenital anomalies of the odontoid process. Orthop Clin North Am 9:901–912, 1978.
32. Hensinger, R.N.; Lang, J.E.; MacEwen, G.D. Klippel-Feil syndrome: A constellation of associated anomalies. J Bone Joint Surg 56-A:1246–1252, 1974.
33. Herndon, W.A. Injuries to the head, neck, and spine. In: Sullivan, J.A.; Grana, W.A., eds. The Pediatric Athlete. American Academy of Orthopedic Surgeons, Park Ridge, IL, 1990.
34. Herzenberg, J.E.; Hensinger, R.N.; Dedrick, D.K.; Philips, W.A. Emergency transport of young children who have an injury of the cervical spine: The standard backboard may be hazardous. J Bone Joint Surg 71-A:15–22, 1989.
35. Horal, J.; Nachemson, A.; Scheller, S. Clinical and radiological long term follow-up of vertebral fractures in children. Acta Orthop Scand 43:491–503, 1972.
36. Jacob, B. Cervical fracture and dislocation (C3–7). Clin Orthop 109:18–32, 1975.

37. Jones, E.T.; Hensinger, R.N. Cervical spine injuries in children. Contemp Orthop 5:17–23, 1982.
38. Jones, E.T.; Hensinger, R.N. C2–C3 Dislocation in a child. J Pediatr Orthop 1:419–422, 1981.
39. Kawabe, N.; Hirotani, H.; Tanaka, O. Pathomechanism of atlantoaxial rotary fixation in children. J Pediatr Orthop 9:569–574, 1989.
40. Kilfoyle, R.M.; Foley, J.J.; Norton, P.L. Spine and pelvic deformity in childhood and adolescent paraplegia. J Bone Joint Surg 47-A:659–682, 1965.
41. Klippel M.; Feil, A. Anomalies de la collone vertebrale par absence des vertebres cervicales; avec cage thoracique remontant jusqu'a la bas du crane. Bull Soc Anat Paris 87:185, 1912.
42. Leventhal, H.R. Birth injuries of the spinal cord. J Pediatr 56:447–453, 1960.
43. Lowrey, J.J. Dislocated lumbar vertebral epiphysis in adolescent children. Report of three cases. J Neurosurg 38:232–234, 1973.
44. Maccartee, C.C., Jr.; Griffin, P.P.; Byrd, E.B. Ruptured calcified thoracic disc in a child. J Bone Joint Surg 54-A:1272–1274, 1972.
45. Mainzer, F. Herniation of the nucleus pulposus; a rare complication of intervertebral disk calcification in children. Radiology 107:167–170, 1973.
46. Marar, B.D.; Balachandran, N. Non-traumatic atlanto-axial dislocation in children. Clin Orthop 92:220–226, 1973.
47. Mayfield, J.K.; Erkkila, J.C.; Winter, R.B. Spine deformities subsequent to acquired childhood spinal cord injury. Orthop Trans 3:281–282, 1979.
48. McClain, R.F.; Clark, C.R.; El-Khoury, G.Y. C6-7 Dislocation in a neurologically intact neonate: A case report. Spine 14:125–126, 1989.
49. Morgan, T.H.; Wharton, G.W.; Austin, G.N. The results of laminectomy in patients with incomplete spinal cord injury. Paraplegia 9:14, 1971.
50. Mubarak, S.J.; Camp, J.F.; Vueltich, W.; et al. Halo application in the infant. J Pediatr Orthop 9:612–614, 1989.
51. Murphy, M.J.; Ogden, J.A.; Bucholz, R.W. Cervical spine injury in the child. Contemp Orthop 3:615–623, 1981.
52. Norman, M.G.; Wedderburn, L.C. Fetal spinal cord injury with cephalic delivery. Obstet Gynecol 42:355–358, 1973.
53. Odom, J.A.; Brown, C.W.; Messner, D.G. Tubing injuries. J Bone Joint Surg 58-A:733, 1976.
54. Ogden, J. Skeletal Injury in the Child. Philadelphia, Lea & Febiger, 1982.
55. Pang, D.; Pollack, I.F. Spinal cord injury without radiologic abnormality in children: The SCIWORA syndrome. J Trauma 29:654–664, 1989.
56. Pang, D.; Wilberger, J.E., Jr. Spinal cord injury without radiographic abnormality in children. J Neurosurg 57:114–129, 1982.
57. Peck, F.C. A calcified thoracic intervertebral disk with herniation and spinal cord compression in a child. J Neurosurg 14:105–109, 1957.
58. Pennecot, G.F.; Gouraud, D.; Hardy, J.R.; Pouliquen, J.C. Reontgenographical study of the cervical spine in children. J Pediatr Orthop 4:346–352, 1984.
59. Pennecot, G.F.; Leonard, P.; Peyrot Des Gachons, S.; et al. Traumatic ligamentous instability of the cervical spine in children. J Pediatr Orthop 4:339–345, 1984.
60. Phillips, W.A.; Hensinger, R.N. The management of atlanato-axial subluxation in children. J Bone Joint Surg 71-A:664–668, 1989.
61. Pueschel, S.M. Atlantoaxial subluxation in Down syndrome. Lancet 1:980, 1983.
62. Pueschel, S.M.; Scolia, F.H. Atlantoaxial instability in individuals with Down syndrome: Epidemiologic, radiographic, and clinical studies. Pediatrics 4:555–560, 1987.
63. Pueschel, S.M.; Herndon, J.H.; Gelch, M.M.; et al. Symptomatic atlantoaxial subluxation in persons with Down syndrome. J Pediatr Orthop 4:682–688, 1984.
64. Rang, M.C. Children's Fractures, 2nd ed. Philadelphia, J.B. Lippincott, 1983.
65. Ribeiro, R.L.; Qui, C.H.; Schell, M.J. Vertebral compression fracture as a presenting feature of acute lymphocytic leukemia in children. Cancer 61:589–592, 1988.
66. Roaf, R. A study of mechanics of spinal injuries. J Bone Joint Surg 42-B:810–823, 1960.
67. Sherk, H.H.; Schut, L.; Lane, J. Fractures and dislocations of the cervical spine in children. Orthop Clin North Am 7:593–604, 1976.
68. Shulman, S.T.; Madden, J.D.; Esterly, J.R.; Shanklin, D.R. Transection of the spinal cord. A rare obstetrical complication of cephalic delivery. Arch Dis Child 46:291–294, 1971.
69. Sim, F.; Svien, H.; Bickel, W.; Jones, J. Swan neck deformity following extensive cervical laminectomy. J Bone Joint Surg 56-A:564–580, 1974.
70. Special Olympics Bulletin. Participation by Individuals with DS Who Suffer From Atlantoaxial Dislocation. Washington, D.C., Special Olympics, Inc., March 31, 1983.
71. Steel, H.H. Anatomical and mechanical consideration of the atlanto-axial articulation. J Bone Joint Surg 50-A:1481–1482, 1968.
72. Sullivan, C.R.; Bruwer, A.J.; Harris, L.E. Hypermobility of the cervical spine in children; A pitfall in the diagnosis of cervical dislocation. Am J Surg 95:636–640, 1958.
73. Swischuk, L. Anterior displacement of C2 in children. Physiologic or pathologic. Radiology 122:759–763, 1977.
74. Tawbin, A. CNS Damage in the human fetus and newborn infant. Am J Dis Child 119:529, 1970.
75. Taylor, J.A.; Eggli, K.D. Lap belt injuries of the lumbar spine in children: A pitfall in CT diagnosis. AJR 150:1355–1358, 1988.
76. Techakapuch, S. Rupture of the lumbar cartilage plate into the spinal canal in an adolescent. J Bone Joint Surg 63-A:481–482, 1981.
77. Townsend, E.H., Jr.; Rowe, M.L. Mobility of the upper cervical spine in health and disease. Pediatrics 10:567–573, 1952.
78. VanDyke, D.C.; Gahagan, C.A. Down syndrome: Cervical spine abnormalities and problems. Clin Pediatr 27:415–418, 1988.
79. Wagoner, C.; Pendergrass, E.P. The anterior and posterior "notch" shadows seen in lateral roentgenograms of the vertebrae of infants: an anatomic explanation. AJR 42:663–670, 1939.
80. Weiss, M.H.; Kaufman, B. Hangman's fracture in an infant. Am J Dis Child 126:268–269, 1973.
81. Wholey, M.D.; Bruwer, A.J.; Baker, H.L. The lateral roentgenogram of the neck. Radiology 71:350–356, 1958.
82. Wollin, D.G. The os odontoideum. A separate odontoid process. J Bone Joint Surg 45-A:1459–1471, 1963.
83. Yasuoko, F.; Peterson, H.; MacCarty, C. Incidence of spinal column deformity after muliple level laminectomy in children and adults. J Neurosurg 57:441–445, 1982.
84. Yngve, D.A.; Harris, W.P.; Herndon, W.A.; et al. Spinal cord injury without osseous spine fracture. J Pediatr Orthop 8:153–159, 1988.

Marc F. Swiontkowski, M.D.

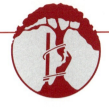

10

Fractures and Dislocations About the Hip and Pelvis

Fractures and dislocations of the pelvis and proximal femur in children are the result of high-energy trauma and therefore are thankfully rare. Because of treatment implications, these injuries are best grouped as pelvic fractures and dislocations (including acetabular fractures), proximal femur fractures, and hip dislocations.

Pelvic Fractures and Dislocations

PATHOLOGY

Relevant Anatomy

Pelvic anatomy in the child differs very little from that in the adult. The pelvis consists of the ilium, ischium, and pubis, together with their apophyseal growth centers, and the sacrum (Fig. 10–1A). The acetabular cartilage complex is a unit, flat and triradiate medially and cup-shaped laterally, that is interposed between the ischium, ilium, and pubis (Fig. 10–1B).[24] These then are the critical differences between child and adult—the epiphyseal growth centers and apophyseal growth regions. This cartilaginous volume as well as the fact that the bones are less brittle[7] provides a greater capacity for energy absorption than that available to adults. When fractures do occur, they can occur within the cartilaginous regions, making diagnosis more difficult. Fractures in these regions can result in growth disturbances from direct trauma or result in misdirected biomechanical forces from bony malunion. Osseous vascular anatomy is also important, as it may be disturbed by direct or indirect trauma.[23, 36, 41] The major area of vulnerability is that of the femoral head.

Incidence

The true incidence of fracture of the pelvis or acetabulum in children is difficult to determine.[9] Watts stated that ten injuries (pelvic fractures) per year could be expected in a large children's hospital, that 97% of these would be of the "stable" type, and, furthermore, that acetabular fractures were "rare."[38] Quinby identified 255 children under the age of 14 years admitted to the pediatric surgery service of the Boston City Hospital for blunt trauma to the trunk over a 4-year period.[25] Of this group, 20 (7.5%) had an identifiable pelvic fracture. There were 6 girls and 14 boys, with an age range of 2.5 to 13 years and a mean age of 8 years. Of 1438 musculoskeletal injuries treated at the State of Washington's Level I trauma center in 1 year, five (0.5%) were pelvic or acetabular fractures in children under the age of 18 years. Associated head injuries with neurologic sequelae are more common in children than in adults.[27] In a recent study, 2.4% of 2248 children admitted to a regional trauma center were identified as having a fracture of the pelvic ring.[2]

Mechanism of Injury

Pelvic and acetabular fractures in children are always the result of high-energy trauma for reasons outlined above. In Quinby's 20 cases, 19 patients were injured by impact with an automobile, truck,

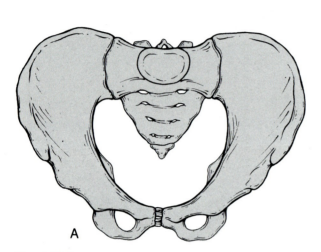
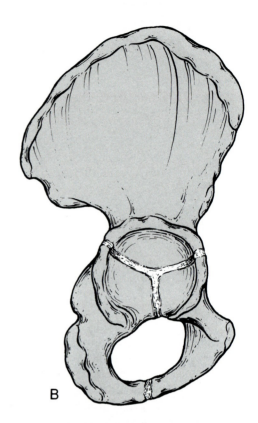

Figure 10–1

Pediatric pelvic osseous anatomy. *A,* The inlet orientation illustrates the two innominate bones, the sacrum, and the pubic symphis. *B,* The lateral orientation reveals the triradiate cartilage as the confluence of the iliac, ischial, and pubic apophyses.

or train; one fell from a roof.[25] Of trauma produced by collisions with motor vehicles, in 8 of the 19 cases it was suspected that the vehicle ran over or crushed the child. In an 8-year review of children under the age of 16 years treated at the University of Manitoba, 84 cases of pelvic fracture were identified. Of these, 58% were due to car versus pedestrian; 17% of patients were passengers in motor vehicle accidents; 7% of injuries were due to impacts or falls from bicycles, and 8% were due to crush injuries.[26] High-energy impact with rigid structures produces these injuries. Rarely, these injuries occur in newborns and toddlers.[17, 40]

Consequences of Injury

Because of the significant energy involved in producing fractures of the pelvis, the major consequences are due to associated visceral injuries. Nineteen percent of patients in Reed's large series had associated visceral injuries,[26] most commonly involving the viscera within or just superior to the pelvic brim. Seven of the total of ten associated visceral injuries involved the lower urinary tract, and seven involved intraabdominal structures. There were three each of significant intrathoracic, intracranial, and soft tissue injuries, again pointing to the velocity involved with this blunt trauma. Of Quinby's 20 patients, 9 required laparotomy for visceral injury and another 5 had severe hemorrhage with visceral injury requiring laparotomy in addition to a significant vascular injury.[25] Three of this latter group eventually died. The major consequences of a pelvic fracture, then, are hemorrhage, shock, and death; bladder/urethral injury (particularly in males); neurologic injury (in particular, injury to the lumbosacral plexus with sacroiliac disruptions or sacral fractures); and infection following open fractures that involve the perineum, rectum, or vagina.[27] The severity of the pelvic fracture is correlated with the risk of visceral injury. In the recent Children's National Medical Center series, 80% of children with "multiple pelvic fractures" had concomitant abdominal or genitourinary injury compared with 33% of children with fractures of the "ilium or pelvic rim" and 6% of children with isolated pubic fractures.[2] In adults, the mortality from major pelvic fractures has been recorded to be in the range of 5 to 20%. In children, the rate has been reported to be 1.4 to 9.0%.[4, 27] Published mortality rates for a severely traumatized group of adult patients with open pelvic fractures are in the range of 8 to 50%; death results from hemorrhage acutely and pulmonary failure and sepsis on a delayed basis. The incidence of lower urinary tract and neurologic injury in combined large series is in the range of 12 to 15% in adults. Owing to small numbers, comparable data do not exist in literature for children.

Systemic consequences aside, there remain serious sequelae from the pelvic fracture itself. When the triradiate cartilage is involved, growth arrest can result in the "mini," shallow acetabulum described by Rodrigues (Fig. 10-2).[28] Six of 15 cases reported by McDonald[21] had injury to the triradiate acetabular cartilage; fortunately, of the four patients followed long term, none developed the deformity described by Rodrigues[28] that results in femoral head subluxation. Acetabular fracture can also result in lateral subluxation of the hip, heterotopic ossification, and ankylosis.[11, 12] Other reported consequences of extra-acetabular pelvic fracture include delayed union, sacroiliac fusion with pelvic distortion, leg length discrepancy, and pelvic obliquity.

Commonly Associated Injuries

As noted earlier, the injuries commonly associated with pelvic fractures are both visceral and skeletal. The visceral injuries directly related to the pelvic injury are bladder and urethral injuries, traction injury to the lumbosacral plexus, and injury to the major and minor arterial and venous systems with resultant hemorrhage. Those associated with high-energy blunt trauma are to the pulmonary, cardiac, gastrointestinal, and central nervous systems (see Chapter 4). The most commonly associated fractures are those of the femur, skull, ribs, tibia and fibula, clavicle, facial bones, and humerus, in that order.[26] The identification of a pelvic injury in the primary phase of the resuscitation and injury survey should

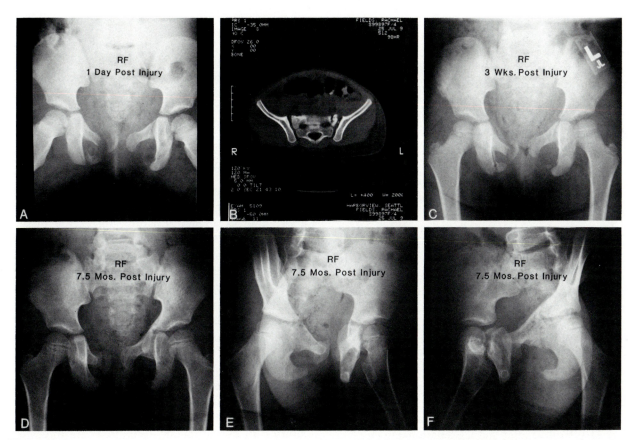

Figure 10-2

A 4-year-old girl was the unrestrained passenger in a motor vehicle accident. *A*, Postinjury pelvic x-ray reveals bilateral rami fractures. *B*, The CT scan confirms this to be a lateral compression injury with a left-sided sacral injury. *C*, At 2 weeks there is evidence of healing of all rami fractures. *D–F*, At 7.5 months, however, there is evidence of triradiate cartilage arrest on the left side on the AP, iliac, and obturator oblique x-rays.

alert the physician to the possibility of these associated injuries.

Classification

Because of the severe nature of the associated injury, Quinby suggested dividing pelvic fractures into those that do not require laparotomy, those that do, and those associated with severe vascular injury.[25] While this system reflects an increasing severity of injury, complication, and mortality rate, it does not help the physician. Many classification systems exist for adult pelvic fractures. The one developed by Trunkey and co-workers has been applied to a series of 84 pediatric pelvic fractures.[37] This system divides pelvic fractures into stable and unstable categories. The stable injuries include pubic fractures, "isolated" fractures, and avulsion fractures. The unstable injuries include pubic diastasis, acetabular fractures, and diametric fractures (fractures on the sides of the pelvic ring). Watts felt that pediatric pelvic fractures are better classified according to the severity of skeletal injury as follows:[38] (1) avulsions, e.g., epiphysiolyses (secondary to violent muscular activity); (2) fracture of the pelvic ring (secondary to crushing injury), stable and unstable; and (3) fractures of the acetabulum (associated with hip dislocation.

In their 1985 report on a series of 141 pelvic fractures, Torode and Zieg improved upon the Watts classification and expanded it as follows:[35]

Type I—Avulsion fractures.

Type II—Iliac wing fractures.

Type III—Simple ring fractures. Includes pubic symphysis diastasis without disruption of the posterior sacroiliac (SI) joint.

Type IV—Any fracture pattern that creates a free bony fragment. Includes bilateral pubic rami fractures, fractures of the anterior pelvic ring with an acetabular fracture, pubic rami fractures or a pubic symphysis disruption with a fracture through the posterior bony elements or disruption of the SI joint.

In a useful addition to the literature, these authors also proposed a classification of complication based on increasing severity: type I, none; type II, occasional altered growth with subsequent remodeling; type III, occasional delayed union; and type IV, nonunion, malunion, triradiate cartilage injury, closure of sacroiliac joint and leg length inequality.

Tile modified Pennal's original classification of pelvic fracture in adults.[34] This system, based on mechanism of injury, has the most widespread application. The types are anteroposterior (AP) compression, lateral compression, and vertical shear. This system has recently been placed into the A, B, C code system of increasing severity used by the AO/ASIF (Fig. 10–3 and Table 10–1).[34]

Because of anticipated future use in the literature, both the Torode-Zieg and the Pennal-Tile systems will be referred to here.[34, 35]

For acetabular fracture, the classification of Letournel and Judet is summarized in Figure 10–4.

DIAGNOSIS

History

Because of their skeletal flexibility,[7] pelvic and acetabular fractures in the pediatric age group occur secondary to "children" being struck by automobiles or as a result of their being unrestrained passengers. The history of high-energy trauma will direct the Emergency Medical Service team to an appropriate response in the field and transfer of the patient to a regional trauma hospital. If shock is a part of the initial presentation, transportation is frequently by air ambulance. The same history of violent injury will dictate a full-scale primary and secondary survey, institution of large-bore venous access, and other measures as outlined in Chapter 4. Minor apophyseal avulsion injuries, usually occurring in those 12 to 15 years of age, are generally due to athletic injury.[29]

Physical Examination

The evaluation procedure for a trauma patient is outlined in Chapter 4; the following comments are directed toward those patients with a potential for a pelvic or acetabular fracture. Inspection of the body surface is the initial step, observing anteriorly and coordinating a "logrolling" of the patient so that the spinal examination can be conducted at the same time. Contusions, abrasions, and areas of degloving where the subcutaneous fat has been sheared off the fascia (the Morel-Lavale lesion) should be identified and recorded. Patients with acetabular fractures frequently have large peritrochanteric ecchymoses, reflecting the orientation of the force that produced the fracture. Lacerations, especially anteriorly, are not uncommon in pediatric patients and are frequently associated with vascular injury.[25] In the perineum, lacerations are often the result of open fractures, with ischial fragments producing the wound.[27] Vaginal lacerations are not unusual,[13] and a digital pelvic examination should be done in all female patients with a displaced

Figure 10–3

The Pennal-Tile classification of pelvic fractures as applied to children. Type A-1: An avulsion fracture of the anteroinferior iliac spine (the straight head of the rectus femoris muscle). Type A-2: A minimally displaced fracture of the ischium and pubis without posterior ring injury. Type B-1: An anteroposterior force has produced an open-book injury with more than 3 cm of symphyseal disruption. By definition, the anterior portion of the sacroiliac joints has been disrupted. Type B-2: A lateral compression mechanism has produced an ipsilateral anterior sacral alar crush and displaced ischial and pubic rami fractures. Type B-3: The same force vector (laterally applied oriented toward the midline in the coronal plane) has produced contralateral disruption of the sacroiliac joint (with a minor ipsilateral anterior sacral impaction) and displaced pubic and ischial rami fractures. C, A Pennal-Tile IIIC$_1$ injury: total disruption of the sacroiliac joint with posterior vertical and rotational displacement of the hemipelvis associated with symphyseal disruption.

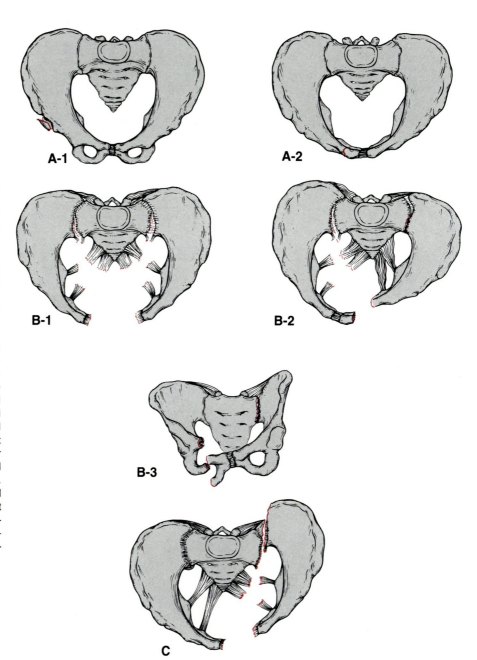

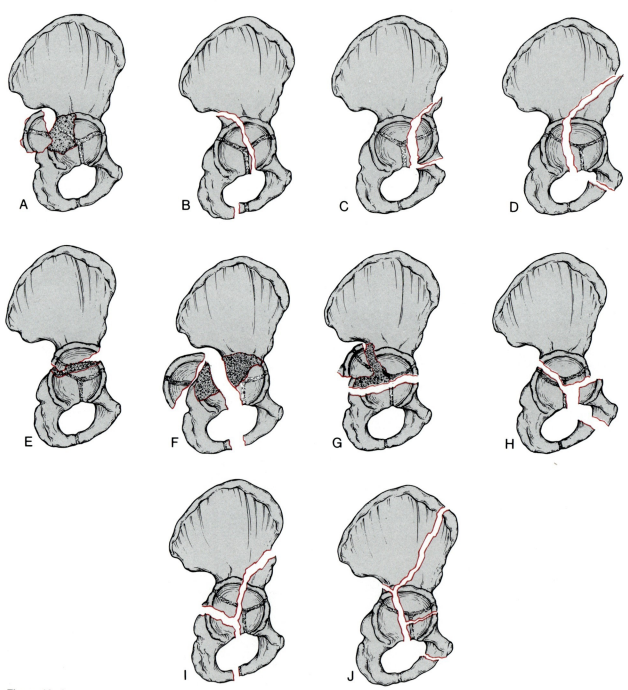

Figure 10–4

The acetabular fracture classification of Letournel. *A,* The posterior wall fracture; this fracture is often associated with impaction of the intact side of the fracture margin. *B,* The posterior column fracture. *C,* The anterior wall fracture; an atypically large fragment size is shown. *D,* The anterior column fracture; the most posterior location of the fracture line through the acetabulum is shown. *E,* The transverse fracture pattern; this location is the transtectal. The fracture may cross the acetabula either higher (juxtatectal) or lower (infratectal). *F,* Associated posterior column and posterior wall fractures. *G,* Associated transverse and posterior wall fractures. *H,* The T-shaped fracture. *I,* Associated anterior column and posterior hemitransverse fractures. *J,* The both-column fracture; note that no segment of acetabulum remains attached to the intact ilium.

Table 10-1 Tile Classification of Pelvic Disruption	
Type	Characteristics
A	Stable
	A1—Fractures of the pelvis not involving the ring
	A2—Stable, minimally displaced fractures of the ring
B	Rotationally unstable, vertically stable
	B1—Open-book
	B2—Lateral compression, ipsilateral
	B3—Lateral compression, contralateral (bucket-handle)
C	Rotationally and vertically unstable
	C1—Unilateral
	C2—Bilateral
	C3—Associated with an acetabular fracture

anterior ring fracture; preferably this should be done with the patient under sedation or with use of an anesthetic in prepubescent children.[22] Similarly, a digital rectal examination should be done to check for gross blood, indicative of a rectal perforation or sphincter injury.

With inspection completed, pelvic stability should be evaluated, preferably while the patient is still on the backboard. Anteroposterior stability is evaluated by the clinician's placing the palms of the hands on the anterior iliac crests and applying posterior-directed pressure (Fig. 10–5A). Placing the palms on the lateral aspect of the anterior crests and applying pressure directed toward the midline, the examiner checks for rotational instability, such as that created by an open-book fracture (Fig. 10–5B). Pain on anteroposterior or medially directed pressure in the conscious patient should be carefully noted. Palpation along the posterior iliac spine, SI joint, and sacrum should be performed, looking for pain consistent with posterior pelvic ring injury. A final check on vertical/rotational instability can be made by assessing the relative height of the antero-superior iliac spines and the relative leg lengths.

With the inspection and palpation phases completed, a thorough evaluation of the arterial circulation should be made. The femoral, popliteal, dorsalis pedis, and posterior tibial pulses should be palpated; if these are nonpalpable, an ultrasound Doppler examination should be done to check for biphasic pulsatile flow. Limb temperature should be assessed by palpation. Finally, in the alert and cooperative patient, a gross motor examination of all major muscle groups in the lower extremity should be completed bilaterally, in addition to a sensory examination to light touch and pinprick. The latter should include the perirectal area because of the frequent involvement of the sacral plexus with sacral fractures. Rectal tone should already

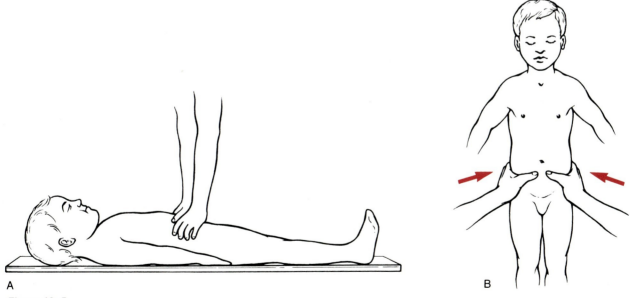

Figure 10–5

The clinical examination of pelvic stability. A, Examining for anteroposterior instability by applying force on the anterior iliac crests directed posteriorly. The examination is most effective when done early with the patient in the emergency department still on the backboard used for transport. B, Examining for external rotation instability (such as that which occurs in the open-book fracture, B_1 type) by applying force on the external aspect of the pelvis and directing it toward the midline.

have been assessed with the digital rectal examination.

Radiographic Evaluation

An important part of the initial evaluation of a multiply injured child is the AP radiograph of the pelvis. Gonadal shielding should not be used, as it may obscure the anterior pelvic ring.[38] Two additional views are indicated if a fracture of the anteroposterior pelvic ring is identified on the initial radiograph. These are the 30 to 45 degree (aimed distally) "inlet" view or "down shot," which demonstrates posterior pelvic ring injury more clearly, and the 40 to 45 degree (aimed toward the head of the patient) "tangential" or "brim shot" or "up view," which delineates the anterior pelvic ring (Fig. 10–6 A and C).[32] Both are helpful for delineating internal or external rotation of one of the hemipelves relative to the other. These three-plane radiographs can help determine the mechanism of injury and the form of treatment in the majority of fractures.[42] Sacral fractures and SI joint injuries are frequently missed with standard x-ray technique. If suspicion is high, based on clinical examination, hemorrhage, shock, or examination of the inlet/tangential view, a computed tomography (CT) scan of the pelvis is indicated. CT is helpful in diagnosing pelvic hematoma, an important factor in the initial management of the patient. Cut intervals of 2.5 to 3.0 mm are generally sufficient to delineate the skeletal injury. Images are obtained from L5 to the lower pelvic region in the axial plane, utilizing contiguous sections with soft tissue and bone window technique.[14]

Because of the complex anatomy of the innominate bone, fractures of the acetabulum require a different approach for radiographic evaluation. The 45 degree oblique views described by Judet are

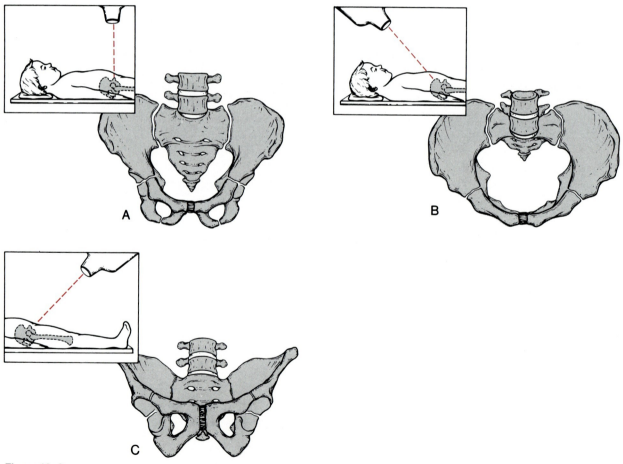

Figure 10–6

The three radiographic views for pelvic fracture assessment. *A,* Standard anteroposterior pelvis view. *B,* The 40 degree distally oriented inlet view; this demonstrates posterior ring pathology optimally. *C,* The 40 degree cephalically oriented tangential view; this demonstrates anterior ring pathology optimally.

indicated when the scout AP pelvis film demonstrates involvement of the acetabulum (Fig. 10–7). The iliac oblique view shows the posterior column in profile as well as the iliac ring. The obturator oblique view places the anterior column in profile and shows the obturator foramen clearly. The two views combined with the AP pelvis view allow the physician to classify the fracture according to the scheme of Letournel (see Figs. 10–4 and 10–7). CT is an important adjunct to the conventional radiographic views described above but is not a substitute. It is especially helpful for detecting intraarticular loose fragments, which occur commonly when there has been an associated hip dislocation.[1] CT also helps define acetabular margin (posterior wall) fragments and occult posterior pelvic ring fractures. Finally, with unduly displaced associated acetabular fracture patterns, three-dimensional reconstructions of the CT data may prove useful. Fractures with less than 2.0 mm of displacement may not be demonstrated with sufficient resolution on three-dimensional CT.[14]

In the case of young children (under 8 years) in whom fracture or dislocation of the proximal femur is suspected, hip arthrography is useful.[27] Ultrasound is being promoted for evaluating treatment for congenital hip dislocation and may prove useful in the case of hip trauma in very young children.

Special Studies

When injury to the lower urinary tract is suspected, either by blood at the penile meatus or by widely displaced anterior ring fractures, a retrograde urethrogram should be performed. By continuing the examination with larger contrast volumes once a Foley catheter has been definitely placed with appropriate urologic consultation, a cystogram can be obtained in order to rule out bladder rupture. If renal or urethral injury is suspected based on physical examination or other diagnostic tests (if shown on abdominal CT scan), an intravenous pyelogram (IVP) may be indicated to define renal and urethral anatomy and determine function.[27]

In the case of posterior pelvic ring injury in which sacral fracture or SI joint disruption has produced a sacral plexus injury, an electromyogram at 3 weeks post injury will help define the extent and depth of damage to neurologic function. Patients who present in shock, especially those with unimpressive pelvic fractures, may benefit from diagnostic angiography and therapeutic embolization with Gelfoam, blood clot, or coils.[27] This study may not be of use when open wounds are associated with major proximal femoral arterial or venous injury if immediate exploration and repair is indicated.[25]

MANAGEMENT

Evolution of Treatment

In the literature, treatment of pediatric pelvic fractures has been nearly universally conservative.[4, 27] Stable avulsion injuries of the anterior iliac spines, ischial hamstring origin, or iliac crests remain best treated by conservative means. "Open-book" AP compression injuries have been generally treated by pelvic slings or spica casts. When these injuries are widely displaced or associated with severe hemorrhage or intraabdominal injury, treatment is evolving toward external fixation or open reduction and internal fixation with small plates.[13, 38] Stable injury to the anterior ring (isolated fractures of the pubis or ischial rami) and more severe four-rami or straddle fractures have been and continue to be best treated by bedrest or spica casts (Fig. 10–8). It is in the area of the most severe unstable pelvic fractures that the most recent developments in treatment recommendations have occurred. The standard treatment regimen for the vertical shear pelvic fracture (ipsilateral or contralateral fracture of both pubic and ischial rami or symphysis disruption anteriorly associated with a displaced fracture of the posterior iliac crest, sacrum, or SI joint) recommended in the literature has been skeletal traction with a traction pin through the distal femur.[38] With more widespread use of external fixation, pediatric pelvic fractures of this nature have also been treated in this fashion (see Fig. 10–10). Both treatments frequently result in SI joint fusion or malunion and leg length inequality. The optimal treatment for displaced fractures of the SI joint, posterior iliac ring, and sacrum is now thought to be open reduction and internal fixation (Fig. 10–9).

Acetabular fractures in children historically have also been treated conservatively. Specifically, this consists of bedrest or non–weight bearing treatment for minimally displaced fractures and 4 to 6 weeks of skeletal traction for displaced fractures. Poor results have been reported, particularly for comminuted fractures and those for which traction did not improve the position of the fragments.[11, 38] When poor radiographic results have not been associated with poor clinical results, inadequate length of follow-up is generally involved.[4] Children with these injuries need to be followed to midadulthood before one can be assured of the functional results.[11] The excellent results published for adults with displaced

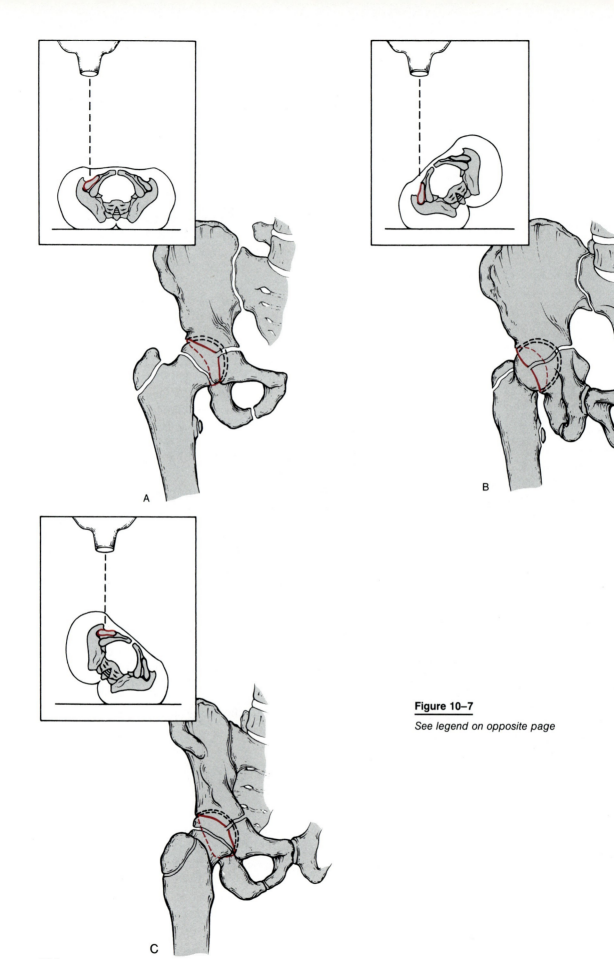

Figure 10–7

See legend on opposite page

316

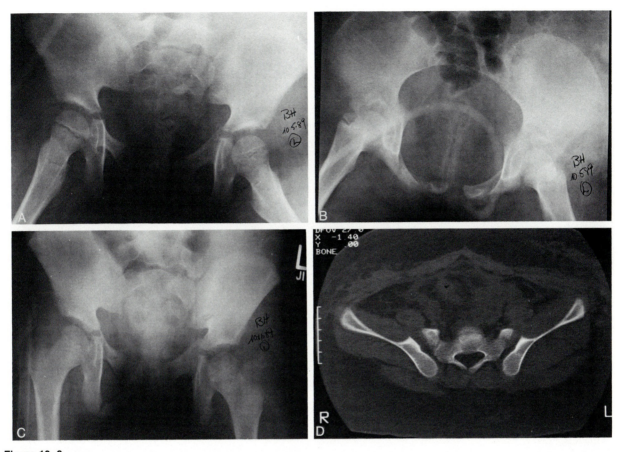

Figure 10–8

A type B_2 injury in an 8-year-old boy struck by a car. A, Admitting AP pelvis radiograph showing ipsilateral ischial and pubic rami fractures moderately displaced. B, The inlet view suggests mild widening of the sacroiliac joint on that side. C, The tangential view confirms the anterior ring displacements. D, The CT scan confirms the mild widening of the right sacroiliac joint. The patient was treated with bedrest. The fractures have healed, and there is no residual pain or dysfunction at 1 year post injury.

acetabular fractures have influenced the treatment of pediatric fractures; the current recommendation for fractures involving the major weight-bearing surface with greater than 2.0 mm displacement and for unstable posterior wall fracture-dislocations is open reduction and internal fixation (Table 10–2).[16, 19]

Special Considerations for Polytrauma Patients

Pelvic fractures associated with significant hemorrhage or concomitant intraabdominal injury requiring laparotomy may benefit from more aggressive treatment. Pelvic hemorrhage will frequently re-

Figure 10–7

The three radiographic views necessary for assessment of acetabular fractures. A, The AP pelvis (or hip) view; this allows assessment of the iliopectineal line, the ilium, the anterior and posterior walls, and the pubis. B, The iliac oblique view of Judet; this allows optimal assessment of the ischial spine and the posterior column and wall as well as the iliac fossae. C, The obturator oblique view of Judet; this view allows optimal assessment of the iliac wing, anterior column, and anterior wall.

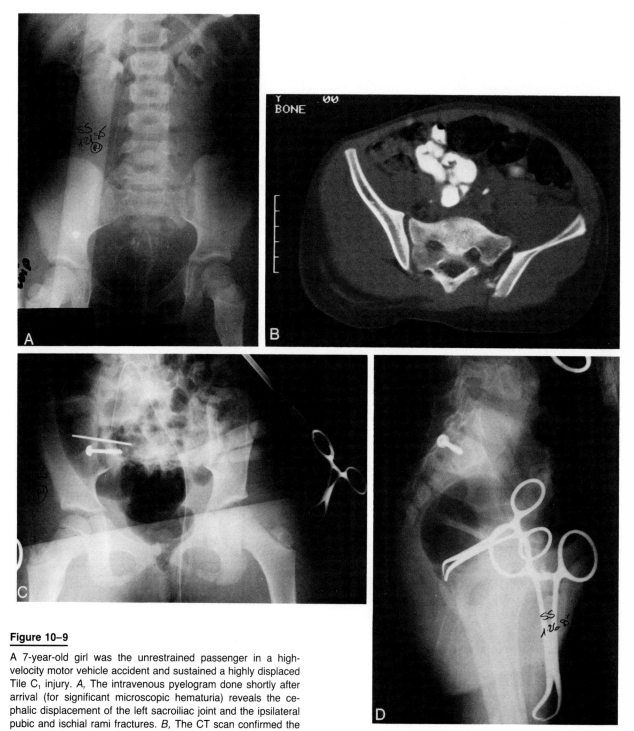

Figure 10-9

A 7-year-old girl was the unrestrained passenger in a high-velocity motor vehicle accident and sustained a highly displaced Tile C_1 injury. A, The intravenous pyelogram done shortly after arrival (for significant microscopic hematuria) reveals the cephalic displacement of the left sacroiliac joint and the ipsilateral pubic and ischial rami fractures. B, The CT scan confirmed the posterior and cephalic displacement of greater than 1 cm. C–D, Intraoperative AP pelvis and lateral sacral x-rays confirming the position of the implants. Open reduction using a posterior approach was done on the fourth day post surgery.

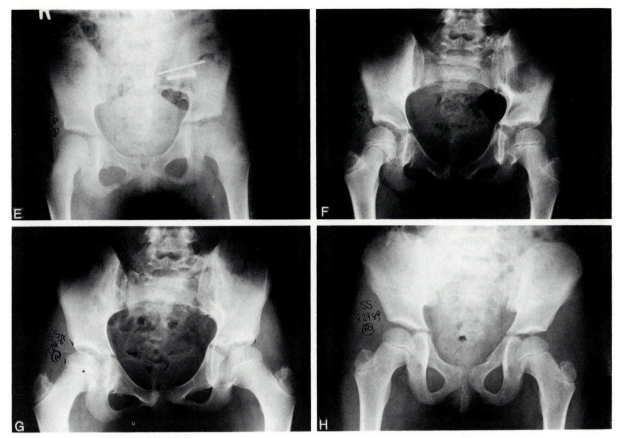

Figure 10–9 Continued

E, At 6 months post injury the reduction was maintained and fracture healing was apparent; the implants were removed 1 month later. *F,* At 1 year the patient was asymptomatic; the radiograph was done in order to evaluate the possiblity of sacroiliac joint fusion. *G,* At 2 years there was concern that premature acetabular triradiate cartilage closure had occurred; watchful waiting was elected. *H,* At 4 years the patient remains asymptomatic; the sacroiliac joint and acetabular apophyses remain open.

Table 10–2
Management of Pelvic and Acetabular Fractures

Fracture Type	Description	Treatment
Pelvic Fractures		
A_1, A_2	Fractures not involving the pelvic ring Isolated avulsions (ASIS, AIIS, ischium, ilium) Isolated pubic rami fractures	Conservative management
B_1	Open-book, isolated	Conservative management *Exception:* When associated with major hemorrhage or laparotomy or with displacement of more than 3.0 mm External fixation versus open reduction and internal fixation
B_2, B_3	Lateral compression Isolated Displaced less than 5.0 mm	Conservative care *Exception:* When associated with laparotomy: Open reduction and internal fixation (if anterior ring is amenable) *Exception:* When widely ($>$ 1 cm) displaced: Attempted closed reduction. Open reduction and internal fixation if not reducible
C_1	Vertical shear, displaced	Open reduction and internal fixation of posterior complex $+/-$ internal or external fixation anteriorly (see Fig. 10–9)
Acetabular Fractures	Displaced $<$ 2.0 mm	Conservative management
	Displaced $\geq$ 2.0 mm	Open reduction and internal fixation

spond to closing down the pelvic volume. This is done easily with simple external fixation frames with one or two pins in each iliac wing and a connecting bar (Fig. 10–10). In cases of an open-book pelvic fracture with diastasis of 3.0 cm or more, in which a laparotomy is being done, a simple open reduction and internal fixation can be performed with a two-hole 3.5 mm dynamic compression (DC) plate and a cortical screw in each pubis. In situations in which the patient is hemodynamically very unstable and no laparotomy has been performed, a pelvic fracture of any pattern can be stabilized by a bilateral long leg spica cast with distal femoral pins incorporated.[6] In all other settings of multiple injury (not involving associated blood loss from the pelvic fracture), pelvic fracture management is best delayed 3 to 5 days and initiated after the full diagnostic evaluation is complete. Acetabular fractures should be managed similarly with a short delay (1 or 2 days) to optimize preoperative planning.

Treatment Options

For pelvic fractures, treatment options are as follows: (1) bedrest/non–weight bearing, (2) skeletal traction, (3) pelvic sling, (4) spica cast, (5) external fixation, (6) closed reduction, and (7) open reduction and internal fixation. Acetabular fractures are amenable to (1) bedrest/non–weight bearing, (2) skeletal traction, and (3) open reduction and internal fixation.

Pelvic Fractures

Bedrest/Non–Weight Bearing

Indications/Contraindications. Bedrest treatment is indicated for all avulsion fractures of the pelvic ring and for stable pelvic fractures. These include avulsion fractures of the anterosuperior (sartorius origin) and anteroinferior (rectus femoris) iliac spines, the iliac apophysis (external oblique origin) and the ischial rami (hamstring origin), and isolated or bilateral pubic rami fractures. Probably the most severe injury that can be treated in this fashion is the straddle fracture (four rami). Other AP compression variants, including the minimally displaced open-book injury (less than 3.0 cm) can be treated in this manner. Unstable pelvic injuries of the B_1, B_2, or C_1, C_2 types should not be treated in this fashion.

Timing. Treatment should begin as soon as all other injuries have been diagnosed and stabilized.

Technique. The muscle associated with the avulsion injury should be relaxed. Therefore, patients with ASIS and AIIS avulsions or iliac apophysis avulsions and those in whom the rectus abdominis muscles are attached to pubic segments adjacent to fractures should be placed in the semi-Fowler position with the hips flexed 30 to 45 degrees. Lower extremity exercises (ankle and foot) should be encouraged. Those with hamstring avulsion injuries should be treated with bedrest with the hip extended and the knee flexed as much as possible. If the patient cannot be positioned in this way and made comfortable, a spica cast should be considered. The child should be treated in this position for 3 to 4 weeks and then advanced to crutch ambulation.

Skeletal Traction

Indications/Contraindications. The remaining indication for distal femoral pin traction is a vertical shear injury through the iliac wing, SI joint, or sacrum that is shown to be *reduced* in traction. This generally will be in children younger than 8 to 10 years. The contraindications for this treatment are lateral compression injuries, open-book A_2 injuries, and stable avulsion type fractures. Additionally, fractures that do *not* reduce in traction should not be maintained with this form of treatment, as leg length inequality will result.

Timing. After complete diagnosis of all injuries and institution of appropriate management, the child should be sedated or given an anesthetic, have the skeletal traction pin inserted proximal to the

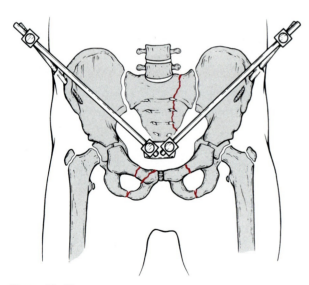

Figure 10–10

A simple two-pin external fixator for resuscitation of a child with hemodynamic instability from pelvic hemorrhage. The 4.0 mm or 5.0 mm Schanz pins are inserted through small stab wounds. Two single adjustable clamps and a tube-to-tube clamp connect two 250 mm carbon fiber rods. With the assistant compressing the pelvis externally to close down the volume, the surgeon tightens the clamps.

distal femoral physis, and placed in skeletal traction. The best chance for reduction is when the traction treatment is instituted as soon as possible after injury, preferably within 24 hours.

Technique. A distal femoral Steinmann pin is inserted proximal to the physis by 2.0 to 3.0 cm, using fluoroscopic control. A Böhler traction bow should be used to help prevent pin loosening with the child's increasing motion in bed. The opposite leg is held in skin traction to prevent significant abduction; this is more often necessary in younger children (under age 8 years). Balanced skeletal traction with a Thomas splint and Pearson attachment is helpful for toileting in older children. Inasmuch as 10 to 20 lb may be necessary to reduce the fracture, depending on the child's age, it is helpful to elevate the foot of the bed on blocks.[38] If a reduction that is within 2.0 mm is not obtained within 5 days, despite increasing weight, traction should be discontinued and consideration given to open reduction. The older the child, the more frequently this will be the case. Traction should continue for 4 weeks in children under age 10 years and continue for 6 weeks in those aged 10 to 14 years. Consideration should be given to open treatment for displaced vertical shear fractures in adolescents 15 years and older. The progression is from traction for 4 to 6 weeks to several days of bedrest out of traction and, following radiographic confirmation of continued reduction, initiation of partial weight bearing with crutches.

Pelvic Sling

Indications. This relatively dated form of treatment is appropriate only for B_1 type open-book closed pelvic injuries that are not associated with shock or hemodynamic instability. Symphyseal displacements of greater than 3.0 cm should be reduced, and a pelvic sling accomplishes a reduction in most instances. Injuries with anterior displacements of this degree will have, by definition, an anterior sacroiliac disruption on one or both sides and warrant reduction.[32] This form of treatment is contraindicated for B_2 and C injuries, as compression directed toward the midline will not accomplish reduction.

Timing. This treatment should be instituted as soon as all other injuries have been diagnosed and stabilized. Early reduction is most likely to succeed, as there is less resistance to bringing the hemipelvis together in the midline before the pelvic hematoma begins to organize.

Technique. A canvas sling 6 in to 9 in in width is placed underneath the supine patient. The ends are connected to traction rope and laterally directed pulleys with sufficient weight to suspend the patient's pelvis, generally 5 to 10 inches for most children. Greater compressive forces can be obtained by crossing the traction ropes over the patient's midline. Reduction should be confirmed by a radiograph obtained within 24 hours of initiating treatment. If the symphyseal gap is not closed down to within 1.0 cm or less, another form of treatment should be considered.

Spica Cast

Indications. The use of a spica cast is indicated in patients who are hemodynamically unstable, so much so that internal or external fixation is not possible. Patients with severely displaced pelvic fractures with posterior ring involvement will benefit from immobilization of the lower limbs in a double long leg spica cast.[6] For definitive management of pelvic injuries, the spica cast is helpful in minimally displaced pelvic fractures or avulsion injuries to allow the patient to be treated at home. Other than in the case of an B_1 open-book pelvic disruption, in which the spica cast should be applied in the lateral position to allow reduction by gravity, these casts do not reduce displaced pelvic fractures. If the displacement is not acceptable, another form of treatment should be selected.

Timing. Spica casts can be applied at any point during the treatment of pelvic fractures to allow mobilization of the patient. The cast should be applied emergently in the case of hemodynamic instability. If the purpose is to reduce and hold an open-book type of injury, the cast should be applied in the lateral position as soon as the patient's general status permits.

Technique. For general treatment purposes, the cast is applied in the supine position—on a spica board for children 10 years and under and on a fracture table equipped for casting for older children. For applying the cast in the lateral position, a fracture table or spica box with a peroneal post that can be removed is most useful. In this instance, the reduction should be confirmed with the patient in the lateral position before the cast is completed. If reduction is not confirmed and the residual symphyseal gap is greater than 1.0 cm, another form of treatment should be considered. These casts should be left in position for a total of 6 to 8 weeks if the cast is applied after initial bedrest or traction treatment.

External Fixation

Indications. The indications for this form of treatment are nearly identical to those for a spica cast. External fixation is also a useful management technique for open pelvic fractures. Patients who are hemodynamically unstable will benefit from closing down the intrapelvic volume (see under Pelvic Sling Technique). External fixation provides definitive treatment only for A_2 type open-book injuries. This method of treatment cannot hold reductions of displaced posterior ring injuries.[13]

Timing. Placement of the frame in circumstances of hemodynamic instability or associated open wounds must be done emergently. If the external fixator is chosen as definitive treatment for an open-book injury, the earlier it is applied, the easier it will be to achieve reduction—for reasons of moving the hemipelvis medially before the intrapelvic hematoma begins to organize.

Preoperative Planning. Depending on the size of the patient, the surgeon must check to be sure of the availability of an external fixation system with pins that are appropriate for the width of the iliac crest and with connecting bars small enough for the intrailiac dimensions. The pin sizes most commonly used are 4.0 mm and 5.0 mm Schanz pins, but 2.5 mm pins are available for infants and toddlers. Connecting rods of 4.0 mm and 10.0 mm are available; the larger size is generally used.

Anesthesia/Positioning. General anesthesia is the technique of choice for either resuscitative application or definitive reduction. The patient is positioned supine for the application of the frame.

Technique. In general, a modular system with a minimum number of components is prepared (see Fig. 10–10). Open wounds must be irrigated and debrided (left open) prior to placement of the frame.[20, 30] Schanz pins or pins specific for the external system of the appropriate diameter are selected. For children older than 6 to 8 years, standard 4.0 to 5.0 mm pins are not too large. In younger children, pins of 2.5 mm diameter are more suitable. If the clamps are flexible enough to close down to this size, threaded Steinmann pins can be used. One or two pins in each ilium are introduced through 1.0 cm stab wounds (see Fig. 10–10). The pins should be introduced through a predrilled hole of slightly smaller diameter. The hole should just penetrate the superior iliac ring cortex, and the pin should be placed by a hand chuck to minimize the chances of perforation. Smooth Kirschner wires (K-wires) can be placed on the inner and outer cortices of the iliac ring as directional guides. The bar or bars can be loosely applied, and then the assistant pushes the two sets of pins to the midline while the surgeon tightens the clamps. Reduction should be confirmed by radiograph. Adequate room should be allowed between the bars and the abdomen to allow the patient to sit up and to permit repeated abdominal examinations.

Closed Reduction

Indications. The two primary indications for attempting closed reduction by manipulation are a lateral compression injury with a locked symphysis and the "tilt" fracture described by Kellam and Tile.[33] In the former, the goal is to unlock the displaced symphysis from posterior to the intact side. In the latter, the goal is to get the displaced free floating pubic segment away from the vaginal wall in the female patient. Because of the lack of stability post reduction of a vertical shear or AP compression injury, closed reduction in this setting is not indicated.

Timing. In order to optimize the chances of a complete reduction, manipulation should be performed as soon as possible after injury.

Anesthesia. For both fracture patterns, a general anesthesia is preferable, with the patient in the supine position.

Technique. For the lateral compression injury, the displaced iliac ring should be grasped on its inner aspect and lateral traction applied while pushing away the intact ring. If the patient's body habitus does not allow a firm grasp in the iliac ring, two Schanz screws of appropriate size (2.5, 4.0, or 5.0 mm) can be inserted to use as manipulation handles. These are removed after the reduction maneuver. The reduction after manipulation of this injury will nearly always be stable. The patient should be kept at bedrest for 3 to 4 weeks and then mobilized with touch-down weight bearing on the injured side.

For the tilt fracture, in female patients a bimanual pelvic examination is performed. If the bony fragment is palpable along the vaginal wall, a reduction is indicated. Using the intravaginal digit, the pubic segment is lifted anterior and superior. The external hand grasps the pubis in an attempt to pull the segment anteriorly. If the reduction is obtained, it should be radiographically confirmed and the stability tested by putting lateral compression on the pelvis. If the segment is not stable, consideration should be given to placing a Steinmann pin across the medialmost fracture line through a small incision to hold the reduction. This pin is removed as soon as callus is evident on follow-up radiographs.

Open Reduction

Indications. The indications for open reduction and internal fixation of pelvic fractures are as follows: an open fracture with massive displacement of the fragments, and widely displaced fractures of the A_2, B_1, B_2, C_1, and C_2 types. Failed closed reduction is a relative indication, as no other means of reduction will be successful if the fracture is more than 5 days old.

Timing. Open reduction of displaced pelvic fractures is optimally done at 48 to 72 hours post injury. Active hemorrhage will have ceased by then, and preoperative studies, such as CT scans, can be obtained and carefully reviewed. Delaying operative reduction further increases the difficulty of obtaining anatomic reduction.

Preoperative Planning. The surgical approach is selected based on the location of the posterior ring injury. The plain radiographs and CT scans are studied to determine optimal positioning of implants. In patients under the age of 10 years, frequently the 3.5 mm cortical screw is the optimal implant. These must be available (special order) in lengths up to 120 cm for pediatric application. An experienced pelvic fracture surgeon should be consulted.

Anesthesia/Positioning. A general anesthetic is appropriate for all pelvic open reductions. The patient is positioned supine for anterior ring approaches; the SI joint or posterior iliac ring injuries are addressed with the superior aspect of the ilioinguinal approach. For posterior approaches to the SI joint and for displaced sacral fractures, the patient is positioned prone. In both instances the patient should be on a radiolucent table; the C-arm is used to confirm placement of hardware intraoperatively.

Technique. For anterior ring injuries, a Pfannenstiel approach is made to the symphysis and medial pubis. This incision is extended laterally to a formal ilioinguinal approach if more lateral displacements must be addressed. It is extended proximally to the posterior aspect of the iliac fossa for posterior iliac fractures and simple SI joint disruptions. For symphysis disruptions, two- or four-hole simple 3.5 DC plates or 3.5 mm reconstruction plates are used with 3.5 mm cortical screws (Fig. 10–11). The 3.5 mm reconstruction plates are useful for posterior iliac fractures if long 3.5 mm cortical lag screws will not suffice. Disruptions of the SI joint may be stabilized in children with one to two two-hole 3.5 mm DC plates with one screw in the sacrum and one in the iliac wing. When the posterior approach is selected for an SI joint disruption, the screws are placed across the iliac ring and into the body of the SI joint. One screw is relatively easy to place if the indirect and tangential views are observed under the fluoroscope during the procedure. This approach, if adequate intraoperative visualization can be achieved, is preferred. A second screw can then be placed posterior to the sacrum into the opposite

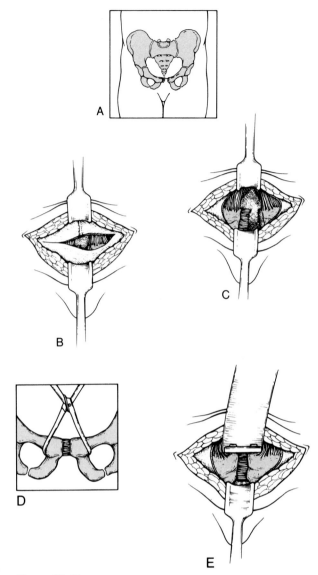

Figure 10–11

A simple two-hole plate is optimal for closing the "open-book" deformity. *A,* If the child has (or is having) a laparotomy through a midline incision, this plate is easily applied by exposing the superior aspect of the pubis bilaterally. If not, the Pfannenstiel approach is preferred. *B,* With this approach, one side of the rectus abdominis is generally seen to be avulsed from the pubis. *C,* With the periosteal elevator, the opposite pubis is exposed. *D,* A reduction forceps is then applied to the anterior aspect of the pubis bilaterally, closing the deformity. A Schanz pin of 4 or 5 mm diameter can be used through a percutaneous insertion incision into the iliac crest to help with this reduction. *E,* Generally, 3.5 mm cortical screws with a two-hole 3.5 mm dynamic compression plate are adequate for children under 12 years of age.

intact iliac wing and capped with a washer and nut to prevent loss of compression. This screw must not be overcompressed, in order to prevent opening of the anterior SI joint. Neither should it be overcompressed when dealing with a transforaminal sacral fracture, in order to avoid crushing of the sacral nerve roots. These techniques are nicely outlined by Matta and colleagues.[18, 19]

Acetabular Fractures

Bedrest/Non–Weight Bearing. Bedrest or non–weight bearing ambulation with crutches is appropriate only for nondisplaced or extremely minimally displaced (1 mm or less) fractures. There is nothing specific about the bedrest treatment other than avoidance of pushing off with the injured limb. The patient must be closely supervised to prevent ambulation. Similarly, patients treated with touch-down weight bearing with crutches on the injured side must be carefully supervised so as to avoid weight-bearing forces being transmitted across the fracture surface, with subsequent displacement.

Skeletal Traction. Traction treatment is appropriate only for acetabular fractures that are reducible to less than 2 mm of displacement. Because of the elastic nature of skeletal tissue in children, this is *rarely* the case. A traction pin should be inserted in the distal femur with fluoroscopic control under anesthesia. The fracture must be demonstrated to be reducible with follow-up AP and obturator and iliac oblique x-rays (with gonadal shielding) within the first 5 days. Fracture patterns that may be reducible with traction include the both-column fracture and associated variants. Isolated columnar injuries or posterior wall fractures are generally not reducible with traction.

Open Reduction and Internal Fixation. All displaced acetabular fractures (with 2 mm or greater displacement documented on CT scan) should undergo operative reduction and internal fixation. The surgical approach will vary according to the pattern of the fracture and the nature and direction of the displacement based on the preoperative AP, iliac, and obturator views and on the CT scan. All posterior wall injuries will be amenable to reduction through the Kocher-Langenbeck approach. When the posterior wall fracture is combined with posterior column injuries, this surgical approach is generally effective as well. We prefer to make the Kocher-Langenbeck approach with the patient in the lateral decubitus position. Anterior column injuries are best managed with the ilioinguinal approach of Letournel.[16] The associated injuries are best dealt with on an individual basis. When the posterior wall is not involved, we generally prefer the ilioinguinal approach because of the lower incidence of heterotopic ossification, better range of motion, and earlier return to function. Some transverse fractures and transverse fractures with associated posterior wall injuries may require the extended iliofemoral approach or combined Kocher-Langenbeck incision with iliofemoral approaches.[31] Internal fixation devices for children's fractures are generally of the 3.5 mm (small fragment) and 2.7 mm family. Extra-long screws must be specially ordered. We generally prefer 3.5 or 2.7 mm reconstruction plates for posterior wall fractures to allow early unrestricted motion of the hip (particularly unrestricted hip flexion). As a general rule, most children's fractures can be treated with lag screws alone. Multiple assistants, Schanz pins with universal chucks, femoral distractors, specialized pelvic clamps, and so forth, are all useful. A surgeon well versed in acetabular fracture approaches and fixation in adults should be consulted for all operative children's fractures.

Follow-Up Care

Immobilization. The duration and type of immobilization differ based on fracture type and selection of treatment, but the treating physician should bear in mind these general rules: 6 to 8 weeks' healing time for pelvic and acetabular fractures, about 2 weeks less for children under age 7 years, and 2 to 4 weeks more for adolescents older than 14 years. If the initial treatment has been bedrest, traction, or pelvic sling, the patient may be placed in a spica cast for the remaining healing time.

Beginning at about 4 to 5 weeks, cooperative children may be mobilized with crutches; this is possible only if there is an intact posterior pelvic ring complex on one side. The intact side is made fully weight bearing, and the injured side partially weight bearing, for the 3 to 4 weeks necessary for complete healing. Care must be taken when mobilizing patients who have suffered significant posterior iliac wing injuries treated by reduction in traction. Since significant leg length inequality has resulted from this form of treatment,[21] the patient should be taken out of bed cautiously and only when there is confirmed radiographic healing and no clinical tenderness. If in doubt, the physician should err on the side of conservatism, leaving the child in traction longer than is strictly necessary. Patients who have been managed operatively with anterior ring open reduction and internal fixation may be treated with bedrest or spica cast for the necessary healing time and then mobilized to full weight bearing. Children and adolescents who have been managed with anterior or posterior iliac reconstruction plating, anterior SI joint plating, or transiliac sacral screws with or without fixation to the initial posterior iliac crest can be treated with bedrest or spica cast for the 6 to 8 weeks' healing time and then mobilized with crutches gradually with progressive weight bearing.

Finally, patients who have been treated with external fixation may be converted to internal fixation if this is done within the first 1 or 2 weeks. Fractures older than this, especially in younger children, must be considered to be malunion, as operative reduction will require removal or osteotomy of the fracture callus. If the anterior ring disruption is to be managed definitively with external fixation, it must be left in place for the required 6 to 8 weeks' healing time. The patient generally can be safely converted to a spica cast after 4 weeks of external fixation but should not be left at bedrest, as external rotation forces in the pelvis may cause significant discomfort or late displacement.

Patients with acetabular fractures also require 6 to 8 weeks of healing time before weight bearing can be allowed without fear of displacement of the fracture. Younger children may be mobilized at 5 to 6 weeks; adolescents older than 12 years should be treated with partial weight bearing for 3 to 4 weeks longer (total of 10 to 12 weeks). Fractures that are minimally displaced and those treated with internal fixation will tolerate partial weight bearing on the injured side with crutches, beginning at 2 to 3 weeks after injury. Fractures reduced in traction should be held there for the full 5 to 6 weeks.

Mobilization. Four to five weeks following injuries, children with radiographically documented healing pelvic fractures can be mobilized with crutches (full weight bearing on the intact side of the pelvis, partial on the injured side). Caution must be exercised in patients who have significant posterior pelvic ring displacement. Similarly, minimally displaced or operatively fixed acetabular fractures can be mobilized (partial weight bearing on the injured side) beginning at 2 to 3 weeks post injury.

Physical Therapy. Other than in crutch ambulation instruction, physical therapy is not generally required for children with pelvic or acetabular fractures. Swimming is excellent rehabilitative therapy for both pelvic and acetabular fractures and can be initiated at 6 weeks post injury.

Disabilities. Barring complications, children and adolescents with pelvic fractures will be fully functional by 4 to 6 months post injury. The same general figure is valid for acetabular fractures that have been anatomically reconstructed. Patients with significant residual posterior pelvic ring displacements and those with remaining acetabular articular incongruities may have permanent disability.[11, 26]

Implant Removal. Removal of implants need be considered only in children with significant remaining growth (see Fig. 10–9). Children under age 10 years should have implants transfixing the sacroiliac joint or symphysis pubis removed at 4 to 6 months post injury. Those implants placed in the ilium, ischium, or pubis to fix anterior ring or acetabular fractures may be removed in children younger than 8 to 10 years to prevent encasement in bone and the great difficulty removing them should later reconstructive surgery be required.

ASSESSMENT OF RESULTS

Functional and Anatomic Parameters

Anatomic parameters, important to consider for pelvic fractures, are based on radiographic evaluation alone. For pelvic ring injury the reconstruction of normal anterior and posterior pelvic ring anatomy is the goal. The SI joint should not be fused, and the symphyseal cartilage space must be maintained. For acetabular fractures there must be the maintenance of a symmetric joint space with no evidence of acetabular or femoral head osteophytes or lateral extrusion of the femoral head as with premature closure of the triradiate cartilage.

Anatomic assessment of results influences the total outcome only minimally. The critical result is patient function. An appropriate functional assessment for both pelvic and acetabular fractures in children must include an evaluation of pain, limp, motion of hip, leg length inequality, activities of daily living, and sports performance as well as an evaluation of altered activities.

Rating Scales

Heeg and co-workers suggested that the rating scale of Harris be used to assess functional results for acetabular fractures.[11] Until an alternative specific to these injuries is designed, this is the best scale available. No rating scale has been published which was used to assess a population of children with pelvic or acetabular fractures.

EXPECTED RESULTS

The mortality figure for children with pelvic fracture is in the range of 2 to 12%, not significantly different from figures published for adult pelvic fractures. Open pelvic fractures and those with significant major vascular injury carry the highest risk.[25] Patients with avulsion injuries and minor anterior pelvic disruptions can be expected to have no residual disability, although, rarely, nonunion results.[8]

On follow-up at maturity, two thirds of patients with serious pelvic displacements will have no significant functional disability, and one half will have normal radiographs to accompany this result. One third will have residual limp and pain and will have had to alter their activities.[21] Growth arrest deformities may be related to triradiate cartilage injury, but these are seen much more rarely than growth arrest due to proximal femoral physeal injury.[5, 15]

Of the 23 patients with acetabular fractures followed by Heeg and colleagues, 18 were treated conservatively.[11] Good to excellent functional results were achieved in 21, and radiographic results were good to excellent in 10. These investigators reported no improved results with operative management over nonoperative treatment in patients with "comminuted" fractures or type V triradiate cartilage injuries.[11, 12] Excellent long-term results have been reported with widely displaced transverse fractures[3] managed operatively. As more experience is gained with the operative management of acetabular fractures in general, good to excellent functional results can be expected in 80 to 90% of children and adolescents with acetabular fractures.

COMPLICATIONS

Complications in the early phase of management of significant pelvic injury are bladder rupture, urethral injury, vaginal or rectal laceration, vascular injury, lumbosacral plexus injury, deep venous thrombosis, hemorrhage, and death. The more general of these complications and their prevention are covered in Chapter 4. The other associated injuries are a result of the primary trauma, and little can be done to prevent them, short of preventing the initial injury.

The long-term complications of pelvic fractures include delayed union, nonunion, malunion, fusion of the SI joint, and leg length inequality. Delayed union and malunion can generally be prevented by an adequate period of immobilization. Fusion of the SI joint is probably a result of the severe trauma producing the fracture, but the rate of this complication may be favorably influenced by anatomic reduction. To this extent, no less than an anatomic reduction of an SI joint should be accepted in a child. Similar standards and an adequate period of immobilization will prevent leg length inequality. Adherence to these high standards will require a high percentage of open reductions for severe displacements in the posterior pelvic ring.

The long-term complications of acetabular fractures are premature closure of the triradiate cartilage,[10, 28] joint space narrowing and sclerosis, femoral head subluxation, and avascular necrosis. Acceptance of no more than 2.0 mm of displacement in the acetabulum and careful surgical exposure will minimize their incidence.

Treatment

The treatable long-term complications of pelvic fracture include leg length inequality, malunion, and nonunion. Leg length inequality in the young child is best managed by properly timed contralateral epiphysiodesis. In the older child, closed femoral shortening as developed by Winquist is appropriate after it has been determined that there is a functional significance to the inequality.[39] Symptomatic nonunion is best managed by stabilization with internal fixation and bone grafting. Malunion of the anterior pelvic ring may require osteotomy and stabilization if it proves to be disabling in terms of sexual function, especially in females.

The most severe long-term complications of acetabular fractures—avascular necrosis, loss of joint space, and degenerative arthritis—are treatable only with drastic surgical measures. With these complications, temporizing with weight loss, canes, modification of activity, and antiinflammatory medications is the wisest course. Ultimately, the choice will come—in most cases between arthrodesis and arthroplasty. The latter is best delayed as long as possible. Premature closure of the triradiate cartilage may be optimally managed by bridge resection and fat interposition, but the difficulty of surgical access and visualization makes this hard to recommend. The misshapen growth and lateral femoral head extrusion must be well defined and documented by CT scan, three-dimensional CT, or MRI before such a procedure is undertaken. The safer course may be a lateral coverage procedure, such as an acetabular osteotomy, in early adolescence.

Proximal Femur Fractures

PATHOLOGY

Relevant Anatomy

The relevant osseous anatomy of the proximal femur can be divided into osseous and vascular anatomy. In terms of osseous anatomy, there are two growth centers of importance in the proximal femur. The proximal femoral epiphysis is responsible for 13% of the overall growth in length of the femur. The greater trochanter apophysis contributes significantly to the growth in shape of the proximal femur.

Damage to this apophysis before the age of 8 years produces a short greater trochanter and a coxa valga.[47]

The vascular anatomy of the growing child's proximal femur plays a central role in the outcome of a proximal femur fracture. Trueta[70] and Ogden[63] have investigated the immature patient's proximal femoral vascular system by injection studies. The metaphyseal and epiphyseal blood supplies remain functionally separate until physeal closure at age 14 to 17 years.[63, 70] Ogden did, however, find some small penetrating vessels bridging the physis in the periphery of the neck.[63] These may play a contributing role in supplying the femoral head until age 4 years.[48] The lateral circumflex system branches supply a significant anterior portion of the femoral head until the age of 5 to 6 years.[63] The lateral epiphyseal branches supply the majority of the femoral head throughout childhood and into adult life; this is the terminal branch of the medial femoral circumflex system. The artery of the ligamentum teres generally arises from the obturator arterial system but supplies only a small amount of the femoral head.[63] This specific arrangement of the dominant medial femoral circumflex system, which Ogden identified as the posterosuperior and posteroinferior arteries, as opposed to Trueta's lateral epiphyseal artery,[70] makes the child's femoral head highly susceptible to avascular necrosis following femoral neck fracture or fracture through the physis.

Incidence

Proximal femur fractures represent less than 1% of pediatric fractures and less than 1% of all hip fractures. Most published series are compilations from orthopaedic societies or regional hospital systems or represent decades of a single institution's experience. There have been less than 1000 total cases reported; specifically, there were 755 cases as of 1982.[62]

Mechanism of Injury

Except when they occur through pathologic bone (usually, simple bone cysts or fibrous dysplasia), fractures of the proximal femur are produced by high-energy trauma. Causes include falls from significant heights (trees), car versus pedestrian accidents, bicycle or motorcycle collisions, passenger injury in motor vehicle accidents, and child abuse, especially in children under age 2 years[45, 53] (see Chapter 15).

Consequences of Injury

Fractures of the proximal femur, particularly those proximal to the base of the femoral neck, carry a poor prognosis. A fracture in this region will frequently result in limb shortening, deformity of the femoral head, and degenerative arthritis. These problems arise from the complications of avascular necrosis and premature physeal closure,[50, 59, 65] complications that may occur more frequently in older children and adolescents (aged 8 to 16 years).[65] Fortunately, these injuries are rare.

Commonly Associated Injuries

Thirty percent of patients will have significant associated injuries. Because of the high-energy nature of the trauma, chest, head, and abdominal injuries are the most common nonmusculoskeletal injuries. Fractures of the femur, tibia-fibula, and pelvis are most commonly associated skeletal injuries.[58]

Classification

Whitman was the first to report fractures of the neck of the femur in children.[71] Delbet published the still standard classification of proximal femur fractures in 1907.[49] This was not widely recognized until Colonna's 1929 report of 12 cases in which he used the classification.[46] Although other systems have been recommended,[60] Delbet's system remains versatile, predictive, and useful for treatment decisions.[46, 49] The Delbet classification is depicted in Figure 10–12.

DIAGNOSIS

History

The history of injury associated with these fractures is that of high-energy trauma in 90% of cases. The nature of the violence by history will direct the physical examination as for that of a multiply injured patient (see Chapter 4).

Physical Examination

The examination must be thorough and cover all organ systems, as established in Chapter 4. The surface of the anterior and posterior aspects of the pelvis must be inspected for contusion, abrasion, and laceration. The affected limb will generally be shortened and in external rotation. The pulses at the inguinal ligament, popliteal fossae, and dorsalis

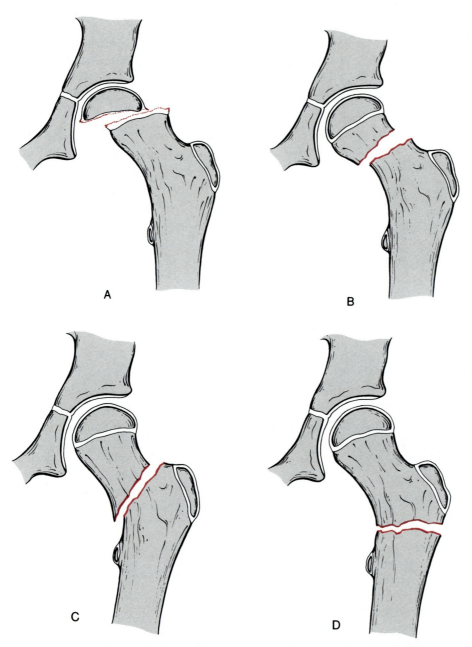

Figure 10–12

The Delbet classification of proximal femur fractures in children. *A*, Type I: transepiphyseal fracture. *B*, Type II: transcervial fracture. *C*, Type III: cervicotrochanteric fracture. *D*, Type IV: intertrochanteric fracture.

pedis and posterior tibialis locations must be assessed and compared with those of the normal limb. Finally, a screening examination for motor strength and light touch and pinprick sensation must be completed. Results of all these examinations are generally normal in these fractures.

Radiographic Evaluation

The AP pelvis radiograph is part of the screening examination for an unconscious, multiply injured patient. In a conscious patient, the complaint of groin or buttock pain generally warrants an AP pelvis radiograph, which confirms the diagnosis for each type of proximal femur fracture. In cases of severe shortening, a traction x-ray will be helpful to establish the fracture anatomy. A cross-table lateral radiograph, with the well leg flexed out of the way, is also useful for planning treatment.

Special Studies

In cases of severe trauma to the pelvis, in which the pulses of the affected limb are not moved by palpation or Doppler examination, an arteriogram is indicated. Currently there is no evidence that a preoperative bone scan or MRI scan is helpful for predicting avascular necrosis or in planning treatment.[99] In children under 18 years, an arthrogram aids in diagnosing a proximal femoral epiphyseal (type I) injury.[56]

MANAGEMENT

Evolution of Treatment

Carrell and Carrell reviewed the recommended treatment for fractures of the proximal femur prior to 1941.[44] The treatment to this point was primarily spica casting after closed reduction in an abducted position. In his review of 71 cases from the British Orthopaedic Association reported in 1962, Ratliff pointed out the higher incidence of nonunion when type II or type III fractures were treated conservatively.[67] Lam, in his review of 75 fractures treated in Hong Kong (57 treated personally), recommended an attempt at closed reduction and spica casting of types I–IV fractures in "younger" children and fixation with threaded pins in "older" children.[54] He advocated open reduction if closed reduction was not adequate. Canale and Bourland, in 1977, reported the Campbell Clinic experience with 61 fractures, the majority of which were treated with Knowles pin fixation.[43] These authors felt that the type of treatment did not affect the incidence of avascular necrosis. Swiontkowski and Winquist reported on ten cases of displaced type I–type III fractures treated with urgent capsulotomy and screw or pin fixation.[69]

Capsulotomy has been advocated and used in this series[69] to evacuate intracapsular hematoma, which has been shown to have a detrimental effect on femoral head blood flow in adults with femoral neck fractures as well as in animals with intact femoral necks. While it is unclear whether hematoma plays a major role in posttraumatic avascular necrosis in children, evacuation via an anterior capsulotomy produces no detrimental effect and may, in fact, help. It may play the most critical role in minimally displaced or nondisplaced fractures.[51,52]

The current protocols are as follows:

Type I   Urgent anterior capsulotomy reduction and fixation with smooth Steinmann pins; postoperative spica cast.

Type II   (Displaced or nondisplaced). Urgent anterior capsulotomy and fixation with two to three lag screws short of the physis; postoperative spica cast.

Type III   (Displaced or nondisplaced). Urgent anterior capsulotomy and fixation with two to three lag screws short of the physis; postoperative spica cast.

Type IV   Children under age 6 years: closed reduction and spica cast. Children aged 6 to 12 years: skeletal traction for 3 to 4 weeks, followed by spica cast.
Children over age 12 years, and for failed closed or traction reduction: open reduction and internal fixation with pediatric hip screw or blade plate.

Special Considerations for Polytrauma Patients

A displaced type I, II, or III fracture represents an orthopaedic emergency. Because of vascular compromise, which is potentially reversible, these fractures need to be reduced urgently. Therefore, this injury should be managed immediately after life-threatening injuries to the head, chest, and abdomen have been ruled out or definitively treated. Intracapsular hematoma occludes veins draining the femoral head and contributes to ischemia and should be emergently evaluated. As noted above, this may be most critical for minimally displaced fractures. Displaced femoral neck fractures may leave the critical lateral epiphyseal artery complex intact but kinked, thereby occluding flow to the femoral head. An emergent reduction, therefore, will return inflow to the femoral head. Open fractures with significant contamination should be irrigated and debrided rapidly before surgery is performed on the femoral neck fracture. All other musculoskeletal injuries should take a secondary position in the hierarchy of treatment.

Individual Treatment Modalities

Treatment options are given in Table 10–3.

Type I—Closed Reduction and Spica Casting

Indication. The indication for this treatment is a displaced type I fracture. I feel that this is contraindicated because of the near-impossibility of obtaining an anatomic reduction. Revascularization is enhanced by stable fixation.

Timing. To achieve the best reduction, the procedure should be done as soon as the patient's general condition allows.

Anesthesia/Positioning. A general anesthetic

Table 10–3
Treatment Modalities for Fractures of the Proximal Femur

Type	Treatment Options	Recommended Treatment
I	Closed reduction and spica casting in an abducted, externally rotated position[54, 60] Closed reduction and smooth Steinmann pin fixation	Open reduction and smooth Steinmann pin fixation
II	Traction treatment in abduction and external rotation Closed reduction and spica cast application Closed reduction and pin or screw fixation	Open reduction and pin or screw fixation
III	Traction treatment in abduction and external rotation Closed reduction and spica cast application Closed reduction and screw fixation	Open reduction and pin or screw fixation
IV	Skeletal traction Closed reduction and spica cast application	Closed reduction and pinning or open reduction and internal fixation

should be used in order to provide maximum muscle relaxation.

Technique. The patient is positioned supine on the operating table. The limb is flexed and externally rotated, and gentle traction is instituted and a radiograph obtained. If the reduction is anatomic, a spica cast can be applied after the patient is carefully transferred to the spica board. Nothing short of an anatomic reduction can be accepted. If after a second attempt, this is not the case, an alternative treatment should be instituted.

Type I—Closed Reduction and Pin Fixation

Indication. The indication is a displaced type I fracture.

Timing. The reduction, as above, should be performed as soon as is feasible to optimize the reduction and minimize reversible vascular injury.

Anesthesia/Positioning. The patient is positioned supine on a radiolucent table, and a general anesthetic is given. For larger children and adolescents, a fracture table is prepared.

Technique. After induction of anesthesia, the closed reduction is performed by simple internal rotation with gentle traction. The reduction is evaluated in the AP and lateral planes with the C-arm, and, if necessary, the reduction is repeated. If the reduction is anatomic, two or three smooth Steinmann pins of appropriate size are placed across the physis through a small lateral approach to the femur. If the reduction is not adequate (anatomic), an open reduction via an anterior capsulotomy should be performed.

Type I—Open Reduction and Smooth Pin Fixation (Author's Preferred Treatment)

Indication. A displaced type I fracture warrants this procedure.

Timing. As above, this procedure should be performed emergently.

Anesthesia/Positioning. See above.

Technique. After induction of anesthesia, a closed reduction is performed as described above. If it is anatomic on both views with the fluoroscope, a small linear capsulotomy is made in line with the femoral neck through a Watson-Jones approach, and the reduction is visually confirmed. Two or three smooth pins of an appropriate size are then used to fix the fracture. If the reduction is not anatomic, the capsulotomy is extended to the acetabular labrum and then transversely along the intertrochanteric ridge. Sutures are used to retract the capsule edges, and the reduction can be done under direct vision. A curved clamp is inserted into the hip joint posterior to the femoral head, and the posterior angulation is corrected by lifting the femoral head onto the femoral neck. In order to facilitate this maneuver, a bone hook can be placed around the medial aspect of the femur and lateral traction applied to disimpact the fracture. Once the reduction is performed, fixation is carried out in the same manner. Because this approach evacuates potential intracapsular hematoma and the reduction can be fully evaluated, this approach is favored.

Type II—Traction in Abduction and External Rotation

Indication. An isolated displaced type II fracture is an indication for this procedure.

Timing. The traction should be instituted as soon as the patient's initial evaluation is completed in order to minimize further vascular damage and to provide the best chance for an anatomic reduction.

Anesthesia. For children under age 12 years who are awake and alert and in whom there are no contraindications, a general anesthetic should be instituted.

Technique. The distal femoral pin is inserted with fluoroscopic control to avoid distal femoral physeal injury. The child is then placed in traction until the limb is abducted, externally rotated, and flexed. The reduction should be confirmed radiographically; if nonanatomic, the weight should be increased or the position altered. If the reduction in terms of the neck-shaft angle is nonanatomic, another form of treatment should be instituted. This is especially critical in older children. I believe that because of the increased risk of malunion and nonunion, and since a potential intracapsular hematoma is not released, this treatment should not be used.

Type II—Closed Reduction and Spica Cast Application

Indication. The indication is a displaced type II fracture in a child younger than 6 years.

Timing. Closed reduction, in order to produce the best reduction, should be done as soon as is practical.

Anesthetic/Positioning. The patient is positioned supine, and a general anesthetic with relaxation is instituted.

Technique. The child is placed on the spica table, and traction is applied as the limb is flexed, abducted, and externally rotated. If the intraoperative radiograph confirms an anatomic neck-shaft relationship, the cast is applied (a double long leg cast) with the limb in that position. A post-cast radiograph must confirm the reduction. If an perfect reduction cannot be obtained, alternative treatment must be selected. For reasons noted above, this form of treatment is not recommended.

Type II—Closed Reduction and Internal Fixation

Indications. A displaced type II fracture in a child older than 8 years or failure of a closed reduction in a younger child warrants this treatment.

Timing. Operation should be done as soon as other injuries are ruled out or treated.

Anesthesia/Positioning. A general anesthetic is required, and the patient is positioned supine on the fracture table with the C-arm available.

Technique. After induction of anesthesia, a closed reduction maneuver, as described above, is performed. If the reduction is confirmed to be anatomic, a midlateral approach to the proximal femur is made. The fracture is fixed using implants of appropriate length. Cortical lag screws of 3.5 mm or 4.5 mm are preferred, or alternating cannulated 3.5, 4.0, or 4.5 mm cancellous screws. If the reduction is nonanatomic, the surgeon should proceed with an open reduction.

Type II—Open Reduction and Internal Fixation (Author's Preferred Treatment)

Indication. The indication is a type II fracture in a child—nondisplaced as well for release of intracapsular tamponade.[51, 52]

Timing. Same as above.

Anesthesia/Positioning. Same as above.

Technique. The closed reduction maneuver as detailed above is performed. If the reduction is confirmed to be anatomic, the lateral approach is extended by detaching the vastus lateralis from the intertrochanteric ridge; the capsule is opened linearly along the femoral neck. The reduction is confirmed by direct vision and the internal fixation placed as noted above. This is the procedure for nondisplaced fractures as well, because of the definitive management of intracapsular tamponade. If the reduction is nonanatomic, the capsule is opened to the anterior acetabular labrum and taken off the intertrochanteric ridge 1.0 cm medially and laterally. With retracting sutures in place, a bone hook is placed around the medial aspect of the femur and lateral traction initiated by the assistant. The proximal fragment is then manipulated into position with a curved instrument. The rotation of the limb will have to be adjusted by a nonscrubbed assistant. Once the reduction is accurate, two to three implants are placed short of the physis as noted above.

Type III—Traction Treatment

Indications. Indications are isolated displaced type III fractures in children aged 4 to 12 years. Contraindications include multiple injuries (especially head injury, in which traction is poorly tolerated).

Timing. As with other proximal femoral fractures with potential of vascular injury to the femoral head, these should be reduced as soon as the patient can be cleared for anesthesia or sedation.

Anesthesia/Positioning. General anesthesia is administered in children under age 12 years whenever it is possible. The patient is positioned supine on the operating table.

Technique. A distal femoral pin is inserted using fluoroscopic control to avoid the distal femoral physis. The child is then placed in 5 to 10 lb of traction in a position of abduction, flexion, and external rotation. The position of the fracture is confirmed. If the reduction is nonanatomic, more weight may be necessary, or a closed reduction maneuver should be performed. If anatomic reduction is not obtained, an alternative treatment must be selected.

Type III—Closed Reduction/Spica Casting

Indication. The indication is a displaced type III fracture in a child under 6 years of age.

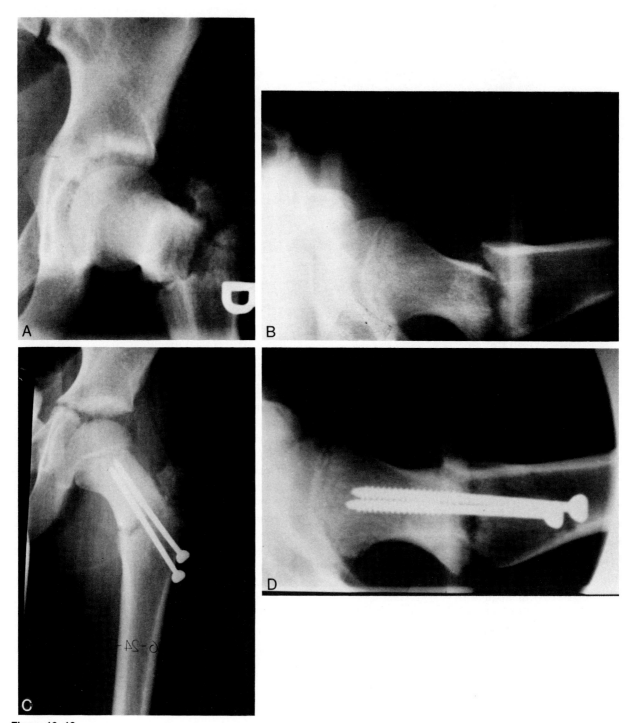

Figure 10–13

A 6-year-old boy is struck by an automobile and sustains a displaced type III fracture. The patient was taken emergently to the operating room, where, using a Watson-Jones approach, a capsulotomy and open reduction were performed. *A–B,* Preoperative radiograph. *C–D,* Postoperative radiograph; the patient was treated for 6 weeks in a one and one-half hip spica cast.

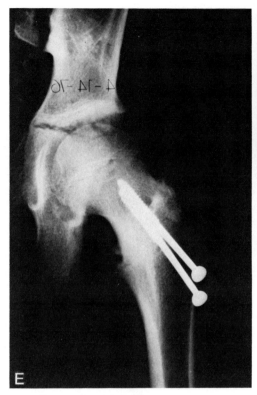
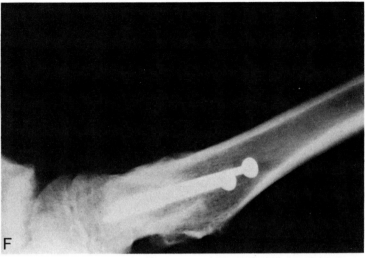

Figure 10–13 *Continued*

E–F, At 8 months the screws were removed. The child is asymptomatic but must be followed for a minimum of 3 years.

Timing. See above.

Anesthesia/Positioning. General anesthesia should be administered to a supine patient positioned on the spica board/table.

Technique. After induction, the fracture is reduced by flexing the limb while applying gentle traction and putting the limb in external rotation and abduction. The reduction is evaluated by two plain radiographs, and a double long leg spica cast is applied. The reduction is confirmed after placement of the cast radiographically. If the reduction is not acceptable, the maneuver can be repeated using fluoroscopy to evaluate limb position relative to reduction. If an anatomic reduction cannot be obtained, an open reduction should be performed.

Type III—Closed Reduction and Screw Fixation

Indications. Indications include type III fracture in a child or failure of closed treatment.

Timing. See above.

Anesthesia/Positioning. General anesthesia is administered to the patient positioned supine on the fracture table.

Technique. The technique is identical to that outlined for type II fractures. Coming near to the physis with the internal fixation is not as critical because of the larger medial (proximal) fragment. The same implants are recommended.

Type III—Open Reduction and Screw Fixation (Author's Preferred Treatment)

Indications. Type III fracture in a child and failure of closed reduction are the indications. The same treatment is recommended for release of intracapsular tamponade.[51, 52]

Timing. See above.

Anesthetic/Positioning. General anesthesia is given with the child in the supine position on the fracture table.

Technique. The technique is identical to that outlined for type II injuries (Fig. 10–13). As noted above, the same implants are used (those able to compress the fracture site). I recommend this treatment for nondisplaced type III fractures, as intracapsular tamponade may play a role in the production of avascular necrosis.

Type IV—Skeletal Traction

Indications. Displaced type IV fractures in children 6 to 12 years of age warrant this procedure.

Timing. Although there are no vascular considerations with this distal fracture, the best reductions are obtained when surgery is performed in the first 24 hours.

Anesthesia/Positioning. General anesthesia is preferred, with the patient in the supine position on the standard operating table.

Technique. The distal femoral pin is inserted under fluoroscopic control to avoid the distal femoral physis. The limb is then placed in 10 to 15 lb of traction with the limb flexed 60 to 70 degrees in an externally rotated and abducted position. The neck-shaft position can be controlled by increasing the weight and distal pull. This angle should be within 3 to 5 degrees of the opposite normal hip. Significant varus should not be accepted. If an adequate reduction cannot be obtained, an open reduction and fixation should be considered.

Type IV—Closed Reduction and Spica Cast

Indication. A displaced type IV fracture in a child under 6 years of age is the indication.

Timing. See above.

Anesthesia/Positioning. General anesthesia is administered, with the child in the supine position on a spica board.

Technique. After induction of anesthesia, the fracture is reduced by longitudinal traction, flexion to 70 degrees, and external rotation. The reduction should be confirmed by fluoroscopic or plain film prior to double leg spica casting. If a neck-shaft angle within 5 degrees cannot be obtained and held, open reduction or closed percutaneous pinning should be considered.

Type IV—Closed Reduction and Percutaneous Pinning

Indications. Indications include failure to maintain a reduction in a cast or in traction, multiple trauma, and irreducible type IV fracture in a child aged 6 to 12 years.

Timing. See above.

Anesthesia/Positioning. General anesthesia is required. The patient is placed in the supine position on the fracture table with the C-arm available.

Technique. A closed reduction is performed, and the limb is placed in traction on the fracture table with flexion of 20 to 30 degrees and external rotation. If the reduction is satisfactory (within 5 degrees of the intact femoral neck-shaft angle and good opposition on the lateral view) on fluoroscopic evaluation, the fracture can be stabilized with two to three threaded pins, either percutaneously or through a small lateral approach to the lateral proximal femur. If the patient is large or the stability of the fixation is in question, a one and one-half spica cast should be added.

Type IV—Open Reduction and Internal Fixation (Author's Preferred Treatment)

Indications. Indications include failure to obtain an adequate reduction in a child of any age by any closed technique, multiple-system trauma, and a displaced type IV fracture in a child 12 years or older.

Timing. If open reduction is selected as the course of treatment, the patient can be placed in skin or skeletal traction for 3 to 5 days prior to operation. If the general condition of the patient allows, reduction and fixation within the first 24 to 48 hours is preferred.

Anesthesia/Positioning. General anesthetic is required. The child is positioned supine on the fracture or radiolucent table with the C-arm available.

Technique. After the patient is anesthetized and placed on the fracture table, traction is placed on the limb in slight external rotation. A standard lateral approach to the proximal femur is made. The fragments are reduced under direct vision. In children under 6 years of age, two to three threaded pins can be used for fixation (Fig. 10–14). In children aged 6 to 12 years, limited fixation with two to three lag or cancellous screws is recommended. In both age groups the fixation should not cross the physis and should be supplemented with a one and one-half spica cast. In patients 12 years and older, a sliding hip screw or angled blade plate should be used, taking care to keep the fixation proximal to the physis. No supplemental casting is indicated under normal circumstances for this type of fixation.

Follow-Up Care

Immobilization. The period of immobilization depends upon the age of the child and the type of fracture. For types I to III fractures treated in spica cast or in traction, a period of 8 to 10 weeks is required for healing; this approaches 6 to 8 weeks for children 6 years and under, and 12 weeks for adolescents. If the initial treatment is in traction, the final 2 to 4 weeks can be in a spica cast. Type IV fractures have similar healing times. Types I to IV fractures managed with smooth pin or threaded Steinmann pin fixation should have supplemental one and one-half spica casts applied for the 8- to 10-week course of treatment. Children with type II and type III fractures, internally fixed with lag screws, will frequently benefit from supplemental spica casting if their ability to cooperate with non–weight bearing regimens is suspect (in ages 1 to 12 years). Adolescents with rigidly fixed type IV fractures can be mobilized with crutches beginning 10 to 14 days postoperatively.

Mobilization. Children from 6 years of age to adolescence will benefit from a transitional period of partial weight bearing with crutches. This should

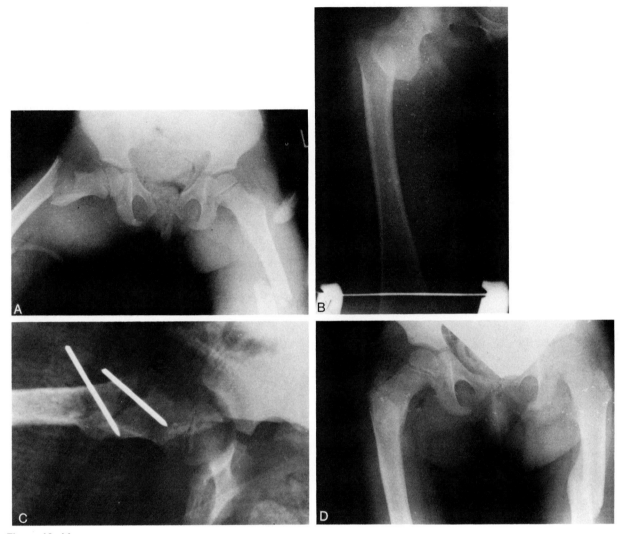

Figure 10–14

A 5-year-old girl was the unrestrained front seat passenger in a high-speed motor vehicle accident. *A–B,* An initial attempt was made to treat this type IV fracture in traction. The neck shaft angle could not be adequately controlled. *C,* Via a limited open reduction, threaded Steinmann pins were inserted. The child was kept in a spica cast for 6 weeks. *D,* Radiographs taken at the time of pin removal.

be instituted beginning at 8 to 10 weeks and should continue for 2 to 3 weeks. Younger children should be mobilized as tolerated. Swimming pool therapy is a helpful transition technique.

Physical Therapy. Formal physical therapy, other than that required for crutch ambulation and possible water therapy, is not necessary for children. Adolescents (age 15 years and older) may benefit from gait training or muscle strengthening programs beginning at 12 weeks post injury.

Disability. Type I to type III injuries that heal and do not develop proximal physeal arrest or avascular necrosis will have a period of functional disability for 4 to 6 months. Type IV fractures that heal without coxa vara will have similar periods of disability. If growth arrest develops in a child under age 10 years, significant leg length inequality may result, leading to limp and altered gait mechanics. Avascular necrosis at any age will ultimately lead to limb length inequality (and deformity in younger children), pain, and altered lifestyle in the vast majority of patients.[54, 58] In every case the disability will be progressive and permanent.[55]

Implant Removal. When pin fixation is selected, the pins should be left long for easy retrieval and should be removed at 4 to 6 months post injury.

Lag screws and larger implants used for type II, type III, and type IV fractures should be removed at 6 to 12 months (see Figs. 10–13 and 10–14).

ASSESSMENT OF RESULTS

Ratliff's assessment of functional and anatomic results includes the parameters of pain, motion, activity, and radiographic findings and has been the most widely used. His guidelines are presented in Table 10–4 and are recommended for use in the future.

EXPECTED RESULTS

Type I. Well over 80% of these injuries develop avascular necrosis with poor functional results. Urgent open reduction may affect the results positively, but a 50% minimum incidence of avascular necrosis in displaced type I fractures should be expected.[59, 69]

Type II. Fifty to sixty percent of displaced type II fractures will develop avascular necrosis, 15% will develop nonunion, and 50 to 60% will develop premature physeal closure following closed treatment or pin fixation.[43, 54, 60, 64] Urgent capsulotomy and internal fixation *may* favorably influence the rates of these complications[69] but will not reduce their incidence to zero, as initial displacement is the critical factor in producing the vascular injury. Avascular necrosis can result from nondisplaced fractures not treated with capsulectomy.[51, 52]

Type III. Thirty to forty percent of displaced type III fractures will develop avascular necrosis; these rates are favorably affected by urgent capsulotomy and fixation.[52] Ten percent of these patients will develop nonunion; this can be minimized by optimal lag screw fixation. If the fracture is not reduced anatomically, coxa vara will result in 20% of cases.[43]

Type IV. Coxa vara will be the result if anatomic reduction is not obtained by whatever treatment is used. This has been reported in 10 to 30% of cases and is most common with traction treatment. Avascular necrosis and physeal closure are not anticipated in type IV injuries. This deformity may rarely correct with time.[50]

In general, if avascular necrosis, premature closure, nonunion, and coxa vara can be avoided, an excellent result will be apparent. Owing to the nature of these injuries, this can be expected only in 40 to 50% of types I and II fractures.[66] Again, urgent capsulotomy and anatomic reduction may significantly influence the rate of these complications. When these complications develop, even though the results at 2 to 4 years may be functionally good, the status of the limb will deteriorate with time.[54, 55, 64]

COMPLICATIONS

The complications of avascular necrosis, preoperative physeal closure, nonunion, and coxa vara are generally apparent on x-ray within 6 to 9 months after injury. These have more severe consequences in adolescents and older children.[65] Avascular necrosis of the metaphyseal region, as described by Ratliff, is not of functional significance.[67, 68]

Treatment

Avascular Necrosis. There is no recognized treatment for posttraumatic avascular necrosis. This complication may have the least long-term significance in children under 6 years of age because of the biologic plasticity of the bone. Acetabular and femoral osteotomies to "contain" the femoral head have been recommended by some authors, but their effect on functional outcome remains in question.[66–68]

Premature Physeal Closure. This complication rarely results in a leg length discrepancy of greater than 1.5 cm.[52] The leg length inequality should be followed by scanograms and distal femoral epiphysiodesis performed on the normal leg if the discrepancy is projected to be greater than 1.5 cm.

Nonunion. If associated with varus deformity, this complication can be effectively treated by subtro-

Table 10–4
Ratliff's Classification of the Results of Treatment for Fracture of the Hip

	Good	Fair	Poor
Pain	None or patient ignores it	Occasional	Diabling
Movement	Full or only terminal restriction	Greater than 50%	Less than 50%
Activity	Normal or patient avoids games	Normal or patient avoids games	Restricted
X-ray	Normal or some deformity of femoral neck	Severe deformity of femoral neck and mild avascular necrosis	Severe avascular necrosis, degenerative arthritis; arthrodesis

chanteric valgus osteotomy and internal fixation across the nonunion. If a normal neck-shaft angle has been maintained, internal fixation with compression and bone grafting is indicated.

Coxa Vara. This complication is avoidable by adherence to a high standard for the initial reduction of type IV fractures. It can be successfully treated, when severe enough to result in effective limb shortening (less than 130 degree neck-shaft angle) with a subtrochanteric or intertrochanteric valgus osteotomy with internal fixation.

Hip Dislocations

PATHOLOGY

Relevant Anatomy

The relevant osseous and vascular anatomy of the acetabulum and proximal femur has been described previously.

Incidence

Traumatic hip dislocation in children is rare, constituting 5% or less of all pediatric dislocations.[77, 90-92, 102] There is no significant peak age of incidence.[77, 83] While the majority of hip dislocations are posterior, anterior dislocations have been reported in children.[75, 79]

Mechanism

In contrast to other injuries presented in this chapter, hip dislocation can occur with relatively trivial injuries. In the detailed report of the Pennsylvania Orthopaedic Society, there were four groups of mechanisms.[96] These are trivial falls (slippery surfaces or "the splits"), athletic injuries (wrestling, football, or baseball), falls from significant heights, and being struck by a vehicle or injuries sustained as a passenger in a motor vehicle accident. Of the 25 cases reported, 15 were in the first two groups (low energy) and 10 were in the latter two groups (high energy). The prognosis has been shown to be related to the amount of energy involved in the dislocation.

Consequences

Hip dislocations in children and adolescents may result in avascular necrosis or degenerative arthritis with resultant pain, limp, and loss of motion, with necessary adjustment in work and recreational activities.[81, 89, 96]

Commonly Associated Injuries

In dislocations that occur in trivial falls or with athletic activities, there rarely are associated injuries. Of the 67 dislocations discussed by Gartland and Benner, 9 of these had an associated fracture of the acetabulum, femoral head, or greater trochanter.[85] All of these were due to high-energy trauma. Fracture of the ipsilateral femur has been a relatively frequent association and often leads to a missed diagnosis of the hip dislocation.[74, 97] In the more severely injured patients, careful evaluation for head, chest, abdominal, and vascular trauma must be performed as for any multiply injured individual (see Chapter 4). Associated fractures of the pelvis and upper and lower extremities in several locations have been reported.

Classification

Pediatric hip dislocations traditionally have been grouped according to age at injury (0 to 5 years, 5 to 10 years, 10 to 15 years), violence of mechanism (see above), and direction of dislocation (anterior versus posterior). Recently, Hougaard and Thomsen[90] suggested using the Stewart-Milford[100] classification of hip dislocations to report associated acetabular fractures. There is no published classification specifically for hip dislocation in children.

The current classification is as follows: anterior (obturator, anteroinferior inguinal, anterosuperior) and posterior. The Stewart-Milford classification is as follows:

Grade I	No acetabular fracture or only a minor chip.
Grade II	Posterior rim fracture, but stable after reduction.
Grade III	Posterior rim fracture with hip instability after reduction.
Grade IV	Dislocation accompanied by fracture of the femoral head and neck.

I feel that when an acetabular fracture exists the classification of Letournel[16] should be applied.

DIAGNOSIS

History

The history associated with hip dislocation generally follows one of three lines. The accident that produces the complaint of groin and buttock pain will be a minor fall, such as on a slippery surface or doing "splits"; an athletic collision in football, wrestling, or baseball; a high-energy fall from a height;

being struck by a car; or being injured as a passenger. Two thirds of cases belong to the former groups of low-velocity injuries, which have the best associated prognosis.

Physical Examination

Children who are the victims of high-energy trauma should be evaluated as outlined in Chapter 4. Ninety percent of hip dislocations are posterior, and the patient will present with the affected limb shortened, flexed, adducted, and internally rotated. In the more rare anterior dislocation, the limb will generally be abducted, flexed, and externally rotated. An inspection is performed of the skin anteriorly and posteriorly for contusions, abrasions, and open wounds. The femoral, popliteal, dorsalis pedis, and posterior tibial pulses should be palpated, since common femoral arterial injury has been associated with hip dislocation.[75] In the alert and cooperative child, motor function should be evaluated in the limb; the presence or absence (palpable contraction) of function in each major muscle group must be recorded. Finally, the sensory function in response to light touch and pinprick should be recorded, especially in the distal sciatic nerve distribution. This examination should be systemically repeated following attempted closed reduction.

Radiographic Evaluation

The AP pelvis examination should be a part of the initial evaluation in all patients who have sustained high-energy trauma with other injuries. The hip dislocation will be apparent on this radiograph. The pelvis radiograph should be requested for all children who present with the aforementioned physical abnormalities. The radiograph should be carefully studied for fractures of the femoral head, neck, and acetabulum. If an acetabulum fracture is present, the 45 degree oblique views of Judet should be obtained (see Fig. 10–7). Following closed reduction, generally under general anesthetic, the AP pelvis x-ray should be repeated to confirm a concentric reduction with symmetric joint space. A postreduction CT scan should be obtained to rule out intraarticular loose bodies and fractures of the acetabulum and femoral head. In certain settings, when the closed reduction has failed, it may be possible to obtain the CT scan prior to open reduction. This is helpful to delineate loose bodies that need removal and acetabulum fractures that may need stabilization. The reduction of the hip should never be delayed for more than an extra 45 to 60 minutes and should always be done within the first 6 hours after injury, whenever possible.[82]

Special Studies

A digitized technetium bone scan may be helpful for predicting avascular necrosis.[101] While this technique has proven value in adult patients with femoral neck fractures, it has never been applied to a group of patients with hip dislocation, and its predictive value has yet to be defined. While MRI has not been proved to be of value as a predictor of avascular necrosis following femoral neck fracture in adults,[99] its role in diagnosing avascular necrosis and following the biologic progress of revascularization following pediatric hip dislocation, is yet to be proven. Arthrography of the hip may be useful to differentiate hip dislocation from type I proximal femur fracture in children under 18 months. If there is an associated sciatic nerve injury, electromyography (EMG) is helpful in defining the nature and severity of the injury at 3 weeks post injury. Arteriography is indicated when screening physical examination with Doppler backup indicates a major proximal arterial injury.[94]

MANAGEMENT

Evolution of Treatment

Once sufficient experience was published regarding the management of hip dislocation in children,[79] the current standard of care was established—that is, a closed reduction under general anesthesia and confirmation of a concentric reduction radiographically. If the reduction is not attainable or is unstable or nonconcentric, open reduction is indicated. There has been some evolution in the postreduction evaluation, as a postreduction CT scan is now recommended to rule out loose bodies and femoral head and acetabular fracture. There have been developments in technique of reduction, with some preferring skin traction to a formal closed reduction maneuver of the hip in young children. The majority favor a manipulative reduction for posterior dislocations utilizing traction with the leg in a flexed position. There is no consensus regarding postoperative care. Bedrest, skin traction, skeletal traction, and spica cast have all been recommended, with no clear advantage of any method. Traumatic dislocations that present late should also generally be reduced.[76] The complication of recurrent dislocation has not been associated with any one method of postreduction treatment. Concerning the management of dislocations associated with displaced acetabular fractures, with more than 2.0 mm displacement of the articular surface, most centers would now recommend surgical reduction and stabilization (see under Pelvic Fractures and Dislocations).

Current treatment of pediatric hip dislocation dictates (1) closed reduction under general anesthesia; and (2) postreduction check of stability with postreduction AP pelvis radiograph and CT scan. If reduction is not attainable, is unstable, or is associated with loose bodies or with a displaced acetabular fracture, an open reduction is recommended.

Special Considerations for Polytrauma Patients

The dislocated hip, like the displaced femoral neck fracture, represents a surgical emergency. Once the patient has been fully evaluated and life-threatening head, chest, abdominal, and vascular injuries have been addressed, the hip must be reduced. This should take precedence over all other orthopaedic problems, as it can be done rapidly, especially if the child is under an anesthetic for any other reason. Urgency is appropriate, as it has been shown that there is an increase in posttraumatic avascular necrosis associated with hips that remain dislocated for more than 6 hours.[82]

Individual Treatment Modalities

Closed Reduction

Indications. An anterior or posterior dislocation noted on an AP pelvis x-ray is an indication for closed reduction. There are no absolute contraindications, but if an associated displaced femoral neck fracture is noted, the closed reduction will probably not succeed. If there is a nondisplaced femoral neck fracture, the closed reduction must be gentle and done with fluoroscopic control to prevent displacing the fracture.

Timing. Whenever possible, the reduction should be performed within 6 hours of injury. This will minimize the risk of avascular necrosis.[82, 96]

Preoperative Planning. If there is an associated acetabular fracture, preoperative Judet views and a CT scan (if they can be done without causing significant delay) are helpful if the closed reduction is unsuccessful and open reduction is required.

Anesthesia/Positioning. A general anesthetic with muscle relaxation is required. The patient should be positioned supine. The older or larger the patient is, the more important it is to have a surgical assistant.

Technique. If the child is older than 5 years or more than 50 lb, an assistant will definitely be required. The assistant should apply countertraction by applying pressure with the palms of the hand on the anterior iliac crests. The surgeon flexes the hip 60 to 90 degrees and applies traction with gentle internal and external rotation. In large adolescents, the increased force required can be provided by standing on the operating table flexing the patient's knee between the surgeon's legs, grasping the limb just distal to the popliteal fossae with the knee bent and using the surgeon's quadriceps and triceps surae to provide the traction necessary. The larger the patient, the more critical it is that the anesthesiologist provide excellent muscle relaxation. For the posterior dislocation, the limb is in neutral position or is slightly adducted when the traction is applied. The reduction maneuver differs for anterior dislocation in that the traction is applied with the limb in the abducted position, and therefore the vector is somewhat lateral.

Open Reduction

Indications. Indications include failed closed reduction, closed reduction that is nonconcentric,[78, 93] dislocation with an associated displaced femoral neck fracture, and displaced acetabular fracture. (See under Pelvic Fractures and Dislocations and Proximal Femur Fractures for details.)

Timing. Open reduction should be performed within 6 hours, as soon as possible after the failed closed reduction.

Preoperative Planning. See above.

Anesthesia/Positioning. The patient should be positioned on a beanbag in lateral decubitus position with the injured hip up. General anesthesia is required.

Technique. A posterolateral approach, the Kocher-Langenbeck, is made to the hip. Great care must be taken in identifying the sciatic nerve distally and following it proximally, especially when neurologic deficits have been identified preoperatively. The nerve should be carefully inspected in this setting and will generally appear contused. The external rotators should be inspected and, if intact, divided 1.0 cm from their femoral insertion. Occasionally, if failure of closed reduction is the reason for the exploration, the piriformis tendon will be displaced across the acetabulum, blocking the reduction.[78, 93] The capsule is then inspected along with the labrum. Most commonly, the femoral head will be buttonholed through the capsule, or there will be an inverted labrum. Once the soft tissue block is identified, the acetabulum must be inspected for osteocartilaginous loose bodies. A bone hook is helpful in laterally displacing the femoral head, and a headlamp helps with visualization. Small pituitary rongeurs make excellent grasping forceps. In older adolescents, a 5.0 mm Schanz screw can be inserted distal to the greater trochanter physis and a universal chuck attached to the pin to provide lateral traction. At this point, posterior column or posterior wall fractures should be reduced and internally fixed with smooth K-wires (with the ends bent to 90 degrees to prevent migration) or small lag screws in younger children; and with 3.5 mm lag screws and 3.5 mm reconstruction plates as buttresses in older children (Fig. 10–15).

Follow-Up Care

Immobilization. Children under age 6 years should be immobilized in a one and one-half spica cast for 4 to 6 weeks. Older, cooperative children should be placed at bedrest for 3 weeks and then can be mobilized with crutches for 3 to 4 additional weeks. Hip flexion greater than 60 degrees should be avoided, especially in the presence of posterior wall fractures.

Mobilization. Following the 4 to 8 weeks of immobilization in a cast or with crutches, the patient may be mobilized with progressive weight bearing as tolerated. Casting is generally more appropriate for children under 10 years of age. There is no evidence that prolonged non–weight bearing affects the incidence or severity of avascular necrosis.[85]

Physical Therapy. Other than the institution of crutch ambulation and hip flexion precautions, physical therapy probably does not influence the final functional result.

Expected Duration of Disability. Barring associated sciatic nerve injury or the complications of avascular necrosis or heterotopic ossification, one can expect the return of full function in children under age 10 years by 3 months post injury. Adolescents, especially those who have undergone open reduction and internal fixation of an associated acetabular fracture through a posterolateral approach, may take 6 months to optimize function postoperatively.

Timing of Implant Removal. Although not absolutely mandatory, implants in young children should probably be removed within 6 months of operation. In adolescents, the implants, plates, and screws can be safely left in place unless there is concern about intraarticular hardware or the possibility of a later reconstructive procedure.

ASSESSMENT OF RESULTS

Functional and Anatomic Parameters. Functional status should include an evaluation of pain, fatigue, gait, weakness, and motion.[90] Radiographic analysis must include a direct evaluation of the hip for joint space, avascular changes in the femoral head, and osteophytes or sclerosis.[90]

A suggested rating scale follows:

Excellent—Full motion. No pain, weakness, or fatigue. Normal x-ray.

Good—No appreciable pain in hip (except after prolonged work/weight bearing). No greater than 25% loss of motion. Slight osteoarthritic changes on x-ray. Normal joint space; no avascular necrosis.

Fair—Mild to moderate pain. Moderate limp. Moderate osteophytes; moderate narrowing of joint space.

Poor—Pain; limp; moderate to extreme limitation of motion; ± adduction deformity; advanced osteoarthritis; avascular necrosis; narrowing of joint space or sclerosis of the acetabulum.

EXPECTED RESULTS

There are very few reported patients in the literature who have been followed for more than 5 years. Fifty

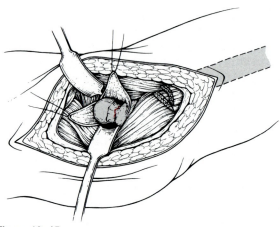

Figure 10–15

The Watson-Jones approach for open reduction of femoral neck fractures. The incision curves gently toward the interval between the tensor fascia lata and the gluteus medius muscles from the tip of the greater trochanter and extends distally along the midlateral line of the femur. The vastus lateralis is elevated off the intertrochanteric ridge, and a T-shaped capsulotomy is done by elevating the anterior hip capsule off the intertrochanteric ridge and extending the capsulotomy toward the center of the acetabulum, exposing the femoral neck fracture. By placing sutures in the edges of the capsulotomy and inserting a Holman retractor along the anterior aspect of the acetabulum, excellent visualization of the femoral neck fracture can be achieved.

patients out of 248 children were followed to skeletal maturity in Gartland and Benner's review.[85] Thirty-four were normal; 16 were not. Thirteen of the 16 had either a fracture about the hip or a delay in reduction of greater than 24 hours. The incidence of avascular necrosis in numerous published series is 8 to 10%. This complication is more common in older children, with delay in reduction, and with greater severity of injury.[84, 85] Twelve of 13 patients followed from 5 to 26 years by Hougaard and Thomsen underwent reduction within 6 hours of injury and had normal hips.[90] One patient with a reduction at 37 hours developed osteoarthritis.

COMPLICATIONS

Complications include (1) sciatic nerve injury, (2) avascular necrosis, (3) osteoarthritis, and (4) recurrent dislocation.

Treatment

Sciatic Nerve Injury. An incidence of 24% of this complication was reported by Pearson and Mann.[95] All involved sensory or motor deficiency, or both. All five patients had improvement in function, and in one, function returned to normal. No effective treatment has been published. There may be a role for neurolysis if improvement is not forthcoming by 3 to 6 months post injury.

Avascular Necrosis. This is the most common complication.[81, 89] It is generally apparent by 3 to 6 months post injury. Patients must be followed quarterly for the first year and then annually if they are asymptomatic, until 4 years post injury. Early weight bearing does not influence the rate of this complication. Younger patients with this complication fare better than older ones.[84, 85] There is no effective treatment available, but acetabular or femoral osteotomy should be considered.

Osteoarthritis. This complication appears to be associated with a delay in reduction.[74] It is apparent only with follow-up in the 5- to 20-year range. Treatment is symptomatic whenever possible: weight control, modification of activity, walking aids, and antiinflammatory medications. Surgical management should be delayed as long as possible. Options include arthrodesis, osteotomy, and arthroplasty.

Recurrent Dislocation. This complication has been reported in 12 children; it generally occurs in those under the age of 8 years[74] and has always been posterior in orientation.[72, 80] There is no clear increase in incidence with more severe trauma or an inadequate period of immobilization. While surgical exploration with repair of the posterior capsule is effective (with follow-up of less than 2 years),[86, 98] conservative care has been effective as well.[73, 88] The recommendation, therefore, is for a postoperative/postreduction CT scan following the first recurrence and subsequent reduction. If there is a symmetric reduction with no loose bodies, a spica cast should be applied for 6 weeks with the hip abducted 20 to 30 degrees and flexed 45 degrees. Patients who have a recurrence thereafter should have a posterior capsular reefing.

REFERENCES

Pelvic Fractures and Dislocations

1. Barrett, I.R.; Goldberg, J.A. Avulsion fracture of the ligamentum teres in a child. J Bone Joint Surg 71-A:438–439, 1989.
2. Bond, S.I.; Gotschall, C.S.; Eichelberger, M.R. Predictors of abdominal injury in children with pelvic fracture. J Trauma 31:1169–1173, 1991.
3. Brooks, E.; Rosman, M. Central fracture-dislocation of the hip in a child. J Trauma 28:1590–1592, 1988.
4. Bryan, W.J.; Tullos, H.S. Pediatric pelvic fractures: Review of 52 patients. J Trauma 19:799–805, 1979.
5. Compere, E.L.; Garrison, M.; Fahey, J.J. Deformities of the femur resulting from arrestment of growth of the capital and greater trochanteric epiphyses. J Bone Joint Surg 22:909–915, 1940.
6. Cotler, H.B.; LaMont, J.G.; Hansen, S.T. Immediate spica casting for pelvic fractures. J Orthop Trauma 2:222–228, 1988.
7. Currey, J.D.; Butler G: The mechanical properties of bone tissue in children. J Bone Joint Surg 57-A:810–814, 1975.
8. Elton, R.C. Fracture-dislocation of the pelvis followed by nonunion of the posterior iliac spine. J Bone Joint Surg 54-A:648–649, 1972.
9. Godfrey, J.D. Trauma in children. J Bone Joint Surg 46-A:422–447, 1964.
10. Harrison, T.J. The influence of the femoral head on pelvic growth and acetabular form in the rat. J Anat 95:12–26, 1961.
11. Heeg, M.; Klasen, H.J.; Visser, J.D. Acetabular fractures in children and adolescents. J Bone Joint Surg 71-B:418–421, 1989.
12. Heeg, M.; Viser, J.D.; Oostvogel, H.J.M. Injuries of the acetabular triradiate cartilage and sacroiliac joint. J Bone Joint Surg 70-B:34–37, 1988.
13. Heinrich, S.D.; Sharps, C.H.; Cardea, J.A.; Gervin, A.S. Open pelvic fracture with vaginal laceration and diaphragmatic rupture in a child. J Orthop Trauma 2:257–261, 1988.
14. Kricun, M.E. Fractures of the pelvis. Orthop Clin North Am 21:573–589, 1990.
15. Laurent, L.E. Growth disturbances of the proximal end of the femur in the light of animal experiments. Acta Orthop Scand 28:255–261, 1959.
16. Letournel, E.; Judet, R. Fractures of the Acetabulum. Berlin, Springer Verlag, 1981.
17. Lindseth, R.E.; Rosene, H.A., Jr. Traumatic separation of

the upper femoral epiphysis in a new born infant. J Bone Joint Surg 53-A:1641–1644, 1971.
18. Matta, J.M.; Saucedo, T. Internal fixation of pelvic ring fractures. Clin Orthop 242:83–97, 1989.
19. Matta, J.M.; Mehne, O.K.; Roff, R. Fractures of the acetabulum: Early results of a prospective study. Clin Orthop 205:241–250, 1986.
20. Maull, K.I.; Sachatello, C.R.; Earnst, C.B. The deep perineal laceration—An injury frequently associated with open pelvic fractures: A need for aggressive surgical management. J Trauma 17:685–696, 1977.
21. McDonald, G.A. Pelvic disruptions in children. Clin Orthop 151:130–134, 1980.
22. Niemi, T.A.; Norton, L.W. Vaginal injuries in patients with pelvic fractures. J Trauma 25:547–551, 1985.
23. Ogden, J.A. Changing patterns of proximal femoral vascularity. J Bone Joint Surg 56-A:941–950, 1974.
24. Ponsetti, I.V. Growth and development of the acetabulum in the normal child. J Bone Joint Surg 60-A:575–585, 1978.
25. Quinby, W.C., Jr. Fractures of the pelvis and associated injuries in children. J Pediatr Surg 1:353–364, 1966.
26. Reed, M.H. Pelvic fractures in children. J Can Assoc Radiol 27:255–261, 1976.
27. Reichard, S.A.; Helikson, M.A.; Shorter, N.; et al. Pelvic fractures in children: Review of 120 patients with a new look at general management. J Pediatr Surg 15:727–734, 1980.
28. Rodrigues, K.F. Injury of the acetabular epiphysis. Injury 4:258–260, 1973.
29. Rogge, E.A.; Romano, R.L. Avulsion of the ischial apophysis. J Bone Joint Surg 38-A:442, 1956.
30. Rothenberger, D.A.; Velasco, R.; Strate, R. Open pelvic fractures: A lethal injury. J Trauma 18:184–187, 1978.
31. Routt, M.L., Jr.; Swiontkowski, M.F. The treatment of complex acetabular fractures using combined simultaneous anterior and posterior surgical approaches. J Bone Joint Surg 72-A:897–904, 1990.
32. Slatis, P.; Huittinen, V-M. Double vertical fractures of the pelvis: A report on 163 patients. Acta Chir Scand 138:799–807, 1972.
33. Tile, M. Fractures of the Pelvis and Acetabulum. Baltimore, Williams & Wilkins, 1984.
34. Tile, M. Pelvic ring fractures: Should they be fixed? J Bone Joint Surg 70-B:1–12, 1988.
35. Torode, I.; Zieg, D. Pelvic fractures in children. J Pediatr Orthop 5:76–84, 1985.
36. Trueta, J. The normal vascular anatomy of the femoral head during growth. J Bone Joint Surg 39-B:358–393, 1957.
37. Trunkey, D.D.; Chapman, M.W.; Lim, R.C.; et al. Management of pelvic fractures in blunt trauma injury. J Trauma 14:912–923, 1974.
38. Watts, H.G. Fractures of the pelvis in children. Orthop Clin North Am 7:615–624, 1976.
39. Winquist, R.A.; Hansen, S.T.; Pearson, R.C. Closed intramedullary shortening of the femur. Clin Orthop 136:54–61, 1978.
40. Wojtowycz, M.; Starshak, R.J.; Sty, J.R. Neonatal proximal femoral epiphysiolysis. Radiology 136:647–648, 1980.
41. Wolcott, W.E. The evolution of the circulation in the developing femoral head and neck. Surg Gynecol Obstet 77:61–68, 1943.
42. Young, J.W.R.; Burgess, A.R.; Brumback, R.J.; Poka, A. Lateral compression fractures of the pelvis: The importance of plain radiographs in the diagnosis and surgical management. Skeletal Radiol 15:103–109, 1986.

Proximal Femur Fractures

43. Canale, S.T.; Bourland, W.I. Fracture of the neck and intertrochanteric region of the femur in children. J Bone Joint Surg 59-A:431–443, 1977.
44. Carrell, B.; Carrell, W.B. Fractures in the neck of the femur in children with particular reference to aseptic necrosis. J Bone Joint Surg 23:225–239, 1941.
45. Chong, K.C.; Chaca, P.B.; Lee, B.T. Fractures of the neck of the femur in childhood and adolescence. Injury 7:111–119, 1975.
46. Colonna, P.C. Fracture of the neck of the femur in children. Am J Surg 6:793, 1929.
47. Compere, E.L.; Garrison, M.; Fahey, J.J. Deformities of the femur resulting from arrestment of growth of the capital and greater trochanteric epiphyses. J Bone Joint Surg 22:909–915, 1940.
48. Craig, C.L. Hip injuries in children and adolescents. Orthop Clin North Am 11:743–754, 1980.
49. Delbet M.P. Fractures du col de femur. Bull Mem Soc Chir 35:387–389, 1907.
50. DeLuca, F.N.; Keck, C. Traumatic coxa vara—a case report of spontaneous correction in a child. Clin Orthop 116:125–128, 1976.
51. Durbin, F.C. Avascular necrosis complicating undisplaced fractures of the neck of femur in children. J Bone Joint Surg 41-B:758–762, 1959.
52. Gerber, C.; Lehmann, A.; Ganz, R. Femoral neck fractures in children: A multicenter follow-up study. Z Orthop 123:767, 1985.
53. Honton, J.L. Les fractures transcervicales récentes du femur. Rev Chir Orthop 72:3–51, 1986.
54. Lam, S.F. Fractures of the neck in the femur in children. J Bone Joint Surg 53-A:1165–1179, 1971.
55. Leung, P.C.; Lam, S.F. Long-term follow-up of children with femoral neck fractures. J Bone Joint Surg 68-B:537–540, 1986.
56. Lindseth, R.E.; Rosene, H.A., Jr. Traumatic separation of the upper femoral epiphysis in a new born infant. J Bone Joint Surg 53-A:1641–1644, 1971.
57. Manninger, J.; Kazar, G.; Nagy, E.; Zolczer, L. Phlebography for fracture of the femoral neck in adolescence. Injury 5:244–254, 1973.
58. McDougall, A. Fractures of the neck of femur in childhood. J Bone Joint Surg 43-B:16–28, 1961.
59. Milgram, J.W.; Lyne, E.D. Epiphysiolysis of the proximal femur in very young children. Clin Orthop 110:146–153, 1975.
60. Miller, W.E. Fractures of the hip in children from birth to adolescence. Clin Orthop 92:155–188, 1973.
61. Morrissy, R. Hip fractures in children. Clin Orthop 152:202–210, 1980.
62. Niethard, F.U. Pathophysiologie und Prognose von Schenkelhalsfrakturen im Kindesalter. Unfallheilkunde 158:221–279, 1982.
63. Ogden, J.A. Changing patterns of proximal femoral vascularity. J Bone Joint Surg 56-A:941–950, 1974.
64. Ovesen, O.; Arreskov, J.; Bellstrom, T. Hip fractures in children: A long-term follow-up of 17 cases. Orthopedics 12:361–367, 1989.
65. Pforringer, W.; Rosemeyer, H. Fractures of the hip in children and adolescents. Acta Orthop Scand 51:91–108, 1980.
66. Ratliff, A.H.C. Traumatic separation of the upper femoral epiphysis in young children. J Bone Joint Surg 50-B:757–770, 1968.

67. Ratliff, A.H.C. Fractures of the neck of the femur in children. J Bone Joint Surg 44-B:528–542, 1962.
68. Ratliff, A.H.C. Fractures of the neck of the femur in children. Orthop Clin North Am 5:903–921, 1974.
69. Swiontkowski, M.F.; Winquist, R.A. Displaced hip fractures in children and adolescents. J Trauma 26:384–388, 1986.
70. Trueta, J. The normal vascular anatomy of the femoral head during growth. J Bone Joint Surg 39-B:358–393, 1957.
71. Whitman, R. Observations on fracture of the neck of the femur in children with special reference to treatment and differential diagnosis from separation of the epiphysis. Med Rec 43:227, 1893.

Hip Dislocations

72. Aufranc, O.E.; Jones, W.N.; Harris, H.H. Recurrent dislocation of the hip in the child. JAMA 190:291–294, 1964.
73. Barquet, A. Recurrent traumatic dislocation of the hip in childhood. J Trauma 20:1003–1006, 1980.
74. Barquet, A. Traumatic hip dislocation in childhood: A report of 26 cases and a review of the literature. Acta Orthop Scand 50:549–553, 1979.
75. Bonnemaison, M.F.E.; Henderson, E.D. Traumatic anterior dislocation of the hip with acute common femoral occlusion in a child. J Bone Joint Surg 50-A:753–755, 1968.
76. Bunnell, W.P.; Webster, D.A. Late reduction of bilateral traumatic hip dislocations in a child. Clin Orthop 147:160–163, 1980.
77. Byram, G.; Wickstrom, J. Traumatic dislocation of the hip in children. South Med J 60:805–810, 1967.
78. Canale, S.T.; Manugian, A.H. Irreducible traumatic dislocations of the hip. J Bone Joint Surg 61-A:7–14, 1979.
79. Choyce, C.C. Traumatic dislocation of the hip in childhood and relation of trauma to pseudocoxalgia: Analysis of 59 cases published up to Jan., 1924. Br J Surg 12:52–59, 1924.
80. Dall, D.; McNab, I.; Gross, A. Recurrent anterior dislocation of the hip. J Bone Joint Surg 52-A:574–576, 1970.
81. Elmslie, R.C. Traumatic dislocation of the hip in a child aged seven with subsequent development of coxa plana. Proc R Soc Med 25:1100–1102, 1932.
82. Epstein, H.C. Traumatic dislocations of the hip. Clin Orthop 92:116–142, 1973.
83. Freeman, G.E. Traumatic dislocation of the hip in children. J Bone Joint Surg 43-A:401–406, 1961.
84. Funk, F.J. Traumatic dislocation of the hip in children: Factors influencing prognosis and treatment. J Bone Joint Surg 44-A:1135–1145, 1962.
85. Gartland, J.J.; Benner, J.H. Traumatic dislocations in the lower extremity in children. Orthop Clin North Am 7:687–700, 1976.
86. Gaul, R.W. Recurrent traumatic dislocations of the hip in children. Clin Orthop 90:107–109, 1973.
87. Glass, A.; Powell, H.D.W. Traumatic dislocation of the hip in children: An analysis of 47 patients. J Bone Joint Surg 43-B:29–37, 1961.
88. Graham, B.; Lapp, R.A. Recurrent post-traumatic dislocation of the hip: A report of two cases and review of the literature. Clin Orthop 256:115–119, 1990.
89. Haliburton, R.A.; Brockenshire, F.A.; Barber, J.R. Avascular necrosis of the femoral capital epiphysis after traumatic dislocation of the hip in children. J Bone Joint Surg 43-B:43–46, 1961.
90. Hougaard, K.; Thomsen, P.B. Traumatic hip dislocation in children: Follow-up of 13 cases. Orthopedics 12:375–378, 1989.
91. MacFarlane, I.J.A. Survey of traumatic dislocation of the hip in children. J Bone Joint Surg 58-B:267, 1976.
92. Mason, M.L. Traumatic dislocation of the hip in childhood: Report of a case. J Bone Joint Surg 36-B:630–632, 1954.
93. Nelson, M.C.; Lauerman, W.C.; Brower, A.C.; Wells, J.R. Avulsion of the acetabular labrum with intraarticular displacement. Orthopedics 13:889–891, 1990.
94. Nerubay, J. Traumatic anterior dislocation of hip joint with vascular damage. Clin Orthop 116:129–132, 1976.
95. Pearson, D.E.; Mann, R.J. Traumatic hip dislocation in children. Clin Orthop 92:189–194, 1973.
96. Pennsylvania Orthopaedic Society. Traumatic dislocation of the hip joint in children. J Bone Joint Surg 42-A:705–710, 1960.
97. Piggot, J. Traumatic dislocation of the hip in childhood. J Bone Joint Surg 43-B:38–42, 1961.
98. Simmons, R.L.; Elder, J.D. Recurrent post-traumatic dislocation of the hip in children. South Med J 65:1463–1466, 1972.
99. Speer, K.P.; Spritzer, C.E.; Harrelson, J.M.; Nunley, J.A. Magnetic resonance imaging of the femoral head after acute intracapsular fracture of the femoral neck. J Bone Joint Surg 72-A:98–103, 1990.
100. Stewart, M.J., Milford, L.W. Fracture dislocation of the hip. J Bone Joint Surg 36-A:315–342, 1954.
101. Strömqvist, B. Femoral head vitality after intracapsular hip fracture—490 cases studied by intravital tetracycline labeling and Tc-MDP radionuclide imaging. Acta Orthop Scand (Suppl) 200:1–71, 1983.
102. Wilson, D.W. Traumatic dislocation of the hip in children: A report of four cases. J Trauma 6:739–743, 1966.

M. L. Chip Routt, Jr., M.D.

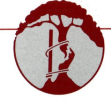

11

Fractures of the Femoral Shaft

Femoral shaft fractures in children continue to challenge the orthopaedic surgeon. Conservative management has historically been advocated, with good results in most cases. The strategies employed have included traction, splinting, and spica casting.[1, 6, 7, 12, 23, 24, 31, 32, 57] As knowledge of physiology, biomechanics, and skeletal development has expanded, the healing of pediatric femoral fractures and thus the foundation for these good results have become better understood. The orthopaedic literature is replete with reports of the outcomes of specific treatment protocols.[1, 2, 7, 9, 12, 23, 24, 26, 31, 32, 36, 39, 40, 42, 50, 51, 55, 61, 66] Other authors have noted the complications of both the fracture and different treatment methods.[4, 8, 11, 25, 28, 47, 49, 52, 54, 56, 63] Skin problems, Volkmann's ischemia, pin track infections, malunions, and others have been identified. Operative treatment has historically been condemned.[6, 12]

Improvement in operative technology has begun to influence the management of the injured child. In general, children with isolated, low-energy pediatric femoral shaft fractures are treated according to accepted conservative methods, whereas the polytraumatized child with a femur fracture is managed more aggressively. Operative methods must also be considered in the child with numerous bony injuries to avoid prolonged immobilization.

Anatomy and Development

Embryonic growth of the femur begins during the fourth week of gestation with the appearance of the limb bud. Rapid mesenchymal growth ensues, and enchondral ossification occurs during the eighth gestational week. Fetal development may be monitored using ultrasound to assess femoral growth sequentially. The femoral shaft serves as the primary ossification center, progressing circumferentially and producing trabecular bone. Ossification of the secondary centers of growth begins in the upper epiphysis at 6 months of gestational age. The distal femoral ossification center develops in the seventh month, and longitudinal and peripheral growth continues. Owing to its trabecular nature and cartilage content, the femur is sufficiently malleable to accommodate passage through the birth canal. With maturation and development, the composition of the femur changes. The bone becomes more like adult bone in being less flexible and containing more mineral. The trabecular bone is remodeled along lines of stress into lamellar bone. This increases the rigidity of the femur and its tensile strength. The greater trochanteric apophysis ossifies by age 4 years. The lesser trochanteric apophysis usually is seen radiographically by 10 years of age. Longitudinal and peripheral growth continues until skeletal maturity. The femur contributes approximately 26% of the adult height.

The femoral shaft blood supply consists of endosteal (medullary) and periosteal vessels. The large muscular cuff of the thigh, together with the thick periosteum of the child's femur, provides excellent vascularity. There are generally two nutrient arteries to the femoral diaphysis, both entering posteromedially. These enter the medullary canal of the femur at the junction of the proximal and middle thirds and the distal and middle thirds of the femoral shaft. This abundant blood supply aids both in growth and in the healing of the skeletally immature femur. Biologically active periosteum and osseous vascularity promote rapid formation and remodeling of callus in pediatric femoral shaft fractures.

Along with growth and vascular changes in the femur during development go architectural changes. Both the neck-shaft orientation and anteversion of the neck decrease with growth. In early childhood, neck-shaft angles are typically 150 degrees, and femoral anteversion begins at about 40 degrees, decreasing by the end of adolescence to 130 ± 7 degrees of neck-shaft angle and 10 ± 4 degrees of anteversion. The anterior curvature (mean 2.2 M radius of curvature) of the femur is maintained during development. These unique features of the developing femur are vital to remember when planning the management of pediatric femoral shaft fractures.

Injury

Most fractures in children are the result of accidents. Accidents are the leading cause of childhood mortality and rank second to acute infections as the cause of morbidity and visits to a physician throughout childhood.[3, 21, 22, 33, 41, 44] Almost half of all deaths in childhood are the result of an accident, compared with about 10% in adults, according to Gratz.[21] Between the ages of 1 and 15 years, accidents are the number one cause of death and injury to children.[21] Izant and Hubay stated, "Accidental injury is one of the poorest understood and most serious social, economic, and medical phenomenon of current times."[33] Unfortunately, minimal funding is directed to accident prevention research in children; therefore, accidents will probably continue to be responsible for high numbers of pediatric femoral shaft fractures in the future.[33] In 1990, 237,000 children under the age of 15 years were treated at hospital emergency rooms for injuries related to playground equipment. Most of these injuries (58%) occurred after falls from swings or monkey bars.[3] Accidents of this type can be responsible for femoral shaft fractures, but these injuries also occur in auto-pedestrian, auto-bicycle, unrestrained auto passenger, and other high-energy mishaps. Minor associated injuries rarely complicate the management of the femoral shaft fracture. Incidental, low-energy accidents may cause femoral shaft fractures in those children with pathologic bone lesions.[13, 14] Blount stated, in his classic text on fractures in children, that approximately 70% of pediatric femur fractures are diaphyseal.[6]

Femoral shaft fractures commonly are isolated injuries or are associated with minor trauma, such as abrasions and contusions. High-velocity trauma in the child will produce unstable fracture patterns with a constellation of other more severe and often life-threatening injuries. Blount recognized that fracture patterns, and concomitant injury patterns, reflect the mechanism of injury.[6] Treatment algorithms, therefore, are different for these two populations of children with femoral shaft fractures.

Child abuse comprises a spectrum of injuries, including fractures of the femoral shaft. The incidence of child battering is estimated at 500,000 new cases annually.[48] According to Green and Haggerty, an abused child has a 50% chance of further battering and a 10% chance of death when returned to his or her home without proper therapeutic intervention.[22] Direct and indirect loads applied to the pediatric femur produce fractures that are often typical of abuse. The radiographic image identifies the fracture type or pattern and may also reveal more subtle findings to alert the physician to a potential child abuse situation. These cases should be fully explored using a team approach. Ignoring these warning signs may result in more severe injury and even death of the child.[5, 18]

Diagnosis

HISTORY/BEHAVIOR

The history of the injury is important in formulating an accurate diagnosis. The parent or accompanying adult usually provides details of the traumatic event. In situations of vehicular trauma, an uninjured adult or emergency medical technician at the scene may furnish vital information to the physicians. Apparent speed of the automobile, tire skid marks, number of people injured or dead, patient presentation at the scene, use of passenger restraints or car seats, and extrication times should be reported accurately. These factors are related directly to the energy of trauma and consequently to the severity and type of potential injury. High-energy trauma forces the clinician to rule in or rule out associated life-threatening injuries, which are less likely in lower velocity accidents.

Children with isolated femoral shaft fractures should be interviewed privately in a calm and quiet environment. A busy emergency room is a poor locale to obtain the history because the patient may be distracted and frightened by the surrounding activities. A private treatment room must be reserved for these instances. Such a setting allows the child to tell his or her own story without parental involvement or active influence. Clues to potential abuse situations may be offered by the child when interviewed alone. The presence of the abuser may force the patient to alter the story in a characteristic attempt to shield the abuser for fear of retribution. The parent or accompanying adult is interviewed separately in order to assess discrepancies in the history. The parental history should be consistent with that of the child and the facts coincident with developmental milestones. For example, a 3-month-old infant does not "fall down while *walking* on the bed." Parental (or accompanying adult) behavior is likewise observed critically. Abnormal adult behavior, such as excessive comforting of a stoic child or refusal to leave the child, can typify abuse situations and must be further evaluated using the team approach. The patient is admitted to the hospital not only for fracture care but for further investigation of the family situation. Potential abuse should not be forgotten in children with metabolic bone diseases, neurologic disorders, and other chronic afflictions that predispose them to fractures. Often these patients place high demands on the caregiver, which can be stressful and lead to abuse of the child.[35]

PHYSICAL EXAMINATION

The physical examination is done individually based on the child's developmental skills, such as the ability to communicate, as well as on the impact of the injury on the child. Infants, young children, and even older polytraumatized children are unable to provide subjective complaints to aid in localizing the physical examination. A meticulous physical examination may be the most important step in disclosing important information relevant to the injury. The patient should be reassured and informed regarding the details of the examination. This not only comforts the already apprehensive child but also secures trust so that he or she may cooperate more fully. The examination must not be limited to the involved extremity. The patient should be disrobed carefully and examined thoroughly. Orthopaedically, this includes palpation of each and every bone in its entirety. Deformed, painful, or swollen areas should be avoided until after all other normal-appearing regions have been evaluated. The obviously injured extremity is checked carefully for both neurologic and vascular function prior to manipulative reduction and splinting. The reduction should be gentle, and the splint should not be circumferential. The extremity is then retested for neurologic and vascular functions to assure that no harm was done by the manipulation. A gentle reduction and comfortable splint should provide pain relief. A difference in the neurovascular status of the extremity after reduction or splinting mandates immediate release of all bandages and removal of the splint.

High-energy trauma changes the focus of the physical examination, which is divided into two phases: (1) the primary resuscitative, and (2) the secondary definitive, injury-specific examination. Initial efforts are directed at resuscitation of the child. Airway, breathing, and circulation take priority (see Chapter 4). The unobstructed airway is secured and the presence of breathing established. Hemodynamic instability in the polytraumatized child may stem from numerous sources. All potential bleeding sources are carefully evaluated during the resuscitation phase. Hemorrhage can occur as a result of a fractured femur, especially from high-energy trauma, and should be a preventable cause of death. A team approach to the resuscitation effort, including the presence of the orthopaedist, is vital to improve survivability in these patients. All members of the team work together simultaneously, rather than in a sequential or staged manner. The team approach allows evaluation, resuscitation, and initial treatment to proceed and is recommended in polytraumatized children. For example, once a patent airway is assured and intravenous lines are placed, the orthopaedist rapidly palpates each extremity and the spine. The child must be logrolled into the lateral decubitus position in order to accomplish the latter examination. Crepitus, deformity, and open wounds are indicative of potential underlying bony injury. Obvious fractures can be reduced and splinted, and open wounds are covered with sterile dressings while other team members work to fully treat the child. The team leader, usually a trauma surgeon, is responsible for the resuscitation effort while prioritizing the injuries. Once stabilized, the patient is evaluated more carefully by the orthopaedist during the second phase of the examination.

Missed diagnoses may be catastrophic or produce a lifelong disability and should be preventable. Head-injured children pose a challenge and warrant repeated daily examinations, ideally by different physicians, to detect occult fractures. Femoral shaft fractures can mask an ipsilateral femoral neck fracture or hip dislocation; therefore, ecchymosis and asymmetry of the buttock must be sought during the physical examination. Fifty percent of these injuries are late diagnoses in some reported series. Femoral head viability is affected by both missed hip dislocations and femoral neck fractures in association with ipsilateral femoral shaft fractures.[16, 27, 30, 45, 58, 62]

RADIOLOGIC EVALUATION

High-quality anteroposterior (AP) and lateral plain radiographs of the femur, including both the hip and the knee joints, generally yield the information necessary to diagnose a pediatric femoral shaft fracture. Poor-quality images must not be accepted but rather x-ray studies must be repeated until satisfactory. The physician or parent may assist in positioning and holding the extremity as well as comforting the child during the process. These biplanar radiographs demonstrate the fracture pattern and displacements. Unopposed muscle contractions across the fracture produce deformities and displacements. In proximal third shaft fractures the typical deformity is flexion, external rotation, and abduction of the proximal fragment due to the forces of the iliopsoas, gluteus medius, and gluteus maximus muscles. Shaft fractures at other levels also produce predictable deformities based on muscle attachments. Similarly, an associated ipsilateral posterior hip dislocation is heralded by adduction and internal rotation of the proximal fragment of the femoral shaft.[62] Imaging the joint both above and below the shaft fracture is mandatory so that ipsilateral associated fractures and dislocations, including physeal injuries, are not missed. Bone quality and preexisting bony abnormalities should be apparent on the plain radiographs.

Computed and plain tomography may be useful in certain situations to better identify associated physeal and intraarticular fractures. Bone scans aid in diagnosing stress fractures, pathologic fractures, and other more occult problems related to the femoral shaft. Bone scans and skeletal surveys are also important in cases of child abuse to demonstrate the extent of injuries. Magnetic resonance imaging is being investigated to assess its value in trauma but has no routine indications at this time. Arteriography is indicated when the femoral shaft fracture is associated with absent distal pulses, knee dislocation, proximal tibial physeal fractures, or an ipsilateral tibial fracture (floating knee). Gonadal shielding for the child should be used, especially when numerous imaging studies are necessary.

Classification

The classification of a femoral shaft fracture should provide information, guide treatment, be easy to remember, and allow communication between physicians. Shaft fractures of the femur are usually classified based on (1) skin integrity, (2) etiology or energy, (3) fracture pattern, (4) preexisting bony or neurologic abnormalities, and (5) displacements.

A fracture is open (or compound) when the normal skin envelope is violated. The soft tissue barrier may be disrupted by sharp bony fragments from within or by external factors. Both allow communication of the fracture with environmental pathogens, thereby increasing the potential for bone infection. Open femoral shaft fractures in children reflect high-energy trauma. The thick periosteum and muscular cuff of the thigh usually contain the bony fragments at the time of injury. Greater energy produces greater deformation of the fragments, which increases the risk of open fracture. Contamination, comminution, and soft tissue violation determine the severity of the open fracture. Ballistic fractures are rare in young children but seem to be increasing in frequency among inner city adolescents. Ballistic fractures are open injuries in which the severity is dependent on the missile energy. Rifle and shotgun blasts cause high-velocity injuries producing extensive bony and soft tissue damage as well as contamination due to cavitation effects.

The origin of most pediatric femoral shaft fractures is accidental blunt trauma. Knowing the energy of the injury is important in order to predict the "behavior" of the fracture. This behavior is reflected in the difficulty of obtaining and maintaining the reduction and in healing times. Comminuted shaft fractures reflect high energy and respond differently to conventional management than low-energy fractures with minimally disrupted periosteal sleeves. High-energy trauma should alert the physician to potential associated diagnoses. Another low-energy type of femur fracture is the "birth fracture," produced by forced traumatic vaginal delivery.[53]

The femoral shaft fracture pattern is best classified by descriptive terms. Spiral, oblique, transverse, greenstick (or unicortical), and comminuted—descriptive terms that are related to the direction and energy of the applied load—are familiar and easy to remember.

Femoral shaft fractures may be seen in situations of incidental, minimal trauma. These cases alert the orthopaedist to the possibility of underlying bony abnormalities. Weakened or pathologic bone may result from metabolic, inflammatory, neurologic, or other disorders. Certain pharmacologic agents interrupt normal bone calcium-phosphorus homeostasis, which may affect the strength of the diaphyseal bone. In this setting, fractures of the femoral shaft may be the result of trivial trauma, and the history must alert the physician to this possibility. The underlying cause should be treated as well as the fracture. Potential primary or metastatic tumors mandate a multidisciplinary evaluation by a pediatrician, a pediatric oncologist, and an orthopaedist with special training. Femoral shaft fractures in children with neurologic disorders may present on a delayed basis, since the fractures are not associated with the typical pain response, and the clinical picture may be more suggestive of infection. Injury can result simply from rolling over in bed with minor associated trauma being the rule.[10, 13, 14, 34]

Femoral shaft fractures are also classified according to their displacement patterns. Shortening is quantified on the lateral radiograph. Angular and rotatory deformities reflect the action of unbalanced muscle forces across the fractured shaft. Angulation is described using the apex of the deformity as a reference. Terms such as varus and valgus usually confuse physicians other than orthopaedists. Apex angulation is more precise and more easily remembered.

Decision Making

The orthopaedic literature on pediatric femoral shaft fractures consists primarily of noncontrolled retrospective case series focused on treatment alternatives.[1, 2, 6, 7, 9, 12, 19, 20, 23, 24, 26, 29, 31, 32, 36, 37, 39, 40, 42, 43, 49–51, 53, 55, 57–61, 65, 66] All seem to have excellent outcomes, yet these are inadequately defined. Many factors affect the ultimate treatment plan which includes considerations of patient, physician, and institution, among others, as well as financial concerns. Humberger and Eyring advocated, "the simplest, safest, and most effective method should be the treatment of choice."[31] Dameron and Thompson outlined seven principles of pediatric femoral shaft fracture care:[12]

1. The simplest form of satisfactory treatment is the best.
2. Initial treatment should be permanent treatment whenever possible.
3. Perfect anatomic reduction is not essential for perfect function.
4. Restoration of alignment is more important than the position of the fragments with respect to one another.
5. More potential growth equals more likely restoration of normal architecture due to remodeling.
6. Overtreatment is usually worse than undertreatment.
7. The injured limb should be immobilized in a Thomas splint before definitive therapy is begun, until there is no danger to the patient or limb. Prolonged elevation of the limb of a child with incipient shock should be avoided owing to the potential for contribution to compartmental syndrome.

Most authors recommend treatment based upon patient age. Younger children with isolated femoral shaft fractures are managed by a variety of closed techniques, whereas the older, or polytraumatized, child receives more aggressive intervention. The remodeling potential of the child justifies such a decision. The family or social situation of the child affects the treatment plan. Potentially abused children require admission to the hospital while the team investigates the case, whereas children with favorable family environments may be candidates for immediate casting and discharge home. These patient-family issues can complicate management.

Physician experience and training affect the treatment plan. Physicians with little experience may feel overwhelmed tackling these injuries. Pediatric femoral shaft fractures require strict attention to detail and frequent, meticulous follow-up. Parental education regarding the injury is also time-consuming. These demands may overly challenge some busy practitioners. Early patient referral is advised in these situations. The hospital or institution may likewise urge the transfer of the patient, especially when lack of accreditation or facilities to care for children exists. Immobilization in a spica cast with early discharge to home, when indicated, is less expensive.[1] Given equivalent results, this method may be the treatment of choice when local inpatient pediatric services or familial resources are lacking.

Management

Treatment alternatives include both invasive and less invasive methods. Most authors use the terms "operative" and "conservative." Some forms of conservative treatment, however, are quite aggressive both to the child and to the family, so the term "less invasive" is preferred. Spica casting, either immediate or after a period of traction, is representative of the less invasive approach. Some less invasive treatment methods may require hospitalization, with social, educational, and financial implications. Invasive treatments include skeletal traction, pins and plaster, external fixation, intramedullary nailing procedures, and plating for femoral shaft fractures. The invasive methods all necessitate hospitalization. Combinations of methods are occasionally indicated, as in spica casting to augment or protect internal fixation.

LESS INVASIVE TREATMENT

Less invasive techniques preserve the soft tissue envelope of the thigh. These methods currently are the predominant treatment for pediatric femoral shaft fractures. Uniformly reproducible, good outcomes can be expected. The decision of how to treat the fracture is based on numerous factors, with patient age, mechanism of injury, and associated injuries being the most important. Although this injury rarely occurs in utero, the youngest patient with a femoral shaft fracture is the newborn infant.[10] "Birth fractures" are incurred during a traumatic delivery and can be difficult to diagnose. The infant may have minimal deformity and crepitus. The fractured femur may be noticed by the neonatologist or intensive care nurse as pseudoparalysis of the extremity. In this setting, septic arthritis of the hip and other systemic causes must be ruled out. Plain radiographs of the femur demonstrate the fracture. Robinson in 1938 described an overhead traction apparatus for the infant with a femoral birth fracture, but this is not necessary and may be risky.[53] Today, simple splinting is the treatment of choice to prevent excessive angular or rotational deformities. The splint is discontinued when the fracture is clinically nontender. Rapid consolidation within 3 weeks is the rule. Longitudinal growth corrects the residual minor deformities. In utero fracture or more than one birth fracture should alert the physician to a potential bone disease, such as osteogenesis imperfecta.[10, 13]

Skin Traction

Skin traction requires initial hospitalization. In cooperative family situations, home traction can be used. Skin traction is usually reserved for younger children, although it can be used in the older child as temporary immobilization prior to casting. Various techniques are advocated, with the common goals being fracture union, alignment and length maintenance, and avoidance of skin problems. Obviously, this method is not indicated in children with insensate skin regions or open wounds of the affected extremity.

Technique. The patient should be sedated during the procedure to provide comfort, especially during transport from stretcher to bed. The skin is cleansed and then prepared with a nonallergenic adherent dressing to prevent skin irritation. The prominences of the malleoli and heel are well protected with cast padding, and the leg is wrapped. Adhesive straps are applied to the cotton padding both medially and laterally and secured with an overwrap of Ace bandage. The straps are attached to a footplate, which is connected to the desired weights through a pulley system. The pulley system is adjusted to obtain the necessary angle of traction. Hip flexion is secured using a folded blanket posterior to the thigh, or a sling about the thigh attached to a weight through a pulley system. The contralateral extremity is likewise padded, wrapped, and placed in traction. Wooden blocks or other stable items are placed beneath the foot of the bedposts. Elevation of the foot of the bed prevents the child from slipping down the bed because of the traction pull.

Accurate AP and lateral radiographs are obtained to assess alignment and distraction of the fracture. Only the lateral x-ray is reliable in assessing length, since the proximal fragment may be flexed by the iliopsoas muscle. Apex anterior angulation (flexion) at the fracture site may give a false impression of adequate, or even excessive, distraction on an AP radiograph. The traction weight amount is adjusted accordingly. The patient should be comfortable in traction. Any complaint related to the lower extremities, especially the contralateral normal side, is thoroughly investigated. This may require frequently removing the skin wraps to assess the skin. Failure to recognize a skin pressure problem can be catastrophic. Skin traction is maintained until early clinical or radiographic union is noted. Early clinical union is reflected as a nontender fracture site with palpable callus. Radiographic signs of early union are callus formation and incorporation. The patient is usually casted at this point. The spica cast is maintained for a total of 6 to 8 weeks, depending on the clinical and radiographic healing response. Younger patients may require a shorter immobilization period, and each child is treated individually.

Immediate Spica Casting

Casting of pediatric femoral shaft fractures should be limited to spica casting techniques. Staheli and Sheridan[57] identified five requisites for spica casting: (1) reliable parents; (2) uncomplicated femoral shaft fractures; (3) otherwise, normal children less than 8 years of age; (4) anesthesia possible; and (5) an initial period of traction. Allen and co-workers advocated early reduction and cast application without initial traction. They reported better results than after initial traction, lower cost, and less hospitalization with such treatment.[1]

Technique. The patient must be adequately sedated during cast application, and general anesthesia is frequently necessary. A pediatric fracture table affords access to the patient and simplifies the procedure (Fig. 11–1A). The cast can be applied either immediately or following a period of traction. Casting strategies vary. Both Irani and associates[32] and Allen and colleagues[1] advocated placement of a long leg, well-molded cast initially. The patient is then transferred to the fracture table, and the remainder of the spica cast is applied. Alternatively, the patient is positioned on the table; the reduction is secured by an assistant (who should be slow to fatigue); and the spica cast is applied. Staheli and Sheridan[57] advocate placement of the patient on the fracture table followed by casting. An assistant applies "fixed skin traction" at the child's ankles (Fig. 11–1A). Prior to finishing the cast, radiographs are obtained to assess reduction and alignment. Distraction is evaluated on the lateral x-ray. Wedging of the cast to perfect any residual deformity is completed. Repeat films confirm the reduction, and the cast is finished.

The spica cast begins at the nipple level and extends to include various portions of the extremities. A small towel temporarily placed on the chest beneath the padding permits full respiratory excursion while in the cast. Bony prominences are well protected using extra layers of cotton padding or thick self-adherent foam cushions applied over the cotton padding. The anterior superior iliac crest, femoral condyles, patella, malleoli, Achilles tendon, and calcaneus are the regions of concern. The groin, buttock, and knee areas are reinforced using splints to avoid cast breakdown. A wooden or plaster connecting bar placed anteriorly between the thighs (applied as necessary after wedging is completed) helps reinforce the construct and also can serve as a handle for patient transport. Some authors advocate inclusion of the ipsilateral foot in the cast, while others advocate removing the footplate on the affected side. Irani and colleagues reported displace-

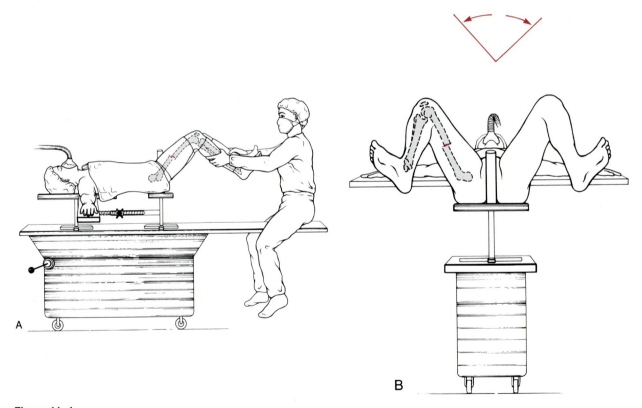

Figure 11–1

A, Spica casting for femoral shaft fractures. The reduction is maintained by the surgeon. Excellent condylar and buttock molding avoids the complication of shortening in the cast. Biplanar x-rays reveal deformities. Shortening and rotational deformities are not corrected by wedging. Wedging to correct angular deformities should be done before the crossbar is added. *B,* Hip abduction should allow perineal hygiene. Excessive abduction can injure the femoral head blood supply. The hip and knee flexions are adjusted to slightly suspend the heels from the bed.

ment of the fracture in those whose cast included a footplate.[32] The position of the extremities in the cast provides fracture reduction and adequate perineal/toileting access for the parent. Insufficient hip abduction prevents good perineal hygiene, which is required for the casted child (Fig. 11–1B). Excessive maximal hip abduction should be avoided owing to the presumed effects on blood flow to the femoral head. The hip and knee should each be flexed so that the heel is slightly suspended from the bed. Excessive knee flexion will transfer pressure to the heel. Attention to details during cast application averts many problems that are due simply to positioning or plastering errors.

Immediate spica casting is a more demanding technique. Without the benefit of initial traction and early healing, the fracture remains unstable. Controlling the fracture reduction during cast application becomes a real challenge. The assistant works hard to maintain the proper distraction, rotation, and position of the lower extremities as the cast is applied. Even in younger, smaller children this is difficult. Heavy children require more than one assistant to secure the extremities. Maintenance of distraction is critical to avoid excessive shortening or collapse of the fracture in the cast. Minor angular deformity is correctable with wedging; excessive shortening is not. Relaxation of muscular spasm is important to the reduction, and the anesthesiologist must therefore be informed. Cast molding at the femoral condyles and buttock region is critical if shortening is to be avoided. Frequent follow-up radiographs are mandatory. Both Allen and co-workers[1] and Staheli and Sheridan[57] define excessive shortening as more than 15 mm. Excessive shortening is unacceptable and is treated with cast removal and traction. Repeat casting is done when the fracture becomes length stable. Allen and co-workers have provided guidelines to acceptable deformities; no rotational malalignment is accepted. Ten degrees or less of apex medial (valgus) or apex lateral (varus) angulation and less than 15 degrees of procurvatum or recurvatum may be tolerated.[1] Irani and associates had similar guidelines for accepted deformities.[32] Most angular deformities can be prevented with precise closed reduction and can be corrected with accurate cast wedging (Fig. 11–2).

INVASIVE TREATMENT

Skeletal Traction

Skeletal traction is generally reserved for older children with isolated fractures. The specific technique of skeletal traction varies. Distal femoral or proximal tibial sites are most frequently used for pin placement. Which bone is chosen depends on four considerations: (1) the status of the knee ligaments, (2) the level of the femoral shaft fracture, (3) ipsilateral extremity trauma, and (4) the age of the patient. Proximal tibial pins are not recommended in children under the age of 10 years owing to the potential for proximal tibial physeal injury.[6] A distal femoral traction pin is used when the knee joint is injured or its stability is unknown. Likewise, an ipsilateral tibial fracture usually precludes placement of a proximal tibial traction pin. The femoral shaft fracture should be more easily controlled with a femoral pin.

Technique. The pin is placed using aseptic technique. The pin size, location, and orientation are planned. Pin placement is critical to optimize the vector of traction pin pull and to avoid growth plate injury. The size is dependent on the type of traction bow to be used. A narrow-diameter pin tensioned adequately (Kirschner bow) is more effective than a larger pin placed in a neutral bow (Boehler bow). The pin may be smooth or threaded. Smooth pins tend to loosen within the bone over a prolonged period. The physician considers the local anatomy carefully prior to pin insertion. The proximal tibia has an unusual apophysis that can easily be injured by errant pin placement. Proximity to the physis is avoided during insertion, and the pin is placed slowly using a hand drill. Heat generated during rapid pin advancement results in thermal injury to the pin track and adjacent physis. This should be avoided to prevent ring sequestrum or physeal bar development. The pin orientation helps correct angular deformity if properly planned. The physician controls the point of insertion, and care is taken to avoid pin bending, especially when narrow-diameter pins are used. Bending may cause the pin to exit the bone in a potentially dangerous area. For this reason, the distal femoral pin is inserted medially and exits laterally. Medial insertion avoids popliteal vascular damage. The opposite holds true in the proximal tibia. The peroneal nerve is most at risk so that the pin is inserted laterally and advanced to exit medially. Fluoroscopic imaging during pin placement provides a safe physeal margin and detects misdirection (Fig. 11–3).

The anesthetic chosen may be local, regional, or general. In younger and less cooperative patients, adequate sedation should supplement the local anesthetic. Liberal local anesthesia should include the periosteum and skin at the point of exit. Biplanar radiographs confirm the pin location. The skin pin

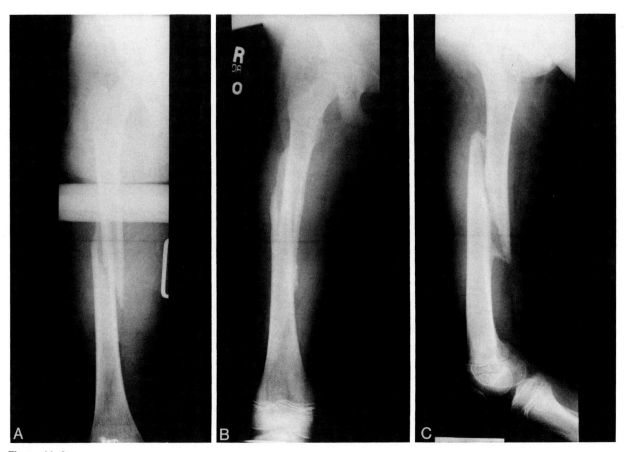

Figure 11–2

A, Plain radiograph of an 8-year-old female after a low-level fall. A temporary splint maintains length and alignment while providing comfort. B, After 8 weeks in an immediately placed spica cast, the femoral fracture demonstrates early healing in a position of varus. C, The lateral image reveals the amount of shortening. The poor cast contour allowed collapse. A period of adjusted skeletal traction, until early consolidation, avoids this situation.

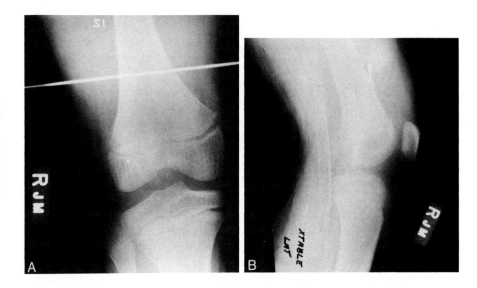

Figure 11–3

A, The traction pin appears to be located safely away from the physis on this AP radiograph. B, A lateral x-ray demonstrates the extraosseous location of the pin. Adequate sedation and fluoroscopic imaging during pin placement allow accurate and safe pin insertion.

sites are treated with frequent cleansing and antiseptic dressings to avoid infection. The amount of initial weight applied as traction depends on the size of the patient. An easy guide is to apply that amount of weight which slightly elevates the ipsilateral buttock from the mattress when using 90/90 traction. The amount of shortening at the fracture site is followed using serial *lateral* plain radiographs. AP images are inaccurate in assessing length because of the usual anterior bowing of the femur as well as the difficulty in obtaining a *true* AP image. The traction weight is adjusted according to the findings on these frequent radiographs. The frequency, determined by the fracture pattern and the difficulty with obtaining the initial reduction, is generally every third or fourth day, at a minimum, during the first 10 to 14 days of treatment.

Pins and Plaster

Pins and plaster techniques have also been used effectively to treat femoral shaft fractures.

Technique. The skeletal traction pin is placed as described earlier, and the patient is immobilized in a spica cast. The skeletal pin is incorporated into the cast and helps maintain the fracture reduction. Unfortunately, the cast denies access to the exit sites of the pin. Systemic signs of inflammation may indicate superficial or deep pin track infection, and pin inspection requires cast removal. Routine femoral condylar molding of the spica cast should provide similar fracture control, thereby avoiding pin site problems in most instances. Because of the inability to observe the pin sites, I do not advocate this method.

External Fixation

External fixation systems have more recently been enthusiastically recommended for pediatric femoral shaft fractures. Quintin and associates[50] recommended external fixation for children with (1) open fractures, (2) fractures associated with neural or vascular damage, (3) fractures associated with central nervous system damage, (4) polytrauma, and (5) fractures that fail more traditional traction/casting treatment. Alonso and Horowitz[2] added burn patients with fractures to the list. In their series they treated five femur fractures with external fixation.[2] Most authors report good results using a variety of frame constructs. The quadriceps muscle mass is spared when the frame is applied laterally (Fig. 11-4). Lateral half-pin frames allow control of the fracture as well as mobilization of both the hip and the knee joints. Pin placement must avoid physes. With external fixation treatment the polytraumatized patient can be placed upright to restore more normal pulmonary function without jeopardizing fracture stability. Head-injured children with combativeness, seizure activity, or spasticity are more easily cared for by the nursing staff when the femoral shaft fracture is controlled by an external fixation device. The frame half-pins should be capped with soft pads to prevent injury to the patient or medical staff by the pins. External fixation systems, which are simple to apply and have few parts, are advantageous. These simple frame constructs can be applied rapidly with minimal blood loss—important factors when dealing with severely injured or clinically unstable children. Prolonged anesthesia and significant blood loss are avoided. The frame can often be applied at the same time as other procedures, such as intracranial pressure monitor placement and diagnostic peritoneal lavage, are ongoing. Fluoroscopic imaging aids pin placement and improves fracture reduction. The reduction can be "fine-tuned" in a forgivable frame system later, when the child is stable, but should not be delayed too long, as head-injured children tend to heal fractures rapidly. Delay in adjusting the frame may result in a malunion. When possible, the initial reduction in the frame should be optimized in all but critical situations. Serial biplanar radiographs evaluate the fracture for changes, especially in the combative or restless patient, and remanipulation is done early. The connecting nuts should be tightened at intervals to prevent frame loosening. The half-pins are cleansed with antiseptic twice daily to avoid pin track problems.

Technique. The patient is generally positioned supine for management of head, chest, or abdominal trauma or for debridement of the open wounds associated with the fracture. For the latter, the skin edges must be sharply cut back, all debris removed, and all nonbleeding crushed or contaminated fat and muscle debrided. This is followed by pulsatile lavage using a minimum of 9 L of fluid; topical antibiotics may be added. The wound is then reinspected for the conditions noted above, and all nonviable (with no significant soft tissue attached) bone is removed. Irrigation may then be repeated.

Based on the study of the injury films, a pin is placed in the longer of the two fracture fragments. The pin will be either a 5 mm standard adult pin or a 4.0 mm (or even 2.5 mm) for smaller children. The pin is placed through a 1 cm stab wound through

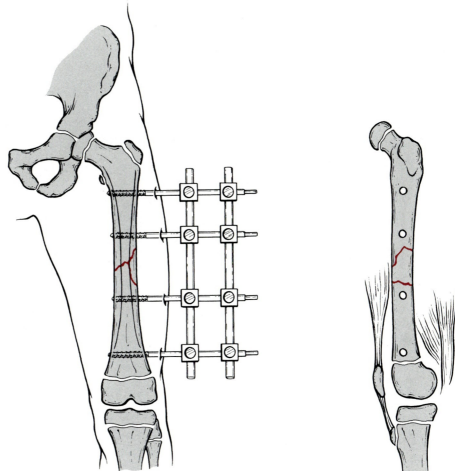

Figure 11–4
A double-bar, unilateral frame construct is shown. The pins are placed posterior to the vastus lateralis muscle belly.

a sleeve system that allows saline cooled predrilling. The length of connecting bar is then selected; a carbon fiber rod is preferred for radiolucency. Two bars are appropriate for length-unstable patterns. Four pin-bar clamps are placed on each bar to be used. The proximal or distal clamp is attached to the pin in the long fragment, and manual traction is applied. The most distal or most proximal pin is then applied through the series of sleeves. This is the crucial step; in order to avoid the use of a bar-to-bar clamp (and maintain the greatest stability), care must be taken to keep the bar directly over the reduced femur throughout its length. This is so the pins placed closest to the fracture hit the bone without being inserted at an angle. This is critical when two connecting bars are stacked, as an angled pin will not be captured by the most external clamp. If this is the case, a pair of bar-to-bar clamps attached to a short intermediate connecting bar will salvage the situation. This configuration also allows for adjusting of the fracture reduction after the frame has been applied (Figs. 11–5 and 11–6).

Intramedullary Nailing

Medullary nailing of pediatric femoral shaft fractures is an excellent treatment method. Reamed nailing in adults was popularized during World War II by Küntscher. The North American experience reported by Winquist and colleagues[64] reproduced excellent clinical results with low rates of infection and malunion. The medullary nailing procedures in the early clinical series were limited to adult patients. Medullary nailing techniques evolved, with nails placed in an antegrade fashion after reaming of the femoral canal. Reaming to the inner cortical diameter provided excellent fit and allowed the nail to function as an internal splint, avoiding the need for external splinting. The traditional method of Küntscher utilized placement of the medullary, antegrade nail through a greater trochanteric starting site. In children, trochanteric apophyseal arrest can occur, producing growth irregularities of the proximal femur, typically a valgus femoral neck deformity. Aseptic necrosis of the femoral head also

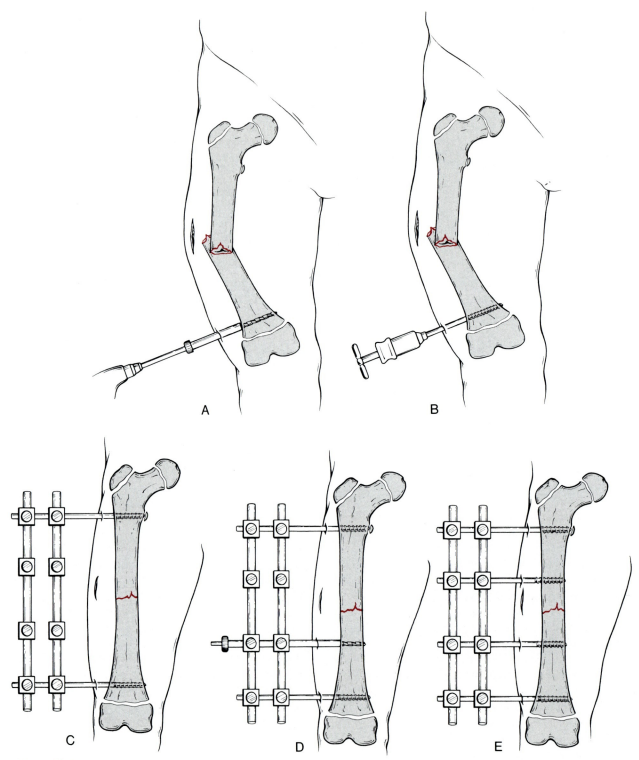

Figure 11–5

A, Schematic representation of pin placement and frame assembly. With the patient anesthetized and using fluoroscopy, the saline cooled drill is used to place the first pin through a stab wound. *B,* The distal far pin (No. 4 pin) is seated adequately, avoiding overpenetration. The fracture is reduced and temporarily manually secured. *C,* The proximal far pin (No. 1 pin) is then placed after predrilling, using the desired frame construct as a guide. The frame must be assembled as needed at this stage. *D,* The distal near pin (No. 2 pin) is placed, again using the frame as a guide. *E,* The unilateral, double-bar frame provides wound access while maintaining fracture stability.

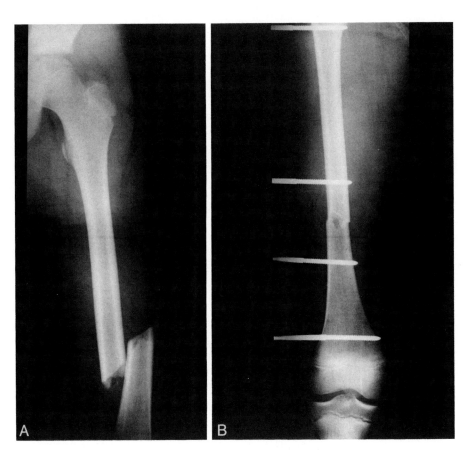

Figure 11–6

A, This 12-year-old male pedestrian was struck by an automobile, sustaining this closed femur fracture and a severe head injury. His intracranial pressure readings were extremely variable, and he demonstrated spasticity. The neurosurgeon requested bone stability with minimal blood volume shift. *B*, An external fixator was placed and used to treat the fracture to union at 10 weeks. The head injury resolved without residua.

rarely occurred after antegrade nailings, most likely as a result of disruption of the delicate vascular supply adjacent to the trochanteric apophysis.

The lateral ascending artery supplies most of the blood to the developing proximal femur between the ages of 3 and 10 years. This artery is located posteriorly in the trochanteric notch. The ascending branches nourish the capital femoral epiphysis, while the descending metaphyseal arteries supply the apophyseal region. Interference with this vascular network about the femoral neck may produce valgus neck deformity and aseptic necrosis of the femoral head. Because of these concerns, femoral nailings in children and adolescents were historically condemned.

Kirby and co-workers[36] compared traction and casting with closed nailing in adolescents with femoral shaft fractures. In this study, the piriformis fossa (the starting point advocated by Winquist and co-workers[64]) was utilized, thereby avoiding the above-noted risks. Remodeling potential is less in the adolescent age group than in the younger patient. These authors found that the casted group had stiffness of the knee as well as rotational and angular deformities of the femur when compared with the group of adolescents treated by nailings. The nailed group had few complications, and this method was especially advocated in those children aged 10 to 15 years with ipsilateral fracture of the tibia or multiple systemic injuries. Kirby and colleagues recommended that the nail be placed antegrade and left just short of the distal femoral physis to allow for remaining longitudinal femoral growth (Fig. 11–7.)[36]

In 1984, Ziv and associates[66] reported their results of open Rush pinning and Küntscher medullary nailing in growing, polytraumatized children. Two incisions were used to place the implant. The lateral approach to the femur fracture provided canal access to allow retrograde reaming. The trochanteric exit point was found using a medullary guide. Retrograde identification of this point avoided injury to the femoral head blood supply, according to the authors. A second buttock incision was made to afford access to the proximal fragment and enable antegrade nail passage. An open reduction was performed as the implant passed across the fracture site. These investigators stated that these methods were reliable and safe in the child but stressed that single Rush pinning provided no rotational control

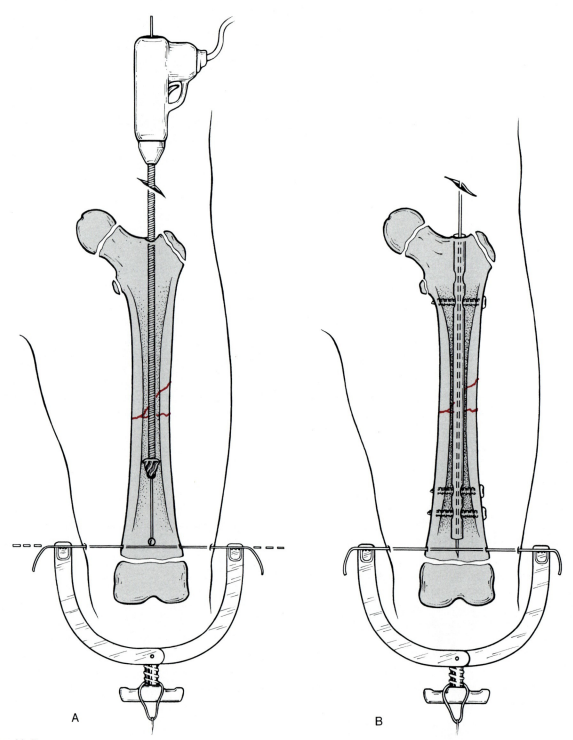

Figure 11–7

A, The piriformis fossa starting point avoids injury to the femoral head blood supply and trochanteric apophysis. Length is determined using the ball-tipped guide wire. Medullary reaming proceeds over the guide wire, avoiding the distal physis. B, The straight-tipped guide wire is exchanged for nail placement after reaming is completed. The guide wire must be removed before interlocking the nail.

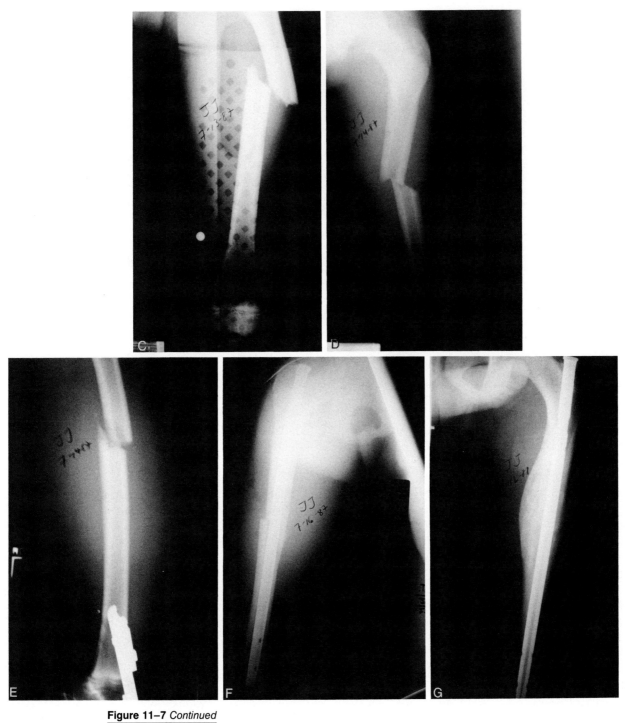

Figure 11-7 *Continued*
C–G, X-ray of a femoral shaft fracture in an adolescent treated with medullary nailing.

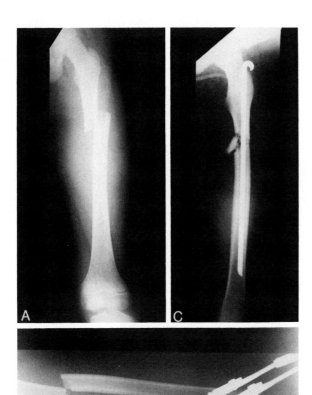

Figure 11–8

A–E, A percutaneous Rush pin technique was used for this fractured femur in a 6-year-old male. The patient was injured in a car crash and clinically was a T10 paraplegic. Spica casting augmented both the spine and femur fixation.

of the fracture, therefore necessitating supplemental casting (Fig. 11–8). Only 10 of the 16 patients were available for direct follow-up. Since growth arrest of the proximal femur is a potential problem with reamed nailings, Ziv and colleagues advised against reaming the proximal fragment in the growing child.[66]

This series, as well as that of Kirby and coworkers, identified no difference in femoral overgrowth with nailings as compared with casting techniques.[36, 66] Femoral nailing has also been advocated in polytraumatized patients and in those with head injuries. This has similar advantages to external fixation but cannot be done percutaneously. Femoral nailing procedures require fluoroscopic imaging for accurate nail placement. The supine or lateral position may be used. The lateral position usually provides better access to the starting point but is contraindicated in patients with pelvic, spinal, or other unstable injuries. A fracture table simplifies the reduction, and therefore the procedure, but is not mandatory.

Flexible or elastic medullary implants have been used to treat pediatric femoral shaft fractures. Mann and associates[42] reported excellent results with Ender nailing techniques in 15 patients between the ages of 9 and 15 years. Ender nails were indicated in polytraumatized or head-injured patients. These authors advocated Ender nailing in those fractures that failed routine closed management.[42] Ligier and co-workers[40] defined "elastic stable intramedullary nailing" in 1988. They treated 123 pediatric femoral shaft fractures with flexible rods introduced retrograde through two incisions in the distal metaphyseal area (Fig. 11–9). Early patient mobilization was possible, and no delayed unions occurred. The complications were minimal, consisting of skin breakdown or knee discomfort caused by the ends of the rods.[40] These results have been reproduced by Kissel and Miller.[38]

Technique. For the hemodynamically stable patient or the one with isolated injuries we favor the lateral decubitus position on the radiolucent fracture table. Fresh fractures can generally be nailed without inserting a skeletal pin. The foot on the injured side is stabilized with the traction boot, and gentle longitudinal distraction is applied. If large forces are required to reduce the fracture, a distal femoral

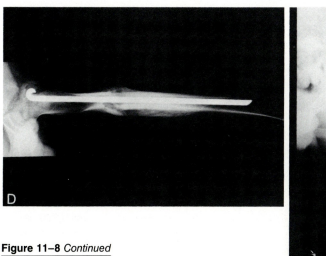
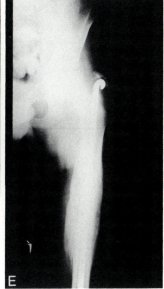

Figure 11–8 *Continued*

traction pin should be inserted in the anterior 1 cm of the femur a minimum of 1 cm proximal to the distal femoral physis under radiographic control. The knee can then be flexed to take the traction off the sciatic nerve. The pelvis must be oblique to the surface of the fracture table so that the femoral necks do not overlie one another on the lateral fluoroscopic view. This is critical for an accurate placement of the starting point; the medial femoral neck and the greater trochanteric apophysis must not be injured.

For unstable or multiply injured patients we prefer the supine position on the fracture table. If there is concern for speed in management of the fracture, the femoral distractor can substitute for the fracture table. The traction pin is inserted in the same position noted above if large traction forces are required, using fluoroscopic control. The injured limb must be adducted to allow better access to the proximal femur for the starting point. If this is made particularly difficult by a very proximal fracture, a percutaneous 4.0 mm pin can be inserted to push the proximal fragment toward the midline. It is inserted through the lateral cortex only, in order to leave the medullary cavity open for the reaming guide rod. Distal locking is done using the free hand method for either position; generally only one distal screw is required unless the fracture is distal to the femoral isthmus. The details regarding the sequence of instruments required to accomplish placement of the intramedullary rod are presented in Figure 11–7.

Plate Fixation

Plating techniques are rarely advocated in the orthopaedic literature for femoral shaft fractures in children. A high infection rate, extensive dissection, and the need for plate removal are concerns that accompany compression plating.[15] Ziv and Rang[65] noted a 60% incidence of infection in four patients with five femoral shaft fractures treated using compression plates. They felt that these polytraumatized patients had a decreased resistance to infection and were more susceptible to nosocomial sepsis.[65] Two recent reports, however, found compression plating to be safe and reliable with low rates of complication.[39, 51] Kregor and co-workers noted excellent results using plating for femoral shaft fractures in polytraumatized children.[39] Fourteen fractures healed without infection, and overgrowth of the femur was not significant. The implant size was dependent on the size of the femur and consequently the age of the patient, yet all were dynamic compression plates applied using proper technique at a Level One trauma center. Postoperative spica casting was reserved for those patients with associated pelvic or spinal trauma requiring immobilization. Hypertrophic scarring on the lateral thigh recurred, even after formal scar revision at the time of plate removal, in the majority of patients.[39]

Technique. The patient is positioned supine with a towel bump under the ipsilateral buttock. If required, a sterile tourniquet of a diameter appropriate for the patient works best. A straight lateral

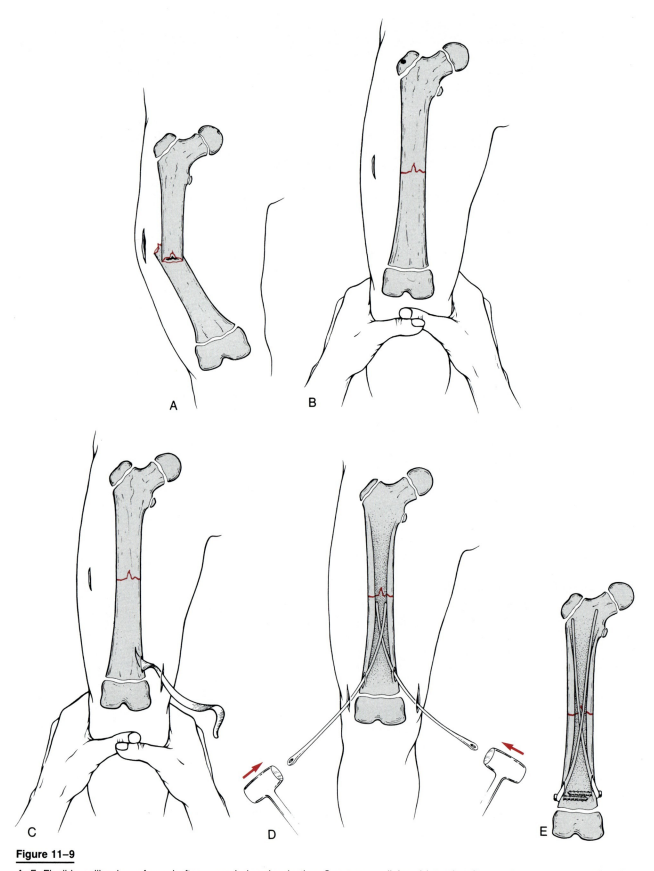

Figure 11–9

A–E, Flexible nailing is performed after manual closed reduction. Separate medial and lateral stab wounds are made, avoiding the distal femoral physis. The implants are advanced simultaneously. Additional implants are used to fill the medullary canal as needed.

incision is made through the fascia lata. The quadriceps is retracted anteriorly, and great care is taken to identify and ligate the perforating arteries and veins. Only the smallest amount of periosteum should be stripped on the proximal and distal fragments—generally the width of the plate. For children age of 12 years and under, the 4.5 mm narrow system is used. We prefer low-contact dynamic compression plates (Fig. 11–10). Plates of six to eight-hole length are adequate. Children under the age of 8 years generally require the 3.5 mm system; the same plate lengths apply. The femoral distractor is helpful in regaining the length needed to perform the plating (Fig. 11–10). Other details regarding the technique are provided in Figure 11–10. We advocate plate removal from the femur for all children. This is generally done, based on the age of the patient, at 6 to 18 months post fracture.

The Multiply Injured Child

The aggressive treatment of pediatric femoral shaft fractures, especially in the polytrauma setting, has many advantages. In 1983, Marcus and co-workers[43] reported on 34 polytraumatized children with 61 total fractures. There were 16 femur fractures. Four patients had residual disabilities as a result of their femoral fractures. All four were treated with closed reduction and spica casting. Three had limb length inequalities, and one had a flexion contracture at the knee. These authors concluded that rigid adherence to the concept of closed management in pediatric fractures may be counterproductive in the polytraumatized patient and may result in increased morbidity. The residual morbidity in these conservatively managed patients was related to their orthopaedic and neural injuries. Marcus and associates felt that acceptance of inadequate fracture alignment because of the severity of associated injuries should be avoided.[43] Because of the reports of excellent function with low rates of infection using operative methods of stabilization, including external fixation, reamed nailing, flexible (Ender) nailing, and plating, in multiply injured children, these approaches are being more widely advocated for isolated fractures. This aggressive approach in the polytraumatized child is in contrast to the advice of Dameron and Thompson[12] regarding isolated femoral shaft fractures. These authors stated that "overtreatment is usually worse than undertreatment."[12] Hansen has stated that although children are more tolerant of severe injury, an aggressive approach saves time, money, disability, and occasionally lives.[26]

Timmerman and colleagues[60] and Reeves and associates[51] demonstrated that operative treatment decreased hospitalization. The latter investigators also estimated conservative management of femur fractures in children to be approximately 46% more expensive than operative management. A shortened hospital stay may well have psychologic, social, educational, and economic benefit.[51]

OUR PREFERRED TREATMENT

The following guidelines are presented according to the age of the child.

Neonate—Splinting for 2 to 3 weeks until united.

1 to 5 years:

   Isolated—Immediate spica casting with close follow-up to limit shortening to 1.5 to 2 cm; wedging as indicated.

   Multiple injuries (especially moderate to severe head injury)—Consider external fixation with small external fixation system for 3 to 4 weeks until callus length stable. Convert to spica cast for additional 3 to 4 weeks.

6 to 10 years:

   Isolated—Spica casting either immediate or after a 10 to 21 day period of traction. Generally, distal femoral pin skeletal traction is necessary in larger/older children. In larger 9- and 10-year-olds closed intramedullary nailing may be offered to the family as an alternative.

   Multiple injuries—Internal or external fixation. The latter is favored when there is severe head injury. The more hemodynamically stable the patient, the more we advocate plating or nailing. Medullary nailing is not done on patients aged 7 years or under because of the potential for trochanteric apophyseal arrest. External fixation with 4 to 5 mm pins is favored for higher grade open fractures.

10 to 15 years:

   Isolated—Initially patients 10 and 11 years of age are placed in skeletal traction to allow the family time to consider the option of nailing. In patients 12 years and older, closed intramedullary nailing utilizing the piriformis fossa as a starting point, leaving the nail short of the distal femoral physis, is the procedure of choice.

   Multiple injuries—Hemodynamically unstable patients or those with moderate to severe head injuries are treated with external fixation or plating. We favor plating when both routes for stabilization of the fracture are acceptable to the anesthesia and trauma teams. More physiologically stable multiply injured patients are treated with closed intramedullary nailing.

14 years and older—Treat as adults.

364 11 / Fractures of the Femoral Shaft

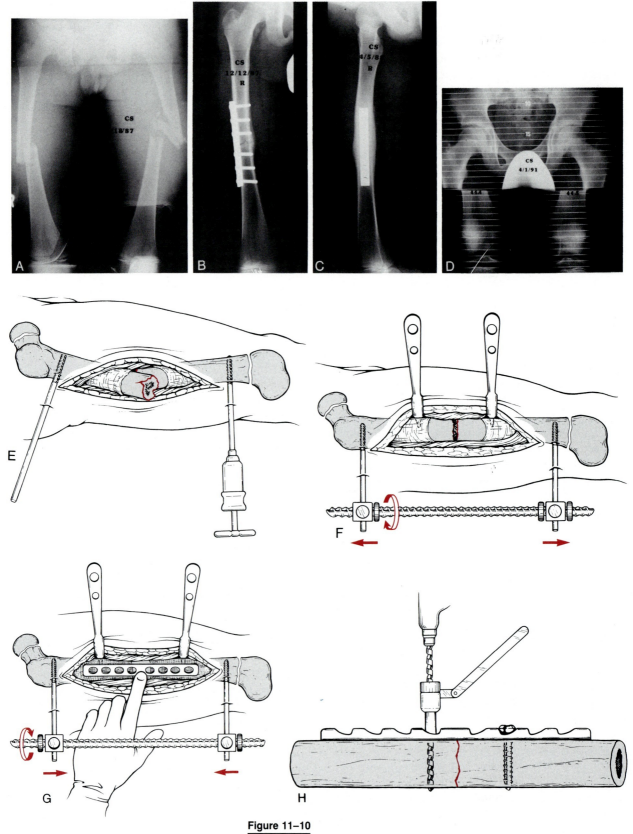

Figure 11–10

See legend on opposite page

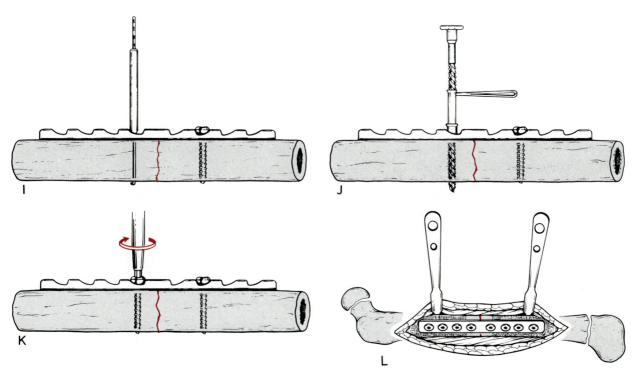

Figure 11–10

A, This 8-year-old polytraumatized male sustained bilateral femoral shaft fractures in an automobile accident. He was treated with open reduction and internal fixation using bilateral compression plates. B, Two months later, periosteal new bone formation is evident bilaterally. C, X-rays at 6 months demonstrate consolidation. D, Scanograms at 3½ years confirm equal limb lengths. E, With the patient supine and the buttock elevated on a bump, a lateral surgical exposure is used. Pins are placed after predrilling. Periosteal stripping is minimized. F, A femoral distractor can be used to grossly align and secure the fracture. Narrow retractors are used to limit soft tissue stripping medially. The retractors should be placed in the same positions throughout the operation. Manipulation of the distractor allows perfect reduction. The distractor can then be reversed to compress the fracture. G, The compression plate is prebent and contoured. A template may be used. H, Eccentric drilling produces fracture compression when the DC plate is used. I, A depth gauge measures length. J, The hole is tapped. K, The eccentrically placed screw is tightened. As the screwhead engages the plate, the fracture is compressed. The plate must be prebent to prevent compression adjacent to the plate and distraction of the opposite cortex. L, Final plate appearance with the distractor removed. Notice the intact periosteum, which was preserved using careful technique.

COMPLICATIONS

Remodeling and Overgrowth

Remodeling will *never* correct rotational malunion. In children older than 9 years, remodeling should not be relied upon to correct angular deformity. The likelihood of correction with remodeling depends on patient age and proximity of the fracture to the physis as well as other factors.[11]

Overgrowth of the fractured femur seems to be most prominent in patients treated between the ages of 8 and 10 years, and therefore some shortening in the original reduction (in the range of 1.5 to 2 cm) is allowable. This phenomenon is variable in older children and adolescents, and it does not seem to be prominent with open reduction. The site of fracture, fracture pattern, and age are not related to overgrowth, but several authors suggest that overgrowth is seen more frequently in more proximal fractures.[31] It may be related to handedness, as identified by Meals,[46] as nondominant-side fractures overgrew more than did dominant-side fractures. Limb length inequality is the most frequent complication of femoral shaft fractures in children, producing limp and compensatory scoliosis. The surgeon should assure equal leg lengths at injury and not accept more than 1.5 to 2 cm of shortening. Growth acceleration is likely related to the amount of osseous and soft tissue disruption, which translates to fracture hyperemia.[56]

Conservative Management of the Multiply Injured Child

Spasticity and restlessness are the main problems in children with moderate to severe head injuries. The head-down position should be avoided because of effects on intracranial pressure. Operative fixation provides immediate stability and simplifies nursing care. Malunion occurred in 6 of 34 fractures treated nonoperatively. None of the 16 patients treated with medullary nailings developed malunion. There were no overgrowth problems in the open-treatment group.[65]

Of 292 children with head injuries in coma for more than 1 week, 39 had 44 femoral shaft fractures. All healed, and 32 of the 39 eventually ambulated. There were no complications in the operatively treated group. Conservative management led to malunion, osteomyelitis, skin breakdown, excessive shortening, and rotational deformities. Open reduction and internal fixation, when feasible in the brain-injured child with a femoral shaft fracture, is an attractive solution to the overall management of this complicated injury.[17]

External Fixation—Pin Track Infection/Refracture

In most series, refracture after frame removal and pin track infections are the most common problems. In 13 patients, one case of refracture and six cases of infection of the pins were recorded in the series of Quintin and co-workers.[50] Kirschenbaum and associates treated ten high-energy femur fractures in children using a variety of lateral frames.[37] All ten healed, with minor deformity noted. Pin track infections occurred in three of the ten patients; all resolved with local care. One patient had spastic cerebral palsy and suffered a refracture after frame removal. The authors recommended brace protection after frame removal, especially in patients with spasticity.[37]

Infection

Infection following closed management of closed fractures is a rare but identified phenomenon. It must be considered when pain of a different character becomes a complaint. An increase in local tissue reaction and erythema when all signs and reactions should be diminishing also brings this possibility to mind. Patients in the series of Canale and colleagues[8] all had a primary source of infection and had a persistent febrile course.

Volkmann's Contracture

Compartment syndrome of the leg can result from prolonged elevation in Bryant's traction, even in the uninjured leg; therefore, this is not advocated as a form of traction treatment.[49] Compartment syndrome can also result from elevation of the injured limb when the patient is hypotensive.[12] When high-velocity trauma produces the fracture, compartment syndrome of the thigh must be considered as a possibility. This is generally manifest by a rigid thigh, severe pain (in the alert patient), and elevated intracompartmental pressures. Fasciotomy on an emergent basis is indicated.

Refracture

Refracture following femoral shaft fracture in children is a rare phenomenon. It is generally associated with highly comminuted fractures with extensive stripping of the bone and is related to manipulation of stiff knees. There does not seem to be a correlation with treatment, deformity, or shortening, since it is seen so seldom.[54]

Traction Pin Complications

Traction pins may produce problems when their position is not radiographically defined. These problems include skin lacerations and disruptions of the knee capsule. When a proximal tibial pin is used and there is an ipsilateral knee injury, ligamentous injuries and physeal disruptions can be made more severe. Finally, poor placement of a proximal tibial pin or multiple passes can result in premature tibial tubercle apophyseal closure and resultant knee recurvatum, which is a very difficult problem to manage. We therefore recommend a distal femoral pin placed under radiographic control for most femoral shaft fractures in the 7- to 12-year-old child.

REFERENCES

1. Allen, B. L.; Kant, A. P.; Emery, F. E. Displaced fractures of the femoral diaphysis in children. J Trauma 17:8–19, 1977.
2. Alonso, J. E.; Horowitz, M. Use of the AO/ASIF external fixator in children. J Pediatr Orthop 7:594–600, 1987.
3. American Academy of Orthopaedic Surgeons. Play It Safe. Chicago, 1991.
4. Beals, R. K. Premature closure of the physis following diaphyseal fractures. J Pediatr Orthop 10:717–720, 1990.
5. Beals, R. K.; Tufts, E. Fractured femur in infancy: The role of child abuse. J Pediatr Orthop 3:583–586, 1983.
6. Blount, W. Fractures in Children. Baltimore, Williams & Wilkins, 1955, p. 129.
7. Burton, V. W.; Fordyce, A. J. W. Immobilization of femoral shaft fractures in children aged 2–10 years. Injury 4:47–53, 1972.
8. Canale, S. T.; Puhl, J.; Watson, F. M.; Gillespie, R. Acute osteomyelitis following closed fractures. Report of three cases. J Bone Joint Surg 57-A:415–418, 1975.
9. Celiker, O.; Cetin, I.; Sahlan, S.; et al. Femoral shaft

fractures in children: Technique of immediate treatment with supracondylar Kirschner wires and one-and-a-half spica cast. J Pediatr Orthop 8:580–584, 1988.
10. Christensen, E.; Dietz, G. A radiographically documented intrauterine femoral fracture. Br J Radiol 51:830–831, 1978.
11. Connolly, J. F. Fractures in children: When the growth plate is damaged. J Musculoskeletal Med 82–97, 1991.
12. Dameron, T. B.; Thompson, H. A. Femoral shaft fractures in children. Treatment by closed reduction and double spica cast immobilization. J Bone Joint Surg 41-A:1201–1212, 1959.
13. Dent, J. A.; Paterson, C. R. Fractures in early childhood: Osteogenesis imperfecta or child abuse. J Pediatr Orthop 11:184–186, 1991.
14. Drennan, J.; Freehofer, A. Fractures of the lower extremity in paraplegic children. Clin Orthop 77:211–217, 1971.
15. Eikenbary, C.; Lecoq, J. F. Fracture of the femur in children. J Bone Joint Surg 14:801–804, 1932.
16. Fardon, D. F. Fracture of neck and shaft of same femur. Report of a case in a child. J Bone Joint Surg 52-A:797–799, 1970.
17. Fry, K.; Hoffer, M. M.; Brink, I. Femoral shaft fractures in brain injured children. J Trauma 16:371–373, 1976.
18. Galleno, H.; Oppenheim, W. L. The battered child syndrome revisited. Clin Orthop 162:11–19, 1982.
19. Gibson, J. M. C. Multiple injuries: The management of the patient with a fractured femur and a head injury. J Bone Joint Surg 42-B:425–431, 1960.
20. Glenn, J.; Miner, M.; Peltier, L. The treatment of fractures of the femur in patients with head injuries. J Trauma 13:958–961, 1973.
21. Gratz, R. R. Accidental injury in childhood. Literature review on pediatric trauma. J Trauma 19:551, 1979.
22. Green, M.; Haggerty, R. J. Ambulatory Pediatrics. Philadelphia, W. B. Saunders, 1968.
23. Gross, R. H.; Davidson, R.; Sullivan, J. A.; et al. Cast brace management of femoral shaft fracture in children and young adults. J Pediatr Orthop 3:572–582, 1983.
24. Guttman, G. G.; Simon, R. Three-point fixation walking spica cast: An alternative to early or immediate casting of femoral shaft fractures in children. J Pediatr Orthop 8:699–703, 1988.
25. Haller, J. Problems in children's trauma. J Trauma 10:269–271, 1970.
26. Hansen, S. T., Jr. Internal fixation of children's fractures of the lower extremity. Orthop Clin North Am 21:353–363, 1990.
27. Helal, B.; Skevis, X. Unrecognized dislocation of the hip in fractures of the femoral shaft. J Bone Joint Surg 49-B:293–300, 1967.
28. Henry, A. N. Overgrowth after femoral shaft fractures in children. J Bone Joint Surg 45-B:222, 1963.
29. Herndon, W. A.; Mahnken, R. F.; Yngve, D. A.; Sullivan, J. A. Management of femoral shaft fracture in the adolescent. J Pediatr Orthop 9:29–32, 1989.
30. Hoeksema, H. D.; Olsen, C.; Rudy, R. Fracture of femoral neck and shaft and repeat neck fracture in a child. J Bone Joint Surg 57-A:271–272, 1975.
31. Humberger, F. W.; Eyring, E. J. Proximal tibial 90-90 traction in treatment of children with femoral shaft fractures. J Bone Joint Surg 51-A:499–503, 1969.
32. Irani, R.; Nicholson, J. T.; Chung, S. M. K. Long-term results in the treatment of femoral shaft fractures in young children by immediate spica immobilization. J Bone Joint Surg 58-A:945–951, 1976.
33. Izant, R.; Hubay, M. The annual injury of 15 million children. J Trauma 6:65–74, 1966.
34. Katz, J. Spontaneous fractures in paraplegic children. J Bone Joint Surg 35-A:220–226, 1953.
35. King, J.; Diefendorf, D.; Apthorp, J.; et al. Analysis of 429 fractures in 189 battered children. J Pediatr Orthop 8:585–589, 1988.
36. Kirby, R. M.; Winquist, R. A.; Hansen, S. T., Jr. Femoral shaft fracture in adolescents: A comparison between traction plus cast treatment and closed intramedullary nailing. J Pediatr Orthop 1:193–197, 1981.
37. Kirschenbaum, D.; Albert, M. C.; Robertson, W. W., Jr.; Davidson, R. S. Complex femur fractures in children: Treatment with external fixation. J Pediatr Orthop 10:588–591, 1990.
38. Kissel, E. U.; Miller, M. E. Closed Ender nailing of femur fractures in older children. J Trauma 29:1585–1588, 1989.
39. Kregor, P. J.; Song, K.; Routt, M. L., Jr.; et al. Plate fixation of femoral shaft fractures in polytraumatized children. Transactions of 7th Annual Meeting of the Orthopaedic Trauma Association. Seattle, November 1991.
40. Ligier, J. N.; Metaizeau, J.; Prevot, J.; Lascombes, P. Elastic stable intramedullary nailing of femoral shaft fractures in children. J Bone Joint Surg 70-B:74–77, 1988.
41. Mann, D. C.; Rajmaira, S. Distribution of physeal and nonphyseal fractures in 2,650 long-bone fractures in children aged 0–16 years. J Pediatr Orthop 10:713–716, 1990.
42. Mann, D. C.; Weddington, J.; Davenport, K. Closed Enders nailing of femoral shaft fractures in adolescents. J Pediatr Orthop 10:651–655, 1986.
43. Marcus, R. E.; Mills, M. F.; Thompson, G. H. Multiple injury in children. J Bone Joint Surg 65-A:1290–1294, 1983.
44. Mayer, T. Causes of morbidity and mortality in severe pediatric trauma. JAMA 245:719–721, 1981.
45. McDougall, A. Fracture of the neck of the femur in childhood. J Bone Joint Surg 43-B:16–28, 1961.
46. Meals, R. A. Overgrowth of the femur following fractures in children: Influence of handedness. J Bone Joint Surg 61-A:381–384, 1979.
47. Mubarak, S.; Carroll, N. C. Volkmann's contracture in children: Aetiology and prevention. J Bone Joint Surg 61-B:285–293, 1979.
48. Newberger, E. The myth of the battered child syndrome. Curr Med Dialogue 40:327, 1973.
49. Nicholson, J. T.; Foster, R. M.; Heath, R. D. Bryant's traction. A provocative cause of circulatory complications. JAMA 157:415–418, 1955.
50. Quintin, J.; Evrard, H.; Gouat, P.; et al. External fixation in child traumatology. Orthopedics 7:463–467, 1984.
51. Reeves, R. B.; Ballard, R. I.; Hughes, J. L. Internal fixation versus traction and casting of adolescent femoral shaft fractures. J Pediatr Orthop 10:592–595, 1990.
52. Reynolds, D. A. Growth changes in fractured long-bones. A study of 126 children. J Bone Joint Surg 63-B:83–88, 1981.
53. Robinson, W. Treatment of birth fractures of the femur. J Bone Joint Surg 20:778–780, 1938.
54. Seimon, L. P. Refracture of the shaft of the femur. J Bone Joint Surg 46-B:32–39, 1964.
55. Spiegel, P. G.; Mast, J. W. Internal and external fixation of fractures in children. Orthop Clin North Am 11:405–421, 1980.
56. Staheli L. T. Femoral and tibial overgrowth following femoral shaft fractures in childhood. Clin Orthop 55:159–163, 1967.
57. Staheli, L. T.; Sheridan, G. W. Early spica cast management

of femoral shaft fractures in young children. A technique utilizing bilateral fixed skin traction. Clin Orthop 126:162–166, 1977.
58. Swiontkowski, M. F.; Hansen, S. T., Jr.; Kellam, J. Ipsilateral fractures of the femoral neck and shaft. A treatment protocol. J Bone Joint Surg 66-A:260–263, 1984.
59. Thompson, G. H.; Wilber, J. H.; Marcus, R. E. Internal fixation of fractures in children and adolescents: A comparative analysis. Clin Orthop 188:10–20, 1984.
60. Timmerman, L. A.; Rab, G. T. Closed reamed intramedullary nail versus traction and casting in treatment of femoral shaft fractures in the 10 to 14 year old. J Pediatr Orthop 10:693, 1990.
61. Tolo, V. T. External skeletal fixation in children's fractures. J Pediatr Orthop 3:435–442, 1983.
62. Wadsworth, T. G. Traumatic dislocation of the hip with fracture of the shaft of the ipsilateral femur. J Bone Joint Surg 43-B:47–48, 1961.
63. Williamson, R. V.; Staheli, L. T. Partial physeal growth arrest: Treatment by bridge resection and fat interposition. J Pediatr Orthop 10:769–776, 1990.
64. Winquist, R. A.; Hansen, S. T., Jr.; Clawson, D. K. Closed intramedullary nailing of femur fractures. A report of five hundred and twenty cases. J Bone Joint Surg 66-A:529–539, 1984.
65. Ziv, I.; Rang, M. Treatment of femoral fracture in the child with head injury. J Bone Joint Surg 65-B:276–278, 1983.
66. Ziv, I.; Blackburn, N.; Rang, M. Femoral intramedullary nailing in the growing child. J Trauma 24:432–434, 1984.

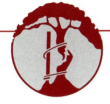

Vernon Tolo, M.D.

12

Fractures and Dislocations Around the Knee

Fractures in the vicinity of the knee in the growing child have characteristics peculiar to this age group. The presence of the physes and secondary ossification centers and an abundance of cartilage compared with the adult knee are the key features implicated in these fracture patterns. As with other long bones in the growing child, one must always be cognizant that the cartilaginous structures are the weak links in the bone-joint-tendon-ligament complex of all extremities, particularly the knee region.[55]

Distal Femoral Metaphyseal and Physeal Fractures

Anatomy

Several anatomic features of the knee region must be considered in evaluating and managing fractures of the distal femoral area. The muscle attachments of the gastrocnemius and the adductor magnus may lead to angulation at the distal femoral fracture site. If the distal femoral fracture is cephalad to the distal adductor insertion, varus angulation of the distal fracture fragment will occur. The medial and lateral heads of the gastrocnemius originate on the posterior aspect of the distal femoral metaphysis and will lead to a flexion angulation of the distal fracture fragment with any fracture cephalad to these origins.

Ligaments of importance in fractures of the distal femur are primarily the medial and lateral collateral ligaments of the knee. Although involvement of the cruciate ligaments may coexist with distal femoral fractures, the relationship of the anterior and posterior cruciate knee ligaments with distal femoral fractures is less direct than for the collateral ligaments. The proximal attachment of both the collateral ligaments is onto the distal femoral epiphysis. When valgus or varus force is exerted on the knee, these ligaments most commonly remain uninjured because the force is transferred to the distal femoral physis, leading to a physeal fracture. The distal femoral physis is more undulated anatomically than many other physes, and this feature may help explain why growth arrest following distal femoral physeal injury is so common.

Important neurovascular structures are positioned in close approximation to the distal femur, primarily posteriorly and laterally. The femoral artery moves from a medial position to a posterior location in the popliteum as it courses through the adductor canal just above the distal femoral metaphysis. In the popliteal region, just above the joint line, the popliteal artery trifurcates, sending three vessels toward the lower leg. While arterial collateral circulation is present around the knee, this collateral arterial supply is less abundant than in the elbow region and often is insufficient to allow continued viability of the lower leg if the popliteal artery is occluded or disrupted. The posterior tibial nerve lies adjacent to the popliteal artery in the posterior part of the knee. The peroneal nerve, which has separated from the sciatic nerve in midthigh, becomes superficial on the posterolateral aspect of the knee as this nerve surfaces at the posterior border of the biceps femoris insertion and wraps around the lateral fibular head.

DISTAL FEMORAL METAPHYSEAL FRACTURE

Mechanism of Injury. The most common causes of this fracture are a direct blow on the anterior or lateral distal thigh or a fall from a high place. When a young child is struck by a car bumper, the height of the bumper reaches to the femoral region, whereas in an adult a similar bumper injury usually results in a tibial fracture.

In a child under 3 years of age, child abuse should be considered. At this age, fractures most commonly occur in the diaphyseal region; if a metaphyseal fracture is present, child abuse is a strong possibility.[6] Child abuse can be confirmed if the radiographs demonstrate a "corner" fracture or "bucket-handle" lesion characteristic of child abuse. Nondisplaced fractures or stress fractures with periosteal new bone in an older child should raise the possibility of a pathologic fracture at this site.[16]

Consequences of Injury. The distal fracture fragment will generally displace posteriorly, often with exaggerated flexion of the distal fragment due to the pull of the medial and lateral heads of the gastrocnemius. If the fracture line is just cephalic to the distal insertion of the adductor magnus, the distal fracture fragment will also angulate into a varus position.

Associated Injuries. With this posterior bony displacement, the femoral artery may be injured, either at the region of the adductor canal or in its position in the upper popliteal region. Arterial injury here is less common than with a proximal tibial physeal fracture, but vascular injury and compartment syndromes of the lower leg may occur and require careful monitoring after a distal femoral fracture.

The peroneal nerve is more likely to be injured with a distal femoral fracture than is the posterior tibial nerve. The peroneal nerve may be damaged either by a direct blow to the posterolateral side of the knee (e.g., from a car bumper) or from a stretch injury to this nerve at the time of fracture angulation and displacement.

Diagnosis. Generally, the diagnosis of this fracture is made easily. The history usually consists of a description of the accident. As with other fractures resulting from significant trauma, the presence of transient head injury or trunk complaints should be investigated.

The physical examination will demonstrate swelling, pain, and deformity in the distal thigh and knee region. The skin must be carefully inspected for a possible open fracture. The presence and strength of the pedal pulses should be documented. Neurologic function of the peroneal and posterior tibial nerves is noted. Ongoing evaluation of the lower leg for a developing compartment syndrome is essential during the first few days following fracture.

Imaging evaluation with plain radiographs of the distal femur and knee will confirm the suspected diagnosis. As with other long bone fractures, radiographs of the entire bone, including the hip in this case, should be obtained at the initial evaluation. The only relevant special imaging study is arteriography, but this is reserved for cases in which positive physical findings in the lower leg indicate possible associated arterial injury.

Management. The distal metaphyseal femoral fracture can present problems both in obtaining proper alignment and in determining what that proper alignment is. The primary treatment options for this fracture include traction followed by hip spica casting, external fixation, open reduction and internal fixation, and cast-brace management.

Traction and Casting. The classic treatment involves the initial application of traction to facilitate fracture reduction. In the young child, skin traction on the lower leg may be used, but I prefer skeletal pin traction for femoral fractures in children over the age of 3 years.

Skeletal traction is applied through either the proximal tibia or the distal femur, keeping the knee flexed to relax the pull of the gastrocnemius muscle and to allow appropriate sagittal plane alignment. The skeletal traction pin is either a Kirschner wire (K-wire) or a Steinmann pin applied under local anesthesia in the emergency room or on the patient floor. If a proximal tibial site is chosen for pin placement, one must ensure that the pin insertion avoids the proximal tibial physis, particularly where this physis courses distally in the anterior tibia at the site of the tibial tubercle (Fig. 12–1). A proximal tibial pin will allow longitudinal traction, but it may be necessary to insert a second pin into the distal femoral fracture fragment to allow an anteriorly directed force to regain satisfactory position on the lateral radiograph. Similarly, if the distal femoral fragment is long enough, two pins inserted into this fragment (cephalic to the physis) will facilitate reduction. In the distal femur, these pins should be passed aseptically from medial to lateral, parallel to the knee joint, to decrease the chance of injuring the femoral artery in the region of the adductor canal.

Even though this two-pin traction may produce satisfactory fracture reduction on the lateral radiograph, the need to keep the knee flexed to maintain reduction makes accurate evaluation of possible

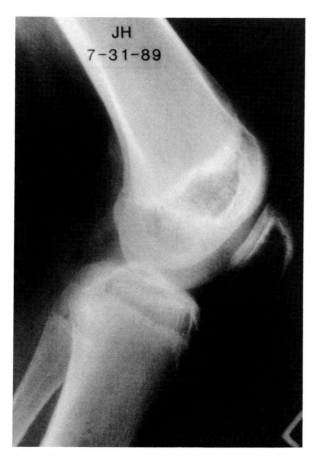

Figure 12–1
Lateral radiograph of the knee of a 17-year-old boy who had sustained a fracture of his femur that was treated with skeletal traction. The smooth traction pin was placed through the proximal tibia. Even though the pin did not penetrate the tibial tubercle, an arrest of its apophysis occurred with resultant distal position of the tibial tubercle. This has produced patella baja. (Courtesy of Dr. Neil E. Green.)

varus or valgus position difficult, if not impossible. An anteroposterior (AP) radiograph of the knee in this position will distort the relationship between the femur and the tibia, while an AP radiograph centered on the distal femur does not allow for evaluation of the femoral-tibial angle. Evaluation of the transverse condylar line in relation to the long axis of the femur will allow some estimate of fracture alignment, but persistence of varus malalignment is common.

If this treatment method is selected, the child can be placed initially in flexed-knee traction using two skeletal traction pins. After the sagittal plane alignment is satisfactory and early callus has formed, the knee can be partially straightened gradually; lateral radiographs are taken to ensure that sagittal plane alignment is maintained. With the knee in a more extended position, the varus and valgus malalignment can be corrected at the time of hip spica cast application, while the callus is still relatively pliable. The duration of cast immobilization varies with the age of the patient, being only a few weeks for the very young and 5 or 6 weeks for the older child.

Once the cast has been removed, rehabilitation is begun. Weight bearing can be full, but crutches are used for protection until knee motion and thigh strength are adequate to allow the patient to walk safely without assistive devices. The quadriceps is extremely weak after cast removal, and this muscle is not strong enough to support the body in a flexed-knee position, so the patient will fall and forcefully flex the stiff knee if crutches are not used initially. As the rehabilitation program strengthens the quadriceps, hamstrings, and hip abductors, the knee range of motion usually will improve rapidly. Although it may be several months before the strength of the hamstrings and quadriceps in the injured thigh are equal to that of the uninjured side, resuming participation in sports is appropriate when full range of knee motion returns and the thigh muscles are graded 5/5 on clinical examination.

The main complications that may result from treating the distal femoral metaphyseal fracture with traction and casting are varus malalignment and premature closure of the anterior part of the proximal tibial physis, which will lead to recurvatum deformity of the proximal tibia (see Fig. 12–1). Both these complications generally can be avoided by meticulous pin insertion and traction management. Malalignment in the sagittal plane, with a posterior apex bowing of the femur at the fracture site, may lead to apparent hyperextension of the knee with limitation of knee flexion, but in the young child this deformity will largely remodel with time.

Cast-Brace Management. If posterior angulation of the distal fracture fragment is not great, a cast-brace may be used after initial traction in selected preadolescents and adolescents. Because knee stiffness after spica cast immobilization is not a major problem in children, cast-brace management is used mainly for patient and family convenience. This treatment method enables the older child to be more active, often allowing school attendance while in the cast-brace.

Initially the patient is treated with skeletal traction, as described earlier. It is preferable to allow resolution of much of the swelling at the site of injury so the thigh mold can be applied more snugly. I prefer to apply this cast-brace in one piece initially, with application of knee hinges after cast hardening. An elasticized knee covering is applied first, followed by thin cast padding. The cast is applied from the toes to the groin, with careful medial and lateral supracondylar molds, in addition to a mold proximally into a quadrilateral socket configuration. After cast hardening and radiographic confirmation of acceptable fracture position, the anterior two thirds of the knee cutout is completed and the hinges are applied. After hinge application is complete, the posterior knee region is cut out and trimmed to allow 90 degrees of knee flexion. The application of a cast-brace in one piece with later knee cutout allows for placement by the orthopaedist without the need for several assistants.

Weight bearing in the cast is encouraged to facilitate fracture healing and is begun once the cast has hardened. Quadriceps and hamstrings are exercised regularly for strengthening. Radiographs are obtained a few days after weight bearing has started to look for possible varus angulation that occurred in the cast-brace. Cast immobilization is continued until radiographic evidence of union is seen.

Besides the social advantages of allowing older children to be out of the home when wearing the cast, this treatment method promotes a quicker return of knee motion. However, since knee stiffness is not a problem with this fracture unless concomitant soft tissue injury has been extensive, the long-term advantage of early knee motion return is arguable.

In general, cast-braces for femoral fractures in preadolescents and adolescents have been used sparingly. Although other methods are superior to the cast-brace in diaphyseal femoral fractures, if a cast-brace is to be used in children and adolescents, the distal femur has been reported to be the best suited to this modality.[23]

External Fixation. External fixation devices are used to reduce and stabilize a distal femoral metaphyseal fracture primarily in instances of open fractures, a floating knee, or polytrauma. In addition, the distal femoral fracture is difficult to treat with traction because of flexion of the distal fragment. Thus, use of an external fixator may be indicated (Fig. 12–2).

In the case of polytrauma with multiple fractures, abdominal injury, or head injury, the child will need to be transported for diagnostic studies or operative treatment and cannot remain in traction. Initially, with an associated head injury, plaster splinting can be used to prevent fracture site motion, since such movement will lead to a rise in intracranial pressure from pain. If the head injury clears readily, the child may be treated with traction and casting, as noted earlier. However, if coma persists, spasticity will ensue, causing excessive shortening at the fracture site, a condition that cannot be handled adequately by traction. With spasticity, reduction and adequate fracture stabilization require either external or internal fixation. As with other fractures in children with head injury, even in the face of prolonged coma, the chance of recovery from the head injury is excellent, and orthopaedic injuries should be treated in a timely fashion, assuming full neurologic recovery.

In open fractures, the use of external fixation for fracture stabilization allows care of the wound, particularly if skin loss or injury has occurred and requires dressing changes and skin grafting. In children with a fractured tibia and a distal femoral metaphyseal fracture, stabilization of this floating knee with an external fixator in the femur allows the tibial fracture to be treated more easily.

If an external fixator is chosen, the surgeon must insert the half pins in such a way as to avoid physeal injury.[63] The pins are inserted laterally when used on the femur. It is recommended that at least 1 cm of metaphyseal bone remain between the most distal pin and the physis. This not only protects the physis from injury during insertion but also helps protect the physis from damage due to an adjacent pin infection. The external fixator pins should be applied in parallel while an assistant holds the fracture site in a reduced position. This fracture reduction may be facilitated by transient placement of a Steinmann pin to assist in fracture fragment manipulation. Use of an external fixation frame that allows some adjustment of varus and valgus as well as rotational changes is preferred; this also makes external fixation easier and less dependent on the exact placement of the pins. After placement of the frame, final adjustments are made and radiographic confirmation of adequate reduction is completed before the child is awakened from general anesthesia.

If other factors allow and the child is mature enough to be cooperative and compliant, partial weight bearing with crutch assistance can be begun early. Pin care is taught to the child and the parents in the hospital, and this pin care is continued daily at home. The child may attend school if school officials are in agreement. When healing callus has formed, weight bearing can be increased, and the fixator can be dynamized to allow for improved strengthening at the fracture site. If the external fixator is used for only a few weeks, after removal a long leg cast can be applied until fracture healing is complete. Alternatively, the external fixator can be used for the full course of treatment. The external fixator pins can be removed in the outpatient area,

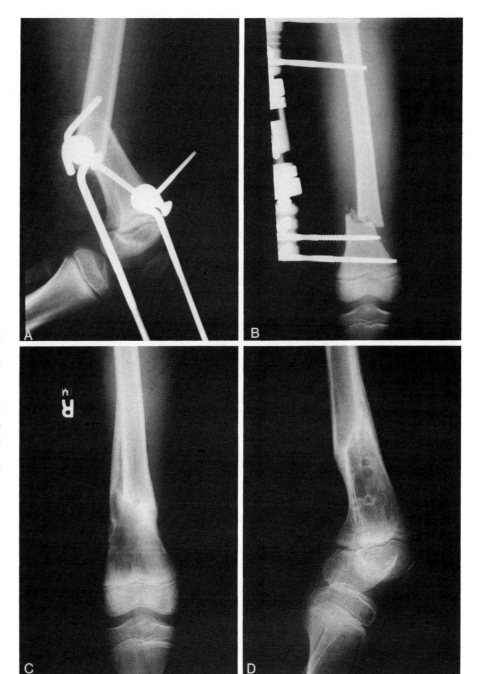

Figure 12–2

Radiographs of an 8-year-old who sustained a fracture of the distal femur. *A*, Lateral radiograph of the distal femur and knee showing a distal femoral fracture with a traction pin in the supracondylar region of the distal femur. The patient is in 90-90 traction, and one can see the posterior angulation of the fracture, which was difficult to control. *B*, Because of the difficulty in controlling it, the fracture was reduced in the operating room and the reduction held with an external fixator. *C*, Anteroposterior radiograph of the knee and distal femur showing healing of the fracture 4½ months after the injury. *D*, Lateral radiograph showing good alignment of the distal femur. (Courtesy of Dr. Neil E. Green.)

but I prefer to administer a short-acting anesthetic for this.

Rehabilitation after healing is similar to that for other distal femoral metaphyseal fractures. Since the fixator pins have pierced the lateral quadriceps, restitution of full range of motion of the knee may take longer but will occur unless there was extensive soft tissue damage at the time of fracture.

Complications from external fixation are primarily due to pin problems and fracture malalignment. Pin infection usually can be avoided by good pin care; if infection appears, however, use of oral antibiotics for a few weeks may be sufficient to eliminate the adjacent cellulitis. The skin should be incised at the pin if skin pressure is noted. If persistent drainage occurs or if erosion around the pin site is noted on radiographs of the femur, either the pin should be changed or the entire device should be removed, a cast applied, and antibiotic treatment continued.

Because the knee can be extended to assess the femoral-tibial angle quite readily, varus or valgus malalignment is not common if care is taken in the initial placement of the fixator. However, there is a tendency to apply this fixator with the distal fragment slightly externally rotated, so rotation should be carefully assessed at initial placement.

Injury to the distal femoral physis is certainly a potential problem, but if the pins are kept at least 1 cm proximal to the physis when inserted, this injury should be avoidable. The pins should always be inserted under fluoroscopic control.

Open Reduction and Internal Fixation. Open reduction with internal fixation is needed if fracture reduction cannot be obtained by other methods or if arterial injury has occurred at the time of fracture. The most common cause of failure to obtain an adequate reduction by other means is the interposition of muscle between the fracture fragments, which blocks reduction. If arterial repair is needed, internal fixation prevents fracture motion and protects the artery.

The surgical approach depends on the reason for the surgery. If an arterial repair is needed, the incision must be posteromedial to allow access to the femoral and popliteal arteries as well as the saphenous vein if vein grafting is needed. If an irreducible fracture necessitates surgery, a straight lateral approach is used, reflecting the quadriceps anteriorly to afford access to the distal femur.

Internal fixation devices used in children and adolescents are usually less rigid than those used in adults, since casts are often applied postoperatively until fracture healing is complete. Once fracture reduction is obtained, crossed Steinmann pins provide acceptable limited fixation. These pins are bent to prevent migration and are cut off just below the skin, so later removal is simple. Compression-plate rigid fixation is rarely needed or indicated in the growing child. Besides requiring a second operation for plate removal followed by a month of casting to prevent fracture through the screw holes, compression plates appear to lead to greater femoral overgrowth than other treatment methods.

After fracture healing is complete, the Steinmann pins can be removed through small skin incisions, using either a local or a short-acting general anesthetic. Rehabilitation is the same as for other healed fractures in this location.

DISTAL FEMORAL PHYSEAL FRACTURE

In a growing child, an injury in the region of the knee is more apt to lead to a physeal fracture than to a collateral ligament injury, although at times both may be present.[7, 26, 56, 60] The proximal attachments of both the medial and the lateral collateral ligaments stabilize the distal femoral epiphysis, transferring valgus or varus force on the knee to the physis, producing a physeal fracture, primarily through the zone of hypertrophy. However, the distal femoral physis is quite undulated, and this fracture line may cross from one physeal zone to another as the fracture moves across the physis.

Between 1 and 6% of physeal fractures occur at this site. Most common in this location are Salter-Harris types I and II, although any of the five types may occur. Almost any mechanism of injury can be seen, and the radiographic appearance of the fracture may help reconstruct the mechanism in individual cases. If hyperextension of the knee occurs, the epiphysis will be displaced anteriorly. If the injury occurs with the knee in flexion, posterior epiphyseal displacement is seen. If varus or valgus stress has resulted in this fracture, minimal displacement may be present, but examination will demonstrate more instability on either the medial or the lateral side. Sports, especially football, are frequently responsible for this injury in adolescence.

Some of the associated injuries that may occur are similar to those seen with a distal femoral metaphyseal fracture. However, arterial injury with later compartment syndrome of the leg must be carefully looked for, particularly with an anteriorly displaced epiphysis. Since this fracture results from forced hyperextension of the knee, popliteal artery stretch occurs and, despite palpable pedal pulses, may result in an intimal injury that will lead to relative ischemia of the lower leg.

If the fracture has resulted from valgus force to the knee, associated intraarticular injury must be considered, particularly if a bloody effusion is present. In that case, the anterior and posterior cruciate ligaments and the menisci should be evaluated by either magnetic resonance imaging (MRI) or arthroscopy following fracture reduction and stabilization.

Diagnosis. A historical description of the accident causing this fracture will often assist the orthopaedist in knowing what problems to look for most urgently. Of primary importance is the direction of the force that produced the injury.

Physical examination begins with observation of the knee region in the splinted position and documentation of intact pedal pulses and neurologic function of the foot and ankle. If obvious deformity is present, no manipulation is performed until after radiographic evaluation. If there is swelling without obvious deformity, the location of maximal tenderness is identified. Principally, it should be determined whether the tenderness is greatest over the distal femoral physis or over the joint line itself. Gentle varus and valgus stress testing is performed to detect instability and to see if such movements elicit pain medially or laterally. No attempt to assess the full range of knee motion should be made at this time.

Radiographic imaging is important early when this fracture is being evaluated. Initially, AP and lateral plain radiographs of the knee are obtained. If these views show the fracture, no further radiographs are needed prior to treatment. If no fracture is apparent and knee instability has been noted on examination, gentle valgus or varus stress AP radiographs of the knee should be obtained. The orthopaedist should personally supervise the positioning for these x-rays to avoid applying excessive force that may turn a nondisplaced physeal fracture into a displaced fracture. If no fracture is seen, even with stress applied, a more thorough knee examination can be done.

Other evaluative studies come into consideration mainly if there is an associated knee effusion, which can be aspirated using aseptic technique. If the effusion is grossly bloody, an associated cruciate or meniscal injury should be suspected. If there is fat in the aspirate, an associated osteochondral fracture may be present and should be further evaluated by either MRI or arthroscopy.

The differential diagnosis essentially involves distinguishing between a physeal fracture and a ligament injury, because these two conditions are treated differently and have different prognoses. Although ligament injuries may occur in the skeletally immature child, physeal fractures are more common and should be first on the list of possible diagnoses when an open physis is present. Even if the knee examination points toward a ligament injury in an immature child, a radiograph must be obtained to rule out a fracture before treatment proceeds.

Management. Accurate and anatomic reduction of this fracture is essential. Prior to attempting reduction, the orthopaedist must evaluate the options because repeated manipulation of physeal fractures increases the risk of later growth disturbance.

Nondisplaced physeal fractures can be treated with long leg cast immobilization for 4 to 5 weeks. Because of its theoretical detrimental effect on an injured physis, weight bearing should be avoided, but crutch walking is allowed. After cast immobilization, rehabilitation is the same as for distal femoral shaft fractures, but growth must continue to be assessed for 1 to 2 years after injury.

If a Salter-Harris I or II fracture is displaced, the treatment choices are closed reduction and casting, closed reduction with percutaneous pinning and casting, and open reduction with limited internal fixation and casting. If fracture manipulation is needed, this reduction should be performed under general anesthesia and repeated manipulation should be avoided. Open reduction and internal fixation is needed for all displaced Salter-Harris III and IV fractures.

Closed Reduction and Casting. This method is not used for intraarticular displaced fractures but is employed only for Salter-Harris I and II injuries. Following general anesthesia, reduction is attempted, reversing the forces that led to the injury. If the epiphysis is displaced anteriorly, hyperflexion of the knee is performed after the fragment has been aligned satisfactorily in the anteroposterior plane on the image intensifier. Extension is used to reduce fractures with the epiphysis posteriorly displaced. After reduction is thought to have been obtained, a lateral image intensifier view is used for confirmation. Because of potential injury to neurovascular structures, extremes of flexion and extension should not be used to maintain reduction. The stability of the reduction is tested under fluoroscopy to see if, on the lateral view, fracture reduction is lost as the knee is placed in less extreme positions of flexion or extension. If the fracture is stable and reduction is maintained, a long leg cast is applied in relative flexion for the anteriorly displaced fracture and in nearly full extension for the posteriorly displaced fracture. The cast is left on for 6 weeks, and rehabilitation is begun.

Closed Reduction, Percutaneous Pinning, and Casting. This method is used for Salter-Harris I and II fractures, and the initial part of this treatment is the same as with closed reduction and casting. After reduction has been obtained, if the fracture is stable only in extreme positions of flexion or extension, the knee area is prepared and surgical drapes applied in the usual fashion. Fracture reduction is obtained and confirmed by fluoroscopy. In type I fractures, two smooth Steinmann pins are placed in a crossed fashion, coursing diagonally from a starting point just above the joint line on the medial and lateral femoral condyles, respectively (Fig. 12–3). This same crossed-pin placement may be needed for Salter-Harris II fractures, but two Steinmann pins placed parallel to the physis in the metaphyseal region may be used if the metaphyseal portion of the distal fracture fragment is sufficiently large. After pinning, the knee is moved through the full range of motion under fluoroscopy to assess stability. If the knee is still not stable, pin replacement is

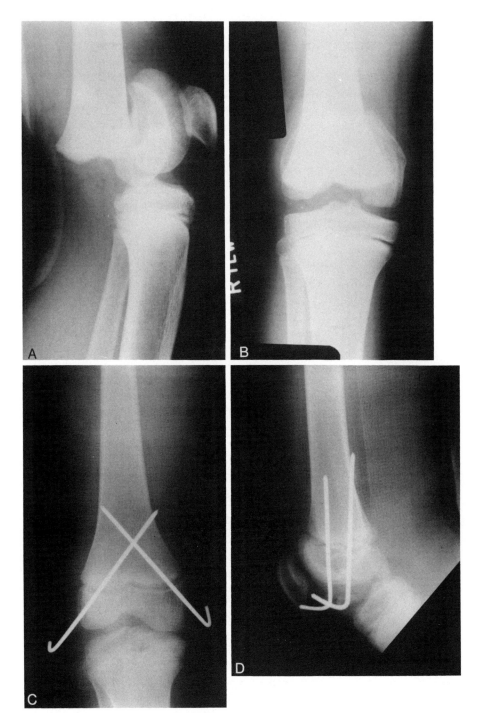

Figure 12–3

Type I fracture of the distal femoral physis of a 13-year-old male. The patient sustained a hyperextension injury of the knee. There was no neurovascular injury. *A*, Lateral radiograph of the knee that shows a completely displaced type I physeal injury of the distal femur with anterior displacement of the femoral condyles. *B*, Anteroposterior radiograph of the same knee demonstrating the displacement of the condyles. *C*, Anteroposterior radiograph after closed reduction and percutaneous pinning showing anatomic restoration of the fracture. Note that the pins are smooth pins that have crossed the physis. *D*, Lateral radiograph of the knee that again shows anatomic reduction of the fracture.

needed. If the knee is stable after pinning, the pins are bent to avoid migration; a dressing is applied around the pins; and a long leg cast is applied in 20 to 30 degrees of flexion. Weight bearing in the cast is avoided. The pins are removed in the outpatient area when the cast is removed after 6 weeks.

Open Reduction, Internal Fixation, and Casting. Open reduction is needed for all displaced Salter-Harris III and IV fractures and in those type I and II fractures that cannot be anatomically reduced by the means just described. The technique used for fixation will vary with the type of fracture encountered.

For types I and II fractures that are irreducible by closed methods, the goal is to remove the impediment to reduction. For type I fractures, I use a medial incision. Once the hematoma and other potential obstructions to reduction are removed, two crossed smooth Steinmann pins are placed, as noted previously. In the case of a Salter-Harris II fracture that requires open reduction, the incision is made on the side with the metaphyseal fragment. Once reduction is obtained, either oblique smooth Steinmann pins or an AO cancellous screw is placed horizontally in the metaphysis if the metaphyseal fragment is large enough (Fig. 12–4). A long leg cast is used postoperatively for 6 weeks, after which the implants are removed.

Since Salter-Harris III and IV fractures are intra-articular, a more extensive operative exposure is needed to visualize both the articular surface and the physis or metaphysis. For a type III fracture, an anteromedial or anterolateral arthrotomy is made, the choice being influenced by the side of the vertical fracture through the epiphysis. After the knee joint is opened, a thorough irrigation eliminates the hemarthrosis and clot from the fracture surfaces. The edge of the physis is exposed, and fracture reduction is completed. One or two AO cancellous screws with a washer are placed transversely through the fracture site under image-intensifier control. It is preferable for the threaded portion of the screw to be short enough to not span the fracture site and thus allow better compression at the fracture surface (Fig. 12–5). A long leg cast is used for 4 to 5 weeks, and no weight bearing is advised. The screw may be removed at any time after fracture healing; removal usually requires general anesthesia in a child.

In type IV fractures, the incision is made on the side of the metaphyseal portion attached to the distal fracture fragment. An arthrotomy is used as for the type III fracture, and thorough evacuation of blood from the joint is attempted. The metaphyseal portion of the femur is exposed, and the periosteum is elevated to allow clear visualization

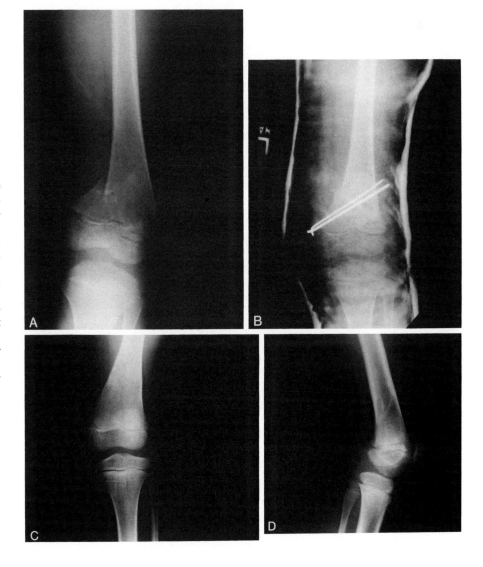

Figure 12–4

A, Anteroposterior radiograph of the left knee of a 10-year-old boy who sustained a displaced Salter II fracture of his distal left femur. *B*, Closed reduction of this fracture was attempted once but was unsuccessful. Limited open reduction with percutaneous pinning was used to obtain realignment, as shown in this AP postoperative radiograph. Pins were removed at 3 weeks, and the cast was removed 6 weeks after fracture. *C–D*, Anteroposterior and lateral radiographs of left knee 18 months after fracture.

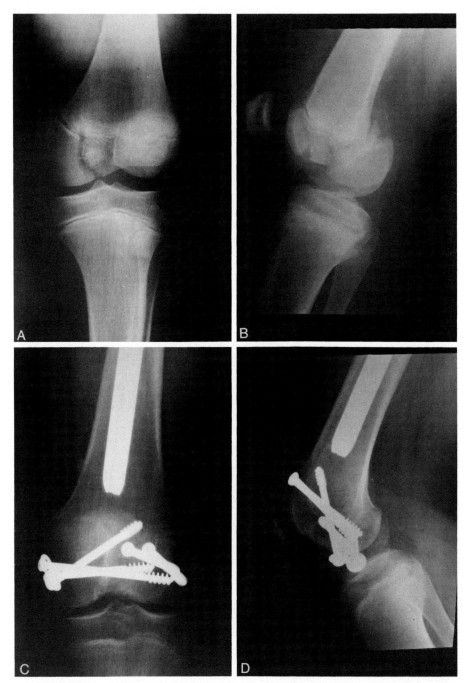

Figure 12–5

A 13-year-old boy sustained a closed midshaft fracture of his right femur and a comminuted type 4 fracture of his distal femoral epiphysis. *A,* Anteroposterior radiograph of the knee showing a comminuted fracture that has split off both sides of the distal femoral epiphysis. *B,* Lateral radiograph showing the comminution of the distal femoral physeal fracture. *C,* Anteroposterior radiograph made postoperatively that demonstrates restoration of the anatomy of the distal femur. The fracture was reduced and stabilized with multiple screws. *D,* Lateral radiograph that demonstrates maintenance of the normal architecture of the femoral condyles. The fracture was very comminuted at the time of the injury, and screws were placed across the physis because the physis had been crushed and a distal femoral epiphyseodesis on the contralateral side was performed a short time later. (Courtesy of Dr. Neil E. Green.)

of the fracture site. Reduction of the fracture is carried out, and a transverse cancellous screw is placed in the metaphysis using fluoroscopy. Unless the metaphyseal fragment is very small and will not hold a screw, no hardware is placed in the epiphysis. Casting is used postoperatively as in the foregoing discussion. The screw can be removed at any point after fracture healing.

Complications. Although neurovascular complications may occur in the acute stage, as noted earlier, the primary later complication involves the arrest of growth in all or part of the distal femoral physis. Even the Salter-Harris I and II fractures, which rarely cause a growth disturbance in most other long bones, have a physeal growth abnormality in 30 to 40% of children with this injury.[52] Some authors have postulated that this high rate of growth disturbance is due to the size of the femur and the corresponding need for extensive force to cause a fracture here. Other possible explanations include the coexistence of a crush injury (type V fracture) with the more obvious type I or II fracture or fracture propagation through more than one zone of the physis due to the undulating anatomy of the physis at this location. Failure to fully reduce these fractures into an anatomic position leads to higher rates of growth disturbance.[52] Even without a known injury to the distal femoral and proximal tibial physes, closure of these growth plates has been reported following fracture of other lower extremity long bones.[34] Children who have had distal femoral physeal fractures require periodic follow-up after injury for 2 to 3 years to detect growth abnormalities early and allow planning for the best way to deal with any projected leg length discrepancy.

The treatment of the complication of distal femoral growth arrest, either partial or complete, will depend on the age at injury and the degree of growth disturbance present. The distal femoral physis furnishes approximately 40% of the longitudinal growth of the lower extremity, contributing approximately 7 to 10 mm of length per year of growth. If growth arrest is complete and the child has more than 5 years of growth remaining, femoral lengthening near the time of skeletal maturity most likely will be indicated. With smaller differences, one must consider the use of a shoe lift or possible contralateral femoral epiphysiodesis alone or in combination with a proximal tibial epiphysiodesis. After distal femoral physeal fractures have healed, it is often useful to obtain a scanogram as a baseline study for use in more accurate plotting of future limb growth on either the Moseley or the Green-Anderson graph.

If only a portion of the distal femoral physis stops growing, an angular deformity will result as the remaining physis continues to grow. Once a physeal bar is identified, consideration should be given to surgical resection to reestablish more normal longitudinal growth. Mapping the extent of the physeal bar, using both AP and lateral tomograms, is the first step in estimating the percentage of physis involved. Results of physeal bar excision are best if less than 50% of the physis is involved and if the bar is located peripherally (Fig. 12–6).

The surgical incision is made either laterally or medially over the physeal area to be resected. The area of resection is planned before the incision is made, on the basis of the tomograms. A high-speed bur is used to resect the physeal bar, the approach being made primarily from the metaphyseal region. Normal physeal cartilage will be seen when the bony bar has been removed, and it is also necessary to visualize physeal cartilage circumferentially within the defect created by the bur to ensure complete bar resection. The area is then packed with either autogenous fat (from the buttock region) or methyl methacrylate (Cranioplast) to prevent the re-formation of the physeal bar. Small metal markers are placed in the metaphysis and the epiphysis to allow for later radiologic evaluation of growth. If the varus or valgus deformity of the distal femur is greater

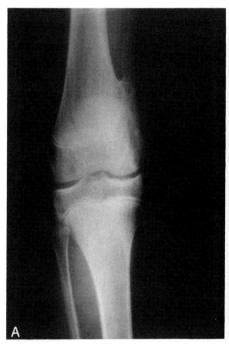
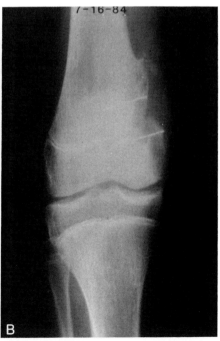

Figure 12–6

Anteroposterior radiograph of the knee of a 14-year-old boy who had sustained a lawn mower injury 4 years before this radiograph was obtained. *A,* This AP radiograph demonstrates a varus deformity of the distal femur with a peripheral growth arrest of the medial side of the distal femoral physis. *B,* After excision of the physeal bar, there has been correction of the varus deformity with subsequent growth. (Courtesy of Dr. Neil E. Green.)

than 10 degrees at the time of physeal bar resection, a distal femoral osteotomy should also be performed to realign the knee joint. In patients with more than 50% involvememt of the physis with a bony bar, realignment osteotomy with epiphysiodesis of the remaining physis will prevent progressive deformity at this site.

Osteochondral Fracture of Femoral Condyles or Patella

The diagnosis of an osteochondral fracture of the knee area may be difficult, particularly if the fracture fragment is small and largely cartilaginous.[21, 32, 62] Patellar osteochondral fractures should be suspected in cases of acute patellar dislocation that have been identified by either history or examination.[2, 27, 57] An osteochondral fracture of the lateral femoral condyle is likely to be secondary to a direct blow on a flexed knee (such as in a soccer player)[58] or associated with a patellar dislocation[61] (Fig. 12–7).

The child will present with a swollen, tender knee after this injury. In a cooperative patient, it may be possible to palpate the site of maximum tenderness as being over the injured articular surface. Radiographic evaluation should include AP and lateral views of the knee as well as tunnel and patellar sunrise views to search for possible areas of injury. If radiographic appearance is normal, particularly when the history suggests an acute patellar dislocation or relocation, the knee joint effusion should be aspirated to confirm the presence of a hemarthrosis. Although in an adult an acute hemarthrosis without fracture often is an indication of a rupture of the anterior cruciate ligament,[17] hemarthrosis in children with normal-appearing radiographs frequently indicates a chondral or osteochondral fracture. If fat globules are present within the aspirated bloody fluid, this is presumptive evidence of an osteochondral fracture somewhere within the knee.

Although an MRI study is useful for localizing occult cartilaginous lesions and osteochondral fractures,[44] I recommend arthroscopy if the aspirate contains fat. If an osteochondral fracture is seen during arthroscopy, the next step consists of either removing the fragment or replacing the fracture fragment, a decision that depends mainly on the size and location of the fragment. A large fracture fragment from the weight-bearing areas of the femoral condyles warrants replacement more often than does a smaller fragment from a non–weight bearing surface.

If the osteochondral fracture fragment is reattached, a number of fixation techniques have been reported, much as for reattachment of a displaced osteochondritis dissecans fragment. Suture, bone pegs,[36] Smillie pins, countersunk AO screws, Herbert screws,[51] K-wires introduced laterally with the tip in the fragment, fibrin and other adhesives,[20, 29] and polyglycolic acid pegs have all been used with similar results (Fig. 12–8).[27] Healing of this fracture is rapid, but if reattachment is used, weight bearing should be avoided for about 1 month after injury.

The important aspect of this fracture is not the type of fixation used but the need for accurate diagnosis. Failure to diagnose this injury will lead to restriction of knee motion, persistent pain, and, if the loose fragment is allowed to remain intraarticular for a prolonged period, the possibility of premature osteoarthritis from continuing articular cartilage injury.[41]

Fractures of the Patella

The patella is a sesamoid bone, incorporated into the quadriceps tendon, and functions to make the quadriceps a more effective extensor of the knee. There are three main facets on its articular surface, which articulates with the distal femur as the patella moves proximally and distally in the patellofemoral

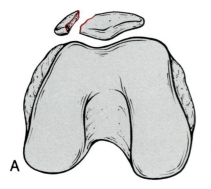
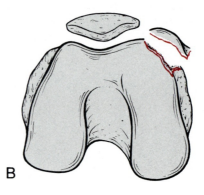

Figure 12–7

Diagrammatic representation of an osteochondral fracture of the lateral femoral condyle (B) and medial pole of the patella (A), both secondary to patella dislocation. Radiographs may appear normal, but the hemarthrosis aspirate will contain fat droplets. Arthroscopy is indicated when these chondral or osteochondral fractures are suspected.

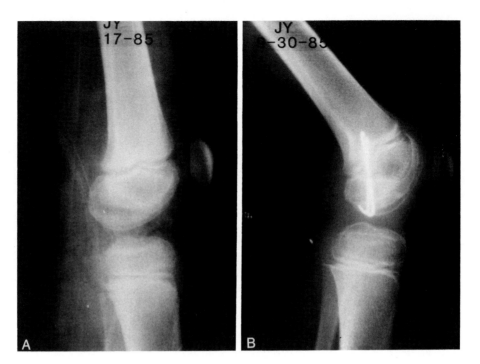

Figure 12–8

A, Lateral radiograph of a 7-year-old child who sustained an osteochondral fracture of the medial condyle of the knee from an open injury. Note the fracture through the inferior portion of the epiphysis. *B*, Lateral radiograph of the knee after open reduction and pinning of the fracture. The smooth pins were removed after healing of the fracture. (Courtesy of Dr. Neil E. Green.)

groove with knee movement. Although a single ossification center for the patella is most commonly seen, various ossification centers that coalesce by skeletal maturity may be present. Incomplete coalescence of these centers may result in a bipartite patella (Fig. 12–9), which may be confused with a fracture in the superolateral portion of the patella.

Transverse or comminuted patellar fractures, which are seen in adults, are relatively unusual in children. Apart from osteochondral fractures of the patella, which are associated with acute lateral dislocation of the patella, as discussed previously, patellar fractures in children are uncommon.[31, 35] Generally these fractures are associated either with a fracture through the cartilaginous portion of a bipartite patella or with a fracture through the cartilage on the inferior pole of the patella; such fractures may result from repetitive stress rather than from a specific injury.

A fracture through the cartilage-bone junction of a bipartite patella presents with pain and tenderness to palpation over the superolateral portion of the patella.[18, 25] No knee effusion is present. An AP knee radiograph will demonstrate a bipartite patella, which may be present bilaterally even though symptoms are unilateral. Displacement rarely occurs, and healing results with activity restriction and a knee immobilizer or cylinder cast. As a rule, no surgery is needed, unless the bipartite fragment is displaced and is causing patellofemoral incongruity and pain with motion.[47]

A fracture through the cartilage on the inferior pole of the patella, the so-called sleeve fracture, occurring in children 8 to 12 years of age, is often difficult to diagnose.[33] Although there can be normal ossification irregularities in the patella from as many as six ossification centers, any tenderness to palpation at the inferior pole of the patella should raise the examiner's suspicion at once.[30] With these sleeve fractures, the distal fracture fragment has a small bony piece from the distal patella, together with a large piece of inferior patellar articular cartilage and

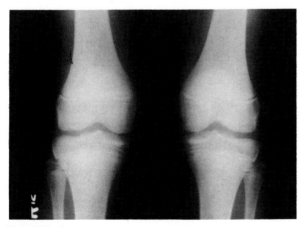

Figure 12–9

Anteroposterior radiograph of both knees demonstrates a unilateral bipartite patellas. Bipartite patellas are commonly bilateral. If tenderness is present at this superolateral location, a fracture should be diagnosed. Operative treatment is rarely indicated.

retinaculum (Fig. 12–10). If the fragments are widely displaced and not treated surgically, the result is significant enlargement of the patella, as the gap created at the time of fracture fills in with healing new bone.

The treatment of pediatric transverse patellar fractures does not differ much from that for adults,[8] although the difficulty in making the diagnosis may be greater. Nondisplaced fractures are well treated with a cylinder cast for a few weeks until tenderness is absent.

When full active knee extension is impossible in a transverse patellar fracture, a cerclage tension-band wire, as described by the AO group, is the treatment of choice.[65] Similarly, with the sleeve fracture, tension-band wiring with close anatomic fracture fragment approximation is the recommended treatment. If a small lateral fragment is present, it is usually best to excise this fragment, depending on the size of the fracture fragment and the extent of involvement of the articular surface. If a large portion of the articular surface is involved, AO screw fixation of the fracture is preferable to excision.

Tibial Spine Fracture

The tibial spine or intercondylar eminence is the point of tibial attachment of the anterior and posterior cruciate ligaments. The former attaches to the anterior intercondylar eminence, while the latter inserts on the posterior aspect of this eminence.

Fracture of the tibial spine is seen primarily in children from the ages of 8 to 14 years. This injury virtually always is to the anterior intercondylar eminence.[19, 22] The posterior intercondylar eminence is rarely fractured, and when this occurs, it is generally in skeletally mature individuals (Fig. 12–11). The anterior intercondylar eminence fracture appears to be analogous to an injury to the anterior cruciate ligament in the skeletally mature individual; it is most likely to be caused by hyperextension of the knee associated with some lateral rotation movement, leading to increased stress on the anterior cruciate ligament.

The most common activity associated with this fracture is bicycle riding[45]; some authors have gone as far as to say that if a knee injury with effusion occurs during a bike ride, a tibial spine fracture is present until proved otherwise. Although previously considered to be caused by the child's leg being hyperextended when the foot is caught in the spokes of the revolving wheel, this fracture also may occur

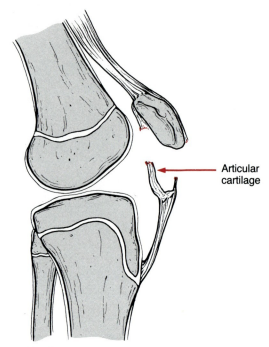

Figure 12–10

Sleeve fracture of the patella. A small segment of the distal pole of the patella is avulsed with a relatively large portion of the articular surface.

from a fall from a bicycle as well as from a wide variety of other sports activities leading to knee hyperextension.

Meyers and McKeever have described three main types of intercondylar eminence fractures in children[42, 43] (Fig. 12–12) based on the amount of displacement and the fracture pattern seen on the initial knee radiographs. Type I is almost nondisplaced and does not generally interfere with knee extension. The type II fracture has a posterior hinge, with the anterior portion being elevated. In this type, knee extension is generally limited, and there is a possibility that the anterior horn of the meniscus (either medial or lateral) is caught under the anterior fracture fragment (Fig. 12–13). A type III fracture is fully displaced, usually with associated rotation of as much as 90 degrees.

The history often involves bicycle riding at the time of injury. Physical examination will demonstrate a knee effusion, usually with the knee held in a mildly flexed position.

Diagnosis. The diagnosis is confirmed by AP and lateral radiographs of the knee. The base of the tibial spine must be carefully inspected on the radiographs for discontinuity of the bony margin; the fracture often is seen more clearly on the lateral

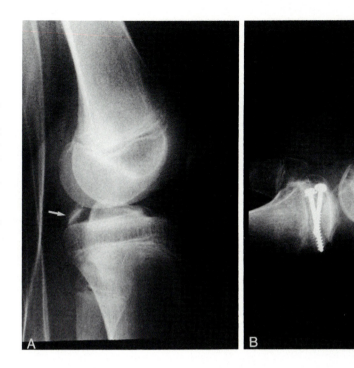

Figure 12–11

A, Lateral radiograph of the knee of a 15-year-old boy who sustained a fracture of the midshaft of his femur plus avulsion of the posterior cruciate ligament of his ipsilateral knee. The arrow points to the avulsion of the posterior tibial spine. *B*, Lateral radiograph of the knee after closed femoral nailing of the fracture of the femur and open reduction and internal fixation of the fracture of the posterior tibial spine through a posterior approach.

radiograph. If an MRI study is done, a concomitant partial tear of the anterior cruciate ligament may be noted in some cases.

Treatment. The treatment will vary with the type of fracture present. In type I fractures, long leg cast immobilization in a few degrees of knee flexion for 5 to 6 weeks leads to satisfactory healing.

In type II fractures, with the child under general anesthesia, the knee is hyperextended to attempt fracture reduction by forcing the elevated anterior portion of the fracture fragment back into place through the contact pressure of the femoral condyles. Afterward the knee is brought back to a position of a few degrees of flexion for long leg cast immobilization. Casting in full extension or hyperextension should be avoided to prevent excessive popliteal artery stretch and a resultant lower leg compartment syndrome. If this closed reduction

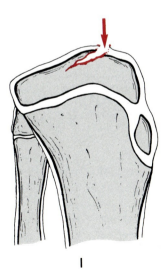
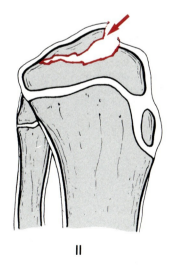
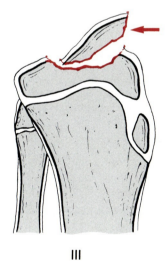

I II III

Figure 12–12

Meyers and McKeever classification of fractures of the anterior tibial spine. *A*, Type 1 fracture with no displacement of the fracture. *B*, A type 2 fracture with elevation of the anterior portion of the anterior tibial spine, but with the fracture posteriorly reduced. *C*, A type 3 fracture that is totally displaced.

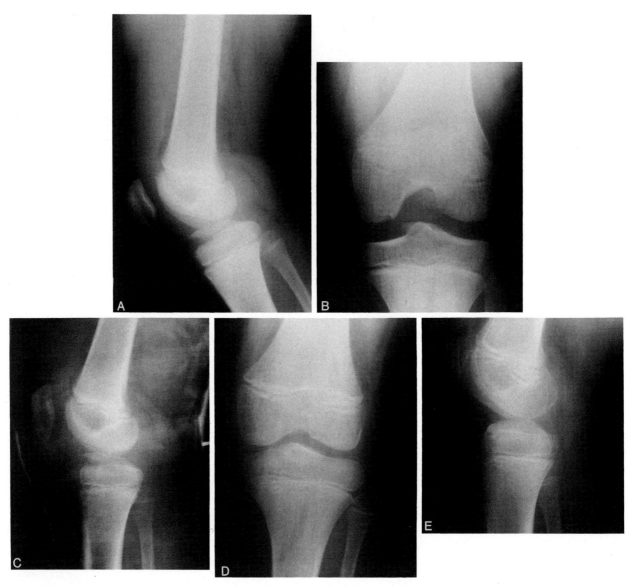

Figure 12–13

A–B, Anteroposterior and lateral radiographs of left knee demonstrate a type II fracture of the tibial intercondylar eminence in this 9-year-old boy. *C,* Lateral radiograph after attempted closed reduction (by knee extension) demonstrates no change from initial radiograph. This generally indicates that the meniscus is blocking fracture reduction. *D–E,* Anteroposterior and lateral radiographs of left knee made 2 months postoperatively show excellent reduction and fracture healing after open reduction and suture fixation of the fracture.

maneuver is unsuccessful, operative reduction is needed for type II fractures (Fig. 12–13). Operative reduction is indicated for all type III fractures.

The goal of operative treatment for this fracture is to remove the soft tissue (usually the meniscus and blood clot) that is blocking reduction and to secure reduction by simple methods. A cast is used following this reduction and minimal internal fixation. This reduction can be accomplished either by arthroscopic means or by a limited anteromedial or anterolateral arthrotomy.

If arthroscopic techniques are used, the standard anteromedial and anterolateral portals are used for introduction of the arthroscope and manipulating instruments. After the blood has been irrigated from the knee, the fracture site is visualized. Any clot between the fracture fragments is evacuated. The anterior horn of the medial or lateral meniscus, which may be displaced between the fracture fragments, is inspected. The meniscus is rarely torn and should not be removed unless obviously injured in a way that precludes repair. The meniscus is retracted out of the fracture site, and the articular surface of the fracture fragment is depressed with a probe to allow reduction. A suture is then passed through the anterior part of the fracture fragment and through the anterior lip of the tibial epiphysis, using the arthroscope for visualization. No drill holes are usually needed, but if they are, care must be taken to avoid injury to the proximal tibial physis. A long leg cast in 10 to 20 degrees of flexion is applied for 6 weeks following reduction to allow healing, after which strengthening and range-of-motion exercises are instituted. Brace protection after cast immobilization is not used.

An equally appropriate approach to types II and III fractures needing operation is through a limited anteromedial or anterolateral arthrotomy. Under tourniquet control, the incision is made adjacent to the patellar tendon, and the knee capsule is opened in line with the skin incision. Under direct vision, the blood is irrigated out of the joint and fracture site. Manual retraction of the meniscus from between the fracture fragments accomplishes reduction—the fracture fragment is pushed down with a finger. An absorbable suture is then passed through the cartilaginous portion of the fracture fragment and the anterior tibial epiphysis and is tied to secure the reduction. After routine closure, a long leg cast in 10 to 20 degrees of flexion is used for 6 weeks, following which rehabilitation begins.

With appropriate treatment of a tibial spine fracture, follow-up results are very good. Nonunion is rare. Provided the meniscus is not allowed to remain between the fracture fragments, functional recovery is excellent. Although mild, asymptomatic laxity of the anterior cruciate ligament is often present after final healing of this fracture,[4,5] excellent function can be expected. If the fracture remains unreduced, late surgery for malunion may be needed[39] to improve functional knee motion.

Tibial Tubercle Fracture

The proximal tibial physis not only contributes to the longitudinal growth of the tibia but also controls the development of the tibial tubercle, with the physis moving distally in its anterior aspect. A secondary ossification center develops in the cartilaginous tibial tubercle, which serves as the primary insertion for the patellar tendon.

Knee pain secondary to Osgood-Schlatter disease is common in active children between the ages of 10 and 14 years. Tenderness directly over the tibial tubercle is the sine qua non of this condition. Although knee radiographs initially may be normal, later studies demonstrate irregular ossification of the anterior portion of the tibial tubercle. This pattern is the result of repeated stress leading to microfractures in the unossified cartilage at this patellar tendon attachment. Though Osgood-Schlatter disease is a self-limiting condition that resolves as the proximal tibial physis closes, the child may require activity restriction in one form or another to allow resolution of symptoms during the earlier stages.

It is thought that if the stress at this site results in failure anterior to the ossified area of the tibial tubercle, the clinical picture will be that of Osgood-Schlatter disease. However, if the failure is deep to the ossified portion of the tibial tubercle, an intraarticular, Salter-Harris III fracture often occurs.[28,46] Some authors have reported an association between Osgood-Schlatter disease and tibial tubercle fracture,[9] but this appears to be related more to the skeletal age or degree of tibial tubercle ossification at the time of injury than to other factors.

The classification of tibial tubercle fractures is based on the amount of displacement seen and the size of the fracture fragment. Although various classifications have been proposed for these fractures, that of Ogden and associates is probably the most useful.[46] Each of Ogden's three types has the fracture line extend up the tibial tubercle cartilaginous apophysis, with the difference in the types being the location of the fracture line. With type I, the fracture line exits through the distal portion of the ossified tibial tubercle. In type II, the fracture exits anteriorly parallel with the proximal tibial physis; in type III, the fracture exits intraarticularly, in many ways similar to a Salter-Harris III fracture at this location (Fig. 12–14). These fractures occur in children in mid- to late adolescence, in whom the posterior portion of the proximal tibial physis has already closed.[38] Basketball is the sport most commonly associated with this injury.

If no displacement of the type I fracture occurs, active knee extension is usually possible, though limited because of pain. Tenderness is present at the fracture site. There is generally no knee effusion. If there is minimal or no displacement of a type I fracture, a long leg cast for 4 to 6 weeks will allow healing.

In types II and III injuries, active knee extension on physical examination is not possible. Operative treatment is needed if displacement is present and should even be considered in nondisplaced fractures to prevent further displacement from the pull of the patellar tendon. Because a portion of the physis has already closed at the time of injury in most of these

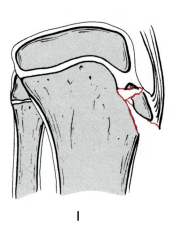 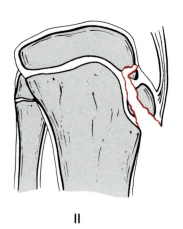 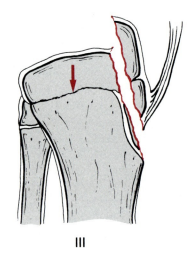

Figure 12–14

Avulsion fractures of the tibial tuberosity. *A*, This is a type I fracture that is through the secondary ossification center. *B*, A type II fracture, which occurs at the junction of the primary and secondary ossification centers. *C*, This fracture is a true Salter-Harris type III fracture that is intraarticular.

children, it is not generally necessary to avoid the physis when placing internal fixation devices to stabilize the fracture reduction. My personal preference for internal fixation is one or two AO cancellous screws placed from anterior to posterior. Washers are used to prevent the screw head from sinking below the cortex with tightening (Fig. 12–15). Other devices, such as Steinmann pins, may be used, but fixation must be strong enough to resist the tendency of the patellar tendon forces to redisplace the fracture.

The surgical incision for reducing and stabilizing displaced types II and III fractures is anterior, parallel with the patellar tendon, either medially or laterally. Hematoma and adjacent soft tissue are removed from the fracture line. With the knee in full extension, the fracture is reduced anatomically and held temporarily in the reduced position with a Steinmann pin through the fracture fragment into the tibial metaphysis. Under image-intensifier control, a cancellous screw with a washer is placed from anterior to posterior through the proximal tibial

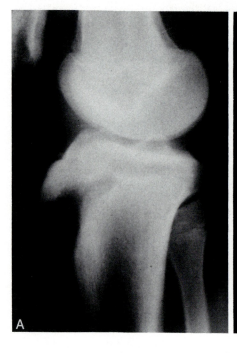 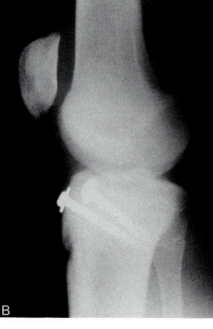

Figure 12–15

A, Lateral knee radiograph of a 14-year-old boy with a displaced fracture of the tibial tubercle. *B*, Lateral knee radiograph of same boy postoperatively after open reduction and screw fixation of fracture. Since these fractures occur usually in adolescents whose proximal tibial physis has already partially closed, no significant growth is lost by screw fixation across the remaining physis.

metaphysis. If solid fixation is not obtained with a single screw, a second screw or a Steinmann pin can be used to prevent rotational displacement. If the fracture fragment is small, only a single cancellous screw is used. In type II fractures, knee arthrotomy is unnecessary, but arthrotomy is needed with type III fractures to remove hematoma and other soft tissue impediments to reduction prior to replacing and stabilizing the fracture fragment.

Following operative reduction, a cylinder or long leg cast in nearly full extension is used for 4 to 6 weeks, with motion exercises and strengthening exercises beginning at the time of cast removal. The screw can be removed a few months later, after motion and strength have been largely regained.

Proximal Tibial Physeal Fractures

Of all the physeal fractures in the long bones of children, that involving the proximal physis of the tibia has the greatest potential for disastrous vascular consequences and permanent neurologic loss.[3, 14, 59] The local vascular anatomy primarily accounts for this high risk of associated injury.

As the popliteal artery passes distally in the posterior aspect of the knee, it divides into three branches: the anterior tibial, peroneal, and posterior tibial arteries. The vessels of this trifurcation pass distally, with the peroneal artery usually terminating in the lower leg, while the anterior tibial (dorsalis pedis) and posterior tibial arteries join to form the vascular plantar arch in the foot. Just below the level of trifurcation, the anterior tibial artery pierces the interosseous membrane as it courses into the anterior compartment of the leg, causing the arteries to be relatively tethered and immobile at this location. Since this trifurcation occurs just distal to the proximal tibial physis, any displacement of the bony structures at this site is often associated with an arterial injury (Fig. 12–16).

Occurring mainly in the 8- to 15-year age group, the proximal tibial physeal fracture is uncommon, accounting for only 0.5 to 2% of physeal fractures. The most common mechanism of injury is hyperextension of the knee. As the knee hyperextends, fracture occurs at either the distal femoral physis or the proximal tibial physis. A similar force in a mature individual would result in a knee dislocation.

As the knee hyperextends the arterial structures posterior to the proximal tibial physis are stretched, with this stretching being worse if the tibia is displaced anteriorly at the physeal level.[53] Depending on the degree of arterial damage, the most common

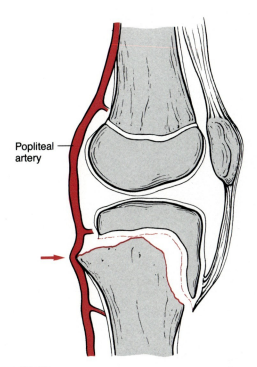

Figure 12–16

Lateral drawing of a knee that shows a displaced proximal tibial physeal injury and demonstrates the risk of arterial injury because of the close proximity of the popliteal artery to the proximal tibia.

sequelae of this injury are total ischemia of the lower leg or development of a compartment syndrome in the lower leg, especially in the anterior and lateral muscle compartments. Failure to diagnose and treat these arterial injuries may result in amputation or permanent muscle and nerve loss in the lower leg.[11]

Although a history of knee hyperextension at the time of injury can be helpful, a careful physical examination at the time of presentation is extremely important. Tenderness, swelling, and often deformity are present at the lower knee level. However, the evaluation of the distal neurovascular status is most important, especially regarding the presence of dorsalis pedis and posterior tibialis pulses and the intact function of the posterior tibial and peroneal nerves. Pain on hyperextension of the toes should be considered a baseline measure in evaluation for possible development of compartment syndrome in the anterior compartment.

Diagnosis. Definitive diagnosis is generally readily accomplished by AP and lateral plain radiographs of the proximal tibia and knee. One must remember that even minimally displaced proximal tibial physeal fractures may have been severely displaced

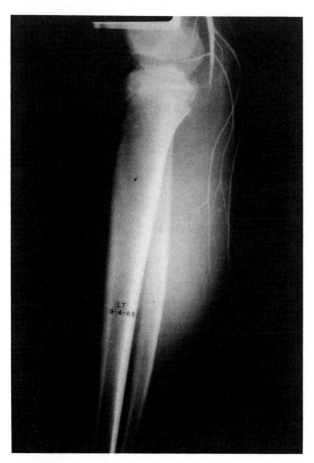

Figure 12–17

Arteriogram of the knee and proximal tibia of a 13-year-old who sustained a complete popliteal artery injury as the result of a displaced proximal tibial type 1 physeal injury that reduced spontaneously. (Courtesy of Dr. Neil E. Green.)

Anatomic closed or open reduction should be the goal of the fracture treatment in order to reduce the risk of later growth abnormality. The fracture site must be well stabilized to prevent further potential vascular insult. Internal fixation needs are generally simple, and Steinmann pins should be adequate to maintain reduction in nearly all cases.

Reduction of this fracture should be completed under general anesthesia, using fluoroscopic control. Since most of these fractures result from hyperextension injury, flexion usually accomplishes reduction. If hyperflexion is needed to maintain reduction, crossed Steinmann pins are placed to secure fixation in type I fractures. In type II fractures, the pins may be passed through the metaphyseal fragment and should not cross the physis. Immobilizing the leg in significant flexion will increase the possibility of vascular compromise in the popliteal space, leading to relative or complete ischemia of the lower

before recoiling to the nearly reduced position often seen on radiographs (Fig. 12–17).

Arteriography to assess popliteal and lower leg arterial flow should be performed in all children with any abnormality of pulses or coolness of the foot on physical examination. Even if the vascular evaluation is normal, an argument can be made for use of arteriography prior to definitive fracture treatment because of the extremely high risk of vascular injury with this fracture (Fig. 12–18).

Treatment. The proximal tibial physeal fracture can be treated definitively after the potential vascular problems have been evaluated. These fractures are usually Salter-Harris types I and II, although type IV fractures are more common if lawn mower injuries are included. Many of these fractures have a component of a type V crush injury as well, since growth disturbances in the proximal tibial physeal area are relatively common sequelae.

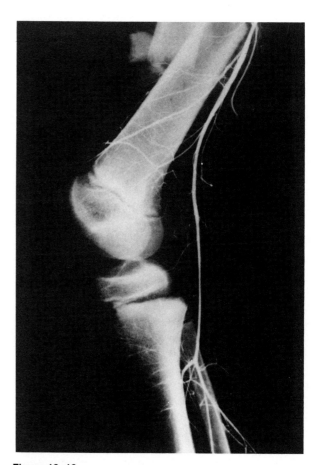

Figure 12–18

Lateral radiograph of the distal femur and proximal tibia of a boy who sustained a closed femoral fracture and a displaced type 1 fracture of the proximal tibia. The arteriogram shows that the popliteal artery is narrow and under spasm, but there is no intimal damage to the artery. (Courtesy of Dr. Neil E. Green.)

leg. Even if moderate flexion is needed to maintain reduction, I prefer to use percutaneous fixation to hold the fracture reduction and allow for postoperative care with the knee in 20 to 30 degrees of flexion.

If one or two (at most) attempts at closed reduction are unsuccessful, open reduction is required. This is more often needed in type II than in type I fractures. The reason that closed reduction of these fractures fails is usually the interposition of soft tissue in the fracture site. If an arterial repair is needed, open reduction is quickly accomplished just prior to arterial surgery to provide bony stability for the repair.

If open reduction is needed, the orthopaedic surgeon must consider doing the procedure without a tourniquet or, at least, using a tourniquet for only a short time to prevent exacerbation of early compartment syndrome that may be developing. The incision for open reduction is anterior, most often directly lateral to the tibial tubercle. In type II fractures, the incision is made over the metaphyseal fragment site. Hematoma evacuation and soft tissue extraction will allow anatomic reduction without knee arthrotomy in types I and II fractures. Steinmann pins are used to stabilize the fracture, and closed suction drainage is placed prior to wound closure.

Because of the proclivity to compartment syndrome with this fracture, the orthopaedic surgeon should measure the compartment pressures prior to leaving the operating room. A Wick catheter (or even an 18-gauge needle) can be readily connected to a saline-filled tube, which is connected to the arterial pressure monitor of the anesthesiologist. As the needle is inserted directly into the anterior, lateral, posterior, and deep posterior compartments, the tissue pressures are read directly off the monitor screen. These readings can be used as a baseline for later measurements on the ward, or, if values are over 40 mm Hg, appropriate fasciotomies can be done while the patient is still in the operating room.

After fracture reduction and stabilization have been completed and compartment pressures have been checked, a long leg splint is applied with the knee flexed at approximately 20 or 30 degrees. Bedrest with the leg slightly elevated is maintained for 24 to 48 hours as the child is carefully and serially evaluated for the development of a compartment syndrome. If the child is cooperative, this monitoring can be performed by assessment of toe sensation, pain on passive toe movement, and pedal pulses. If the child has an associated head injury and is unconscious, sequential compartment pressure readings should be performed until the surgeon is convinced that a compartment syndrome is not developing. If a compartment syndrome is diagnosed at any time after fracture, fasciotomy is needed urgently.

Once it is clear that no compartment syndrome is present or is developing, a long leg cast is applied with the leg in mild flexion. The fracture should be healed in about 4 weeks, at which time the Steinmann pins and cast are removed, with rehabilitation begun at once. Because of the propensity to later angular deformity or leg shortness from physeal arrest at this location,[30, 48, 49] these patients must be followed for at least 2 to 3 years after injury to detect such problems early and plan appropriate management.

Proximal Tibial Metaphyseal Fractures

Fractures of the proximal tibial metaphysis are of two major types. The most common type is found in children under the age of 10 years. Though not difficult to treat initially, these fractures may lead to later valgus deformity in many cases.[15, 54] The initial fracture is relatively nondisplaced but often demonstrates a fracture gap on the medial side of the proximal tibial metaphysis. Often the fibula is not fractured. Neurovascular injury is uncommon.

Although at first presentation this fracture appears relatively benign, treatment should be directed to closing the medial metaphyseal gap at the fracture site. Reduction is best accomplished under general anesthesia. The knee is straightened, and varus stress is applied across the fracture. If fluoroscopy shows that fracture reduction has been obtained, a long leg cast is applied with the knee nearly fully extended. If this medial fracture gap cannot be reduced by closed means, the pes anserinus may be interposed into the fracture site. In this instance, open reduction can be accomplished by a small medial incision over the fracture site and extraction of the interposed soft tissue. Internal fixation is unnecessary, and casting with some varus molding will hold the reduction satisfactorily.

Although healing of this fracture is complete by 5 or 6 weeks, follow-up is needed for 2 to 4 years. Within 12 to 18 months, 10 to 20 degrees of valgus deformity of the tibia commonly develops. The most likely cause of this valgus deformity is asymmetric growth stimulation, with the tibia growing faster than the fibula as a response to this injury and resultant hyperemia. Increased radionuclide activity on the medial aspect of the proximal tibial physis has been reported after this metaphyseal fracture, so some asymmetric growth may take place within the tibia itself.[66] An alternative explanation for this valgus development proposes that a portion of the pes anserinus remains interposed in the fracture site.[64] (As noted previously, if the medial gap persists, open reduction of this fracture should be considered.)

Although the valgus deformity resulting from the proximal tibial metaphyseal fracture is unsightly to the parents, osteotomy to correct this should be deferred for the first 2 or 3 years after fracture healing. Many of these valgus angulations will remodel with continued growth, but it may take as long as 4 years after fracture for return to essentially normal alignment. If it is performed, osteotomy of both tibia and fibula is needed to prevent a valgus recurrence, which may still occur as a result of repeated tibial overgrowth after surgery. The surgeon should be in no hurry to perform osteotomy for valgus deformity after this fracture.

The second type of fracture seen in this location is produced by greater trauma and has a greater risk of neurovascular complication, much like the proximal tibial physeal fractures discussed previously. These displaced fractures often injure the anterior tibial artery and lead to a compartment syndrome of the lower leg. The fibula is generally fractured and displaced with the proximal tibia and may be associated with an injury to the proximal peroneal nerve.

If adequate closed reduction can be obtained and there are no signs or symptoms of compartment syndrome, a long leg cast in slight knee flexion for 6 weeks is adequate treatment. After reduction, continued evaluation in the hospital for 1 to 2 days is needed as ongoing monitoring for compartment syndrome proceeds. If a fasciotomy is needed to treat a compartment syndrome, either external or internal fixation is needed for fracture stabilization. To allow for fasciotomy wound care and effective reduction without opening the fracture site, an external fixator bridging the knee joint can be applied[63] for a few weeks, without excessive concern for residual joint stiffness in a child. If external fixation is not used, limited internal fixation with Steinmann pins can provide fixation, with splint support of the leg until wound healing is sufficient to apply a long leg cast for the final stages of healing.

Proximal Fibular Physeal Fracture

Most proximal fibular fractures coincident with proximal tibial physeal or metaphyseal fractures involve the proximal fibular shaft. Although these fractures do not require anatomic reduction, careful evaluation of peroneal nerve function is needed whenever this injury is seen on the radiographs.

Physeal fracture of the proximal fibula is unusual.[1, 10] This fracture typically occurs during adolescence, so growth disturbance is generally not a problem. If knee ligament instability is not present, long leg cast treatment for 3 to 4 weeks is sufficient for management.

Open Fractures in the Knee Region

Open fractures near a major joint require thorough evaluation to determine whether the joint was entered at the time of injury. Particularly in the knee region, the proximity of major neurovascular structures to the bony structures predisposes the limb to a greater risk of neurocirculatory injury in open fractures.

In open fractures resulting from blunt trauma, compared with management of closed fractures, the primary additional consideration is possible communication of the skin wound with the knee joint. Sometimes the examiner can look into the knee joint through the wound, and the diagnosis is easy. If the radiograph demonstrates air within the knee joint, this can be used as presumptive evidence of communication of the wound into the knee joint. If the diagnosis is less clear, however, 30 to 50 ml of saline or other physiologic fluid is injected aseptically into the knee. If the wound communicates with the knee joint, the injected fluid will be seen to exit the knee through the skin wound. If no fluid extravasation through the wound is seen, the external wound does not communicate with the knee joint. If there is communication with the knee joint, a formal arthrotomy is included with the irrigation and debridement of the open fracture site. The knee joint is closed over a closed suction drain, while the open fracture wound may be closed loosely over drains or left open, depending on the surgeon's evaluation. As with other open fractures, antibiotics are administered for 3 to 5 days after operation.

In open fractures secondary to penetrating trauma, such as a bullet, fracture management is somewhat different. If the bullet is a low-velocity missile with little adjacent soft tissue injury, an open fracture of the femoral or tibial shaft does not usually require formal irrigation and debridement unless adjacent vascular structures are injured. However, if the bullet has lodged in the knee joint or has passed through the knee, arthrotomy of the knee is recommended to remove bony and cartilaginous fragments as well as to remove the bullet. Even if a bullet is not mechanically causing a problem with knee movement, a retained bullet within the knee joint may lead to elevated serum lead levels.

With gunshot wounds of the knee, careful attention must be paid to the path of the bullet, particularly with regard to the popliteal and proximal tibial area vessels. Arteriography or popliteal exploration, or both, should be performed if the bullet trajectory is in the posterior aspect of the proximal tibia. Once the wound and soft tissue injuries have been managed appropriately, the fracture may require external fixation to allow for ease of dressing changes; however, management has to be individualized for each open fracture in this region.

Patellar Dislocation

Dislocation and subluxation of the patella are relatively frequent in children and adolescents. These injuries are more common in females than in males.

Anatomy. The patella is a sesamoid bone situated within the quadriceps tendon itself. It influences the lever arm of the quadriceps muscle by increasing its force. A line drawn through the center of the femur and thigh and then drawn distally along the patellar ligament inferior to the patella shows that the angle of pull of the quadriceps mechanism is in a slightly valgus direction. Its angle, called the Q angle, is increased in patients with recurrent patellar dislocation or subluxation (Fig. 12–19).

Mechanism. Patellar dislocation is most often the result of a forceful twisting injury of the knee while the foot is planted. It can occur in all sports and in many physical activities. Very few dislocations are the result of direct trauma to the patella.

Incidence and Classification. Almost all patellar dislocations are lateral, with the patella moving in a lateral direction. An intraarticular patellar dislocation may occur, but it is extremely rare. Recurrent dislocations may follow an initial dislocation. Cash and Hughston found that in patients under the age of 14 years, up to 60% developed a recurrent dislocation.[12] Over the age of 19 years, 30% of patients sustained recurrent dislocation. In those who were older than 28 years at the time of their first dislocation, recurrent dislocation seemed to be very rare.

Diagnosis. Most acute patellar dislocations reduce spontaneously or with passive extension of the knee prior to the patient's evaluation in an emergency department. Therefore, the diagnosis of acute patellar dislocation should be suspected in most children and adolescents who present with an acute hemarthrosis of the knee.

One must distinguish between a patellar disloca-

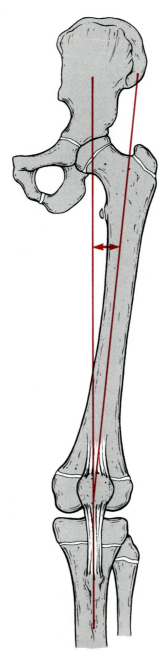

Figure 12–19

The Q angle. The quadriceps mechanism has a normal valgus alignment. This is measured by drawing a line from the anterosuperior iliac spine to the center of the patella. The angle that this line makes with a line drawn along the center of the longitudinal axis of the patella and then from the center of the patella to the center of the tibial tubercle is called the Q angle.

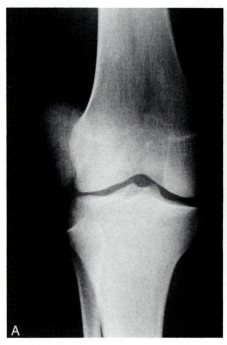
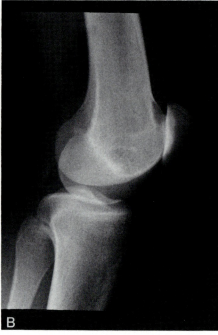

Figure 12–20

A, Anteroposterior radiograph of the knee of a teenaged girl who sustained a patellar dislocation. Note that the patella is laterally displaced. *B*, Lateral radiograph demonstrating that the patella overlies the distal femoral condyle, indicating that the patella is dislocated. (Courtesy of Dr. Neil E. Green.)

tion that reduced spontaneously and an injury to the intraarticular knee ligaments or the physes of the distal femur and proximal tibia. This distinction should be made in the acute care setting, before severe pain is experienced. A knee aspiration may be required to relieve the acute hemarthrosis. Blood will be found, but if fat is also found in the blood aspirated from the knee, one should suspect the presence of an osteochondral fracture. The osteochondral fracture may originate from the medial facet of the patella or from the lateral femoral condyle (see Fig. 12–7), occurring as the patella dislocates laterally. The medial pole of the patella strikes the lateral femoral condyle, and one or the other may be fractured.

Treatment. Because most patellar dislocations reduce spontaneously, reduction in the emergency department is rarely necessary. Nevertheless, the diagnosis is extremely important. Aspiration of the joint may be indicated, both for relief of the tense hemarthrosis and for evaluation of a potential osteochondral fracture. Radiographs of the knee may fail to demonstrate an osteochondral fracture because in the younger child much of the fracture will involve cartilage (Fig. 12–20).

Immobilization in a cylinder cast for approximately 4 weeks is recommended. Afterwards, the cast is removed, and the patient begins rehabilitative exercises to increase the strength of the quadriceps and hamstring musculature.

RECURRENT PATELLAR DISLOCATION AND SUBLUXATION

Chronic subluxation or dislocation of the patella is more common in patients whose first dislocation occurs in childhood.[37] In addition, if the Q angle is large, the incidence of recurrence of the dislocation or subluxation is high. Initial immobilization plus rehabilitation should be undertaken. However, with multiple recurrences of the dislocation or subluxation despite excellent rehabilitative exercises, one should consider surgical correction of the patellar subluxation or dislocation. In children with open physes, tibial tubercle transfer is contraindicated. The mainstay of surgical correction is release of the lateral retinaculum and plication of the medial retinaculum. In addition, the pull of the quadriceps mechanism may be altered by one of two methods.

The Roux-Goldthwait procedure involves splitting the patellar ligament in half and detaching the lateral half from the tibial tubercle without disturbing the apophysis. The lateral half is then transposed medially underneath the medial half of the patellar ligament and sutured to the periosteum on the medial side of the patellar ligament. This will alter the vector force of the quadriceps mechanism, thereby decreasing the Q angle.

A second procedure that is popular is transfer of the semitendinosus. The semitendinosus is detached from its musculotendinous junction but is left attached distally on the tibia. The tendon is then passed through a drill hole in the patella from inferomedial to superolateral, brought out through the superolateral drill hole, and then sutured back to itself inferomedially (Fig. 12–21).

Postoperatively, these patients are maintained in a cylinder cast with the knee straight for approximately 4 to 6 weeks. After that time, they are begun on rehabilitative exercises of the knee to strengthen their quadriceps and hamstring musculature.

DISLOCATION OF THE KNEE

Complete dislocation of the knee is rare in children. It is more common in teenagers and adults.

Mechanism. Complete dislocation of the knee is usually the result of severe trauma to the knee. In a series of patients with complete dislocation of the knee, most injuries were the result of a violent accident, such as a motor vehicle accident or a fall from a significant height.

Diagnosis. The diagnosis should be obvious, and it is certainly obvious radiographically. However, possibility of a vascular injury must also be investigated. The incidence of vascular injury is very high with knee dislocation. Green and Allen found that 32% of patients with an acute dislocation of the knee sustained a popliteal artery injury.[22] They also found that vascular injury resulted in amputation if it was not repaired within 6 to 8 hours of injury.

Management. The treatment of knee dislocation usually requires ligamentous reconstruction. This will not be discussed, as it is beyond the scope of this text. Nevertheless, the most important element of the initial management of the knee dislocation is determination of the vascular status of the popliteal artery. If there is any abnormality in the pulse distally, an arteriogram should be performed. Some have even advocated arteriography routinely with a confirmed knee dislocation because of the possible presence of an intimal flap that may allow vascular flow initially but may clot off later.[22]

It must be remembered that the popliteal artery is essentially an end-artery and that the collateral blood supply about the knee is inadequate to maintain the viability of the musculature of the lower extremity. The skin may remain viable for a period of time with a complete popliteal artery disruption;

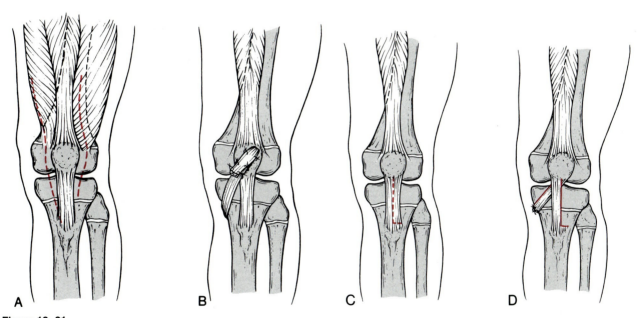

Figure 12–21

Surgical technique for treatment of patellar subluxation or dislocation. *A*, Lateral retinacular release. The lateral retinaculum has been released well up into the vastus lateralis, and the vastus medialis plus the medial retinaculum has been plicated. *B*, Semitendinosus tenodesis. The semitendinosus has been released at its musculotendinous junction and pulled distally. It is passed through a drill hole in the patella and then sutured back onto itself. *C*, Roux-Goldthwait reconstruction. A lateral retinacular release is performed plus plication of the medial retinaculum and advancement of the medialis obliquus. In addition, the lateral half of the patellar ligament is split off from the medial half and detached from the tibial tubercle extraperiosteally. *D*, The lateral half is then transferred medially underneath the medial half of the patellar ligament and sutured to the periosteum of the proximal tibia.

however, the musculature and nerves will die very quickly. Repair of the vascular injury, if performed within 6 to 8 hours, will usually avert the need for amputation.

REFERENCES

1. Abrams, J.; Bennett, E.; Kumar, S. J.; Pizzutillo, P. D. Salter-Harris type III fracture of the proximal fibula. A case report. Am J Sports Med 14:514–516, 1986.
2. Ahstrom, J. P. Osteochondral fracture in the knee joint associated with hypermobility and dislocation of the patella. Report of eighteen cases. J Bone Joint Surg 47-A:1491–1502, 1965.
3. Aitken, A. P. Fractures of the proximal tibial epiphyseal cartilage. Clin Orthop 41:92–97, 1965.
4. Bachelin, P.; Bugmann, P. Active subluxation in extension; radiological control in intercondylar eminence fractures in childhood. Z Kinderchir 43:180–182, 1988.
5. Baxter, M. P.; Wiley, J. J. Fractures of the tibial spine in children. An evaluation of knee stability. J Bone Joint Surg 70-B:228–230, 1988.
6. Beals, R. K.; Tufts, E. Fractured femur in infancy: The role of child abuse. J Pediatr Orthop 3:583–586, 1983.
7. Bertin, K. C.; Goble, E. M. Ligament injuries associated with physeal fractures about the knee. Clin Orthop 177:188–195, 1983.
8. Boestman, O.; Kiviluoto, O.; Santavirta, S.; et al. Fractures of the patella treated by operation. Arch Orthop Trauma Surg 102:78–81, 1983.
9. Bowers, K. D., Jr. Patellar tendon avulsion as a complication of Osgood-Schlatter's disease. Am J Sports Med 9:356–359, 1981.
10. Brendel, I. J.; Prosser, A. J.; Pearse, M. Salter type 2 fracture separation of the proximal epiphysis of the fibula. Injury 18:421–422, 1987.
11. Burkhart, S. S.; Peterson, H. A. Fractures of the proximal tibial epiphysis. J Bone Joint Surg 61-A:996–1002, 1979.
12. Cash, J. D.; Hughston, J. E. Treatment of acute patellar dislocation. Am J Sports Med 16(3):244–249, 1988.
13. Christie, M. J.; Dvonch, V. M. Tibial tuberosity avulsion fracture in adolescents. J Pediatr Orthop 1:391–394, 1981.
14. Ciszewski, W. A; Buschmann, W. R.; Rudolph, C. N. Irreducible fracture of the proximal tibial physis in an adolescent. Orthop Rev 18:891–893, 1989.
15. Dal Monte, A.; Manes, E.; Cammarota, V. Post-traumatic genu valgum in children. Ital J Orthop Traumatol 9:5–11, 1983.
16. Davies, A. M.; Carter, S. R.; Grimer, R. J.; Sneath, R. S. Fatigue fractures of the femoral diaphysis in the skeletally immature simulating malignancy. Br J Radiol 62:893–896, 1989.
17. DeHaven, K. E. Diagnosis of acute knee injuries with hemarthrosis. Am J Sports Med 8:9–14, 1980.
18. Echeverria, T. S.; Bersani, F.A. Acute fracture simulating a symptomatic bipartite patella. Report of a case. Am J Sports Med 8:48–50, 1980.
19. Fyfe, I. S.; Jackson, J. P. Tibial intercondylar fractures in children: A review of the classification and the treatment of malunion. Injury 13:165–169, 1981.
20. Gaudernak, T.; Zifko, R.; Skorpik, G. Osteochondral fractures of the knee and the ankle joint. Clinical experiences using fibrin sealant. Acta Orthop Belg 52:465–478, 1986.
21. Gilley, J. S.; Gelman, M. I.; Edson, D. M.; Metcalf, R. W. Chondral fractures of the knee. Arthrographic, arthroscopic, and clinical manifestations. Radiology 138:51–54, 1981.
22. Green, N. E.; Allen, B. L. Vascular injuries associated with dislocation of the knee. J Bone Joint Surg 59-A:236–239, 1977.
23. Green, W. T., Jr. Painful bipartite patellae. A report of three cases. Clin Orthop 110:197–200, 1975.
24. Groenkvist, H.; Hirsch, G.; Johansson, L. Fracture of the anterior tibial spine in children. J Pediatr Orthop 4:465–468, 1984.
25. Grogan, D. P.; Bobechko, W. P. Pathogenesis of a fracture of the distal femoral epiphysis. A case report. J Bone Joint Surg 66-A:621–622, 1984.
26. Gross, R. H.; Davidson, R.; Sullivan J. A.; et al. Cast brace management of the femoral shaft fracture in children and young adults. J Pediatr Orthop 3:572–582, 1983.
27. Hammerle, C. P.; Jacob, R. P. Chondral and osteochondral fractures after luxation of the patella and their treatment. Arch Orthop Trauma Surg 97:207–211, 1980.
28. Hand, W. L.; Hand, C. R.; Dunn, A. W. Avulsion fractures of the tibial tubercle. J Bone Joint Surg 53-A:1579–1583, 1971.
29. Harper, M. C.; Ralston, M. Isobutyl 2-cyanoacrylate as an osseous adhesive in the repair of osteochondral fractures. J Biomed Mater Res 17:167–177, 1983.
30. Heckman, J. D.; Alkire, C. C. Distal patellar pole fractures. A proposed common mechanism of injury. Am J Sports Med 12:424–428, 1984.
31. Hensal, F.; Nelson, R.; Pavlov, H.; Torg, J. S. Bilateral patellar fractures from indirect trauma. A cast report. Clin Orthop 178:207–209, 1983.
32. Hopkinson, W. J.; Mitchell, W. A.; Curl, W. W. Chondral fractures of the knee. Cause for confusion. Am J Sports Med 15:309–312, 1985.
33. Houghton, G. R.; Ackroyd, C. E. Sleeve fractures of the patella in children. A report of three cases. J Bone Joint Surg 61-B:165–168, 1979.
34. Hresko, M. T.; Kasser, J. R. Physeal arrest about the knee associated with non-physeal fractures in the lower extremity. J Bone Joint Surg 71-A:698–703, 1989.
35. Iwaya, T.; Takatori, Y. Lateral longitudinal stress fracture of the patella: Report of three cases. J Pediatr Orthop 5:73–77, 1985.
36. Johnson, E. W.; McLeod T. L. Osteochondral fragments of the distal end of the femur fixed with bone pegs. Report of two cases. J Bone Joint Surg 59-A:677–679, 1977.
37. Larsen, E.; Lauridsen, F. Conservative treatment of patellar dislocations. Influence of evident factors on the tendency to redislocation and the therapeutic result. Clin Orthop 171:131–136, 1982.
38. Levi, J. H.; Coleman, C. R. Fracture of the tibial tubercle. Am J Sports Med 4:254–263, 1976.
39. Lipscomb, A. B.; Anderson, A. F. Open reduction of a malunited tibial spine fracture in a 12-year-old male. A case report. Am J Sports Med 13:419–422, 1985.
40. Lombardo, S. J.; Harvey, J. P., Jr. Fractures of the distal femoral epiphysis. Factors influencing prognosis: A review of thirty-four cases. J Bone Joint Surg 59-A:742–751, 1977.
41. Mayer, F.; Seidlein, H. Chondral and osteochondral fractures of the knee joint—treatment and results. Arch Orthop Trauma Surg 107:154–157, 1988.
42. Meyers, M. H.; McKeever, F. M. Fracture of the intercondylar eminence of the tibia. J Bone Joint Surg 41-A:209–222, 1959.

43. Meyers, M. H.; McKeever, F. M. Follow up notes. Fracture of the intercondylar eminence of the tibia. J Bone Joint Surg 52-A:1677–1684, 1970.
44. Mink, J. H.; Deutsch, A. L. Occult cartilage and bone injuries of the knee: Detection, classification, and assessment with MR imaging. Radiology 170:823–829, 1989.
45. Nichols, J. N.; Tehranzadeh, J. A review of tibial spine fractures in bicycle injury. Am J Sports Med 15:172–174, 1987.
46. Ogden, J. A.; Tross, R. B.; Murphy, M. J. Fractures of the tibial tuberosity in adolescents. J Bone Joint Surg 62-A:205–215, 1980.
47. Ogden, J. A.; McCarthy, S. M.; Jokl, P. The painful bipartite patella. J Pediatr Orthop 2:263–269, 1982.
48. Olerud, C.; Danckwardt-Lilliestroem, G.; Olerud, S. Genu recurvatum caused by partial growth arrest of the proximal tibial physis: Simultaneous correction and lengthening with physeal distraction. A report of two cases. Arch Orthop Trauma Surg 106:64–68, 1986.
49. Pappas, A. M.; Anas, P.; Toczylowski, H. M., Jr. Asymmetrical arrest of the proximal tibial physis and genu recurvatum deformity. J Bone Joint Surg 66-A:575–581, 1984.
50. Pennig, D.; Baranowski, D. Genu recurvatum due to partial growth arrest of the proximal tibial physis: Correction by callus distraction. Case report. Arch Orthop Trauma Surg 108:119–121, 1989.
51. Rae, P. S.; Khasawneh, Z. M. Herbert screw fixation of osteochondral fractures of the patella. Injury 19:116–119, 1988.
52. Riseborough, E. J.; Barrett, I. R.; Shapiro, F. Growth disturbances following distal femoral physeal fracture-separations. J Bone Joint Surg 65-A:885–893, 1983.
53. Rivero, H.; Bolden, R.; Young, L. W. Proximal tibial physis fracture and popliteal artery injury. Radiology 150:390, 1984.
54. Robert, M.; Khouri, N.; Carlioz, H.; Alain, J. L. Fractures of the proximal tibial metaphysis in children: Review of a series of 25 cases. J Pediatr Orthop 7:444–449, 1987.
55. Roberts, J. M. Operative treatment of fractures about the knee. Orthop Clin North Am 21:365–379, 1990.
56. Robinson, S. C.; Driscoll, S. E. Simultaneous osteochondral avulsion of the femoral and tibial insertions of the anterior cruciate ligament. Report of a case in a thirteen-year-old boy. J Bone Joint Surg 63-A:1342–1343, 1981.
57. Rorabeck, C. H.; Bobechko, W. P. Acute dislocation of the patella with osteochondral fracture. Review of eighteen cases. J Bone Joint Surg 58-B:237–240, 1976.
58. Rosenberg, N. J. Osteochondral fractures of the lateral femoral condyle. J Bone Joint Surg 46-A:1013–1026, 1964.
59. Shelton, W. R.; Canale, S. T. Fractures of the tibia through the proximal tibial epiphyseal cartilage. J Bone Joint Surg 61-A:167–173, 1979.
60. Stephens, D. C.; Louis, D. S.; Louis, E. Traumatic separation of the distal femoral epiphyseal cartilage plate. J Bone Joint Surg 56-A:1383–1390, 1974.
61. Ten Thije, J. H.; Frima, A. J. Patellar dislocation and osteochondral fractures. Neth J Surg 38:150–154, 1986.
62. Terry, G. C.; Flandry, F.; Van Manen, J. W.; Norwood, L. A. Isolated chondral fractures of the knee. Clin Orthop 234:170–177, 1988.
63. Tolo, V. T. External fixation in multiply injured children. Orthop Clin North Am 21:393–400, 1990.
64. Weber, B. G. Fibrous interposition causing valgus deformity after fracture of the upper tibia metaphysis in children. J Bone Joint Surg 59-B:290–292, 1977.
65. Weber, M. J.; Janecki, C. J.; McLeod, P.; et al. Efficacy of various forms of fixation of transverse fractures of the patella. J Bone Joint Surg 62-A:215–220, 1980.
66. Zionts, L. E.; Harcke, H. T.; Brooks, K. M.; MacEwen, G. D. Posttraumatic tibia valga: A case demonstrating asymmetric activity at the proximal growth plate on the technetium bone scan. J Pediatr Orthop 7:458–462, 1987.

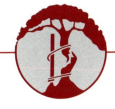

George H. Thompson, M.D.
Fred Behrens, M.D.

13

Fractures of the Tibia and Fibula

Nonphyseal fractures involving the tibia and fibula are among the most common injuries involving the lower extremities in children.[110, 164, 191, 223] The fracture patterns, mechanisms of injury, and anatomic location of these fractures will vary according to the age of the child. Most can be treated conservatively with minimal complications and satisfactory long-term results. However, certain tibial fractures produce unique problems that must be evaluated and treated carefully to avoid complications.

Pathology

Relevant Anatomy. The tibial and fibular shafts consist of the proximal metaphysis, central diaphysis, and distal metaphysis. In this chapter we will not be concerned with fractures involving the proximal or distal epiphyses or the associated physes, as they have been discussed elsewhere. The blood supply to the tibia consists of (1) a nutrient artery, which is a branch of the posterior tibial artery, that enters at the junction of the distal and middle thirds of the tibia and is responsible for the endosteal or medullary blood supply; (2) periosteal vessels, which are segmented and enter from the surrounding tissues; and (3) epiphyseal vessels. The inner two thirds of the cortex are supplied by the endosteal vessels, and the outer third is supplied by the periosteal vessels. Proximally, the epiphyseal and periosteal vessels are branches of the medial and lateral inferior geniculate arteries. The collateral circulation is rich proximally, especially on the medial aspect.[156] Tibial fractures distal to the nutrient artery may deprive the distal fragment of its medullary blood supply, and in such cases that portion must rely on its periosteal and metaphyseal blood supply for healing. This may result in a slower rate of healing. Periosteal and soft tissue stripping of the distal fracture may further slow the healing process.

The blood supply to the fibula arises from the peroneal artery, which gives off a nutrient artery that enters the diaphysis just proximal to the midpoint. This artery supplies multiple segmental musculoperiosteal vessels that pass circumferentially around the fibula, supplying both the fibula and the adjacent muscles.

From the surgical perspective, it must be remembered that the popliteal artery descends between the posterior aspect of the medial and lateral femoral condyles. It passes between the medial and lateral heads of the gastrocnemius and along the distal border of the popliteal muscle before dividing into the anterior and posterior tibial arteries. The anterior tibial artery passes anteriorly between the two heads of the tibialis posterior muscle and enters the anterior compartment of the leg by passing through the proximal aspect of the interosseous membrane at the flare of the proximal tibia and fibular metaphyses.[156] Displaced fractures in this region may damage the anterior tibial artery, but fortunately this is rare.[171] The foramen in the interosseous membrane is long and narrow; this affords some protection, as the anterior tibial artery is allowed to move both proximally and distally. Corrective osteotomies in this region may also potentially damage the anterior tibial artery.[100, 139, 198] This, fortunately, is also rare. Subperiosteal dissection in the region of the proximal tibia will usually allow protection of this vessel.

Fracture Patterns. Nonphyseal fracture patterns involving the tibia and fibula include (1) compression (torus), (2) incomplete tension-compression (greenstick), and (3) complete fractures. Plastic deformities can also occur but involve predominantly the fibula.[119, 131, 204] Complete fractures can be further classified according to the direction of the fracture (spiral, oblique, or transverse) or as comminuted or segmental. Tibia and fibula fractures may also be open or closed, depending on the integrity of the overlying skin and soft tissues.

Pediatric bone, including the tibia and fibula, displays different fracture patterns from adult bone because of its material properties. The lower ash content of pediatric bone indicates less mineralization.[43] Thus, pediatric bones have greater plasticity, and less energy is necessary for bone failure. Bending is the most common mode for failure in long bones. A low-yield stress on the tension side of a bone initiates a fracture followed by compression on the opposite side. As bending continues, the fracture line eventually traverses the entire width of the bone. Currey and Butler[43] demonstrated that pediatric bone is weaker, primarily because it has a greater capacity to undergo plastic deformation than does adult bone. Because the pediatric bone yields at a lower force, the stress on the bone and the energy required to propagate a fracture are both less. These factors account for the compression, greenstick, and plastic deformation fracture patterns seen in children and adolescents but not in adults. The increased porosity of pediatric bone was previously thought to play a role in the different fracture patterns, but this view is no longer accepted. Currey[42] studied impact energy absorption in 39 human femurs ranging in age from 3 to 95 years. He found no relationship between the impact energy absorbed by the specimens and their porosity.

Incidence. Fractures of the tibia and fibula shafts are very common[110, 164, 191, 199, 223] and constitute approximately 15% of all pediatric fractures.[199] Males are more commonly involved than females.[110, 199] The tibia and fibula shaft fractures are the most common long bone fractures of the lower extremity. Parrini and co-workers[164] reported on 1027 long bone fractures in children between 1 and 11 years of age seen between 1976 and 1982; 477 fractures involved the lower extremities, with 157 (33%) isolated fractures of the tibia and 169 (35%) of both the tibia and fibula. The remaining 151 fractures involved the femur. An epidemiologic study by Kärrholm et al.[110] in Lund, Sweden, showed an annual incidence of 190 tibia fractures per 10,000 males between infancy and 18 years of age and 110 tibia fractures per 10,000 females in the same age range. In males, the incidence peaked between 3 and 4 years of age and again between ages 15 and 16. The first peak was due predominantly to spiral or oblique fractures, and the second peak involved primarily transverse fractures. In females the incidence was relatively even up to 11 to 12 years of age, with a tendency toward lower values with advancing age.

Mechanisms of Injury. Fractures of the tibia and fibula may be the result of direct as well as indirect forces. Direct trauma frequently produces a transverse fracture or segmental fracture pattern, while the indirect forces are typically rotational, producing an oblique or spiral fracture.

Steinert and Bennek[199] in 1966 analyzed 263 tibial fractures in children and found that a fall was the most common mechanism of injury. Falls accounted for 45% of the fractures and approximately one half of those involved a fall from a height. Motor vehicle accidents were the most common cause of a complete fracture, which occurred in 42.5% of the cases. Drewes and Schulte[54] analyzed 212 fractures in children less than 14 years of age. The frequency and mechanism of injuries varied according to the age of the child. In 51 children less than 4 years of age, 17 fractures (35%) were caused by bicycle spoke accidents. In 160 children between 4 and 14 years of age, sports and motor vehicle accidents were the major mechanisms of injury.

In the study by Kärrholm and colleagues,[110] a motor vehicle accident, involving a child as a passenger, as a bicycle rider, or as a pedestrian, was the most common mechanism of a tibia fracture. The age range of children in motor vehicle accidents was 8 to 14 years. It was interesting that winter sport activities had almost the same incidence as motor vehicle accidents in females. Similar results regarding winter sports were reported in England, where the risk for tibia fractures in children involved in a skiing accident was ten times higher than for an adult.[85] Falls were the most common mechanism of injury in young children.

In the 1988 study by Shannak[191] of 142 tibial shaft fractures, motor vehicle accidents caused 63% of the fractures; falls caused 18%; direct violence accounted for 15%; and sports caused only 4%.

Consequence of Injury. Considering the frequency of pediatric tibia fracture, the consequences for most children are minimal. These fractures heal readily with minimal complications. Children typically have a rapid return to normal activities, including sports, and minimal disability. However, in a small percentage of cases, especially those involv-

Table 13-1 Classification of Tibia and Fibula Fractures
Fractures of the proximal tibial metaphysis
Fractures of the tibial and fibular shafts
Isolated fractures of the tibial shaft
Incomplete (greenstick)
Complete
Fractures of the tibial and fibular shafts
Isolated fractures of the fibular shafts
Fractures of the distal tibial metaphysis

Adapted from Dias, L.S. Fractures of the tibia and fibula. In: Rockwood, C.A., Jr.; Wilkens, K.E.; King, R.E., eds. Fractures in Children. Philadelphia, J.B. Lippincott, 1984, pp. 983–1041.

ing open fractures or severe soft tissue injury, there may be residual disability.

Associated Injuries. It is not uncommon for children who sustain tibia fractures to have associated injuries. This is especially true for children who are victims of high-energy trauma, such as motor vehicle–related accidents. In the study by Kärrholm and co-workers,[110] 27 of 480 children (6%) with tibia and fibular fractures sustained associated injuries, the most common being head injuries, fracture of the femur, and injury to an upper extremity. However, other body areas (face and neck, chest, and abdomen) may also be injured, depending on the severity of the trauma.

Classification. A classification for nonphyseal fractures of the tibia and fibula is presented in Table 13–1. A modification of the classification of Dias,[50] this classification divides the tibia and fibular shafts into three major anatomic areas—proximal metaphysis, diaphyses, and distal metaphysis. The fractures of the tibia and fibular diaphyses are subdivided according to the location (proximal third, middle third, and distal third) and combination of the bones fractured. Each of these subgroups may be further divided according to the fracture pattern—compression (torus), incomplete tension-compression (greenstick), or complete. This classification is useful in determining treatment methods and understanding the potential long-term results and possible complications.

Diagnosis

History. The typical symptom of a tibia or fibula fracture is pain. However, the severity of discomfort varies, depending on the magnitude of injury, the mechanism, and the age of the child. Frequently, the history may be lacking because the injury was not observed and the child is unable to verbalize the symptoms or mechanism of injury. In these cases, child abuse must also be considered.[158] In young children, the inability to walk may be the only sign or symptom. If the child is able to speak, it is important to ascertain the mechanism of injury.

Physical Examination. Because pain is the major symptom in a tibia or fibular shaft fracture, it is important to have the child point to the most painful area. Palpation in this area may reproduce or increase the child's discomfort. Deformity is not a common finding in children, as many tibia fractures may be nondisplaced. Swelling or edema of the lower leg also varies with the mechanism of injury, the extent of soft tissue injury, and the presence of displacement. Usually the soft tissue swelling is maximal at the fracture site. Stress examination may reveal instability or crepitation but will invariably increase pain. A stress examination is usually unnecessary when a fracture is suspected. Injured extremities with a suspected tibia fracture are best splinted prior to radiographic evaluation, usually with a long leg posterior plaster splint. This will relieve pain, prevent additional injuries to the soft tissues, and allow more accurate positioning of the extremity for the radiographs.

Nerve damage in association with tibia and fibular fractures is uncommon (see discussion of neurologic injury under Complications). In all fractures it is important to check dorsiflexion and plantar flexion of the ankle and toes as well as sensation, especially to touch. Nerve damage, if present, most likely will be the result of a direct injury to the peroneal nerve at the proximal fibula metaphysis. Arterial injuries associated with a tibial shaft fracture are also uncommon. The peripheral pulses of the dorsalis pedis and posterior tibial arteries must be ascertained and recorded at the initial physical examination. However, the presence of pulses does not completely eliminate the possibility of an associated arterial injury (see Vascular Injuries). Arterial injuries, when present, are most likely to be associated with a displaced proximal tibial metaphyseal fracture or an open fracture. Capillary circulation, sensation to the toes, pain on passive stretch, and pain out of proportion to injury must be monitored carefully as compartment syndromes can occur in children following tibial fractures (see Compartment Syndromes).

The soft tissue of the lower leg should also be evaluated. It is important to assess the integrity of the skin at the fracture site. Fractures in association with bicycle spoke injuries may ultimately result in full-thickness skin loss that will require delayed skin grafting. Any evidence of skin penetration at the fracture site is an indication that the fracture is open and contaminated (see Open Tibia and Fibula Fractures).

Radiographic Evaluation. When a tibial or fibular shaft fracture is suspected, radiographs must be obtained. Following splinting of the injured extremity, anteroposterior (AP) and lateral radiographs are made. They must include the knee and ankle joint to rule out a remote fracture. Comparison radiographs may be indicated in difficult situations, but this is unusual. Occasionally, incomplete fractures, such as a torus fracture, may be difficult to visualize. A spiral fracture of the tibial shaft with an intact fibula may be visible on only one view. It is imperative that orthogonal radiographs be obtained. Oblique radiographs may be beneficial if the initial radiographic appearance is normal and a fracture is suspected.

Special Diagnostic Studies. Special diagnostic imaging studies of the tibia and fibula may include (1) technetium bone scans, (2) laminagrams, (3) computed tomography (CT), and (4) magnetic resonance imaging (MRI).

Technetium bone scans may be useful in identifying occult fractures, especially in infants.[136, 162] Park and associates[162] found that bone scans could be used to differentiate between occult fractures of the femur or tibia and early acute osteomyelitis in infants. Images obtained early (1 to 4 days following onset of symptoms) demonstrated a subtle increase along the entire length of the injured bone when an occult fracture was present. The distribution of uptake was similar regardless of the fracture pattern. In early acute osteomyelitis there was focal uptake at the site of infection.

Laminagrams may be helpful in diagnosing occult fractures in older children. A CT scan of the tibia can be beneficial in assessing torsional alignment following complex unilateral fractures.[101] It can also be used in the assessment of pathologic fractures of the tibia to determine the presence, size, and intralesional contours of the lesion.[106]

MRI has been demonstrated to detect early stress fractures accurately. This procedure, although expensive, avoids the high doses of radiation incurred with bone scans, laminagrams, and CT scans.

Management

FRACTURES OF THE PROXIMAL TIBIAL METAPHYSIS

Fractures of the proximal tibial metaphysis are relatively uncommon injuries that generally occur in children between 3 and 6 years of age (range, 1 to 12 years).[44, 96, 105, 156, 177] There is a male:female ratio of approximately 3:1, which closely parallels the incidence by gender of tibial fractures in children.[81] Skak and colleagues[193] reported an incidence of approximately 6 proximal third metaphyseal fractures per 100,000 children per year. Rang[171] recognizes two types of fractures in this region: (1) displaced fractures with a risk for vascular injury to the anterior tibial artery, and (2) greenstick fractures with or without a valgus angulation. The majority of fractures are of the latter type. These fractures are typically the result of a direct injury to the lateral aspect of the extended knee. The primary injury patterns are compression (torus), incomplete tension-compression (greenstick), and complete fractures.[174] The majority of these fractures have minimal or no displacement and appear benign clinically but may, in fact, be followed by a post-traumatic valgus deformity. The incomplete tension-compression, or greenstick, fracture is the most common pattern. In the greenstick fracture the medial cortex (tension side) fractures while the lateral cortex (compression side) remains intact or hinges slightly. If the lateral cortex hinges, a valgus deformity occurs. However, there is usually no displacement and the apposition remains normal. The fibula is typically intact but occasionally may sustain either a fracture or a plastic deformation. Radiographically, the degree of angulation can be difficult to ascertain unless radiographs of both lower extremities symmetrically positioned on a long cassette are obtained and the true angulation measured. Oblique views and occasionally fluoroscopy may be beneficial in defining the fracture and any angulation.

The most common sequela of the fracture of the proximal tibial metaphysis is the development of a transient, progressive valgus deformity and overgrowth of the tibia. Cozen[39] in 1953 reported four cases of valgus deformity following nondisplaced or minimally angulated fractures of the proximal tibial metaphysis. Since then, numerous other reports have been published regarding this complication.[1, 8, 9, 12, 19, 22, 31, 37, 40, 41, 44, 70, 72, 83, 96, 99, 105, 107, 132, 133, 168, 174, 177, 178, 185, 193, 203, 218, 222, 231, 232] Similar valgus deformities have also been observed following other conditions affecting the proximal metaphysis of the immature tibia, including acute and chronic osteomyelitis,[9, 203] harvesting for a bone graft,[113] excision of an osteochondroma,[214] and osteotomy.[203]

The incidence of valgus deformity following proximal tibial metaphyseal fractures is variable. Salter and Best[185] reported 21 cases of proximal tibial metaphyseal fractures in which 13 (62%) showed a valgus deformity between 11 and 22 degrees at the time of cast removal. At follow-up this angle had increased to 18 to 25 degrees. Ten of their patients required surgical correction of the valgus deformity. Robert and associates[174] studied 25 patients with fractures of the proximal tibial metaphysis, 12 of whom (48%) later developed a genu valgum deformity. In a review of 40 consecutive patients by Skak and co-workers,[193] 4 had valgus deformities. These deformities occurred only following greenstick fractures. Boyer and colleagues[29] reported no valgus deformities in seven children, age 2 to 5 years, who sustained fractures while jumping on trampolines with a heavier child or an adult. Valgus deformities seem to be most commonly associated with greenstick and complete fractures.[174, 193] They are unusual after a torus fracture.

The theories regarding the etiology of the valgus deformity have included (1) injury to the lateral aspect of the proximal tibial physis, (2) inadequate reduction, (3) premature weight bearing, (4) hypertrophic callus formation, (5) dynamic muscle action, (6) soft tissue interposition, (7) tethering from an intact fibula, and (8) asymmetric growth stimulation.

Blount[25] initially felt that the lateral aspect of the proximal tibial physis was damaged by the original injury. Goff[70] and Ben-Itzhak and associates[19] supported this concept. However, it has not been substantiated by others.

Best[22] and Salter and Best[185] believed that inadequate reduction of the fracture was the major cause of the initial valgus deformity. Others have concurred.[8, 171] Salter and Best[185] as well as Pollen[167] agreed that early weight bearing in the cast contributed to the valgus angulation due to asymmetric compression in the preexisting valgus position. However, the valgus deformity has also occurred in nonambulatory children with myelodysplasia who sustained nondisplaced bilateral proximal tibial metaphyseal fractures.[107] One of the major reasons for difficulty in obtaining an anatomic reduction has been the interposition of soft tissues such as periosteum, pes anserinus, or medial collateral ligament in the medial fracture gap. Weber[222] explored four acute fractures of the proximal tibial metaphysis and found that the periosteum and the insertion of the pes anserinus were stripped from the medial surface of the tibia and were interposed into the fracture gap. When these soft tissues were removed from the fracture gap, anatomic alignment could be achieved. These fractures then healed uneventfully and without a subsequent valgus deformity. Visser and Veldhuizen also reported a similar case.[218] Weber believed that with soft tissue interposition there was a loss of biomechanical equilibrium between the medial and lateral soft tissues. He felt that traction on the proximal metaphyseal portion from the pes anserinus was lost while traction on the lateral side remained intact, thereby producing a bending moment on the tibia that resulted in a progressive valgus deformity.

Bassey[11] repaired the pes anserinus at the time of corrective osteotomy for a recurrent valgus deformity following proximal tibial osteotomy with a posttraumatic valgus deformity. He claimed that the loss of the pes anserinus medial tether resulted in medial overgrowth due to hemichondrodiastasis (physeal lengthening). The deformity did not recur. Similar observations were made by Potthoff.[168] Brougham and Nicol,[31] however, reported a case in which the pes anserinus was repaired in a 2-year-old child, who still developed an acquired valgus deformity. Coates[37] also reported two cases in which the superficial portion of the medial collateral ligament was interposed in the fracture gap, preventing anatomic alignment. After removal, anatomic alignment was achieved and the fractures healed without vaglus deformity. Others have felt that an intact fibula tethers the tibia, and as mild overgrowth occurs it causes a progressive valgus deformity.[39, 99, 203] However, valgus deformity has been reported following complete fractures of the proximal tibia and fibula.[9, 174]

Currently, most authors attribute the valgus deformity to asymmetric growth in the proximal tibia.[8, 9, 39, 41, 90, 91, 99, 107, 232] Cozen[39] and Jackson and Cozen[99] felt that hypertrophic callus formation resulted in asymmetric growth from the medial aspect of the proximal tibial epiphysis. Bahnson and Lovell[8] studied five children with unilateral genu valgum following a fracture of the proximal tibial metaphysis. All had an average of 6.7 degrees of valgus deformity in their initial cast. The amount of valgus increased during the next 12 to 14 months to 10.8 degrees and then improved to a mean of 8.7 degrees over the next 2 years. These investigators concluded that weight bearing caused compression forces laterally and distraction medially, resulting in asymmetric growth. Houghton and associates,[90, 91] in experimental studies with immature rabbits, found that medial hemicircumferential division of the periosteum resulted in valgus overgrowth. They believed that if the medial periosteum is torn during a proximal tibial metaphyseal fracture, asymmetric overgrowth occurred and produced the valgus deformity. Balthazar and Pappas[9] studied nine patients with an acquired valgus deformity of the tibia in childhood—seven were secondary to an acute fracture and two occurred with osteomyelitis of the proximal tibia. One of the children had an infection that was drained through the medial metaphysis, and another had a pathologic metaphyseal fracture. In all nine children the valgus angulation was associated with longitudinal overgrowth of the tibia. Balthazar and Pappas[9] believed that both the valgus deformity and the overgrowth were due to asymmetric growth stimulation. The maximum deformity (17 to 30 degrees) was attained approximately 18 months after injury. Green[72] demonstrated an asymmetric growth arrest line in the proximal tibia 1 year following a nondisplaced metaphyseal fracture in association with a valgus deformity. This indicated increased growth on the medial aspect of the physeal plate. Bohn and Durbin[26] observed the asymmetric growth arrest line in the proximal tibia in three boys following ipsilateral fractures of the femoral shaft and proximal tibial metaphysis. Herring and Moseley[83] observed similar asymmetry in the proximal tibia in a 2-year-old child following corrective osteotomy for an acquired valgus deformity. The deformity recurred following the osteotomy and then underwent spontaneous correction. MacEwen and Zionts[132] made similar observations in two of seven children with acquired valgus deformities. Zionts and associates[232] demonstrated asymmetric activity of the physeal plate on technetium bone scan 5 months after a metaphyseal fracture with a progressive valgus deformity. They concluded that there was increased stimulation of the physis that was greater in the medial side. It is clear from these publications that the valgus deformity is not secondary to the initial reduction at the time of casting but rather is secondary to differential growth between the medial and lateral aspects of the physis.

Aronson and colleagues[5] in 1990 reported on an experimental model using immature rabbits that confirmed asymmetric growth as the cause of post-traumatic valgus deformity. Twenty-two 8-week-old rabbits were divided into two equal groups. In one group the periosteum on the medial aspect of the proximal tibial metaphysis was excised, and a partial osteotomy involving the medial one half of the metaphysis was performed. In the other group, the same procedure was performed on the lateral side. Parallel Kirschner wires (K-wires) were inserted above and below the partial osteotomy. A valgus deformity (mean of 12 degrees) occurred in the first group and a varus deformity (mean of 10 degrees) developed in the second. In each animal the K-wires remained parallel, indicating that the deformity occurred at the physis. Despite the asymmetric growth the light microscopic appearance of the physes was normal. The deformities were therefore attributed to asymmetric physeal growth, which was not demonstrable histologically. Ogden[156] has demonstrated that collateral circulation to the knee is more extensive along the medial side, especially in the region of the proximal tibia. This may be responsible for transient asymmetric overgrowth. Jordan and co-workers[107] also concluded that the asymmetric growth stimulation was secondary to an increased vascular response.

Evolution of Treatment

It is important to understand the current concepts regarding the natural history of the valgus deformity before beginning a discussion on current treatment. It is now accepted that the valgus deformity will stabilize and then improve with growth and development. The deformity usually develops within 5 months of injury, reaches its maximum within 2 years, stabilizes, and then begins to improve toward the diaphysis by longitudinal growth and physeal (proximal and distal) realignment.[132, 156, 231] Unfortunately, there are no data indicating how much improvement can be anticipated. Salter and Best[185] found no improvement in 21 cases, and 13 later required a proximal tibia varus osteotomy. Visser and Veldhuizen[218] in their series reported no spontaneous improvement in the valgus deformity from the proximal tibial epiphysis but did observe some correction in alignment from the distal tibial epiphysis. Taylor[203] noted improvement in some patients, but not in all. Of the 12 children with valgus deformities reported by Jordan and co-workers,[107] 11 had documented improvement, although 4 subsequently underwent a corrective osteotomy. Two children had their deformity recur, and two also had postoperative compartment syndromes. Six of the children who were observed had complete correction of their deformities.

Jackson and Cozen[99] and later Ippolito and Pentimalli[96] observed that deformities of 15 degrees or less usually remodeled completely, especially in young children. The more severe deformities did not completely correct. Bahnson and Lovell[8] found some improvement in the valgus deformity in the five children who they followed for a minimum of 3 years after injury. Balthazar and Pappas[9] reported that two of nine patients who were treated nonoperatively resolved their valgus deformities over a period of 1 to 3 years. Skak and colleagues[193] reported that the valgus deformities tended to increase during the first year after injury, then to remain constant for 1 to 2 years, and then to improve. Only one of their six patients had a significant residual deformity at final follow-up.

Zionts and MacEwen[132, 231] followed seven children with posttraumatic tibia valga for a mean of 39 months following injury. These children ranged in age from 11 months to 6 years. It was found that the valgus deformity progressed most rapidly during the first year following injury and then continued at a slower rate for as long as 17 months; overgrowth of the tibia accompanied the valgus deformity. The mean overgrowth was 1.0 cm, with a range from 0.2 to 1.7 cm. Clinical correction with subsequent growth occurred in six of the seven patients. These authors recommended a conservative approach to management of both the acute fracture and the subsequent valgus deformity. If the valgus deformity fails to correct satisfactorily by early adolescence, then a tibial osteotomy may be performed. They also recommended that the mechanical tibiofemoral angle, as described by Visser and Veldhuizen,[218] be used to measure the alignment of the lower extremity rather than the metaphyseal-diaphyseal angle of Levine and Drennan.[127] The latter measures only the alignment of the proximal tibia. This is useful in the immediate postinjury stage but not in the follow-up period, as considerable correction of the deformity is due to distal realignment.[132, 193, 218] The distal tibial epiphysis tends to reorient itself perpendicularly to the pressure forces, resulting in asymmetric growth and an S-shaped appearance of the tibia radiographically.[65, 166] In an experimental study in dogs, Karaharju and co-workers[108] observed that the tibial physes changed their direction of growth after an osteotomy and residual valgus angulation.

Current Algorithm

Most proximal tibial metaphyseal fractures can be treated nonoperatively with closed reduction techniques. Treatment consists of correction of any valgus angulation of greenstick fractures and immobilization in a long leg cast with the knee in extension for 4 to 6 weeks or until the fracture is well united. Slight overcorrection, if possible, may be desirable.[156] Displaced fractures require reduction as well as correction of any residual valgus angulation. However, normal apposition is not always necessary. Currently, there are limited indications for operative management of these fractures. Inability to correct a significant valgus deformity under general anesthesia, rather than failure to close the medial fracture gap, is probably the major indication. The latter is usually indicative of soft tissue entrapment.

Following satisfactory fracture reduction and cast application, fracture alignment should be assessed radiographically at least weekly during the first 3 weeks following injury. Any loss of alignment should be corrected. During this initial period the child must avoid weight bearing to minimize compression forces and the possibility of valgus angulation at the fracture site in the cast.

Special Considerations for Multiple Trauma

Children who are victims of multiple trauma may sustain an unrecognized proximal tibial metaphyseal fracture. This is especially true if there is an ipsilateral femoral shaft fracture.[26, 230] Bohn and Durbin[26] reported three boys with proximal tibial metaphyseal and ipsilateral femoral fractures who developed genu valgum and lower extremity overgrowth of 1.8 to 2.2 cm. One resolved a 20 degree deformity over a 5-year period. It is important that during the secondary survey the lower legs be carefully evaluated for occult injuries and radiographs be obtained in suspicious cases. The presence of a proximal tibial metaphyseal fracture may necessitate a change in treatment plans for the other musculoskeletal injuries. If there is an associated femoral shaft fracture, stabilization by either internal or external fixation of this fracture may be necessary so that adequate closed reduction of the proximal tibial metaphyseal fracture can be achieved and maintained.

Treatment Modalities

Proximal tibial fractures may be treated by either nonoperative or surgical management techniques.

Nonoperative Management. The vast majority of angulated or displaced proximal tibial metaphyseal fractures are amenable to closed reduction and immobilization in a long leg plaster cast. This is almost always performed under general anesthesia to ensure adequate relaxation and pain relief. In some instances, the intact lateral cortex of the greenstick fracture must be fractured in order to achieve correct alignment. Once satisfactory alignment is obtained, the leg must be immobilized in a long leg cast with the knee in extension. An AP radiograph of both lower extremities on a long cassette should document correction of the valgus deformity and symmetric alignment with the opposite uninvolved extremity. Slight overcorrection (5 degrees) is desirable to counter any valgus overgrowth. A lateral radiograph of the fractured tibia is also obtained.

Following a satisfactory closed reduction, repeat radiographs are obtained weekly for the first 3 weeks to assess maintenance of alignment. These radiographs usually consist of an AP view of both lower extremities on a long cassette and a lateral view of the fractured extremity. Subtle changes in alignment may not be appreciated unless both extremities are included on the radiograph. Any loss of alignment should be corrected by cast wedging techniques or repeat closed reduction. Closed reduction may require general anesthesia, depending on the age of the child, the amount of correction necessary, and the degree of healing. Immobilization is continued until the fracture is well healed radiographically.

Surgical Management. Surgery is rarely indicated. Usually the best alignment by closed reduction is accepted. Only if there is significant residual valgus deformity, with or without closure of the medial fracture gap (entrapped soft tissue), is open reduction considered. At surgery, after any entrapped soft tissue has been removed, the fracture can typically be reduced anatomically and the periosteum repaired. Internal fixation usually is not necessary, and fracture alignment is maintained by a long leg plaster cast with the knee in extension. The child is then followed as described for nonoperative management.

Open proximal tibial metaphyseal fractures are rare but can occur in children who are victims of polytrauma. They are managed in the same manner as other open tibial shaft fractures (see Open Tibia and Fibular Fractures). An external fixator may be necessary for stabilization, especially if there is segmental bone loss, instability, or other significant fractures or body area injuries.[4, 16] Alonso and Horowitz[3] and Behrens[16] reported on open proximal tibial metaphyseal fractures treated with an external fixator. Epiphyseal pins may be necessary in these fractures to achieve adequate stability.

The final step in management in either method is to advise the families that even though satisfactory or anatomic alignment of the fracture has been obtained, valgus deformity and tibial overgrowth are possible as a natural consequence to this fracture. This will prepare the family for this complication should it occur. The necessity for long-term follow-up should also be emphasized.

Treatment of Valgus Deformities. The treatment of valgus deformities following proximal tibial metaphyseal fractures is controversial. Conservative management with braces has been suggested, but there is no evidence to substantiate the efficacy of this method.[50, 83, 96] Surgical correction was initially believed to be necessary. Salter and Best[185] reported that 10 of 13 patients with valgus deformity required tibial osteotomy for correction. Balthazar and Pappas[9] pointed out that even with osteotomies the valgus deformity can recur. This has been attributed to the same asymmetric overgrowth phenomenon that led to the valgus deformity initially. In their six patients who had osteotomies, the valgus deformity recurred, although to a lesser degree. Similar results were reported by DalMonte and associates,[44] who saw recurrent valgus deformities in 7 of 16 patients (44%) following proximal tibial osteotomies. There was no significant difference in the incidence of recurrence in children less than 5 years of age (60%) and those between 5 and 10 years old (36%) except that the younger children experienced a greater recurrent deformity. These authors concluded that the osteotomy is essentially a second fracture and therefore has the same pathologic factors. Recurrent valgus deformity following a corrective osteotomy has been documented by others.[12, 31, 107, 174]

MacEwen and Zionts[132] now recommend that most valgus deformities be observed until early adolescence. If spontaneous improvement fails to provide sufficient clinical correction, a proximal tibial varus shortening osteotomy and fibular diaphyseal osteotomy may be necessary. They also suggested partial or medial epiphysiodesis as another method for simultaneous correction of both the angular deformity and any remaining lower extremity length inequality. Medial epiphysiodesis also has been recommended by others.[174] Although tibial overgrowth is usually not excessive, it is considered important for both the valgus and the overgrowth to be corrected if surgery is performed.

Follow-up Care and Rehabilitation

Once fracture healing is complete, the long leg cast can be removed. Initially, the child is allowed full weight bearing, and knee range-of-motion exercises are encouraged. Failure to achieve satisfactory knee motion within 2 weeks following cast removal is an indication for supervised physical therapy, but this is rarely necessary. Radiographic follow-up at 3-month intervals is usually performed during the first year. This should be a standing AP view of both lower extremities on a long cassette to assess alignment. Orthoroentgenograms or scanograms may be necessary if a significant tibial overgrowth occurs. It is important that all children be followed for at least 2 years following their fracture. Longer follow-up will be necessary if a valgus deformity or significant lower extremity length inequality occurs.

Results

It appears that approximately 50% of the children who sustain proximal tibial metaphyseal fractures will develop a clinically apparent valgus deformity or tibial overgrowth, or both. Zionts and MacEwen[231] have shown that the maximal deformity induced by overgrowth is present by approximately 18 months after injury. Improvement begins thereafter, and the maximal improvement usually has been achieved by 4 years after injury. Minor residual deformities may continue to correct with subsequent growth and physeal alignment. Significant deformities persisting after 12 years of age may require surgical correction.

Authors' Preferred Method of Treatment

In the initial management of the acute fracture any angular or valgus deformity must be corrected, or even slightly overcorrected, by nonoperative closed reduction techniques under general anesthesia, and the parents must be warned of possible valgus deformity and tibial overgrowth. To evaluate the alignment following closed reduction, adequate radiographs must be obtained. The alignment of the lower extremities should be assessed on the AP view of both lower extremities symmetrically positioned on a long cassette. In this method the true alignment of the tibia can be measured directly and compared with the opposite side. If correction of a valgus deformity cannot be obtained by closing the medial fracture gap or fracturing the lateral cortex, open reduction is indicated. Failure to close the medial fracture site is typically indicative of soft tissue interposition from the periosteum, pes anserinus, medial collateral ligament, or a combination thereof. After satisfactory reduction is achieved, a long leg cast is applied with the knee in extension. Only by having the knee in extension is it possible to radiographically assess the alignment of the tibia. The child is reevaluated radiographically at weekly intervals for the first 3 weeks following injury. Any change in the position of the alignment in the cast is an indication for cast wedging or repeat closed reduction.

Treatment of valgus deformities usually is not considered for 2 to 3 years after injury, depending on the age of the patient and the degree of valgus. We do not believe that the use of orthoses or night splints will be able to correct or alter the growth abnormality. The families are advised that approximately 50% correction of any valgus deformity will occur during the first 3 to 4 years following injury (Fig. 13–1). Only after this time is it possible to determine if treatment will be necessary. If the maximum valgus deformity exceeds 20 degrees, the residual deformity may be too severe to accept, and a proximal tibia varus and shortening osteotomy and a fibular diaphyseal osteotomy may be necessary. Valgus deformities are usually not clinically significant until they are 5 to 10 degrees greater than the normal side.[83]

If a corrective osteotomy is performed, it is important that a fasciotomy of the anterior compartment be performed in order to minimize the risk for a compartment syndrome. The deformity should be slightly overcorrected at the time of surgery because there will be a tendency for recurrence. Internal fixation with staples or crossed Steinmann pins can be utilized. Compression plates can also be considered, but these require a second extensive operative procedure for removal. We recommend stabilization following the osteotomy to maintain alignment and prefer a simple external fixation system consisting of a single threaded Steinmann pin placed above and below the osteotomy and secured with an external fixation clamp. This simple external fixation technique maintains apposition and prevents rotation and angulation. It must be supplemented with a long leg cast, usually with the knee in extension. The child is followed closely radiographically to assess alignment and healing. Once the osteotomy site is healed (usually in 6 weeks), the external fixation clamp and Steinmann pin may be removed.

Following satisfactory healing the child is allowed full weight bearing, and knee range-of-motion exercises are encouraged. If after 2 weeks a satisfactory range of motion of the knee has not been obtained, supervised physical therapy may be beneficial. The child should be followed for at least 2 years to observe for recurrent valgus deformity or tibial overgrowth, or both. Standing radiographs are obtained at 3- to 6-month intervals, and scanograms are taken annually.

FRACTURES OF THE TIBIAL AND FIBULAR SHAFTS

Fractures involving both the tibial and the fibular diaphyses are more common than isolated fractures of the tibia.[164, 191] In the 1988 review by Shannak[191] of 117 children with tibial shaft fractures, 85 (73%) had an associated fracture of the fibula. The most common causes of injury were motor vehicle accidents (63%), falls (18%), direct trauma (15%), and sports (4%). The mean age at fracture was 8 years (range, 1 to 15 years). Males were involved three times more frequently than females. There were 104 fractures (90%) that involved the middle or lower third of the tibial shaft. Oblique (35%) and com-

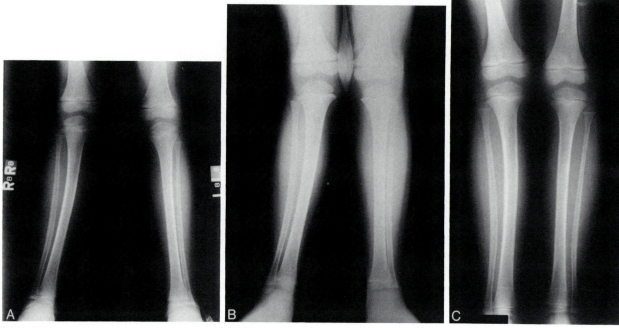

Figure 13-1

A, Anteroposterior standing radiographs of the lower extremities of a 5-year-old male who sustained a nondisplaced fracture of the right proximal tibial metaphysis 15 months previously. The fracture healed uneventfully. The valgus deformity occurred shortly after cast removal. Using the mechanical axis there is a 22 degree valgus alignment of the right knee as compared with 5 degrees on the left. B, Repeat radiographs 1 year later demonstrate an improvement in the right genu valgum to approximately 18 degrees. Overgrowth of the tibia is also occurring. Observe the increased width between the distal tibial physis and the physeal growth arrest line on the right as compared with the left. C, Repeat radiographs 40 months after injury showing further improvement in the alignment of the right tibia. Although the tibia is longer, the genu valgum measures only 12 degrees. A significant proportion of the realignment has occurred in the distal tibia. The articular surface of the right ankle joint is now parallel to the ground and perpendicular to the weight-bearing axis.

minuted (32%) were the most common fracture patterns. Only four fractures were open (3%). Parrini and associates[164] also found that tibial and fibular fractures were more common than isolated tibial shaft fractures in children between 1 and 11 years of age. However, the mechanisms of injury were not presented. Typically, fractures of both the tibia and the fibula require greater energy then does an isolated tibial shaft fracture. They generally result from direct injury rather than from rotation, as occurs in the latter. This accounts for the increased incidence of oblique, transverse, and comminuted fracture patterns.

Evolution of Treatment

The major problems with fractures of the tibia and fibula shafts are shortening, angulation, and malrotation. Valgus deformities are common because of the muscle action in the anterolateral aspect of the lower leg. However, these problems are usually not severe, and almost all fractures are amenable to nonoperative or closed methods of treatment. In the study by Shannak,[191] in which 117 pediatric tibial shaft fractures were followed for a mean of 3.9 years (range, 3 to 10 years), it was determined that satisfactory results can almost always be expected with conservative treatment and that surgery usually is not indicated or justified. Similar results have been reported by others. Shortening of 5 mm or less is compensated by growth acceleration; mild varus angulations undergo spontaneous corrections; however, valgus malalignments and rotational deformities persist.[72, 191, 201] For these reasons the conservative methods of treatment of tibial and fibular shaft fractures have changed little in this century. However, in certain situations surgical management using either internal or external fixation techniques may be advantageous. These selected indications are presented in Table 13-2.

Current Algorithm

Nearly all closed tibial and fibular shaft fractures in children can be managed by conservative or nonoperative methods. Nondisplaced fractures are im-

Table 13–2
Indications for Internal or External Fixation of Pediatric Tibia and Fibula Fractures
Open fractures
Type III and some type II (Gustilo and Anderson)
Segmental bone loss
Unstable closed fractures
Segmental
Neurovascular injuries
Multiple trauma
Severe body area injuries
Head injuries with spasticity or combativeness
Ipsilateral femoral fractures
Multiple fractures
Soft tissue abnormalities
Burns
Skin loss
Compartment syndromes (fasciotomies)

Modified from Thompson, G.H.; Wilber, J.H.; Marcus, R.E. Internal fixation of fractures in children and adolescents. Clin Orthop 188:10–20, 1984.

mobilized in a long leg cast with the knee flexed 20 to 60 degrees.[25, 73, 171, 191] Depending on the fracture pattern, the child is kept from weight bearing for 3 to 4 weeks or until there is initial radiographic healing. A long leg cast with the knee extended may then be applied, and full weight bearing is allowed until complete healing has occurred. In distal one third diaphyseal fractures a patella-tendon-bearing (PTB) or short leg cast may be applied instead.

Displaced fractures require closed reduction with strict attention to maintenance of tibial length and correct angulation and rotation alignment. This can usually be accomplished with manipulation and application of a long leg cast with the knee flexed 20 to 60 degrees. If the tibia fracture is oblique or comminuted, maintenance of length may be difficult, and alternative methods of treatment should be considered. Following application of the long leg cast, the patient must be followed closely, usually weekly, to assess maintenance of fracture alignment. Minor alterations in angulation can be corrected by cast wedging techniques. When the fracture is stable clinically and radiographically, usually at 4 to 6 weeks after injury, a long leg weight-bearing cast with the knee in extension, or possibly a PTB or short leg cast, depending on the fracture type and location, may be applied for an additional 2 or 3 weeks until the fracture is well healed.

Unstable fractures and the child who is a victim of polytrauma may benefit from the more aggressive operative methods of management, especially external fixation.

Special Considerations for Multiple Trauma

Children who are victims of multiple trauma and have additional long bone fractures or significant injuries to other body areas may benefit by having their fractures stabilized surgically (Table 13–2). This will enhance their overall care by improving both stability and mobility. The child is more easily nursed, and other diagnostic studies such as CT and MRI scans are facilitated by allowing the child to be transportable as well as to be properly positioned in the gantry. The most common method of surgical stabilization of pediatric tibia and fibula fractures is by external fixation. A variety of both large-pin cantilever systems and small-pin transfixation rings are available for children. The former is usually the preferred method because of the ease and speed of application and, a decreased risk for neurovascular injury; in addition, this system does not block surgical exposure to any associated wounds. Wires, pins, and screws occasionally may be used. Compression plates and intramedullary rods are not generally recommended because of the extensive dissection necessary for application, the increased risk for infection, and the need for a second extensive procedure for hardware removal.

Treatment Modalities

Fractures of the tibial and fibular diaphyses in children are usually uncomplicated, and their healing is typically rapid and much shorter in comparison with similar fractures in adults. Current treatment methods consist of nonoperative management and surgical management; the latter includes both internal and external fixation techniques.

Nonoperative Management. The majority of closed fractures of the tibial and fibular shafts can be managed by closed reduction and immobilization in a long leg cast.[25, 73, 171, 191]

Displaced fractures usually require reduction under general anesthesia, whereas nondisplaced fractures frequently can be casted following sedation. This first cast usually has the knee flexed 20 to 60 degrees to discourage weight bearing. Once satisfactory alignment has been achieved, the fracture is assessed radiographically at weekly intervals for the first 3 weeks. Minor changes in alignment can be achieved with cast wedging techniques. Significant loss of alignment may require a repeat closed reduction under general anesthesia. In the first weeks after injury most children are kept from weight bearing. After 1 to 4 weeks, depending on fracture type and the degree of radiographic healing, a weight-bearing long leg cast with the knee in extension may be applied.[191] This is worn until fracture healing is complete. In patients with fractures in the lower third of the tibia and fibula a PTB cast, or possibly a short leg cast, may be used instead. A functional brace as described by Sarmiento and associates[186] can also be considered for the older adolescent. Sarmiento's group applied the functional brace approximately 4 weeks after injury and initial treatment with a long leg plaster cast. They reported minimal problems with shortening, angulation, malrotation, and delayed union or nonunions.

The major problem when both the tibial and the fibular shafts are fractured is shortening.[81, 191] Angulation can also develop, as the long flexor muscles tend to produce a valgus rather than a varus deformity at the fracture. Recurvatum may also occur, especially when there is considerable soft tissue swelling at the time of the initial reduction and cast application. Wedging of the cast may be required to correct the angulation.[191] Often, it is best to wait 1 to 2 weeks for the soft tissue swelling to resolve and for the fracture to obtain fibrous stability. If there is considerable swelling initially, it may be better to apply a posterior splint and then perform the definitive manipulative reduction 3 to 4 days later, when the swelling has subsided, the risk for compartment syndrome has subsided, and a more appropriate, well-fitting cast can be applied.

For unstable fracture of the tibial and fibular diaphyses, especially those that are displaced, comminuted, and with appreciable shortening, other methods of closed management have been proposed. Steinert and Bennek[199] recommended an unpadded long leg cast with the foot in mild plantar flexion. After 3 weeks the cast is changed and the foot is brought to the neutral position. Weber and co-workers[223] and Shannak[191] recommended skeletal traction with a Steinmann pin through the os calcis of the heel. After 10 to 14 days sufficient healing has usually occurred to allow application of a long leg cast with the knee in extension. These methods are rarely utilized today. Most authors would prefer surgical stabilization with some type of external fixation.

Surgical Management. The principles of surgical management of pediatric fractures are distinctly different from those used in skeletally mature adults. When surgical management of pediatric fractures is indicated, the general principles of Spiegal and Mast[196] must be considered. These are applicable both in the polytrauma patient and in specific tibial fractures (see Table 13–2). The principles applicable to tibial shaft fractures include the following: (1) Satisfactory, possibly anatomic, alignment is achieved with particular attention to rotation and angular orientation; (2) internal fixation devices, if used, should be easily removable; (3) rigid fixation to maintain fracture alignment rather than to allow immediate mobilization of the lower leg is usually the goal, although a supplemental plaster cast may be required; and (4) external fixators, when used, should be removed as soon as any soft tissue wounds have healed or the fracture is stable and will not displace. Cast immobilization is continued until complete healing has occurred. The three basic surgical techniques of open reduction and internal fixation (ORIF), closed reduction and percutaneous internal fixation (CRIF), and external fixation may be considered for the pediatric tibial shaft fracture.[206] The last is the most common method. Hansen[80] has stated that the choice of surgical treatment of a pediatric tibial fracture should be guided by analyzing the extent of soft tissue injury, the fracture pattern, the location of the fracture, and the extent of other associated injuries.

External Fixation. External skeletal fixation is the surgical procedure of choice for most pediatric tibial and fibular fractures.[3, 80, 206, 208] It is particularly useful in open tibial fractures but may be beneficial in unstable or other specific fractures (see Table 13–2). Techniques include pins above and below the fractures that are incorporated into a plaster cast[11] or a variety of commercial cantilever and ring fixator systems.[3, 16, 208] External fixation is usually maintained until adequate callus formation has been achieved and the fracture is stable. At that time the fixator is removed and replaced by a long leg cast with the knee in extension. It is important that the frames be removed as soon as it is safely possible. Tolo[208] found that the use of external fixators increased healing time, had a significant incidence (50%) of superficial pin tract infections, and had a significant rate of refracture. He reported that 3 of 13 tibia fractures (23%) refractured 5 to 10 months after injury. Whether this was due to stress shielding or relative ischemia from the local trauma was unknown. All three refractures healed with immobilization in a long leg cast. The advantages of external fixation of pediatric tibial shaft fractures include (1) rigid immobilization; (2) direct surveillance of the lower leg and any associated wounds; (3) facilitation of wound dressings and management; (4) patient mobilization for other diagnostic studies and management of other injuries; and (5) possible application under local anesthesia in severely injured children.

Internal Fixation. Closed or open reduction and internal fixation of pediatric tibial and fibular diaphyseal fractures are not commonly performed. Operative techniques include limited internal fixation with K-wires, Steinmann pins, and cortical screws; compression plates and screws; and intramedullary rodding. Although Thompson and colleagues[207] reported that the most common fixation devices for achieving stable fixation in pediatric fractures were Steinmann pins, K-wires, and cortical screws, these are rarely used in tibial shaft fractures. A possible indication would be an unstable segmental fracture that could not be aligned satisfactorily by closed methods or in conjunction with an external fixator. Compression plates and screws may be considered in similar situations. However, compression plates and screws require extensive dissections and occasionally periosteal stripping. This can increase the risk for infection as well as for a delayed union or nonunion due to further disruption of the blood supply to the bone. Highland and LaMont[84] reported on six cases of deep, late infection following internal fixation of proximal femoral osteotomies. They recommended routine removal of internal fixation devices in children, which is a second relatively extensive procedure.

Intramedullary rodding of the pediatric tibia is rarely indicated because of possible injury to adjacent physes or apophyses, especially the tibial tubercle of the proximal tibial epiphysis, which is near the usual entry points.[80] Ligier and associates[128] reported from France on the results of intramedullary rodding using two flexible rods in 19 pediatric tibial fractures. This produced elastic stability at the fracture site. This type of stability enhanced the formation of bridging external callus by eliminating shear forces and providing compression forces across the fracture site. One rod was inserted through the medial and the other through the lateral proximal tibial metaphysis, distal to the physis and posterior to the apophysis of the tibial tubercle, and then passed distally across the fracture site, terminating proximal to the distal tibial physis. These workers reported that no cast immobilization was necessary and all fractures healed within 3 months. The major indications for intramedullary fixation were few, being predominantly for unstable fractures that failed standard conservative care. Verstreken and associates[215] from Belgium also used the technique of elastic stable rodding in children. They recommended its use for tibial fractures with contralateral lower limb injuries in children 6 years of age or older, especially those who were victims of multiple trauma.

Follow-up Care and Rehabilitation

Most children with tibia and fibula fractures do not require physical therapy for rehabilitation. They usually regain full knee and ankle motion within the expected time and wish to return to full activities much sooner than their parents and orthopaedic surgeons would like. Inability to regain full knee and ankle motion within 2 to 3 weeks after the cast is removed is a common indication for physical therapy. Once motion has been regained, muscle strength has returned to normal, and radiographs show a solid union, then normal activities, including sports, can be allowed. This usually occurs 4 to 6 weeks after the last cast is removed. The child is then followed at 3- to 6-month intervals for approximately 2 years to assess function, leg lengths, and resolution of any residual problems, such as angulation.

Results

The results following closed management of uncomplicated tibial and fibular shaft fractures are uniformly satisfactory. The fractures heal rapidly, depending on age, and minor discrepancies in length and angulation may correct spontaneously with subsequent growth.[81, 86, 191, 199] Shannak[191] reported union in a mean of 37 days with or without preliminary traction in children with a mean age of 8 years (range, 1 to 15 years). Hansen and associates[81] reported healing in 2 to 18 weeks in children in the same age group. Young children healed quickly, while adolescents took the longest.

Approximately 25% of children with tibial and fibular shaft fractures will have minor tibial length inequalities and angulatory changes at initial healing.[81, 191] Rotational problems, however, are uncommon. Because the amount of overgrowth of the tibia and fibula secondary to fracture stimulation is small, it is important to maintain adequate length. In tibia fractures in males older than 12 years and in females older than 10 years an attempt must be made to achieve full length. Significant shortening must be avoided if equal leg lengths are to be reached by maturity. The amount of shortening that can be accepted following closed reduction of these fractures is 5 to 10 mm in females between 3 and 10 years of age and in males 3 to 12 years of age.[73, 173, 191, 201] Older children and adolescents require as close to anatomic alignment as is possible. The younger children may have overgrowth in both the tibia and the femur, whereas older children and young adolescents may actually have a growth retardation. The type of fracture and the presence of residual angulation do not appear to affect the amount of overgrowth. The growth stimulation process is usually complete 2 years after injury.[201] Reynolds[173] demonstrated that within 3 months of injury the rate of growth was at its maximum and was 38% in excess of normal. The growth rate then decreased but remained significantly elevated for 2 years and returned to normal in the tibia approximately 40 months after injury.

It is also important to correct any coexistent angular or rotational deformity. Angular deformities may improve with growth, but rotational malalignments usually do not.[73, 191] Varus deformities up to 15 degrees in young children can undergo spontaneous correction.[191] However, valgus and posterior angulation tend to persist, as will rotational deformities, particularly medial rotation. Function, in uncomplicated fractures, can be expected to be normal.

Authors' Preferred Method of Treatment

Because closed tibial and fibular fractures in children usually heal rapidly and with satisfactory long-term results we recommend closed reduction and immobilization in a long leg cast for the vast majority of cases. Only a small percentage of closed fractures require the use of operative management with either external or internal fixation.

Most nondisplaced fractures are usually managed by a long leg cast applied with the knee in 20 to 60 degrees of flexion. Weight bearing is avoided for 2 to 3 weeks, and then a long leg cast is applied with the knee in extension and toe-touch weight bearing allowed. Once callus formation is visible the cast may be changed to either a PTB or a short leg cast, depending on fracture location and the degree of radiographic healing. A long leg cast is always used initially because a PTB or short leg cast will fail to control motion at the fracture site, thus allowing pain and possible displacement of the fracture.

Displaced fractures of the tibia and fibula are reduced under general anesthesia. When displacement is present, there usually has been extensive injury to the surrounding soft tissues. These children are at an increased risk for compartment syndrome and are admitted to the hospital for observation following reduction and immobilization in either a posterior splint or a long leg cast, depending on the degree of soft tissue swelling. If a splint is used initially, the long leg cast may be applied 3 to 4 days later. This allows resolution of the soft tissue swelling and is usually performed under general anesthesia. Following immobilization the patient is evaluated radiographically at weekly intervals for the first 3 weeks. If the alignment has been lost, the need for cast wedging or repeat closed reduction will have to be considered. In the majority of cases the displacement will be minor and can be managed by cast wedging.

For an unstable fracture with unacceptable alignment following closed reduction, an external fixator may be necessary. We prefer the half-pin cantilever systems. These are easy to apply, but care must be taken to avoid injury to the proximal and distal tibial physes. The use of fluoroscopy ensures safe application of these devices. These systems will control length, angulation, and rotation. They are typically supplemented with a posterior splint for the first several weeks in order to immobilize both the knee and the ankle for comfort. Depending on the age and reliability of the child, partial weight bearing may be allowed at 2 to 4 weeks following injury. Once callus is confirmed radiographically and any associated wounds have healed, the external fixation device is removed and replaced with a long leg or PTB cast until fracture healing is complete.

ISOLATED FRACTURES OF THE TIBIAL DIAPHYSIS

Isolated fractures of the tibial shaft can be either incomplete tension-compression (greenstick) or complete. Steinert and Bennek[199] reported that 70% of their 263 fractures were isolated tibial fractures and 30% were complete fractures of both the tibia and the fibula. However, the reverse was reported by Shannak[191] and by Parrini and associates.[164] Shannak found that only 32 (27%) of 117 children with tibia fractures had isolated tibial diaphyseal fractures.

Teitz and co-workers[204] reported on 45 patients less than 20 years of age (range, 3 to 19 years) with isolated tibial shaft fractures. In this group, falls were the most common mechanism of injury, followed by skiing and motor vehicle accidents. Most fractures were spiral, involving the middle or distal third of the shaft or a combination thereof. It appears that fractures of the tibia and fibula are more commonly the result of more severe, high-energy accidents, such as motor vehicle accidents, whereas isolated tibial shaft fractures result from less severe types of trauma, such as falls or sporting accidents.

Steinert and Bennek[199] observed that isolated fractures were caused predominantly by torsional forces and that most were localized in the distal one third or at the junction between the middle and distal one third of the tibia. The most common mechanism for torsion was a lateral rotation of the body while the foot was in a fixed position on the ground. The fracture line began distally on the anteromedial surface of the tibia and progressed proximally to the posterolateral aspect. The intact fibula and periosteum prevent significant displacement or shortening. However, angulation, especially varus, can occur. When the fibula is intact, the tendency toward shortening is converted to a torsional deformity at the fracture line, producing the varus deformity. This is due predominantly to the effects of the long flexor muscles across the fracture site producing a rotational force. Occasionally, a plastic deformation of the fibula may also be present.[119, 131, 204] The degree of deformation is usually minimal. This may present difficulties in realigning the tibia unless the plastic deformation of the fibula is corrected simultaneously.

Teitz and co-workers corroborated clinical observations with biomechanical studies on tibial fractures with an intact fibula.[204] They found that when the fibula remains intact, a tibiofibular length discrepancy develops and causes altered strain patterns in the tibia and fibula. These may lead to delayed union, nonunion, or malunion of the tibia. They found a lower incidence of these complications in children and adolescents and attributed this to greater compliance of their fibulas and soft tissues.

Treatment of the isolated tibial shaft fracture is predominantly nonoperative with immobilization in a long leg cast alone (Fig. 13–2). Occasionally, closed reduction may be necessary, especially if a varus deformity greater than 15 degrees is present and there is coexistent plastic deformation of the fibula. Flexing the knee 70 to 90 degrees and placing the foot in some degree of plantar flexion during the first 2 or 3 weeks may negate some of the deforming force from the long toe flexors. After fracture stability is achieved a long leg weight-bearing cast with the knee in extension is applied. This is usually maintained until healing is complete. A PTB or short leg cast can be used for distal fractures. Indications for surgical intervention in isolated tibial shaft fractures are almost nonexistent. Even in children with multiple trauma these fractures may be treated by simple immobilization with a long leg cast. Severe soft tissue damage, such as with burns or open fractures, may be better managed by an external fixator.

Isolated tibial fractures usually heal uneventfully, and the child quickly returns to normal activities. Tibial length inequality is not a problem, and any associated varus deformity is usually not appreciable clinically. Varus deformities up to 15 degrees remodel during subsequent growth.

SPECIAL TIBIAL SHAFT FRACTURES
Toddler's Fracture

In children between 9 months and perhaps up to 6 years of age, torsion of the foot may produce an oblique fracture of the distal aspect of the tibia shaft without fibular fracture.[55, 145, 146, 158, 205] The term "toddler's fracture" was first used by Dunbar and associates in 1964.[55] These fractures are usually the result of a trivial or innocuous injury, such as tripping while walking or running, stepping on a ball or toy while walking, or falling from a modest height. It is most common in younger children, hence the name "toddler." Dunbar and co-workers reported 76 cases, with 63 occurring in children under 2.5 years of age. Tenenbien and colleagues[205] in 1990 reported 37 cases in children between 1 and 4 years of age.

The physical findings and radiographic appearance are often subtle. These children are typically seen because of failure to bear weight, a limp, or the appearance of pain when forced to stand on the involved extremity. Usually there is no soft tissue swelling, ecchymoses, or deformity. Localized tenderness is the most common physical finding. Local warmth may be noted during palpation at the fracture site.[205] The traumatic episode is typically not witnessed.[158]

AP and lateral radiographs of the entire tibia and fibula are necessary for diagnosis and may demonstrate an obvious spiral fracture of the distal tibia. The characteristic finding is a faint oblique fracture line crossing the distal tibial diaphysis and terminating medially. When the routine radiographs are normal and a fracture is suspected, an internal rotation oblique view may be beneficial.[55] Occasionally, a series of oblique films in various degrees of rotation are of value, with two being made in external rotation and two made in internal rotation.[50] The fracture line may be visualized on only one film. If a fracture is suspected but not visualized, immobilization is still indicated. Technetium bone scan may reveal increased uptake, thereby confirming the fracture; however, this is rarely indicated. Repeat radiographs 7 to 10 days following injury will usually demonstrate subperiosteal new bone formation, thereby substantiating the injury. The

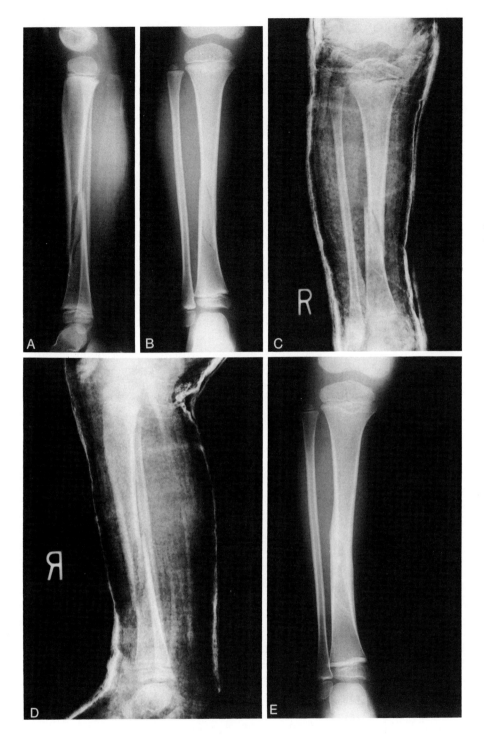

Figure 13–2

A, Anteroposterior radiograph of the right lower leg of a 4-year-old male who fell through a boat hatch. There is an isolated spiral fracture of the distal one third of the tibia. The fibula is intact. B, Lateral radiograph demonstrates that spiral fracture is minimally displaced. C, Slight varus angulation of 5 degrees occurred during immobilization in a long leg plaster cast. There was minimal shortening at the fracture site. D, Lateral radiograph shows no change in alignment from the initial radiographs. E, Three months following injury the fracture is well healed. Despite the slight varus angulation the articular surface of the ankle is parallel to the floor and perpendicular to the weight-bearing axis.

periosteal reaction can vary from slight to abundant. Treatment for this fracture is immobilization in a long leg cast for 2 to 4 weeks (Fig. 13–3). When the fracture is discovered after 2 weeks or more, immobilization may not be necessary, provided there is adequate callus formation and no tenderness to stress examination.

Tenenbien and co-workers[205] differentiated the radiographic features of the typical toddler's fracture from those of child abuse or the battered child syndrome. In the latter, the fracture is usually midshaft and less oblique. It is important to distinguish between these two entities. In the review by Oudjhane and colleagues[158] in 1990, of 500 consecutive radiographic evaluations of children less than 5 years of age with an acute limp, excluding cases

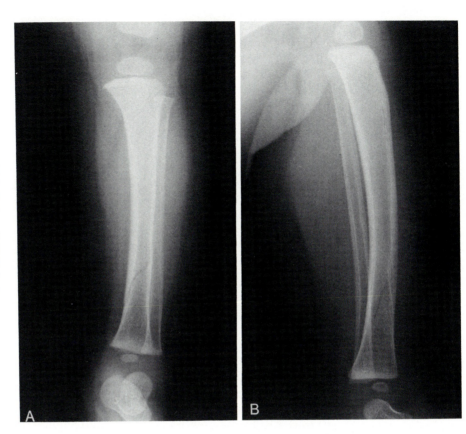

Figure 13–3

A, Toddler's fracture in a 9-month-old female. She fell while taking her first independent steps. There is a faint oblique fracture crossing the distal tibial diaphysis and terminating medially and distally. This fracture healed with 2 weeks of immobilization in a long leg plaster cast. *B,* Lateral radiograph shows that the fracture is barely visible and that there is no displacement.

of child abuse, occult fracture of the tibia or fibula was the most common cause (56 cases). These fractures occurred predominantly in the distal metaphysis, occasionally in the proximal metaphysis, and only rarely in the diaphysis. Similar findings regarding occult tibia fractures in young children have been reported by others.[145, 192]

Battered Child Syndrome

Fractures are second only to soft tissue injuries as the most common presentation in the battered child syndrome.[67] Approximately 25 to 50% of abused children have fractures.[2, 67, 115] The tibial shaft is the second or third most commonly fractured long bone in recent published series.[2, 67, 115, 118, 124, 157] The humeral shaft is typically the most common long bone fractured, followed by the femur and the tibia. In some series, the metaphyseal "bucket-handle" or "corner" fracture is the most frequent type, but in recent publications the diaphyseal fractures were more common. Kleinman and colleagues[116] in 1986, in a combined histologic and radiographic study, demonstrated that the corner fracture is not an avulsion of the metaphyses at the site of attachment of periosteum or ligaments but rather is a subepiphyseal fracture through the most immature portion of the metaphysis. Depending upon the size of the injury, the degree of involvement of the metaphysis, and the radiographic projection, the lesion may appear as a bucket-handle fracture, a corner fracture, or metaphyseal lucency. Thus, these are complete rather than avulsion fractures.

King and associates,[115] in a review of 750 children seen at the Children's Hospital of Los Angeles between 1971 and 1981 who were considered to be victims of battered child syndrome, found that 189 children (25%) sustained 429 total fractures. The median age was 7 months, with the range being from 1 month to 13 years. The majority were 2 years of age or less. In this series the most commonly fractured bones were the humerus, tibia, and femur. However, the most commonly fractured bones per patient were the humerus, femur, and tibia. Of all the long bone fractures, 48% were transverse, 26% spiral, 16% avulsion, 10% oblique, and only 1.5% were comminuted. When fracture combinations were analyzed, the avulsion or metaphyseal corner fractures were the fourth most common pattern involving the proximal one third of the tibia. A similar fracture pattern involving the distal one third was the sixth most common pattern. Twenty-eight percent of the patients had a history of prior fractures. Ultimately, ten of the children (5.3%) died.

The findings of King and associates are similar to those in other studies. O'Neill and associates[157] demonstrated that 29 of 110 (26%) abused children had fractures. In this study, the humerus, femur, and tibia were the most commonly involved long bones. In the 1974 study by Akbarnia and associates,[2] of 74 abused children with fractures, the ribs were the most commonly fractured bones, but the humerus, femur, and tibia were the most common long bones fractured. Also, in 1974, Kogutt and associates[118] reported the tibial fracture to be second only to a femoral shaft fracture. In 1982, Galleno and Oppenheim[67] reported that the metaphyseal corner fracture was the most common fracture pattern occurring in 29 of 36 children with fractures. Of their 24 diaphyseal fractures 17 were transverse and only 5 were spiral or oblique. Their study included 89 fractures in 36 children. Fifteen fractures involved the tibia, the second most common bone fractured. In 1983, Leonidas[124] emphasized that diaphyseal fractures were more common than epiphyseal-metaphyseal fractures.

The diagnosis of battered child syndrome requires a high index of suspicion. Typically, the injuries are unobserved and the parents' descriptions are vague. Physical examination may reveal soft tissue injuries in various stages of healing, failure to thrive, and emotional abnormalities due to deprivation and fear. Another potential problem in the evaluation of the battered child syndrome is distinguishing between nonaccidental injuries and osteogenesis imperfecta. Usually the diagnosis of the latter is not difficult because of the existence of a family history, the presence of fractures at birth, blue scleras, dentogenesis imperfecta, and other characteristic findings. However, these factors may not always be present. In a comparison of fracture patterns between these two disorders, Dent and Paterson[46] found that in osteogenesis imperfecta the peak incidence for fractures was between 2 and 4 years of age; that lower limb fractures, especially the distal femur and tibial diaphysis, were more common than upper extremity fractures; and that severe displacement of the fracture fragments was more common. Metaphyseal, spiral, and transverse fractures were common, while greenstick and torus fractures were not. However, even when the diagnosis of osteogenesis imperfecta is clear, the possibility of nonaccidental injury still must be considered. Knight and Bennet[117] reported a case of a 2-year-old male with osteogenesis imperfecta who was the victim of child abuse. They noted that most children with osteogenesis imperfecta and fractures do not have associated bruising or soft tissue injuries. When soft tissue injuries are present, the possibility of child abuse must be considered.

Care must also be taken in distinguishing the toddler's fracture from fracture in the abused child. Mellick and Reesor[145] recognized another accidental spiral tibial fracture that occurs in children between 2 and 6 years of age. This is similar to the toddler's fracture and overlaps the same age range, although it requires more energy and radiographically the fracture is more visible. The fracture begins more proximally at the middle rather than the distal one third of the tibia. The fibula is not involved. This fracture is usually the result of a fall with a torque or rotational component. The majority of tibial fractures in the abused child are diaphyseal and transverse rather than distal and spiral. Also, concomitant fracture of the fibular shaft is suggestive of an abused child because the energy necessary to fracture both bones is much greater than that which causes a toddler's fracture or the isolated spiral fracture in the older child. Skeletal surveys are necessary in suspected cases to assess for a previous healing fracture and evidence of subperiosteal new bone formation secondary to blunt trauma. If a truly accidental origin cannot be ruled out immediately, the child requires admission to the hospital and evaluation by the child abuse team.

The management of tibia fractures in battered children is similar to that described for the isolated tibia and the combined tibial and fibular shaft fractures. Closed reduction with simple cast immobilization is usually sufficient in these young children. The most important aspect is the diagnosis and appropriate intervention to prevent further injuries and possible death.

Bicycle Spoke Injuries

Bicycle spoke injuries of the lower extremity, especially over the medial malleoli, are relatively common in children. They may be caused by the lower leg becoming trapped between the spokes of the wheel and the frame of the bicycle when the child is being transported as a passenger. They may also result from a bicycling accident. These injuries can produce severe compression or crushing to the soft tissues over the foot and ankle. A fracture may also result[60] (Fig. 13–4). Kärrholm and associates[110] reported that 39 of 462 (8%) pediatric tibial and fibular shaft fractures were due to spoke injuries. Izant and colleagues[98] reviewed 60 cases of bicycle spoke injuries. They found that the most common age was between 2 and 8 years, with a mean of 5 years. In almost every instance the injury occurred

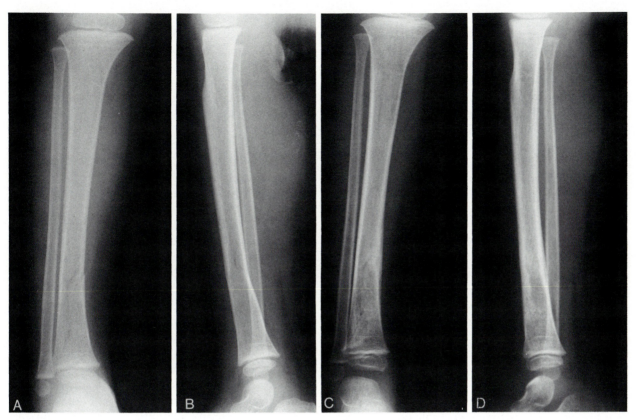

Figure 13-4

A, Anteroposterior radiographs of the right lower leg of a 3-year-old female demonstrating an oblique fracture of the right distal tibia and an intact fibula. This occurred when her leg was trapped between bicycle spokes and a rear fender support while sitting in an unprotected rear passenger seat. The skin and subcutaneous tissues were contused and abraded, but no lacerations occurred. B, Lateral radiograph demonstrated mild anterior angulation of the fracture. C, Two months following injury the fracture is well healed. D, Lateral radiograph demonstrates no change in alignment.

while two children were on a bicycle built for one. The initial appearance of the extremity can be deceiving. The skin may appear to be only abraded. However, over the next 2 to 3 days there may be an area of full-thickness skin loss. These injuries bear a striking similarity to the wringer injuries of the upper extremity. Izant and associates[98] recognized three aspects of this injury: (1) laceration of the tissues from the knifelike action of the spokes; (2) crushing from the impingement between the wheel and frame of the bicycle; and (3) shearing injuries from the coefficient of these two forces. Lacerations usually involve the area over the medial malleoli or the Achilles tendon. Simple suture closure may result in dehiscence of the wound, which may prolong secondary healing. The decision to do a skin graft must await adequate demarcation of the area of necrosis and wide debridement. The most common site for skin necrosis is over the malleoli, where the skin and subcutaneous tissues are thin.

All children with spoke injuries should be admitted to the hospital for observation. Treatment recommendations, after fracture management if necessary, include well-padded dressings, mild elevation, and frequent wound inspections. Debridement is performed as necrosis becomes apparent. This is followed by early split-thickness skin grafting. Closure of initial lacerations is done only after careful debridement, with special attention to defatting the thick skin flaps about the heel.

Stress Fractures

Pediatric stress fractures are uncommon and frequently lead to misdiagnosis, especially in young children. The pattern of stress fractures in children is different from that in adults. The tibia and fibula are the most common pediatric bones to sustain stress fractures.[148] Males are affected more commonly than females. Stress fractures are more common in adolescents and are similar to those in adults. A stress fracture incurred by a young child may resemble osteomyelitis or a malignant process. Roberts and Vogt[175] in 1939 were the first to describe stress fractures of the tibia in children. They found 12 children who had stress fractures, or "pseudofractures," involving the proximal third of the tibia. Since their report, there have been numerous reports of stress fractures involving the tibia in children.[21, 24, 47, 57, 82, 95, 148, 188, 202]

The children typically present with mild pain and a limp that was gradual in onset. Although there is no history of specific injury, frequently the older child has participated in vigorous physical activities, such as sports, to which he is unaccustomed or not properly conditioned.[24, 95, 148, 202] In a review of pediatric stress fractures, Devas[47] confirmed that the proximal tibia is the most common site, with the peak incidence between 10 and 15 years of age. The pain is typically relieved by rest and exacerbated by returning to activities. The most common positive physical finding is local tenderness to palpation over the fracture site. There is usually no soft tissue swelling, erythema, or ecchymoses.

The radiographic diagnosis of a stress fracture of the tibia and fibula is frequently difficult, especially in the young child.[57, 123, 147, 169, 182, 187] Radiographic changes may even be absent. Pediatric tibial stress fractures most commonly involve the posteromedial or posterolateral aspect of the proximal third of the tibia. They do not occur in the anterior aspect. Engh and associates[57] recognized that the typical radiographic changes occur in three phases. Initially, there is a small area of radiolucency in the cortex in the posterior wall of the tibia. This is associated with some metaphyseal and endosteal increase in bone density and a fine haze of periosteal reaction. These findings are usually present 2 to 3 weeks after the onset of symptoms. This phase is often missed in children. No linear fracture is seen radiographically. Follow-up radiographs show a gradual increase in the periosteal and endosteal new bone formation. The second phase is sometimes associated with the appearance of a definite incomplete defect in the posterior cortical wall. If an actual fracture does not occur, the third phase involves the maturation and partial resorption of the periosteal and endosteal new bone formation. If a fracture line becomes apparent, it is typically that of a nondisplaced fracture, and the characteristic radiographic sequence then follows. In difficult cases, technetium bone scans may be of benefit. In 1977, Prather and associates[169] reported on 42 patients suspected of having a stress fracture. Of the 21 who were ultimately so diagnosed, the radiographs were normal in 15, but the bone scans were positive in each case. This included eight stress fractures of the tibia and one involving the fibula. Prather and co-workers felt that bone scans were a highly sensitive technique for the early diagnosis of stress fracture and that the findings on scans can be identified long before radiographic changes. Roub and associates[182] reported that the typical bone scan appearance of a stress fracture of the tibia consists of a sharply marginated oval or fusiform area of increased radiodensity located posteromedially. It occasionally will extend the width of the bone at the area of involvement. The medial aspect of the tibial cortex is more commonly involved. Meurman and Elfving[147] found that the average delay between a positive bone scan and positive radiographs in a stress fracture in adults was 10.5 days. Currently, MRI may also be beneficial in recognizing stress fractures while avoiding the use of ionizing radiation. Lee and Yao[123] described characteristic MRI features for stress fractures that were useful in distinguishing between occult fractures and other subtle abnormalities. These changes included intraosseous bands of very low signal intensity that are continuous with the cortex as well as juxtacortical or periosteal findings of high signal intensity.

Stress fractures of the fibula can also occur.[34, 48, 74, 148] Devas and Sweetnam[48] have stated that the fibula may sustain a stress fracture at a younger age than any other bone. Griffiths[74] reported eight children between 2 and 8 years of age who had stress fractures in the distal third of the fibula. Ingersoll[95] reported three patients with a stress fracture of the lower fibula. All three were ice skaters, but the process may also occur in other children who participate in vigorous physical activities.

Clinical examination usually shows an area of tenderness proximal to the lateral malleolus. The involved area is usually tender to palpation, and there may be mild soft tissue swelling. Plain radiographs may be diagnostic, but in difficult cases a technetium bone scan may be indicated.

The treatment of tibial or fibular stress fractures is usually conservative. In most cases, restriction of physical activities will relieve discomfort and allow healing of the fracture. Occasionally, immobilization in a long- or short leg plaster cast, depending on the involved bone, for 2 to 4 weeks may be necessary if there is significant discomfort. A stress fracture of the distal fibula may also be treated with a removable air splint.

Ipsilateral Femur and Tibia Fractures

Ipsilateral tibial and femoral shaft fractures in children are severe injuries, usually the result of high-velocity accidents, such as motor vehicle collisions.[26, 125, 230] As a consequence, these fractures are commonly open, and the victims often sustain other body area injuries. These fractures produce the so-called floating knee. Letts and co-workers,[125] in a study of 15 children with this combined injury, found the treatment difficult. Results were poor when both fractures were treated nonoperatively, and it was recommended that at least one of the fractures be rigidly stabilized by either internal or external fixation techniques. Stabilization maintains alignment of the knee and minimizes problems with angulation and malrotation.

In a recent study by Yasko and colleagues,[230] 23 children with ipsilateral femur and tibia fractures demonstrated that both conservative and surgical treatment produced satisfactory long-term results. Two children died, and two others ultimately required below-knee amputations for grade IIIC open tibia fractures. Most of the patients were treated by closed reduction and cast immobilization of the tibia fractures and skeletal traction for the femur fractures. Two femur fractures were stabilized surgically (closed intramedullary rod and compression plate and screws), and four tibia fractures received an external fixator (Fig. 13-5). Complications occurred in six children (29%): two malunions, two premature physeal closures, one tibial nonunion (open fracture), and one pin tract infection. Four children required additional surgical procedures other than metal removal: two osteotomies for malunion, bone graft for nonunion, and arthroscopy for lysis of intraarticular knee adhesions. At a mean follow-up period of 5 years (range, 2 to 10 years) the results were based predominantly on the associated soft tissue and neurovascular injuries. At last follow-up all patients had hip, knee, and ankle motion that was symmetric with the uninvolved limb. There were no residual angular or rotational deformities. Three children had anterior laxity of the knee, suggesting unrecognized tears of the anterior cruciate ligaments. Scanograms demonstrated equal leg lengths except in three children who had overgrowth greater than 2 cm. It was recommended that the method of treatment be based on the severity of injuries. Satisfactory results can be achieved with conservative methods, especially in children 10 years of age or less, but internal or external stabilization of one or both fractures may be beneficial, especially in open fractures, unstable fractures, and fractures with neurovascular injuries as well as in adolescents.

Recently, Bohn and Durbin[26] reviewed 44 consecutive ipsilateral femur and tibia fractures in 42 children and skeletally immature adolescents. Thirty patients (32 limbs) studied had a mean follow-up period of 5.1 years (range, 1 to 14 years), and 19 were available for personal examination and radiographs. There were 24 males and 6 females and the mean age was 10.5 years (range, 3.6 to 16.6 years). Twenty-seven of the children sustained their fractures in automobile-related accidents, including 17 automobile-pedestrian accidents. Three injury patterns were identified: double shaft fractures (type I), juxtaarticular fractures (type II), and epiphyseal fractures (type III). Twelve of the 30 children had one or both fractures open, 17 children had at least one additional fracture, and 15 had another body area injury, especially cranial. Closed methods of treatment for both fractures were used in 18 patients. Ten patients had operative stabilization of one fracture, and ten had operative stabilization of both fractures. Eight patients had operative fixation of their femoral fractures (closed intramedullary rod, open intramedullary rod, or compression plate and screws), including one of the three open fractures. Twenty-three patients (24 limbs) had their tibial fractures treated by closed reduction and cast immobilization. External fixation was used in five open fractures, and pins in plaster were used in four unstable fractures. One fracture was treated by open reduction and internal fixation.

These authors found age to be the most important variable related to clinical course. Of the 15 patients who were less than 10 years of age, the mean time to unsupported weight bearing was 13 weeks, and the mean combined femoral and tibial overgrowth was 1.8 cm. Three children had early complications. Of the 15 patients who were more than 10 years of age, eight had early complications, the mean time to unsupported weight bearing was 20 weeks, and there was variable femoral and tibial growth. The younger children were treated successfully with closed techniques, while the older children were more successfully treated with reduction and surgical stabilization of the femoral fracture. The older group had the highest incidence of complications, including four with unrecognized ipsilateral knee ligament injuries. These included four anterior cruciate ligament tear and two medial collateral ligament injuries. Careful elevation of the knee was recommended at the time of initial evaluation. The juxtaarticular injury patterns (type II) in the older children had the highest incidence of early and late complications. Of the 19 patients who were person-

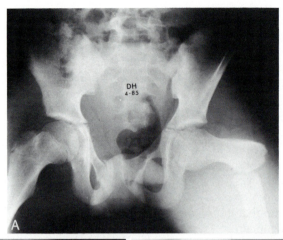
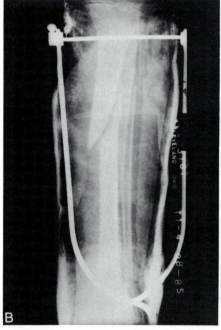
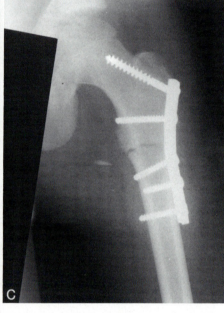

Figure 13–5

A, Anteroposterior radiograph of the pelvis of an 11-year-old male who was struck by an automobile. There is a closed, displaced left subtrochanteric femur fracture. There are minimally displaced fractures of the right superior and inferior pubic rami. This child also sustained an ipsilateral closed, displaced tibia and fibular shaft fracture. The subtrochanteric fracture was initially treated with skeletal traction via a threaded Steinmann pin through the proximal tibia. *B*, The tibia fracture was reduced and immobilized in a long leg plaster cast incorporating the proximal tibial traction pin. Unfortunately, the alignment of both the femur and the tibia fractures was felt to be unsatisfactory. *C*, The left subtrochanteric femur fracture was definitively managed by open reduction and internal fixation using a compression plate and screws.

ally evaluated by the authors, only 7 had normal function. The remainder had compromised results owing to lower extremity length inequality, angular deformity, or knee instability.

Tibial Fractures in Children with Neuromuscular Disorders

Children with neuromuscular disorders, such as myelomeningocele,[30, 64, 69, 71, 78, 102, 129, 135, 163, 170, 195, 200, 209] paraplegia from spinal cord injury or tumors,[135, 143] head injury,[228] spinal muscular atrophy,[135] muscular dystrophies,[135] cerebral palsy,[135, 143] and arthrogryposis multiplex congenita, especially those who are nonambulatory, are at risk for fractures of the tibia and fibula. These fractures must be treated in accordance with the underlying diagnosis and the degree of functional impairment. Although comprehensive care programs, including aggressive orthotic management and appropriately timed surgery, may prevent fractures by increasing the exposure of bone to weight bearing, at the same time maximum function may expose the patient to increased risk for fractures.

The major pathophysiologic change in bone of children with neuromuscular disorders is osteoporosis. Abnormal mechanical properties secondary to lack of weight bearing and normal joint motion result in osteoporosis and inherent fragility and predispose to fracture with minimal trauma. Osteoporotic bone has been demonstrated to be physically soft and therefore has less strength and less stiffness than normal bone.[51] Developing bone deprived of neuromuscular activity has diminished cross-sec-

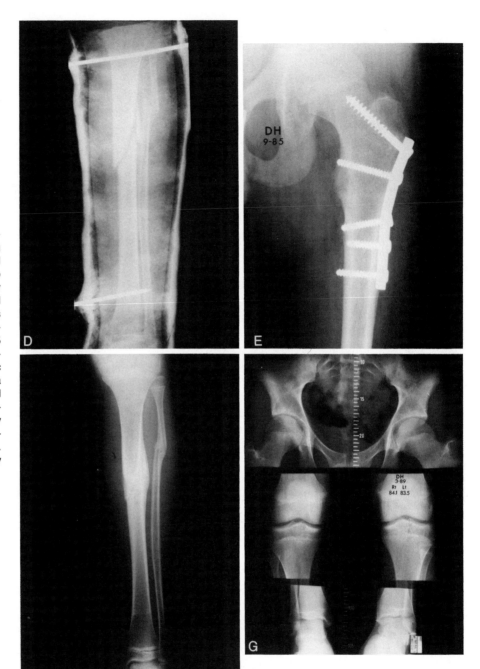

Figure 13–5 Continued

D, The left tibia and fibula fractures were treated with a long leg cast after addition of a second threaded Steinmann pin distal to the tibia fracture. Satisfactory alignment was achieved and maintained. This radiograph was obtained 2 months following injury. *E,* Radiograph taken 5 months following injury demonstrates that the subtrochanteric fracture is well healed. *F,* The tibia and fibula fractures also healed satisfactorily. *G,* Scanograms obtained 47 months following injury demonstrated only 6 mm of shortening in the left lower extremity. The patient is almost skeletally mature and is asymptomatic.

tional area, cortical thickness, and bone circumference, resulting in qualitatively and quantitatively inferior bone.[170] Walton and Warrick[221] correlated the severity of change with the age at onset of the neuromuscular disease, emphasizing the importance of muscle activity in normal growth and development of bone. Although decreased bone mass may result from a loss of motor function, when sensory loss is also present, the bone effects are increased further.[130] In these cases, epiphyseal separations can occur. Stern and associates[200] reported separations of the distal tibia and fibula epiphysis in a child with myelodysplasia. Other cases of unilateral slippage of the proximal and distal tibial epiphyses have been reported.[71, 195] These occurred with minimal or no injury and clinically and radiographically resembled osteomyelitis.

Therefore, neuromuscular disorders in children disturb the normal pattern of bone growth and development in a variety of ways, resulting in bone with thin cortices and decreased mass. Loss of muscle and weight-bearing forces produces abnormal bone and joint shape. Associated soft tissue contractures, resulting from muscle imbalance and weakness, may also predispose to fracture by placing excessive stress on the adjacent metaphyseal regions, especially about the knee. Makin[134] demonstrated that shortening of the lower leg in children secondary to acute poliomyelitis in infancy was asymmetric and that the fibula was shorter than the tibia. This may contribute to deformity of the ankle, the tibia, and the knee. There may also be an association with abnormal stresses and fracture. Similar observations regarding shortening of the fibula were made by Dias in an analysis of 86 children with myelomeningocele.[49]

The clinical features of fractures of the tibia and fibula in a child with a neuromuscular disease are commonly modified. Fractures may occur with no history of trauma or after a trivial injury. Even gentle physical therapy and passive exercises may, unintentionally, cause a fracture. Boytim and associates[30] recognized that infants having myelodysplasia with thoracic and upper lumbar neurologic levels and soft tissue contractures were prone to fractures with physical therapy. The common physical signs include warmth, erythema, and swelling. If sensation is normal, pain is obviously present. However, in the absence of sensation, as occurs in myelomeningocele and spinal cord injury, a fever may also be present. Townsend and associates[209] reviewed a series of myelomeningocele patients with fractures in whom the elevated temperature averaged 38.2°C and the white blood cell count was over 11,000 cells/mm^3. The erythrocyte sedimentation rate may also be elevated, but the calcium phosphorus and alkaline phosphatase values are usually normal.[53] An occasional patient may become toxic and extremely ill, as noted by Freehafer and associates.[64]

Whatever the underlying neuromuscular disorder, the goals of treatment are to achieve satisfactory alignment of the extremity and return the patient to the preinjury level of function. The major principle is to provide minimal immobilization of the patient and the limb compatible with union in a satisfactory position. What constitutes acceptable position is based on the ambulatory abilities of the individual. Functional alignment, including rotation, must be achieved so that standing, walking, use of orthosis, or wheelchair sitting will not be compromised. In displaced fractures in nonambulators, less than perfect alignment may be adequate. The specific method of treatment is individualized for the child, the underlying diagnosis, and the functional level.

Fractures of the tibia and fibula in children with neuromuscular diseases are characterized by rapid healing and the absence of serious displacement. As a consequence, nonoperative methods are usually sufficient as well as desirable.[53] In nonambulatory children, bulky cotton roll dressings or pillow splints may be all that are necessary to maintain satisfactory alignment of the fractured tibia. Plaster or thermoplastic splints may also be utilized. Once acute swelling subsides, the patient's orthosis may be used to support the fracture. If a child is able to stand, this should be allowed as soon as possible after injury. If fracture displacement, angulation, or rotation is too severe, a short leg or a long leg plaster cast may be required.

Matejczyk and Rang[135] reviewed the distribution of fractures in children with neuromuscular disorders at the Hospital for Sick Children in Toronto. They found that the majority of fractures occurred in the region of the knee joint. The femur, followed by the tibia, was most commonly fractured, especially the distal femoral and proximal tibial metaphyses. In children with myelomeningocele, fractures tended to occur predominantly in areas where there were no functioning muscles. Fractures occurred most often after falls and following removal of postoperative hip spica cast or immobilization for other reason. Freehafer and co-workers[64] demonstrated that fractures following immobilization can be minimized by allowing the child to stand in the postoperative spica cast as soon as possible after surgery.

The major problem with fractures in the children with muscular dystrophies was decreased ambulatory ability. Even short periods of immobilization without weight bearing may result in premature loss of walking ability. Falls were the most common cause of fracture, occurring in children who were walking with orthoses or from a wheelchair. Fractures of the tibial shaft and proximal and distal metaphyses were most frequent in children who were still ambulatory.

McIvor and Samilson[143] as well as Matejczyk and Rang[135] found that only the severely involved institutionalized patient with cerebral palsy had an increased risk for fracture of the extremity. McIvor and Samilson reported a 7% incidence of fractured extremities in more than 1000 patients confined to a state hospital. Severe preexisting disuse osteoporoses were associated with fractures and were similar to those seen in other neuromuscular disorders.

Because of spasticity, internal fixation was successful if nonoperative treatment was precluded.

Pathologic Fractures

Fractures through preexisting osseous tumors, benign or malignant, may be the first indication of the pathologic process. These fractures are usually realigned and temporarily immobilized in a long leg posterior splint while a thorough evaluation of the pathologic lesion is performed. Pathologic fractures in the proximal metaphysis may result in the acquired valgus deformity. Jordan and associates reported a 14 degree valgus deformity over a 2-year period in a 4-year-old male following fracture through a large proximal tibial simple bone cyst.[107] The deformity spontaneously corrected to 4 degrees over the next 7 years. Pathologic fractures of the proximal tibial metaphysis resulting in acquired valgus deformities have also been reported following osteomyelitis.[8] Definitive management is based on the diagnosis and natural history of the lesion.

ISOLATED FRACTURES OF THE FIBULAR DIAPHYSIS

The isolated fracture of the fibular shaft is rare and usually the result of a direct blow to the lateral side of the leg. These fractures may be either compression (torus), incomplete tension-compression (greenstick), complete, or plastic deformation (bend). Such fractures typically heal with only simple immobilization (Fig. 13–6). A peroneal nerve palsy may accompany a proximal fibular fracture if there is direct injury to the nerve itself. There are rarely any complications with healing and subsequent growth. However, it is important to rule out the presence of an associated physeal injury of the distal tibia because a high fracture of the fibula can be seen in pronation/eversion/external rotation injuries to the ankle.[50]

FRACTURES OF THE DISTAL TIBIAL METAPHYSIS

The distal tibial metaphysis may sustain fractures similar to those in the proximal tibia. These are predominantly compression (torus) or incomplete tension-compression (greenstick) fractures. Complete fractures may occur, but the thick tibial periosteum and the tendency for the fibula to remain intact or to plastically deform limits major displacement.[156] The most common fracture is the greenstick fracture, in which the posterior cortex is fractured and the anterior cortex impacted and angulated.

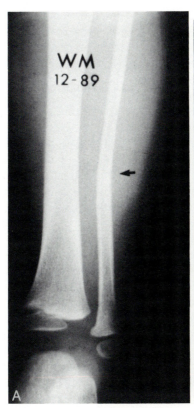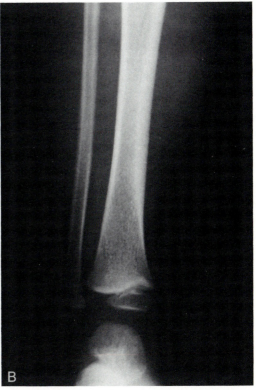

Figure 13–6

A, Anteroposterior radiograph of the left lower leg of a 2-year-old child who was observed to be limping. There was no history of injury. There is a plastic deformation of the distal one third of the fibula, producing a slight valgus deformity. B, Comparison view of the opposite right lower leg. The fibula is normal.

This results in a radiographic and occasionally a clinical recurvatum deformity.

Metaphyseal fractures of the distal tibia are typically visible on standard AP and lateral radiographs. Toddler's fractures occasionally may not be visible on the initial radiographs but should be treated symptomatically if a fracture is suspected. Special radiographic studies, such as technetium bone scans, are usually not indicated.

Treatment of distal tibial metaphyseal fractures depends on displacement or angulation of the fracture. Nondisplaced fractures require only simple immobilization in a long leg cast. A short leg cast may be appropriate in certain cases, depending on the fracture pattern and the child's age and reliability. Any angular deformity should be corrected, especially varus or valgus. If significant recurvatum is present, closed reduction should be performed. This is usually difficult because of impaction and will require general anesthesia. Immobilization in a long leg cast with the foot in plantar flexion for 3 to 4 weeks followed by a short leg walking cast until healing is complete will maintain alignment.

Fractures of the distal tibial metaphysis generally heal quickly and without significant deformity (Fig. 13–7). They are not associated with the problems of asymmetric overgrowth and progressive angular deformity, which occur in fractures of the proximal metaphysis.

OPEN TIBIA AND FIBULA FRACTURES

Open fractures of the tibia and fibula are among the most serious injuries of the musculoskeletal system in children and adults.[13] Despite modern concepts and techniques of prehospital care, wound debridement, antibiotics, and early fracture stabilization—which have saved the lives of many a young patient—amputation after an open tibia fracture is still not uncommon.

Skeletal maturity and preexisting conditions (e.g., osteogenesis imperfecta) have some influence on the injury patterns of open fractures and dislocations. But, more than any other variable, the kinetic energy ($E_k = m \cdot v^2/2$), especially at the level produced by colliding bodies, determines severity and presentation of a particular injury. Thus, closed tibial fractures in children are largely due to low-energy domestic activities and play, whereas violent traffic accidents cause over 80% of open fractures after the age of 2 years.[81, 120, 216, 217] Even in adolescents, athletic activities count for less than 5% of open fractures. Although some open tibia fractures may also involve the proximal or distal tibial physes, most occur in the diaphyses.

Approximately 3 to 19% of all fractures of the tibia and fibula in children are open.[81, 86, 191, 197, 216, 217, 229] Yasko and Wilber[229] reported that 53 (5%) of 1049 consecutive tibia fractures in skeletally immature patients seen between 1972 and 1988 were open. It has been estimated that 1% of open tibia fractures occur before the age of 2 years, 15 to 20% from age 2 to 6 years, and about 40% each in the age groups of 6 to 10 years and 10 to 14 years.[216, 217] The rarity of open fractures in children below school age is related to their small body mass and a large amount of protective subcutaneous fat. Young children also are rarely exposed to massive violence, which, if it occurs in this age group, threatens life rather than limb.

In addition to the communication between the fractured bone and the outside environment, open fractures of the tibia differ in many other characteristics from similar closed lesions. In two thirds of all open fractures of the lower leg in adults, only the tibia or the fibula is fractured, while both bones are involved in one third of the cases. Comminution is seen in about one third of all open tibia fractures but only in about 5 to 10% of those that are closed. From 25 to 50% of open tibia fractures are accompanied by other body area injuries; this number is more than double the ratio seen in closed fractures. The most common additional injuries include other fractures, closed head injuries, and blunt abdominal and chest trauma.[33, 81, 120, 191, 216, 217, 229]

Classification

At this time, most classifications of open musculoskeletal injuries account for size, severity, and extent of the soft tissue disruption but neglect such modifying factors as wound contamination, fracture pattern, and associated injuries. The classification that is currently most popular for both children and adults was developed by Gustilo and Anderson in 1976 and groups fractures into three types. It was further refined in 1984 to allow for better differentiation of the most severe injuries (Table 13–3).[76] In the type I open fracture the wound is less than 1 cm long. It is usually a clean puncture wound in which a spike of bone has pierced the skin. There is little soft tissue damage and no sign of crushing injury. The fracture is usually simple, transverse, or short oblique with little comminution.

In the type II open fracture the laceration is more than 1 cm in length, but there is still no extensive

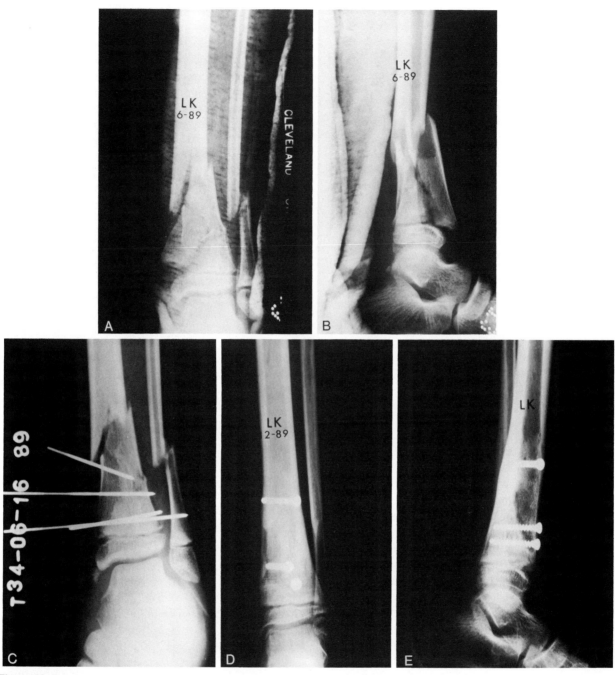

Figure 13-7

A, Anteroposterior radiographs of the left lower leg in a 9-year-old female who was struck by an automobile while riding her bicycle. There is a very comminuted fracture involving the left distal tibial metaphysis. There is also a Salter-Harris type II distal tibial epiphyseal fracture. *B*, The lateral radiograph demonstrates displacement of the anteromedial portion of the metaphysis of the Salter-Harris type II epiphyseal fracture. *C*, Limited internal fixation was performed because the fracture was unstable and satisfactory alignment could not be obtained. Initial alignment was obtained with multiple Kirschner wires followed by cortical screws. *D*, Nine months following surgery. The fractures are healed, and the distal tibial physis remains open. The cortical screws were subsequently removed. *E*, Lateral radiograph also confirmed no evidence of premature physeal closure.

Table 13–3
Classification of Open Fractures

Type I
   Wound 1.0 cm or less (frequently from inside to outside)
   Minimal muscle contusion
   Simple transverse or short oblique fractures
Type II
   Wound greater than 1 cm
   Soft tissue damage, flaps, or avulsion
   Minimal to moderate crushing component
   Simple transverse or short oblique fractures with minimal comminution
Type III
   Extensive soft tissue damage—muscles, skin, and neurovascular structures
   Frequently a high-velocity injury with a severe crushing component
   IIIA: Adequate bone coverage
      Segmental fractures
      Gunshot injuries
   IIIB: Periosteal stripping and bone exposure
   IIIC: Usually associated with massive contamination
      Associated with vascular injury requiring repair

Modified from Gustilo, R.B.; Mendoza, R.M.; Williams, D.N. Problems in the management of type III (severe) open fractures: A new classification of type III open fractures. J Trauma 24:742–746, 1984.

soft tissue damage. There is slight or moderate crushing injury, moderate comminution at the fracture site, and moderate contamination.

The type III injury is characterized by extensive damage to the skin and soft tissues, including muscle and possibly neurovascular structures. There is a high degree of contamination. The fracture is usually caused by high-velocity trauma, resulting in considerable fracture comminution and instability. The type III injuries are subdivided into three additional groups. In type IIIA, soft tissue coverage of the fractured bone is adequate despite the extensive soft tissue injury. This subtype includes segmental and severely comminuted fractures from high-energy trauma regardless of the size of the wound. In the type IIIB injury, there is extensive injury to or loss of soft tissue with periosteal stripping and exposure of bone. Massive contamination and comminution of the fractures are common. After debridement and irrigation are completed and the segment of bone is exposed, a local or free flap is needed for coverage. The type IIIC injury includes any open fractures associated with an arterial injury that must be repaired regardless of the extent of soft tissue injury. The incidence of wound infection, delayed union, nonunion, amputation, and residual disability is directly related to the type of injury. The more severe the injury, the greater the risk of complications.

With advances in prehospital resuscitation and the development of free flaps and microvascular reconstructions,[89, 126] many limbs with extensive open fractures that involve vascular compromise[45, 155] or partial amputation can be salvaged. However, despite the great potential for healing that is so typical of children, some of the most severe open tibial fractures are better managed with a below-knee amputation than with extensive reconstructive procedures that leave the patient with a dubious cosmetic result and only marginal function. In the decision between limb salvage and amputation, a number of investigators have developed severity indices to provide some guidance.[27, 104] Johansen and associates[104] in 1990 developed the mangled extremity severity score (MESS), which is a rating scale for lower extremity trauma based on skeletal and soft tissue damage, limb ischemia, shock, and age of the patient. Applied both retrospectively and prospectively to adult patients, the index has proved highly reliable and predictive. To what extent it can be applied to pediatric lower extremity injuries is, at this time, not known.

It has become increasingly clear that some closed fractures, caused by violent forces, may result in extensive destruction of the soft tissue sleeve surrounding the leg without resulting in an open lesion.[211, 212] Typically, these injuries are characterized by skin contusions, deep abrasions, burns, or frank separation of the cutis from the subcuticular tissue. Even in children, these lesions can result in delayed partial or full tissue loss and secondary infection of the fracture site. To avoid catastrophes, these lesions must be treated as open fractures. Tscherne and Oestern[211] have provided a classification that describes four grades of these treacherous injuries and can prove useful in choosing among different treatment options (Table 13–4).

Treatment Modalities

The objectives of treatment of open tibial fractures in children is the same as for adults: (1) prevention of wound sepsis; (2) healing of soft tissues; (3) achieving bone union; and (4) returning the patient to optimal function.[75–77] The modalities in achieving these goals include (1) emergent initial care; (2) thorough initial evaluation to diagnose other life-threatening injury; (3) appropriate antibiotic therapy; (4) extensive and possible repeat wound debridement; (5) fracture stabilization; (6) local wound

Table 13-4
Classification of Closed Fractures with Soft Tissue Injuries

Classification	Description
Grade 0	Minimal soft tissue damage
	Indirect violence
	Simple fracture patterns
	Example: Torsion fracture of the tibia in skiers
Grade 1	Superficial abrasion or contusion—pressure from within
	Mild to moderately severe fracture configuration
	Example: Pronation fracture-dislocation of the ankle joint with soft tissue lesion over the medial malleolus
Grade 2	Deep contaminated abrasion—localized skin or muscle contusion
	Impending compartment syndrome
	Severe fracture configuration
	Example: Segmental "bumper" fracture of the tibia
Grade 3	Extensive skin contusion or crush
	Underlying muscle damage may be severe
	Subcutaneous avulsion
	Decompensated compartment syndrome
	Associated major vascular injury
	Severe or comminuted fracture configuration

Modified from Tscherne, H.; Oestern, H.J. Die Klassifizierung des Weichteilschadens bei offenen und geschlossenen Frakturen. Unfallheilkunde 85:111–115, 1982.

care; (7) early autogenous cancellous bone grafting; and (8) rehabilitation (Fig. 13–8).

Initial Care. As in adults, open tibial fractures in children are surgical emergencies.[17] The acute care follows the guidelines that have been established for similar lesions in adults.[77] In addition to vigorous acute intervention, the final outcome of these injuries depends on a comprehensive plan of rehabilitation that includes physical therapy as well as educational and socioeconomic support for the family.[27, 53]

At the scene of injury, the open wound is covered with a sterile dressing; the leg and fractures are aligned through gentle manipulation and then are splinted for transport. Profuse bleeding is controlled by local compression.

Initial Evaluation. In the emergency room, the patient's vital functions are assessed and monitored, and all organ systems are systematically reevaluated. If wound dressings are removed at all, mask and gloves are required. Bone fragments causing undue soft tissue compromise are gently reduced. After the history is taken, physical examination is performed, and pertinent radiographs are obtained, blood is drawn for a complete blood count, serum electrolytes, and typing and cross-matching for blood replacement. Tetanus prophylaxis[35] and the first dose of intravenous antibiotics[165] are then given. Any patient with a suspected dysvascular limb is transferred to the operating room without delay for further assessment and possible vascular exploration and repair.

Appropriate Antibiotic Therapy. After specimens are taken for initial aerobic and anaerobic microbial culture, antibiotic therapy is started in the emergency room. The use of antibiotics has been demonstrated to be effective in decreasing the risk for infection in open fractures. Patzakis and Wilkins[165] found the infection rate to be 13.9% in 79 patients who received no antibiotics, compared with 5.5% in 815 patients who were treated with broad-spectrum antibiotics (cephalothin alone or cefamandole plus tobramycin). Approximately 70% of open fractures are contaminated with bacteria at the time of injury. Both gram-negative and aerobic gram-positive bacteria are the major pathogens of infections that are associated with fractures. The risk for infection in an open tibial fracture depends significantly on the severity of the soft tissue injury. Because of the nature of the infecting organisms, combined antibiotic therapy is recommended for treatment of open fractures. Hospital-acquired infections are also a problem. For this reason, limiting the duration of initial antibiotic therapy to 2 to 3 days is important in order to minimize the development of resistant nosocomial bacteria.[165]

A cephalosporin (cefazolin or cefamandole) is currently recommended for patients with an open fracture. For type I open fractures, this therapy is continued for 48 to 72 hours. In type II or III open fractures, combined antibiotic therapy is necessary to cover both gram-positive and gram-negative bacteria. The patient is treated with a cephalosporin as well as an aminoglycoside. This combined antibiotic therapy is also continued for 72 hours. Penicillin is added if the patient sustained the injury on a farm. Antibiotics are repeated when another major operation, such as delayed primary or secondary closure of wound, elective open reduction and internal fixation, or bone grafting, is performed. Prolonged antibiotic therapy (more than 3 days) has been reported not to prevent the development of infection in wounds.

Debridement and Irrigation. In the operating room, all the patient's clothes are removed, and the whole patient is reexamined, particularly as to neurovascular function. Anesthesia is induced. The skin surrounding the wound is shaved, and the injured

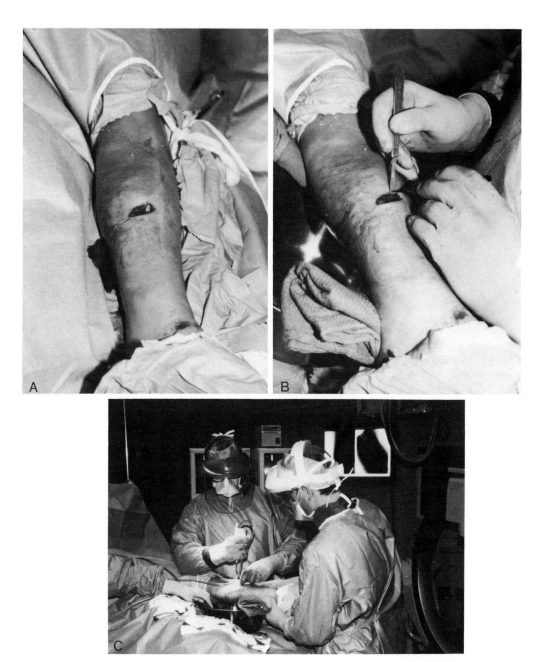

Figure 13–8

A, Intraoperative clinical photograph of a grade IIIB open tibia and fibula shaft fracture in an 11-year-old female who was struck by an automobile. B, Debridement of the skin margins, subcutaneous tissues, and muscle and direct visualization of the fracture and inspection of the bone ends. C, Pulsed irrigation with 7 to 10 L of normal saline.

leg is prepared and draped. A pneumatic tourniquet is applied as a safety measure, but it is not inflated unless massive bleeding occurs. Then follows potentially the most important process in the management of an open fracture: the search for the extent and the severity of the "real injury," which often is greater than the open wound, or "apparent injury," by a factor of 2 to 3. Many clues alert the surgeon to the true extent of the injury zone, including (1) an estimate of the energy involved in the injury event; (2) the size and location of bruises and other skin openings, as noted during the preliminary examination; and (3) such radiographic features as air pockets extending along tissue planes and the relationship of bony fragments to neurovascular structures.

Based on this information, the debridement—a carefully planned and systematic process that re-

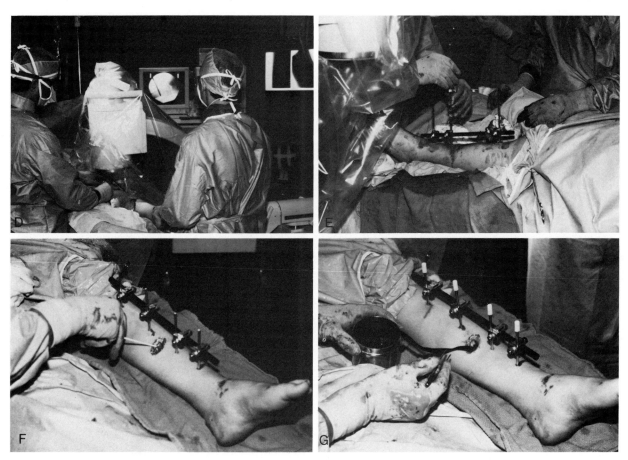

Figure 13-8 *Continued*

D, Application of external fixator under fluoroscopic control. The latter allows proper pin placement and alignment, avoids possible physeal injury, and facilitates the final reduction. *E,* Final adjustments of the half-frame external fixator. *F,* Intraoperative cultures are obtained after debridement, irrigation, and application of the external fixator. *G,* Packing of the wound. In this case Betadine-soaked gauze was utilized. This is followed by the application of sterile dressings and a long leg posterior plaster splint.

moves all foreign and dead material from the wound—is initiated. As the first step, the wound edges are liberally extended to allow an unobstructed access to the entire injury zone. These extensions should be extensile, should not create flaps, and should respect vascular territories. All dead and necrotic skin is resected to a bleeding edge, and necrotic or contaminated subcutaneous tissue and fat are sharply debrided. Contaminated fascia is resected, and prophylactic fasciotomies and epimysiotomies are performed to allow the injured tissue to swell and avoid secondary vascular compromise and tissue necrosis. Ischemic muscle is the principal culture medium for bacteria. It is radically resected where compromised. The four C's—consistency, contractility, color, and capacity to bleed—are classic guides to viability, but unfortunately, they are not always reliable. The capacity to contract after a gentle pinch with the forceps and the presence of arterial bleeding seem to be the best signs of viability. A decision must be made at this time whether primary amputation should be performed. Although no definite criteria for amputation in children exist, Bondurant and associates[27] have utilized the following factors: (1) the presence of protective sensation to the foot; (2) restorable vascular supply; and (3) the presence of substantial viable muscle. When amputation is inevitable, performing early surgery enhances patient survival, reduces pain and disability, and shortens hospitalization. The MESS,[104] discussed previously, can also be applied to help determine which patient is a candidate for limb salvage or primary amputation.

The intramedullary cavity of the principal fracture fragments is carefully inspected and cleansed of any contaminated material. Small devitalized and contaminated pieces of cortical bone are discarded. Cancellous bone, if it can be cleaned sufficiently, may serve as excellent graft material. In adults, large nonviable cortical fragments are often retained, but such fragments can be discarded in children, whose capacity for bony regeneration is so much greater. Major neurovascular structures must be carefully identified and debrided.

Debridement is completed when all contaminated, dead, and ischemic tissue has been resected and the remaining wound cavity is lined by viable and bleeding tissue. Nerves, vessels, tendons, and denuded cortical bone are covered with local soft tissue, and the wound cavity is dressed with a bandage soaked in isotonic saline or an antiseptic. Despite meticulous care, the extent of tissue necrosis is easily underestimated; thus, the wound is left open after the initial debridement. It should be reevaluated in the operating room within 48 to 72 hours. At that time it may be necessary to resect more necrotic tissue and do more extensive fasciotomies. The process of debridement is repeated at intervals of 2 to 3 days, or shorter intervals, until the wound can be closed or covered without the risk of infection.

Following extensive debridement copious pulsed irrigation with 5000 to 10,000 ml of normal saline solution or distilled water is recommended. For final irrigation 2000 ml of bacitracin-polymyxin solution is used. At the completion of the debridement and irrigation, additional aerobic and anaerobic wound cultures are obtained. When positive, these are more likely to represent the infecting organism. Even when the initial debridement of the wound is aggressive, it is difficult to determine the viability of marginal tissues at that time. Repeat debridement in 48 to 72 hours is essential to reevaluate the soft tissues and complete the debridement of any tissues that have subsequently become necrotic or nonviable.

Additional problems that must be assessed at the time of debridement and irrigation include treatment of associated vascular injuries and treatment of the contaminated or infected wound.

Associated Vascular Injuries. In children, vascular injuries associated with tibial fractures are uncommon. In a series of 60 arterial injuries, Navarre and associates[155] reported that 46% were due to extremity fractures and dislocations. Of these, 11% involved the popliteal artery, and 5% the anterior tibial or peroneal arteries distal to the trifurcation. The prevalent clinical findings were a cold extremity, numbness, swelling, and altered pulse amplitude. Distal pulses were absent in 13%, diminished in 23%, and normal to finger palpation in 64% of the limbs. The incidence of vascular injuries in open pediatric tibial fractures (type IIIC) varies between 5 and 10%.[33, 229] If there is only the slightest suspicion of vascular compromise, a careful clinical assessment of vascular and neurologic function must be followed by Doppler flowmetry and possibly arteriography. Once the lesion is diagnosed, an attempt should be made to repair all injuries to the popliteal vessels. Vessel repair below the trifurcation will depend on the severity of associated lesions, the age of the patient, and the number of the vessels involved.[45, 155] It appears that, as in adults, warm ischemia times exceeding 4 hours are accompanied by an amputation rate of 50% or more. Unless the patient with a vascular injury is brought to the operating room early, stabilization of the tibial fracture should follow the vascular repair, or a temporary intraluminal shunt is used.[103] Johansen and associates[103] reported the use of temporary intraluminal shunts for early revascularization of severely injured lower extremities with complex vascular injuries and open fractures in which prolonged warm ischemia time would occur with traditional management. Following or, even better, preceding the vascular repair, compartment pressures (see Compartment Syndromes) should be measured, and fasciotomies of the four compartments of the lower leg should be performed when indicated. Prophylactic fasciotomies have been recommended by Rorabeck[180] when arterial circulation to the leg has been interrupted for 4 hours or longer. The fascial compartments of the foot also should be carefully observed.

Contaminated and Infected Wounds. It is advisable to assume that all open fractures, dislocations, and closed lesions covered with devitalized tissue are contaminated.[165] Frank infections, however, will develop only if necrotic tissue remains in the wound. Despite the use of systemic antibiotics, Dellinger and associates[45] reported that about 16% of all open fractures in adults will become infected eventually. They also reported that the infection rate increases from 7% in type I fractures to 56% in type IIIC fractures.[45] Although infection rates in children are unknown, it is expected that they are somewhat lower. Patzakis and Wilkins[165] in 1989 reported only 1 infection (1.8%) out of 55 open fractures in children. In contrast, they had an overall infection rate of 7.2% in 1049 open adult fractures. Typically, the infecting organisms are *Staphylococcus aureus* and aerobic or facultative gram-negative rods in fractures with less severe soft tissue injuries, while mixed flora prevails in lesions of type IIIB and IIIC severity.[45, 75, 165] Patzakis and Wilkins[165] reported the

Table 13–5 Schedule of Active Immunization Against Tetanus		
Dose	Age/Intervals	Vaccine
Age less than 7 years		
Primary 1	Age 6 weeks or older	DPT
Primary 2	4–8 weeks after the first dose	DPT
Primary 3	4–8 weeks after the second dose	DPT
Primary 4	About 1 year after the third dose	DPT
Booster	4–6 years of age	DPT
Additional boosters	Every 10 years after the last dose	Td
Age 7 years and older		
Primary 1	First visit	Td
Primary 2	4–6 weeks after the first dose	Td
Primary 3	6 months to 1 year after the last dose	Td
Boosters	Every 10 years after the last dose	Td

Abbreviations: DPT = diphtheria and tetanus toxoids and pertussis vaccine absorbed; Td = tetanus and reduced-dose diphtheria toxoids absorbed (for adult use).

From Cates, T.R. Clostridium tetani (tetanus). In: Mandell, G.L.; Douglas, R.G., Jr.; Bennett, J.E.; eds. Principles and Practice of Infectious Diseases. New York, Churchill Livingstone, 1990, pp. 1946–1982.

highest incidence of infection following open tibial fractures. Undoubtedly, the major reason for this is relative ischemia due to injury to nutrient arteries and lack of muscle coverage distally.

The vigorous uncompromising resection of all dead soft tissue is the mainstay in preventing development of an infected wound. However, systemic antibiotics; repeated irrigation with solutions that contain topical antibiotics such as neomycin, bacitracin, and polymyxin; and the use of an antibiotic containing polymethyl methacrylate (PMMA) beads appear to further reduce the development of an infection in open wounds.[17] Intravenous antibiotics are routinely used according to previous guidelines for 2 to 3 days following injury. These are, however, general guidelines, as the choice of the optimal antibiotic depends on the regional prevalence of pathogenetic bacteria, the profile of nosocomial infections in a particular institution, the emergence of resistance, and the development of new chemotherapeutic agents.[165]

CLOSTRIDIAL INFECTIONS. Tetanus is a rare disease; only about 200 cases occur per year in the United States, where the death rate is between 10 and 40%. The causative organism is *Clostridium tetani*, an anaerobic gram-negative rod that grows best under anaerobic conditions and in necrotic tissue. The clinical manifestations are caused by the effects of a neurotoxin on skeletal muscle, peripheral nerves, and spinal cord. Generalized tetanus starts with cramps in muscles surrounding the wounds, neck stiffness, hyperreflexia, and changes in facial expression. Later, contractions of whole muscle groups cause opisthotonos and acute respiratory failure. Local tetanus is rare and usually resolves without sequelae.[35]

Tetanus is preventable through active immunization using a formaldehyde-treated tetanospasmin, known as tetanus toxoid. In children below the age of 7 years, tetanus toxoid is administered combined with diphtheria toxoid and pertussis vaccine (DPT). Completion of a three- or four-dose series will confer humoral immunity to tetanus for at least 10 years in the vast majority of those who receive the vaccine (Table 13–5). A child or adolescent presenting with an open tibia fracture who has not completed the primary series of immunization or has not received a booster dose in 10 years should receive tetanus toxoid and, if the wound is severe, passive immunization with tetanus immune globulin (TIG). Usually 250 to 500 units of TIG are given intramuscularly together with tetanus toxoid, but at a separate site (Table 13–6).[35]

Gas gangrene is most frequently caused by *Clostridium perfringens* and *C. septicum*, anaerobic gram-positive spore-forming bacteria that produce numerous exotoxins. Gas gangrene is most frequently seen following primary wound closure, after

Table 13–6 Guide to Tetanus Prophylaxis				
History of Tetanus Immunization (Doses)	Clean, Minor Wounds		All Other Wounds	
	Td[a]	TIG[b]	Td[a]	TIG[b]
Uncertain or less than 2	Yes	No	Yes	Yes
2	Yes	No	Yes	No[c]
3 or more	No[d]	No	No[e]	No

[a]Tetanus toxoid.
[b]Tetanus immune globulin.
[c]Yes, if wound more than 24 hours old.
[d]Yes, if more than 10 years since last dose.
[e]Yes, if more than 5 years since last dose. (More frequent boosters are not needed and can accentuate side effects.)

From Cates, T.R. Clostridium tetani (tetanus). In: Mandell, G.L.; Douglas, R.G., Jr.; Bennett, J.E.; eds. Principles and Practice of Infectious Diseases. New York, Churchill Livingstone, 1990, pp. 1946–1982.

open crush injuries, and in wounds contaminated by bowel content or soil. Open tibial fracture is one of the most common injuries leading to gas gangrene.[32, 160, 165] The exotoxins produced by these organisms create local edema, muscle and fat necrosis, and thrombosis of local vessels. The clostridia also generate several gases that dissect into the surrounding tissues and facilitate a rapid spread of the infection. In terminal stages, clostridial infections cause hemolysis, tubular necrosis, and renal failure.[32, 59, 160]

The earliest symptoms of gas gangrene following an open fracture of the tibia include excruciating pain in the affected area followed by high fever, chills, tachycardia, contusion, and evidence of toxemia. Initially, the skin about the wound is very edematous and cool but without crepitation. Later, the skin has a brown or bronze coloration, crepitation, and drainage of a thin brownish fluid with a pungent odor. Radiographs will demonstrate gas formation within the muscle and intrafascial planes. Gram stain of the exudate reveals gram-positive rods.

It is important to remember that not all posttraumatic crepitation is due to gas gangrene. It also may be caused by mechanical introduction of air by trauma, surgery, or chemical irrigation.[62] This is especially true for crepitation in the first 12 hours after injury. Crepitation from gas gangrene usually occurs between 12 and 60 hours after injury; initially it is minimal but progresses with time.[160]

The crucial steps in the treatment of early gas gangrene are a radical debridement to remove all necrotic muscle and fasciotomies of all four compartments to relieve pressure from the edema and to enhance blood flow. Repeated debridements are usually necessary. In addition, the patient should receive intravenous penicillin (several million units per day in divided doses). In allergic patients, intravenous clindamycin (Cleocin Phosphate) or Flagyl (metronidazole) are very acceptable substitutes. As clostridial wounds often grow out a mixed flora, cephalosporin and an aminoglycoside are usually added. The efficacy of polyvalent gas gangrene serum, which can cause sensitivity reactions, for the treatment of gas gangrene remains unproved. Hyperbaric oxygen ventilation may also be beneficial.[32, 59, 160] Elevated tissue oxygen tension appears to have an inhibitory effect on clostridial growth and the production of exotoxins.

Fracture Stabilization. Fixation of the principal fracture fragments reduces pain, prevents additional injuries to surrounding soft tissues, decreases the spread of bacteria, and allows for early soft tissue and bone repair.[154] For the initial care, the method of stabilization must allow for free wound and limb access to carry out repeated debridements and assess limb viability. Later, the method must be sufficiently rigid to permit early weight bearing without interfering with range-of-motion exercises in adjacent joints.

Splints and Casts. Plaster splints, reinforcing soft cotton or wool dressings (Robert Jones dressings), are ideal for the early care of stable open tibial fractures of type I and some type II severity.[80, 81, 120, 191] Once the tissue edema has subsided and the soft tissues are closed, more rigid fixation of the bony fragments is needed. In most instances, further immobilization of the fracture can be achieved in a well-padded, long leg cast with about 10 degrees of knee flexion.[81, 86, 197] Younger children, up to 6 to 8 years of age, may be kept in a long leg cast until the fractures are healed, usually 6 to 10 weeks after the initial injury. In older children, the long leg cast may be removed after 4 to 5 weeks and replaced by a snugly fitting patellar tendon bearing cast, which remains until the fractures are healed, generally between 10 and 15 weeks.[73, 86]

External Fixation. For most closed fractures with grade 2 or 3 soft tissue injury (see Table 13–4), and for a majority of the unstable open fractures, cast treatment is not ideal.[3, 80, 216] The more severe lesions (some type II and all type III open fractures) often require repeated debridements with unobstructed wound access. In unstable fractures with more than 25 degrees of obliquity in relation to the transverse plane, fractures with more than minimal comminution, and segmental fractures, casts often inflict additional injury at the fracture site. These injuries are best managed with an external fixator.[3, 13, 14, 16, 80, 112, 172] If properly applied, these devices should allow free access to the wound for initial debridements and, if necessary, secondary flap procedures or bone grafts.[13, 15] They should be of sufficient rigidity to prevent further injuries to the soft tissues, preserve length, and allow full weight bearing without undue delay. A high rate of complications, occasional loss of reduction, and negative perceptions by children and parents have in the past made many surgeons reluctant to use these devices. Today, the introduction of rational concepts, simple designs, and protective instrumentation have made serious complications or rejection of the device by patient or parent a rare event.[17]

In older children and adolescents, devices and components designed for adults are more appropriate. However, for smaller children, fixators used for wrist fractures in adults or a combination of smaller pins with adult clamps and connecting rods have proved to be successful improvisations. The pin diameter should rarely exceed one quarter of the diameter of the bone. Pins with diameters ranging from 2.5 to 4.0 mm are most appropriate for children below the age of 12 years.[16] Small-diameter pins are successfully fitted to a larger clamp with use of shims or small segments of a K-wire, which, if properly fitted, will maintain a tight clamp for long periods.[16]

Out of concern to erect fixator frames of sufficient rigidity, many surgeons use such optimizing methods as a wide pin spread, dual longitudinal bars, and two-plane unilateral or two-plane bilateral designs.[18, 80, 208] With the exception of the athletic or obese teenager, simple one-plane unilateral frames routinely achieve sufficient rigidity for early unsupported weight bearing. Hansen[80] recommends an anterior half-pin device with dual bars for stability as the best method of treatment for the type III open pediatric tibial fractures. Ring fixators (Ilizarov), using wires under tension, which can be ideal to deal with pediatric leg length discrepancies, malalignments, or soft tissue contractures, are rarely used in treating an open tibial fracture in a child.[15] These devices tend to obstruct the wound, can bind the soft tissues, and may impale neurovascular structures.

In order to provide optimal function and prevent serious side effects, three basic criteria pertain when external fixators are applied: (1) They should not damage vital anatomy; (2) they should provide sufficient wound access for the initial debridements and secondary procedures; and (3) the frame should be appropriate to the mechanical demands of patient and injury.[13]

As a limb segment, where the principal long bone lies eccentrically, the tibia is ideally suited for the application of an external frame. The anteromedial third of the tibia represents a safe corridor, where pins are safely inserted without the risk of impaling neurovascular structures or myotendinous units. Occasionally, pins may be inserted into the epiphysis. Great care must be taken when pins are placed periarticularly, as the undulating shape of the physis creates an unsafe zone that varies in width from 1.0 to 2.0 cm.[3] Pins injuring the physis can cause serious growth disturbances, and pins entering the joint may give rise to septic arthritis. With some care and the use of an image intensifier, epiphyseal pins can be placed safely and may prove highly effective in the management of comminuted metaphyseal injuries. Epiphyseal pins also demand meticulous pin care, as an infected pin tract may damage the physis as well as the adjacent joint.

As in adults, the fixator is applied in the operating room under sterile conditions, usually under general anesthesia. The leg is draped so that the knee and ankle joint lie within the operating field, as this aids clinical limb alignment. The most proximal and distal pins are inserted first under image intensification to avoid injuries to the physes. This is followed by inserting the remaining screws, including those for a segmental fragment. An image intensifier is used routinely to check pin location and depth of penetration and overall limb alignment.[3, 16] The pins are predrilled with a sharp drill bit and a trochar sleeve that helps protect the soft tissues and facilitates accurate pin placement. Universal articulations, which allow for easy alignment, are routinely used. If the AO/ASIF fixator is used, care must be taken to avoid malrotation, which is difficult to correct after the insertion of all four pins.[3] Once the frame is applied, final fracture alignment is documented on long films. Pin care is usually performed several times each day with hydrogen peroxide.[3, 208] For younger children this is done by the parents, but responsible teenagers can handle this task independently. Unless there is bone loss, most patients walk, fully weight bearing with little support, within 3 weeks.

Internal Fixation. Although the introduction of well-designed, mechanically effective and biocompatible wires, screws, plates, and intramedullary nails has revolutionized the treatment of tibial fractures in adults, these new implants have had a minimal influence on the care of tibial shaft fractures in children.[84, 207, 216]

Wires, pins, and screws, although common internal fixation devices in children, do not provide sufficient stabilization for most open fractures. Occasionally, they may be used for the approximation of metaphyseal fragments, generally in conjunction with an external fixator in order to neutralize the fracture zone from undue bending and axial forces.[16] In adults and children, compression plates and screws used to stabilize open tibial fractures have been associated with a higher rate of soft tissue complications and infections than have external fixators.[84, 197, 233] At this time their use appears contraindicated. In adults, rigid and elastic intramedullary nails have become the principal means to stabilize closed and some open tibial fractures. Because of the physis their use in pediatric lesions is limited to older adolescents. In the younger child, nails have insufficient working length in the diaphysis, and the insertion creates undue risk of injuries to the proximal or distal physis. Maurer and colleagues[142] have demonstrated an increased rate of infection when changing from an external fixator to a reamed intramedullary nail after satisfactory wound healing if there had been an infection at one or more pin sites. Fortunately, this conversion is not applicable in the pediatric population.

Wound Care. Early in the management of open tibial fractures, the surgeon must judge the means by which soft tissue coverage of the wound will eventually occur. Proper planning is facilitated if the wound is reassessed during the first or second debridement, in conjunction with an expert in soft tissue and microvascular techniques.[89] The goal is to provide soft tissue coverage of open tibial fractures within 5 to 7 days, before the wound is secondarily infected.[165] Prior to soft tissue coverage, the wound must be kept moist with damp saline dressings. In children with degloving injuries of the lower leg associated with a tibia fracture, Letts has recommended that the skin be defatted and grafted to the extremity.[126] In severe cases the skin can be properly stored and reapplied several days later. External fixation is beneficial in stabilizing the fracture during wound care. Additional split-thickness skin grafts are usually necessary for complete wound coverage.

Most open tibial fractures from type I to type IIIA can be covered easily by delayed primary wound closure. Occasionally a split-thickness skin graft is needed to cover a large cutaneous defect overlying muscle or fascia covered with healthy granulation tissue. For larger defects, particularly over the knee and the proximal anteromedial aspect of the tibia, the medial gastrocnemius or other muscle flaps are ideal for children.[89] The soleus muscle flap can be used to provide coverage of the middle third of the tibia, and microvascular free flaps can be used for large defects of the distal one third.[89] Muscle and composite free flaps are also indicated for massive soft tissue and bony defects.[89, 97, 144] In addition to giving excellent coverage, these free flaps eliminate low-grade bacterial colonization in their recipient bed and facilitate union of the associated fractures.

Early Autogenous Cancellous Bone Grafting. Nonunion in pediatric tibial shaft fractures is practically limited to situations with major soft tissue compromise and bone loss. Planned autogenous bone grafting is indicated in all tibial fractures with partial bone loss exceeding more than half the bone diameter. If there is combined soft tissue and bone loss, placement of a muscle flap generally precedes autogenous bone grafting by 4 to 8 weeks to be sure that the recipient side is clean. A large segmental defect in a very young child may simply reconstitute if there is retained periosteum; in the older child a large cancellous bone graft will be needed; and in teenagers the microvascular transfer of free bone segment, such as the fibula, is generally the method of choice. Behrens[16] recommends autogenous bone grafting if no significant callus is visible 10 to 12 weeks after injury. Stabilization of these unstable fractures during the healing process is generally achieved with an external fixator. Fixators can remain in place until the lesions are healed. If large bone defects occur, bone transport using a ring fixator system and callotasis technique can be used.[159]

Rehabilitation. Once soft tissues have healed and bone union has been obtained, rehabilitation of the patient is important. This typically consists of range-of-motion exercises followed by strengthening of the remaining musculature. It is important that these children undergo long-term follow-up to assess ultimate outcome with respect to function and lower extremity length equality.

Results

The results of treatment of open tibial fractures in children have been primarily speculative and correlated with the results of open tibial fractures in adults or closed tibial fractures in children,[81, 86, 191, 197] as no published series until recently dealt solely with this injury. In 1966, Stanford and associates[197] studied 94 pediatric tibial fractures, of which 19 were open. They reported on the results of treatment of 18 children, 16 of whom were treated by closed techniques and healed at a mean of 3.14 months. The two fractures treated by open reduction developed infection. Healing occurred at 11 and 24 months. Hoaglund and States[86] in 1967 reported 43 pediatric tibial fractures. Five fractures were open and were treated with closed techniques without complications, with a union time of 3 months. Alonso and Horowitz,[3] in their report on the use of the AO/ASIF external fixator in children, including 10 of 20 children with tibia fractures, found that only one patient with an open proximal metaphyseal fracture developed a 12 degree progressive valgus deformity and 2.5 cm of overgrowth. Another patient had a refracture 6 months after injury. The external fixator was used for a mean of 7 weeks, when a cast was applied. Union occurred after an average of 16 weeks.

Tolo[208] reported on 13 open tibial fractures treated by external fixation. He reported that one half had superficial pin tract infection, although none developed osteomyelitis. Three patients had refracture 5 to 10 months after injury. Two children had mild angular deformities, and three had overgrowth of 1.0 to 1.4 cm. The fixator was used for a mean of 11 weeks before being removed. Union was achieved at a mean of 21 weeks. This author believed that fracture healing was slightly delayed by the use of the external fixator. Hansen and co-workers[81] in 1976 reported on 14 open fractures in a series of 102 pediatric tibial fractures that healed without complications with cast immobilization. Shannak[191] in 1988 reported on 117 pediatric tibial fractures, of which 4 were open. Three fractures were treated with os calcis traction and one with pin fixation. No complications related to these fractures occurred. Bohn and Durbin reported that 12 of 30 (32 limbs) children or adolescents had one or both fractures open.[26] Other than increased healing time, there were no complications. The mean time to union was 23 weeks.

In 1990, Buckley and associates[33] reported the results of 41 children with 42 open tibial fractures who were followed at least to fracture healing. The mean age at injury was 9 years 9 months (range, 3 to 16 years) and the mean follow-up period was 15 months (range, 3 to 96 months). There were 32 males and 9 females in this series, for almost a 4:1 ratio. The mechanism of injury was predominantly automobile-pedestrian accidents. This occurred in 29 patients (71%). Other mechanisms included bicycle accidents, sports injuries, motor vehicle accidents, gunshot wounds, lawn mower accidents, and crush injuries. Twenty-one fractures (50%) were comminuted, and 33 fractures involved the tibial diaphysis. The fibula was fractured in 38 (93%) of the 42 extremities. According to the classification of Gustilo and colleagues,[76] there were 12 type I, 18 type II, and 12 type III (six type IIIA, four type IIIB, and two type IIIC) fractures. Nineteen children (46%) had other associated injuries—14 other fractures, nine closed head injuries, two abdominal injuries, and one pulmonary contusion.

All patients and all extremities were managed according to the recommendations of Gustilo's group.[76, 77] Twenty-two of the fractures were immobilized in a long leg plaster cast, while 20 had an external fixator applied. The indications for external fixation included severe soft tissue injury, the need for a fasciotomy, and an unstable fracture pattern with tibial shortening. Only two patients had elevated compartment pressures that required a four-compartment fasciotomy. All fractures were immobilized until there was evidence of healing both radiographically and clinically. Three patients developed wound infection, one of whom progressed to osteomyelitis. Pin tract infections developed in 4 of the 20 patients who were treated with external fixation. All pin tract infections resolved with appropriate treatment. Four fractures at the time of healing had developed 10 degrees or more of angulation. Spontaneous correction secondary to growth and remodeling occurred in three patients. Corrective osteotomy was necessary in one patient—the same patient who developed osteomyelitis. Four patients had lower extremity length discrepancies greater than 1 cm (range 1.3 to 2.5 cm). The involved tibia was longer in all four patients. Shortening of more than 1 cm did not occur in any of the involved children. The average time of union of the fractures was 4.8 months (range, 2 to 22 months). Six patients had delayed unions. Most of the delayed unions were directly related to the severity of the soft tissue injury and the pattern of the fracture. The patients with segmental bone loss took the longest time to heal.

The authors felt that their data demonstrated that children with open fractures of the tibia have an incidence of vascular injury, compartment syndrome, infection, and delayed unions similar to that reported for adults. The type I fractures, however, were not associated with these complications and tended to heal relatively quickly in a manner similar to closed fractures. The factors that were unique to open fractures of the tibia in children were tibial overgrowth associated with severe open fractures.

Yasko and Wilber[229] studied 53 open tibial fractures in children with a mean age at injury of 10 years (range, 2 to 15 years) and found similar results. There were 24 type I, 17 type II, and 12 type III (three type IIIA, four type IIIB, and five type IIIC) fractures that were followed for a mean of 5.5 years (range, 6 months to 16 years). In this series, the most common mechanism of injury was motor vehicle accidents (82%). Thirteen children (25%) had other body area injuries, and an additional nine children had other fractures. Treatment was according to the criteria of Gustilo and colleagues.[76, 77] External fixation was used in 18% of type I, 23% of type II, and 40% of the type III injuries (Fig. 13–9). Uncomplicated healing occurred in all type I fractures, while delayed union or nonunion occurred in 12 or 50% of the type II and type III fractures, respectively (Fig. 13–10). The overall sepsis rate was 8%, with 6% and 30% of the type II and III fractures becoming infected, respectively. Two delayed amputations were necessary in type III fractures because of severe sepsis. This study revealed a significant morbidity rate associated with open tibial fractures in children.

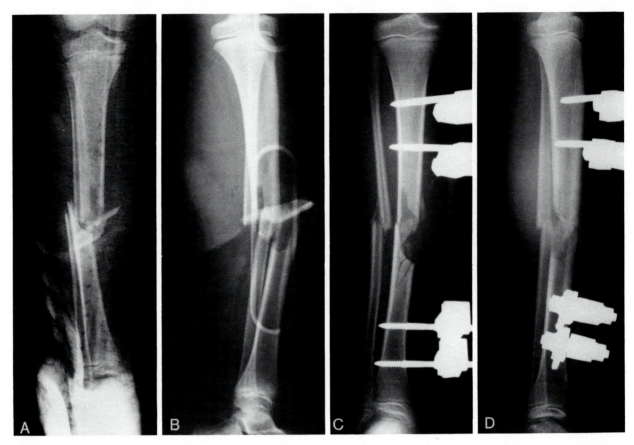

Figure 13–9

A, Anteroposterior radiographs of the right lower leg of a 6-year-old female with a comminuted, displaced grade IIIB open fracture of the tibia and fibular diaphyses. These fractures were sustained when she was struck by an automobile. *B*, The lateral radiograph demonstrates malrotation and a large, transversely oriented tibial fracture segment. *C*, Radiographs obtained 1 month following debridement, removal of devascularized tibial fracture fragment, irrigation, stabilization with an external fixator, and a soleus muscle rotation flap covered with meshed split-thickness skin graft. There is a large residual defect in the tibia. Leg length was maintained owing to reduction of the lateral cortices of the tibia. *D*, Lateral radiograph demonstrates satisfactory alignment.

Authors' Preferred Treatment

We use the classification and initial methods of management described by Gustilo's group.[76, 77] The classification yields prognostic information and guides subsequent treatment. Types I and II open fractures are usually managed by closed techniques and immobilization in a long leg plaster cast. However, children with multiple injuries, those with second- and third-degree burns, and those with unstable fracture patterns may benefit from external fixation. The definitive management for each child must be individualized for optimal results. In type III open fractures, external fixation is utilized, usually with a unilateral frame. The authors have not used compression plates or intramedullary rods. Occasionally, simple screw fixation may be useful to stabilize unstable segmental fractures in conjunction with external fixation.

Complications

The common complications of tibial and fibular diaphyseal fractures include (1) delayed union; (2) nonunion; (3) angular deformity; (4) malrotation; (5) proximal tibial physeal closure; (6) lower extremity length inequality; (7) vascular injury; (8) neurologic injury; and (9) compartment syndromes.

DELAYED UNIONS

Delayed unions (6 months or longer) in pediatric tibia fractures are not common. The total time to satisfactory healing depends on the child's age and the type of fracture. In the series of Steinert and Bennek,[199] the duration of immobilization varied between 8 and 10 weeks. In Hoagland and States'[86] report of 43 tibial fractures in children less than 16

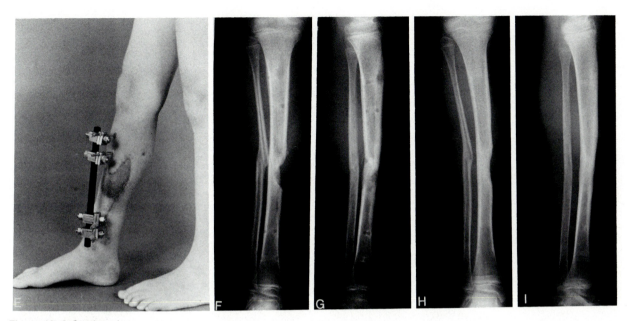

Figure 13–9 Continued

E, Clinical photograph 2 months following injury. The wounds are well healed, and the patient is allowed partial weight bearing with crutches. Cancellous bone grafting of the tibial defect was performed at this time. F, Anteroposterior radiograph 3 months following injury and 1 month after cancellous bone grafting and removal of the external fixator. The tibial defect is healing satisfactorily. The patient then had 2 months of additional immobilization in a short leg, weight-bearing fiberglass cast. G, Lateral radiograph shows maintenance of satisfactory alignment. H, At 6 months following injury there is excellent reconstitution of the tibial defect. The patient was now allowed unprotected weight bearing. I, Lateral radiograph demonstrates excellent healing and alignment.

years of age the mean healing time for 38 closed fractures was 10 weeks, with a range of 6 to 25 weeks. In five open fractures, the mean immobilization period was 12 weeks. In the study by Buckley and associates[33] of open pediatric tibial fractures, the mean time to healing was 5 months (range, 2 to 21 months). The time to union was clinically related to the severity of the soft tissue injury, the fracture pattern, the amount of segmental bone loss, the occurrence of infection, and the use of external fixation. The last-named appeared to significantly increase the time to healing. These investigators reported six delayed unions (15%) in 41 children with open fractures. These occurred in two type II, three type IIIB, and one type IIIC fracture. Yasko and Wilber[229] reported four delayed unions (8%) in 53 children with open tibial fractures. This included one type II and three type III fractures.

Typically, younger children heal faster than older children. Also, comminuted, displaced fractures take longer to heal than do simple nondisplaced fractures in which the periosteum is intact, and type I open fractures heal faster than type IIIC fractures. When healing is delayed, this usually represents inadequate vascularization of the fracture site. This problem may be due to an injury to the nutrient artery, the overlying soft tissue and periosteum, or both. Additional time for revascularization and healing is therefore necessary. Also, inadequate immobilization that allows motion at the fracture site may contribute to a delayed union or possibly to a nonunion.

Delayed unions are usually managed by autogenous bone grafting from the iliac crest and proper immobilization until healing occurs.

NONUNIONS

Nonunions of pediatric tibial fractures are extremely uncommon. Hansen and co-workers[80] reported no nonunions in 99 pediatric tibial fractures followed through fracture union. When present, nonunions are usually associated with severe trauma, such as occurs in open fractures.[26] However, Buckley and associates[33] reported no nonunions, while Yasko and Wilber[229] reported one case in a child with a type IIIC fracture. Union was ultimately achieved at 1 year following two separate bone-grafting procedures.

Autogenous bone graft from the iliac crest and appropriate fracture stabilization form the basis of treatment of pediatric tibial nonunions. In cases

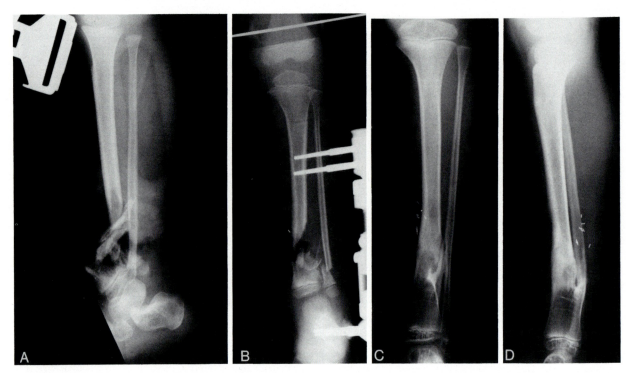

Figure 13–10

A, Anteroposterior radiographs of the left lower leg in a 3-year-old male who sustained an open, comminuted grade IIIC fracture of the distal tibia and fibula when he was struck by an automobile. There was a closed ipsilateral femoral shaft fracture. Circulation to the left foot was compromised. Arteriogram demonstrated occlusion of both the anterior tibial and the peroneal arteries. Blood flow through the posterior tibial artery was intact. *B*, Radiographs 1 month following extensive debridement, irrigation, application of an external fixator, vascular repair, wound coverage with a rotational skin flap, and cancellous bone grafting. The femoral shaft fracture was treated with skeletal traction through the distal femur. *C*, Radiographs 28 months after injury. The child experienced delayed union and required two additional bone grafts. He ultimately had a free microvascular muscle transfer and split-thickness skin grafting to obtain vascularized soft tissue coverage over the fracture. Union ultimately occurred. The patient has equal leg lengths and normal function. *D*, Lateral radiograph confirms satisfactory alignment, although there is a slight posterior angulation.

with inadequate vascularization of the fracture site, a delayed muscle or myocutaneous flap using microvascular techniques as well as cancellous bone grafting may be beneficial in achieving a union. Immobilization can be accomplished either with an external fixation frame or perhaps with compression plate or screws. Ring fixators (Ilizarov) and callotasis have been successfully utilized for tibial nonunions associated with bone loss.[159] We prefer external fixation because it does not require a separate second extensive procedure for metal removal and there is less soft-tissue damage at the time of the initial bone grafting.

ANGULAR DEFORMITIES

Angular deformities following nonphyseal pediatric tibial fractures are due to either inadequate alignment prior to union or transient asymmetric overgrowth. The latter is typically associated with proximal tibial metaphyseal fracture, which has already been discussed. Fractures of long bones, including the tibia, in children with angular deformities may undergo spontaneous correction with growth.[33, 65, 81, 191] Certain generalities can be stated regarding remodeling:[65] (1) the younger the child, the greater the capacity for correction; (2) the closer the fracture to the physis, the more remodeling needed; (3) the smaller the remaining angulation, the more complete the correction should be; and (4) residual angulation in the same plane as the movement of the adjacent joints has a greater capacity for correction. Correction of residual angular deformities is due to a combination of asymmetric epiphyseal growth, both proximally and distally, and remodeling of the fracture site according to Wolff's law. However, the amount of correction is not predictable and varies with each long bone.

Shannak[191] identified several factors associated with spontaneous correction of angulated tibial malunions. These factors included varus and anterior angulation, spiral fractures, and younger age at injury (more remaining musculoskeletal growth). Hansen and associates[81] reported angular deformities in 25 of 85 children (29%) who were followed clinically and radiographically for a mean of 2 years. These deformities were mild, varying between 4 and 19 degrees. They found only a 14% correction of angular deformities of the tibia in children. Correction ceased 18 months after injury and was independent of the child's age. Shannak[191] reported that 43 (41%) of 117 children had residual varus or valgus angulation. In 25 children it was mild and varied from 1 to 10 degrees, and in 18 children it was moderate, being greater than 10 degrees but less than 22 degrees. At follow-up of 3.9 years (range, 1 to 10 years) 91 children had no residual angulation, 20 had 1 to 10 degrees, and only 6 had more than 10 degrees. Thus, one third of the children with greater than 10 degrees of angulation had persistent malunion. This was typically a valgus or anterior angulation, or both. Even when remodeling is incomplete at the diaphyseal level, epiphyseal realignment, both proximally and distally, will compensate for some of the residual deformity.[166, 223] This occurs with varus more than valgus deformities and with posterior more than anterior deformities. Buckley and associates[33] had 4 (10%) of 41 children with open fractures develop an angular deformity of greater than 10 degrees. Three children resolved their deformity with growth, but the maximum deformity was only 14 degrees. One patient required a corrective osteotomy for a 25 degree diaphyseal angulation. The fracture was complicated by both osteomyelitis and a delayed union. Bohn and Durbin[26] reported two femoral and three tibial malunions in 30 children (32 limbs) with ipsilateral femoral and tibial shaft fractures. All occurred after closed treatment of their fractures.

The treatment of angular deformities is prevention. It is important that tibial fractures be followed closely radiographically and that any residual angulation in the frontal and sagittal planes be corrected prior to fracture healing. Angulations of 10 degrees or less at healing should be observed, for many will improve with growth. Deformities greater than 10 degrees may be observed in young children but in the older child and adolescent may require corrective osteotomy.

MALROTATION

Pediatric tibial fractures that are allowed to heal in a malrotated position will not correct or remodel with subsequent growth and development. Lateral rotation of the distal fracture fragment will result in an out-toed gait as well as increase in the stresses along the medial aspect of the knee and pronation of the ankle and foot. Medial rotation of the distal fracture fragment will result in an in-toed gait. It may also produce internal rotation at the knee joint level and a supination of the foot.

Fortunately, the incidence of significant rotational malunion is low. Hansen[81] reported that only 5 of 85 patients (6%) had rotational deformities between 10 and 20 degrees. Shannak[191] had three (3%) of 117 children with rotational deformities—two medial and one lateral. These persisted after 3.9 years of follow-up. All three were 12 years of age or older at injury. Bohn and Durbin[26] reported no rotational malalignments in 30 children (32 limbs) with ipsilateral femoral and tibial fractures followed for a mean of 5.1 years.

It is important that accurate rotational alignment be achieved during closed reduction of a tibial fracture and application of a long leg cast or an external fixator. Any degree of malrotation should be avoided. If adequate radiographic assessment cannot be made, a CT scan, including views of the opposite intact tibia, can be helpful.[101] If the fracture is allowed to heal in excessive rotational malalignment, surgical correction may be necessary. Its location will depend on the level of the deformity. Surgery usually is performed either proximally but inferior to the tibial tubercle or in the supramalleolar area. Concomitant osteotomy of the fibula is always necessary. The risk for compartment syndrome is lower if the osteotomy is performed distally below the origin of calf musculature.

PROXIMAL TIBIAL PHYSEAL CLOSURE

Kestler[114] in 1947 reported on premature cessation of epiphyseal growth about the knee joint. He recognized infectious and noninfectious causes involving the hip but also noted an idiopathic group without hip lesions or other pathologic processes. Morton and Starr,[149] in 1964, reported this complication following a tibial fracture in two children. Both sustained comminuted fractures of the tibial diaphysis with no apparent injury to the knee. The fractures were reduced, and K-wires were used in the proximal fracture segment but were 4 cm distal to the tibial tubercle. Both patients later developed a genu recurvatum deformity secondary to anterior closure of the proximal tibial physis. Subsequently, other similar cases were described following both tibial and femoral shaft fractures.[26, 50, 92, 161, 194] The mean age at injury for children who have an increased risk for this complication is between 10 and 12 years.[92, 161] The clinical deformity is usually noticed 1 to 3 years later.

The cause of the closure of the anterior aspect of the proximal tibial physis is unknown. Fielding and associates[61] reported anterior closure of the proximal tibial epiphysis following tibial tubercle transplantation in 1 of 15 growing children. This was not surprising considering the anatomy of this physis and the tibial tubercle. Hresko and Kasser[92] speculated on two possible mechanisms: (1) direct blunt trauma to the subcutaneous tibial tubercle, resulting in anterior growth arrest and recurvatum, and (2) compression injury to the anterior part of the proximal tibial physis generated by hyperextension of the knee. Pappas and associates[161] recognized trauma, prolonged immobilization, proximal tibial wire traction, a surgical procedure involving the proximal tibial physis, and coexistent Osgood-Schlatter disease as risk factors.

The genu recurvatum deformity is best managed by corrective opening wedge osteotomy of the proximal tibia, iliac crest bone graft, and possible epiphysiodesis of the remainder of the proximal tibial physis, depending on the patient's age at surgery, to prevent recurrence. Since the osteotomy is usually an opening wedge, in order to correct the normal posterior slope to the proximal tibia, care must be taken not to overstretch the anterior skin and predispose to wound dehiscence and necrosis. Subcutaneous fasciotomy of the anterior compartment and closed suction drainage should be performed to minimize the risk of an anterior compartment syndrome. Epiphysiodesis of the distal femoral and or proximal tibial epiphysis of the contralateral extremity may be required in children with significant tibial shortening to achieve equal leg lengths at skeletal maturity.

LOWER EXTREMITY LENGTH INEQUALITY

As with other long bone fractures in children the periosteal stripping, callus formation, and increased blood flow to the involved bone results in stimulation of the adjacent physes and transient acceleration in growth. However, it does not occur with the same magnitude as in femoral shaft fractures except in children with open tibial fractures.[33] Greiff and Bergmann[73] and Swaan and Oppers[201] reported tibial overgrowth of approximately 5 mm in females 3 to 10 years and in males 3 to 12 years of age. Older children and young adolescents may actually have a growth retardation induced by the fracture. Additional overgrowth of 1 to 3 mm can occur in the ipsilateral femur. The overgrowth is not affected by the fracture type or any residual angulation and lasts 1 to 2 years following injury. Shannak,[191] however, found that comminuted fractures, proximal and distal fractures, and fractures with significant shortening had the greatest overgrowth. Similar results were reported in the Italian literature in 1985.[36, 52, 164] DiLeo and associates[52] reported in their study of 121 tibia fractures that the greatest incidence of overgrowth occurred in children 3 to 8 years of age with proximal metaphyseal fractures in which the fracture line encroached on the physis.

Open fractures treated by external fixation also seem to have a greater amount of overgrowth than would normally be anticipated.[3, 26, 33, 199, 208] Tolo[208] reported overgrowth between 1.0 and 1.4 cm in 3 of 13 open tibial fractures. He recommended slight overriding of the fracture fragments in children between 2 and 12 years of age to compensate for this expected overgrowth. Alonso and Horowitz[3] reported overgrowth in 1 of 10 open tibia fractures of 2.5 cm. However, this was a proximal metaphyseal fracture. Buckley and associates[33] reported that four (15%) of 41 open tibial fractures had overgrowth of more than 1 cm (range, 1.3 to 3.5 cm). All were treated by anatomic alignment and application of an external fixator.

Open reduction with intramedullary rod can cause significant overgrowth, provided that the proximal physis is not injured. Steinert and Bennek[199] reported three cases of overgrowth of 2 to 3 cm.

Trotter and Gleser[210] as well as others[4, 10, 213] have demonstrated that there is a mean of 5 mm (range, 5 to 12 mm) length discrepancy in the lower extremities of normal children. Therefore, some degree of luck is involved in obtaining equal leg lengths, especially if the fractured extremity was originally the larger one.

Based on these data it is important that accurate restoration of length be achieved in the management of pediatric tibial shaft fracture. Fortunately, most instances of shortening will not be clinically significant. Most studies indicate that a lower extremity length inequality of 2 cm to be of no importance in adults. If excessive shortening should occur, it must be followed with periodic radiographic measurements and bone age determinations to assess the behavior of the shortening and whether contralateral epiphysiodesis will be necessary in order for the patient to have equal leg lengths at skeletal maturity.

VASCULAR INJURIES

Vascular injuries in association with tibial shaft fractures are uncommon in children.[66, 190, 219] Shaker and associates[190] reported that in only 8 of 118 children (7%) under age 15 years seen between 1965 and 1975 were vascular injuries due to fractures, and most were from supracondylar fractures of the distal humerus. No vascular injuries from tibial fractures were reported. When vascular injuries secondary to tibial fractures are present, they usually are the result of high-velocity injuries and open fractures, such as occur in motor vehicle accidents.[26, 33, 58, 155, 229] Males are more commonly involved than females. From 5 to 10% of open fractures have associated vascular injuries (type IIIC), but such injuries can also occur in closed fractures.[38, 66, 155] Vascular injuries in association with tibial fractures are most often seen with displaced fractures of the proximal metaphysis or diaphysis.[26, 38, 79, 155, 171] Fractures in the proximal tibial metaphysis may damage the anterior tibial artery as it passes from posterior to anterior through the interosseous membrane. The proximal tibial diaphyseal fracture may damage the trifurcation of the anterior tibial, posterior tibial, and peroneal arteries. Another fracture that may involve the anterior tibial artery occurs in the lower aspect of the tibia when the distal fragment is displaced posteriorly. Isolated injuries to the posterior tibial artery as a consequence of a tibial shaft fracture are very rare.

Prompt recognition, evaluation, and vascular reconstruction are critically important in initial limb salvage and avoidance of late complications. The cardinal signs of an arterial injury are known as the five P's: (1) pulselessness, (2) pain, (3) pallor, (4) paresthesias, and (5) paralysis.[150, 219] However, the presence of palpable pulses on Doppler flowmetry does not rule out an arterial injury. If such an injury is suspected, an arteriogram should be obtained. Compartment syndromes can present with many of the same features as an arterial injury and may occur following vascular repair[179, 183] (see Compartment Syndromes). Fasciotomies at the time of vascular repair have been recommended. If fasciotomy is not performed, sequential or continuous compartment pressure measurements need to be taken.

Friedman and Jupiter[66] reported the results of seven children with vascular injuries associated with closed extremity fractures, including three with tibial fractures, who were not diagnosed initially and underwent delayed repair. Early complications included wound infections, below-knee amputation, deep-vein thrombosis, and motor and sensory deficits. Late follow-up revealed two cases of limb overgrowth and one of limb undergrowth. Minor motor and sensory deficits persisted, but the overall function was good. These authors recommended arteriography in all children with a suspected vascular injury following fracture. If the arteriogram revealed a major vascular lesion, it should be repaired immediately, usually after fracture stabilization with internal or external fixation. This is applicable even with adequate collateral circulation to keep the limb viable. This study indicated that as the child grows and places greater functional demands on the extremity, the collateral circulation may be inadequate to meet the increased demands, resulting in altered growth or intermittent ischemia-like symptoms related to activity. However, it is important to remember that arteriography is not without complications and should be used only when there is a high index of suspicion for an associated vascular injury. Thrombosis is a recognized complication following angiography in children.[190] As a consequence, Friedman and Jupiter[66] recommended the use of digital subtraction angiography to evaluate the long-term vascular patency in children.

Another potential vascular complication following tibial fractures is traumatic arterial spasm. Diffuse arterial spasm without a specific arterial injury can occur and result in gangrene. Children appear more susceptible to this condition than do adults. Russo[184] reported a 9-year-old male who sustained a type IIIC open tibial, fibular, and calcaneal fracture and developed traumatic arterial spasm, resulting in gangrene of the lower leg and foot requiring below-knee amputation. Arteriography showed only diffuse arterial spasm. The spasm was not relieved by vasodilating agents. Treatment options for this rare condition, as discussed by Russo,[184] include intraarterial injection of vasodilating agents such as papaverine, sodium nitroprusside, reserpine, tolazoline, and prostaglandin E. Surgical measures may include external irrigation with warm Ringer's lactate solution, application of local anesthetics or 32% papaverine, and adventitial stripping. If these fail, dilation of the artery with mechanical dilators or catheters may be beneficial.

The treatment of fractures associated with arterial injuries in children is controversial. Generally, the fractures are stabilized by an external fixator prior to arterial repair. However, Wolma and associates[227] as well as Friedman and Jupiter[66] have demonstrated satisfactory results with conservative management. Each case must be individualized and the vascularity to the lower leg restored as rapidly as possible. Some fracture patterns may prevent initial vascular repair, necessitating reduction and stabilization prior to repair. If limb viability is in question, the arterial repair should be performed first or an intraluminal shunt used.[103] When limb viability is not in question, the fracture should be stabilized first to allow for more normal anatomic restoration of the soft tissues and bone.

NEUROLOGIC INJURY

Neurologic injuries associated with pediatric tibial fractures are uncommon, even in open fractures. The most common neurologic injury involves the peroneal nerve as it passes around the lateral aspect of the proximal fibula.[81] The nerve is more likely to be damaged by a direct blow rather than by a fracture fragment. It is important when fractures occur in this area that the function of the muscles innervated by the peroneal nerve be well documented. Bohn and Durbin[26] reported two transient, partial peroneal nerve palsies in children with ipsilateral femoral and tibial fractures. One occurred during skeletal traction and the other at the time of injury or during fracture reduction and application of a hip spica cast. Buckley and associates[33] reported only one case of a direct neurologic injury in a child with an open fracture. This was a posterior tibial nerve laceration in a 10-year-old with a type IIIB fracture. Although it was repaired, primary neural function was not restored, and 2 years later a free muscle transfer to the medial aspect of the foot and ankle was necessary to treat a persistent neuropathic ulcer. Yasko and Wilber[229] reported no neurologic injuries in their patients with open tibial fractures.

Perhaps the most common mechanism for a neurologic injury with a pediatric tibial fracture is the posttraumatic compartment syndrome.

COMPARTMENT SYNDROMES

A compartment syndrome due to bleeding and extravasation of tissue fluid into one or more of the four compartments of the lower leg can and does occur in children as well as adults following a fracture of the tibial shaft.[56, 151] It can also be a complication of proximal tibial corrective osteotomies, tibial lengthening procedures, and use of tibia bone graft donor sites in children.[100, 139, 151, 189, 198] Increased tissue pressure results in an increased net force per unit area exerted on the vessel walls within one or more compartments. This force increases local venous pressure, which decreases the local arteriovenous gradient, reducing local blood flow and oxygenation and thus compromising local tissue function (muscle and nerve) and viability.[6] The tolerance for increased compartment pressure varies with the local arterial pressure, the duration of pressure, and possibly the local metabolic needs of the tissues.[137] Prompt diagnosis and surgical decompression are essential to preserve the viability and function of tissues within the compartment. Failure to diagnose and treat either an incipient or an established compartment syndrome may result in irreversible ischemia of the intrinsic and extrinsic muscles of the lower leg and possibly amputation.[121, 151, 181] Mubarak and Carroll[151] in 1979 presented a review of 55 patients with Volkmann's ischemic contractures seen between 1955 and 1975 at the Hospital for Sick Children in Toronto. This series included 11 children with lower leg compartment syndromes, 5 of which were a complication of a tibial shaft fracture. All but one patient had a delay in diagnosis of greater than 3 days. As a consequence, there was one below-knee amputation, in addition to five severe and four moderate cases of residual functional deficit and only one case of mild residual functional deficit.

Although most compartment syndromes occur in closed fractures, the presence of open fracture with supposed compartment disruption does not preclude the possibility. Buckley and associates[33] reported two compartment syndromes (5%) in 42 open pediatric tibial fractures. Both were type II injuries. However, the incidence of compartment syndrome in the more severe open fractures (type III) is very low. Buckley and associates[33] as well as Yasko and Wilber[229] reported no cases of compartment syndromes in a total of 24 type III open fractures.

The clinical findings of a compartment syndrome are subjective, and its detection depends heavily on patient cooperation. In children, this can be difficult because of pain, fear, and anxiety. The physician, therefore, must have a high index of suspicion. Intracompartment pressure measurements, using a variety of techniques, allow a more objective method of evaluating and monitoring compartment pressures. The first and most important symptom of an impending acute compartment syndrome is pain out of proportion to that expected from the fracture.[141, 150, 153, 179, 180] Other symptoms may include extremity swelling, a feeling of tenseness in the involved compartments, and paresthesias of the nerves that traverse those compartments.

The earliest clinical finding is a swollen and tense compartment caused by the increased intracompartment pressure. Pain with passive stretch of the muscles in the involved compartment is a common finding but, again, is subjective.[150, 180] Children with sensory deficits due to a proximal nerve injury may not exhibit stretch pain, even in the presence of elevated intracompartment pressures. Differentiating paresthesias due to a proximal nerve injury rather than a compartment syndrome can be difficult.

The most reliable physical finding for a compartment syndrome is the sensory deficit.[150] Most compartments of the lower leg are traversed by nerves having distal sensory distribution. Decreased sensation to light touch, pinprick, or two-point discrimination in the distal sensory distribution is a common finding.

Except in the presence of major arterial injury, peripheral pulses and capillary filling are usually intact in children with compartment syndromes.[150] As a consequence, the presence of palpable distal pulses and good capillary filling is no assurance that compartment syndrome does not exist.[225]

The most complex differential diagnoses following a tibial shaft fracture arise in distinguishing between compartment syndrome, arterial occlusion, and proximal nerve injury (neurapraxia).[150-152, 189] These conditions can frequently coexist, and their clinical findings can overlap. Mubarak and Hargens[152] developed an algorithm to assist in differentiation and choice of appropriate treatment. Arterial injuries normally have absent peripheral pulses but no increased compartment pressure. In children with neurapraxia, there is no pain with passive stretch muscles within a given compartment, no increased compartment pressures, and normal peripheral pulses. These characteristics are simplified, and each child must be carefully evaluated for these possibilities.

Mubarak and associates[153] have identified three groups of patients in whom difficulties in eliciting and interpreting the physical findings of compartment syndromes are frequently encountered and in whom measurement of intracompartment pressures may be extremely helpful. These groups are (1) patients who are unresponsive; (2) those who are uncooperative or unreliable, especially young children; and (3) those with peripheral nerve deficits attributable to other causes, such as a peroneal nerve palsy. Several methods have been developed for the measurement of compartment pressures.[28, 180, 181] These methods include (1) needle, (2) continuous infusion, (3) Wick catheter, and (4) slit catheter techniques. The last technique appears to be the most popular and affords an accurate method for continuous monitoring of intracompartment pressures.[150] The pressure threshold for diagnosis of a compartment syndrome will vary for each of these techniques. The orthopaedic surgeon needs to be familiar with the advantages, the disadvantages, and the pressure thresholds for each technique. Whitesides and associates,[224] using the needle technique, recommended decompression when compartment pressures rise to within 10 to 30 mm Hg of the diastolic blood pressure. Matsen and associates,[141] using the infusion technique, suggested that fasciotomies be performed in patients with clinical findings of the compartment syndrome who had pressures greater than 45 mm Hg. Using the Wick and slit catheter techniques, Mubarak,[150, 153] Rorabeck,[179, 180] and Rorabeck and MacNab[181] recommended decompression when the intracompartment pressures exceed 30 to 35 mm Hg when combined with the appropriate clinical findings.

The anterior compartment syndrome occurs most often following a fracture of the tibial shaft and is characterized by pain referred to the anterior compartment on passive flexion of the toes and mild weakness of the extensor hallucis longus followed by the extensor digitorum longus. The last sign to appear is hypoesthesia in the first web space.[28, 181] Although the anterior compartment syndrome is the most common, other compartments may be involved concomitantly or individually. A deep posterior compartment syndrome can occur in children. It was initially described by Matsen and Clawson[138] in 1975 as characterized by pain, plantar hyperesthesia, weakness of toe flexion, pain on passive toe extension, and tenseness of the fascia between the tibia and the triceps surae in the distal medial part of the leg. Decompression of the deep posterior compartment within 12 hours of onset of the syndrome prevented permanent sequelae. Karlström and associates[109] as well as Bohn and Durbin[26] have reported on the results of unrecognized deep posterior compartment syndrome. Karlström and coworkers[109] found 23 cases, and 2 occurred in adolescents less than 15 years of age. These patients presented with a clawed foot and limited ankle and subtalar motion secondary to fibrous contractures of the muscles of the deep posterior compartment. The muscle changes were attributed to vascular damage, soft tissue swelling, or severe muscle laceration. Because of the involvement of multiple compartments, it is now recommended that (1) during the initial evaluation, pressure measurements be made in all four compartments; and (2) if a fasciotomy is required, all compartments be released simultaneously.[181]

Incipient compartment syndromes can also exist. This problem may occur in children who are complaining of inordinate pain under the cast but in whom no frank signs of a compartment syndrome are present. The first step in management of the incipient compartment syndrome involves bivalving the cast and splitting the underlying padding. Garfin and associates[68] demonstrated that univalving a cast of a hind limb of an experimental animal reduced compartment pressures by 30% and that bivalving the cast and cutting the underlying padding will further reduce the pressure by an additional 55%. Thus, by removing a cast and associated soft dressings it is possible to decrease compartment pressures by as much as 85%. Rorabeck[179] has stated that bivalving a long leg cast in a patient with a fracture of the tibial shaft and cutting underlying padding may reduce compartment pressures by as much as 50%. Bingold,[23] in an experimental model, made similar observations. Elevation of an extremity with incipient compartment syndrome is not recommended. It was noted both experimentally and clinically that elevation of the limb reduced the mean arterial pressure and therefore reduced blood flow to the compartment.[6, 140, 151] In addition, elevation reduces the arteriovenous gradient and hence increases the susceptibility of the limb to compartment syndrome by reducing oxygen perfusion to the muscles. An extremity with an incipient compartment syndrome should be positioned to be level with the heart to promote arterial inflow.

In an established compartment syndrome the patient has the clinical signs and symptoms of a compartment syndrome coexisting with elevation of intracompartment pressures. Rorabeck[179] identified the indications for surgical decompression for patients with established compartment syndromes. They include (1) clinical signs of an acute compartment syndrome with demonstrable motor or sensory loss; (2) elevated compartment pressures above 35 mm Hg, using either the slit or Wick catheter technique, or above 40 mm Hg, with the needle technique in a conscious or unconscious patient; and (3) interrupted arterial circulation to an extremity for more than 4 hours. Mubarak and Carroll[151] also recommended prophylactic fasciotomies, especially of the anterior compartment, for all elective tibial operations in children. The most common methods for decompression of all four compartments of the lower leg include (1) fibulectomy, (2) perifibular fasciotomy, and (3) double-incision fasciotomy.

Fibulectomy as a method of decompression has been popularized by Kelly and Whitesides.[111] It is particularly useful for a deep posterior compartment syndrome. However, it is usually contraindicated in children because of the risk for residual pseudoarthrosis of the fibula, which may result in fibular shortening due to asymmetric growth and a valgus deformity of the ankle as well as lateral tibial torsion.[93, 94, 226] This risk is especially great when fibulectomy is performed in children 10 years of age or less. Friedman and Jupiter[66] utilized either a fibulectomy, which leaves the periosteum intact, or multiple-incision fasciotomies for their pediatric patients who had fractures associated with vascular injuries. The former allowed re-formation of the fibula. They also performed fasciotomies only when clinically indicated. Hsu and associates[94] and Wiltse[226] recommended bone grafting for fibular pseudoarthrosis following partial fibulectomy. Perifibular fasciotomy, which was recommended by Matsen and associates,[141] has the advantage of allowing access to all four compartments through a single lateral incision. This technique is useful provided the anatomy of the extremity has not been distorted. The double-incision technique has been suggested by Mubarak and colleagues[153] and was studied extensively by Rorabeck and Bourne.[28, 179, 180] The procedure is easy to perform, and no structures are likely to be damaged, with the exception of the saphenous vein medially. This technique allows easy access to all four compartments.

Once the diagnosis of a compartment syndrome has been made, it is imperative that decompression be performed immediately. Rorabeck and MacNab[181] reported complete recovery when fasciotomies were performed for anterior compartment syndrome within 6 hours of the onset of symptoms. In 18 patients who underwent fasciotomies after 6 hours or more (mean, 18 hours) 14 had persistent weakness of dorsiflexion, complete foot drop was seen in three, and a below-knee amputation was required in one. A follow-up study of 18 patients with various acute compartment syndromes demonstrated that acceptable results could be obtained up to 24 hours following onset of symptoms.[180]

Fracture management following fasciotomies in children is controversial. In the adult, Rorabeck[179] recommends rigid stabilization with an external fixator, intramedullary nail, or compression plate. Mubarak and Carroll[151] recommended either internal or external fixation of pediatric tibial fractures associated with compartment syndromes to allow for easier management of the fasciotomy wounds. One of the major reasons for stabilization is that fasciotomies convert a closed fracture into an open fracture that, in most cases, must be left open and later closed secondarily. In a child this may not always be necessary. The decision regarding fracture stabilization must be made on the basis of associated injuries and fracture stability. If rigid stabilization is necessary, this involves predominantly the use of an external fixator. However, young children may, in certain cases, be managed by conservative techniques with a long leg posterior splint followed by a long leg plaster cast.

REFERENCES

1. Aadalen, R. J. Proximal tibial metaphyseal fractures in children. Minn Med 62:785–788, 1979.
2. Akbarnia, B.; Torg, J. S.; Kirkpatrick, J.; Sussman, S. Manifestations of the battered child syndrome. J Bone Joint Surg 56-A:1159–1166, 1974.
3. Alonso, J. E.; Horowitz, M. Use of the AO/ASIF external fixator in children. J Pediatr Orthop 7:594–600, 1987.
4. Anderson, M.; Messner, M. B.; Green, W. T. Distribution of lengths of the normal femur and tibia in children from one to eighteen years of age. J Bone Joint Surg 46-A:1197–1202, 1964.
5. Aronson, D. D.; Stewart, M. C.; Crissman, J. D. Experimental tibial fractures in rabbits simulating proximal tibial metaphyseal fractures in children. Clin Orthop 255:61–67, 1990.
6. Ashton, H. The effect of increased tissue pressure on blood flow. Clin Orthop 113:15–26, 1975.
7. Bach, A. W.; Hansen, S. T., Jr. Plates versus external fixation in severe open tibial fractures. Clin Orthop 241:89–94, 1989.
8. Bahnson, D. H.; Lovell, W. W. Genu valgum following fractures of the proximal tibial metaphysis in children. Orthop Trans 4:306, 1980.
9. Balthazar, D. A.; Pappas, A. M. Acquired valgus deformity of the tibia in children. J Pediatr Orthop 4:538–541, 1984.
10. Barfod, B.; Christensen, F. Fractures of the femoral shaft in children with special reference to subsequent overgrowth. Acta Chir Scand 116:235–250, 1959.
11. Bassey, L. O. The use of P.O.P. integrated pins as an improvisation on the Hoffmann's apparatus: Contribution to open fracture management in the tropics. J Trauma 29:59–64, 1989.
12. Bassey, L. O. Valgus deformity following proximal metaphyseal fractures in children: Experiences in the African tropics. J Trauma 30:102–107, 1990.
13. Behrens, F.; Searls, K. External fixation of the tibia. Basic concepts and prospective evaluation. J Bone Joint Surg 68-B:246–254, 1986.
14. Behrens, F. A primer of fixator devices and configurations. Clin Orthop 241:5–14, 1989.
15. Behrens, F. General theory and principles of external fixation. Clin Orthop 241:15–23, 1989.
16. Behrens, F. External fixation in children: Lower extremity. Instr Course Lect 39:205–208, 1990.
17. Behrens, F. Fractures with soft tissue injuries. In: Browner, B. D.; Jupiter, J. B.; Levine, A. M.; Trafton, P. G., eds. Skeletal Trauma. Philadelphia, W. B. Saunders, 1991.
18. Behrens, F.; Johnson, W. Unilateral external fixation: Methods to increase and reduce frame stiffness. Clin Orthop 241:48–56, 1989.
19. Ben-Itzhak, I.; Erken, E. H. W.; Malkin, C. Progressive valgus deformity after juxta-epiphyseal fractures of the upper tibia in children. Injury 18:169–173, 1987.
20. Bennek, J.; Steinert, V. Knochenwachstam nach Derform Verheilten Unterschenkelschaftfrakturen bei Kindern. Zentralbl Chir 91:633–639, 1966.
21. Berkebile, R. D. Stress fracture of the tibia in children. Am J Roentgenol 91:588–596, 1964.
22. Best, T. N. Valgus deformity after fracture of the upper tibia in children. J Bone Joint Surg 55-B:222, 1973.
23. Bingold, A. C. On splitting plasters. A useful analogy. J Bone Joint Surg 61-B:294–295, 1979.
24. Blatz, D. Bilateral femoral and tibial shaft fractures in a runner. Am J Sports Med 9:322–325, 1981.
25. Blount, W. P. Fractures in Children. Baltimore, Williams & Wilkins, 1955, pp. 183–194.
26. Bohn, W. W.; Durbin, R. A. Ipsilateral fractures of the femur and tibia in children and adolescents. J Bone Joint Surg 73-A:429–439, 1991.
27. Bondurant, F. J.; Cotler, H. B.; Buckle, R.; et al. The medical and economic impact of severely injured lower extremities. J Trauma 28:1270–1273, 1988.
28. Bourne, R. B.; Rorabeck, C. H. Compartment syndromes of the lower leg. Clin Orthop 240:97–104, 1988.
29. Boyer, R. S.; Jaffe, R. B.; Nixon, G. W.; Condon, V. R. Trampoline fractures of the proximal tibia in children. AJR 146:83–85, 1986.
30. Boytim, M. J.; Davidson, R. S.; Charney, E.; Melchionni, J. B. Neonatal fractures in myelomeningocele patients. J Pediatr Orthop 11:28–30, 1991.
31. Brougham, D. I.; Nicol, R. O. Valgus deformity after proximal tibial fractures in children. J Bone Joint Surg 69-B:482, 1987.
32. Brown, P. W.; Kinman, P. B. Gas gangrene in a metropolitan community. J Bone Joint Surg 56-A:1145–1451, 1974.
33. Buckley, S. L.; Smith, G.; Sponseller, P. D.; et al. Open fractures of the tibia in children. J Bone Joint Surg 72-A:1462–1469, 1990.
34. Burrows, H. J. Fatigue fractures of the fibula. J Bone Joint Surg 30-B:266–279, 1948.
35. Cates, T. R. Clostridium tetani (tetanus). In: Mandell, G. L.; Douglas, R. G., Jr.; Bennett, J. E., eds. Principles and Practice of Infectious Diseases. New York, Churchill Livingstone, 1990, pp. 1946–1982.
36. Cigola, F.; Rega, A. N.; Lotito, F. M. Growth disturbances following fractures of the femur and tibia in children. Ital J Orthop Traumatol 11:121–125, 1985.
37. Coates, R. Knock-knee deformity following upper tibial "greenstick" fractures. J Bone Joint Surg 59-B:516, 1977.
38. Cofer, J. B.; Burns, R. P.; Clements, J. B. Popliteal artery injury associated with tibial fracture in a five year old. J Tenn Med Assoc 79:430–432, 1986.
39. Cozen, L. Fracture of the proximal portion of the tibia in children followed by valgus deformity. Surg Gynecol Obstet 97:183–188, 1953.
40. Cozen, L. Knock knee deformity after fracture of the proximal tibia in children. Orthopedics 1:230, 1959.
41. Currarino, G.; Pickney, L. E. Genu valgum after proximal tibial fractures in children. AJR 136:915–918, 1981.
42. Currey, J. D. Changes in the impact energy absorption of bone with age. J Biomech 12:459–469, 1979.
43. Currey, J. D.; Butler, G. The mechanical properties of bone tissue in children. J Bone Joint Surg 57-A:810–814, 1975.
44. DalMonte, A.; Manes, E.; Cammarota, V. Post-traumatic genu valgum in children. Ital J Orthop Traumatol 11:5–11, 1985.
45. Dellinger, E. P.; Miller, S. D.; Wertz, M. J.; et al. Risk of infection after open fracture of the arm or leg. Arch Surg 123:1320–1327, 1987.
46. Dent, J. A.; Paterson, C. R. Fractures in early childhood:

Osteogenesis imperfecta or child abuse? J Pediatr Orthop 10:542–544, 1990.
47. Devas, M. B. Stress fractures in children. J Bone Joint Surg 45-B:528–541, 1963.
48. Devas, M. B.; Sweetnam, R. Stress fractures of the fibula. J Bone Joint Surg 38-B:818–829, 1956.
49. Dias, L. S. Ankle valgus in children with myelomeningocele. Dev Med Child Neurol 20:627–633, 1978.
50. Dias, L. S. Fractures of the tibia and fibula. In: Rockwood, C. A., Jr.; Wilkens, K. E.; King, R. E., eds. Fractures in Children. Philadelphia, J. B. Lippincott, 1984, pp. 983–1041.
51. Dickenson, R. P.; Hutton, W. C.; Stott, J. R. R. The mechanical properties of bone in osteoporosis. J Bone Joint Surg 63-B:233–238, 1981.
52. DiLeo, P.; Lispi, A.; Marciano, R. Growth disturbances following fractures of the femur and tibia in children. Ital J Orthop Traumatol 11:127–131, 1985.
53. Drennan, J. C.; Freehafer, A. A.: Fractures of the lower extremities in paraplegic children. Clin Orthop 77:211–217, 1971.
54. Drewes, J.; Schulte, H. D. Brüche im Bereich des Unterschenkels bei Kindern infolge von Fahrradspeichenverletzungen. Chirurg 36:464–468, 1965.
55. Dunbar, J. S.; Owen, H. F.; Nogrady, M. D.; McLesse, R. Obscure tibial fracture of infants—The toddler's fracture. J Can Assoc Radiol 25:136–144, 1964.
56. Ellis, H. Disabilities after tibial shaft fractures with special reference to Volkmann's ischemic contracture. J Bone Joint Surg 40-B:190–197, 1956.
57. Engh, C. A.; Robinson, R. A.; Milgram, J. Stress fractures in children. J Trauma 10:532–541, 1970.
58. Fabian, T. C.; Turkleson, M. L.; Connelly, T. L.; Stone, H. H. Injury to the popliteal artery. Am J Surg 143:225–228, 1982.
59. Fee, N. F.; Dobranski, A.; Bisla, R. S. Gas gangrene complicating open forearm fractures. J Bone Joint Surg 59-A:135–138, 1977.
60. Felman, A. H. Bicycle spoke fractures. J Pediatr 82:302–303, 1973.
61. Fielding, J. W.; Liebler, W. A.; Tambakis, A. The effect of a tibial-tubercle transplant in children on the growth of the upper tibial epiphysis. J Bone Joint Surg 42-A:1426–1434, 1960.
62. Filler, R. M.; Griscom, N. T.; Pappas, A. Post-traumatic crepitation falsely suggesting gas gangrene. N Engl J Med 278:758–761, 1968.
63. Freehafer, A. A.; Mast, W. A. Lower extremity fractures in patients with spinal-cord injury. J Bone Joint Surg 47-A:683–694, 1965.
64. Freehafer, A. A.; Anscheutz, R. H.; Shaffer, J. W. Fractures of the lower limbs in patients with myelomeningocele. Inter-Clin Information Bull 18:11–12, 1982.
65. Friberg, S. Remodeling after fractures healed with residual angulation. In: Houghton, G. R.; Thompson, G. H., eds. Problematic Musculoskeletal Injuries in Children. London, Butterworths, 1983, pp. 77–100.
66. Friedman, R. J.; Jupiter, J. B. Vascular injuries and closed extremity fractures in children. Clin Orthop 188:112–119, 1984.
67. Galleno, H.; Oppenheim, W. L. The battered child syndrome revisited. Clin Orthop 162:11–19, 1982.
68. Garfin, S. R.; Mubarak, S. J.; Evans, K. L.; et al. Quantification of intracompartmental pressures and volume under plaster casts. J Bone Joint Surg 63-A:449–453, 1981.
69. Gillies, C. L.; Hartung, W. Fracture of the tibia in spinal bifida vera. Radiology 31:621–623, 1938.
70. Goff, C. W. Surgical Treatment of Unequal Extremities. Springfield, IL, Charles C Thomas, 1960.
71. Golding, C. Museum pages. III: Spina bifida and epiphyseal displacement. J Bone Joint Surg 42-B:387–389, 1960.
72. Green, N. E. Tibia valga caused by asymmetrical overgrowth following a nondisplaced fracture of the proximal tibial metaphysis. J Pediatr Orthop 3:235–237, 1983.
73. Greiff, J.; Bergmann, F. Growth disturbance following fracture of the tibia in children. Acta Orthop Scand 51:315–320, 1980.
74. Griffiths, A. L. Fatigue fracture of the fibula in childhood. Arch Dis Child 27:552–557, 1952.
75. Gustilo, R. B. Principles of the management of open fractures. In: Gustilo, R. B., ed. Management of Open Fractures and their Complications. Philadelphia, W. B. Saunders, 1982.
76. Gustilo, R. B.; Mendoza, R. M.; Williams, D. N. Problems in the management of type III (severe) open fractures: A new classification of type III open fractures. J Trauma 24:742–746, 1984.
77. Gustilo, R. B.; Merkow, R. L.; Templeman, D. Current concepts review. The management of open fractures. J Bone Joint Surg 72-A:299–304, 1990.
78. Gyepes, M. T.; Newbern, D. H.; Neuhauser, E. B. D. Metaphyseal and physeal injuries in children with spina bifida and meningomyeloceles. Am J Roentgenol 95:168–177, 1965.
79. Haas, L. M.; Staple, T. W. Arterial injuries associated with fractures of the proximal tibia following blunt trauma. South Med J 62:1439–1448, 1969.
80. Hansen, B. A.; Greiff, J.; Bergmann, F. Fractures of the tibia in children. Acta Orthop Scand 47:448–453, 1976.
81. Hansen, S. T. Internal fixation of children's fractures of the lower extremities. Orthop Clin North Am 21:353–363, 1990.
82. Hartley, J. B. Fatigue fracture of the tibia. Br J Surg 30:9–14, 1942.
83. Herring, J. A.; Moseley, C. Post-traumatic valgus deformity of the tibia. Instructional case. J Pediatr Orthop 1:435–439, 1981.
84. Highland, T. R.; LaMont, R. L. Deep, late infections associated with internal fixation in children. J Pediatr Orthop 5:59–64, 1985.
85. Hill, S. A. Incidence of tibial fractures in child skiers. Br J Sports Med 23:169–170, 1989.
86. Hoaglund, F. T.; States, J. D. Factors influencing the rate of healing in tibial shaft fractures. Surg Gynecol Obstet 124:71–76, 1967.
87. Holderman, W. D. Results following conservative treatment of fractures of the tibial shaft. Am J Surg 98:593–597, 1959.
88. Hoover, N. W. Injuries of the popliteal artery associated with fractures and dislocation. Surg Clin North Am 41:1099–1112, 1961.
89. Horowitz, J. H.; Nichter, L. S.; Kenney, J. G.; Morgan, R. F. Lawnmower injuries in children: Lower extremity reconstruction. J Trauma 25:1138–1146, 1985.
90. Houghton, G. R.; Dekel, S. The periosteal control of long bone growth. Acta Orthop Scand 50:635–637, 1979.
91. Houghton, G. R.; Rooker, G. D. The role of the periosteum in the growth of long bones: An experimental study in the rabbit. J Bone Joint Surg 61-B:218–220, 1979.
92. Hresko, M. T.; Kasser, J. R. Physeal arrest about the knee associated with non-physeal fractures in the lower extremity. J Bone Joint Surg 71-A:698–703, 1989.

93. Hsu, L. C. S.; O'Brien, J. P.; Yau, A. C. M. C.; Hodgson, O. B. E. Valgus deformity of the ankle resulting from fibular resection for a graft in subtalar fusion in children. J Bone Joint Surg 54-A:585–594, 1972.
94. Hsu, L. C. S.; O'Brien, J. P.; Yau, A. C. M. C.; Hodgson, A. R. Valgus deformity of the ankle in children with fibular pseudarthrosis. J Bone Joint Surg 56-A:503–510, 1974.
95. Ingersoll, C. F. Ice skater's fracture. A form of fatigue fracture. Am J Roentgenol 50:469–479, 1943.
96. Ippolito, E.; Pentimalli, S. Post-traumatic valgus deformity of the knee in proximal tibial metaphyseal fractures in children. Ital J Orthop Traumatol 10:103–108, 1984.
97. Iwaya, T.; Kiyonori, H.; Yamada, A. Microvascular free flaps for the treatment of avulsion injuries of the feet in children. J Trauma 22:15–19, 1982.
98. Izant, R. J.; Rothman, B. F.; Frankel, V. Bicycle spoke injuries of the foot and ankle in children: An underestimated "minor" injury. J Pediatr Surg 4:654–656, 1969.
99. Jackson, D. W.; Cozen, L. Genu valgum as a complication of proximal tibial metaphyseal fractures in children. J Bone Joint Surg 53-A:1571–1578, 1971.
100. Jackson, J. P.; Waugh, W. The technique and complications of upper tibial osteotomy. J Bone Joint Surg 56-B:236–245, 1974.
101. Jakob, R. P.; Haertel, M.; Stüssi, E. Tibial torsion calculated by computerized tomography and compared to other methods of measurements. J Bone Joint Surg 62-B:238–242, 1980.
102. James, C. C. M. Fractures of the lower limbs in spina bifida cystica: A survey of 44 fractures in 122 children. Dev Med Child Neurol (Suppl) 22:88–93, 1970.
103. Johansen, K.; Bandyk, D.; Thiele, B.; et al. Temporary intraluminal shunts: Resolution of a management dilemma in complex vascular injuries. J Trauma 22:395–401, 1982.
104. Johansen, K.; Daines, M.; Howey, T.; et al. Objective criteria accurately predict amputation following lower extremity trauma. J Trauma 30:568–573, 1990.
105. Johnson, P. H. Beware: Greenstick fractures of the proximal tibial metaphysis. J Arkansas Med Soc 80:215–218, 1983.
106. Jones, E. T. Use of computed axial tomography in pediatric orthopaedics. J Pediatr Orthop 1:329–338, 1981.
107. Jordan, S. E.; Alonso, J. E.; Cook, F. F. The etiology of valgus angulation after metaphyseal fractures of the tibia in children. J Pediatr Orthop 7:450–457, 1987.
108. Karaharju, E. O.; Ryöppy, S. A.; Mäkinen, R. J. Remodeling by asymmetrical epiphyseal growth. J Bone Joint Surg 58-B:122–126, 1976.
109. Karlström, G.; Lönnerholm, T.; Olerud, S. Cavus deformity of the foot after fracture of the tibial shaft. J Bone Joint Surg 57-A:893–900, 1975.
110. Kärrholm, J.; Hansson, L. I.; Svensonn, K. Incidence of tibio-fibular shaft and ankle fractures in children. J Pediatr Orthop 2:386–396, 1982.
111. Kelly, R. P.; Whitesides, T. E., Jr. Transfibular route for fasciotomy of the leg. J Bone Joint Surg 49-A:1022–1023, 1967.
112. Kendra, J. C.; Price, C. T.; Songer, J. E.; Scott, D. S. Pediatric applications of dynamic axial external fixation. Contemp Orthop 19:477–486, 1989.
113. Kessel, L. Annotations on the etiology and treatment of tibia vara. J Bone Joint Surg 52-B:93–99, 1970.
114. Kestler, D. C. Unclassified premature cessation of epiphyseal growth about the knee joint. J Bone Joint Surg 29:788, 1947.
115. King, J.; Diefendorf, D.; Apthorp, J.; et al. Analysis of 429 fractures in 189 battered children. J Pediatr Orthop 8:585–589, 1988.
116. Kleinman, P. K.; Marks, S. C.; Blackbourne, B. The metaphyseal lesion in abused infants: A radiologic-histopathologic study. AJR 146:895–905, 1986.
117. Knight, D. J.; Bennet, G. C. Nonaccidental injury in osteogenesis imperfecta. A case report. J Pediatr Orthop 10:542–544, 1990.
118. Kogutt, M. S.; Swischuk, L. E.; Fagan, C. J. Patterns of injury and significance of uncommon fractures in the battered child syndrome. Radiology 121:143–149, 1974.
119. Komara, J. S.; Kottamasu, L.; Kottamasu, S. R. Acute plastic bowing fractures in children. Ann Emerg Med 15:585–588, 1986.
120. Kurz, W.; Vinz, H. Zur Epidemiologie und Klinik der geschlossenen diaphysaren Unterschenkelfraktur im Kindesalter. Zentralbl Chir 104:1402–1409, 1979.
121. Leach, R. E.; Hammond, G.; Stryker, W. S. Anterior tibial compartment syndrome. J Bone Joint Surg 49-A:451–462, 1967.
122. Lehner, V. A.; Dubas, J. Sekundäre Deformierungen nach Epiphysenlosungen und Epiphysenliniennahen Frakturen. Helv Chir Acta 21:388–410, 1954.
123. Lee, J. D.; Yao, L. Stress fractures: MR imaging. Radiology 169:217–220, 1988.
124. Leonidas, J. C. Skeletal trauma in the child abuse syndrome. Pediatr Ann 12:875–882, 1983.
125. Letts, M.; Vincent, N.; Gouw, G. The "floating knee" in children. J Bone Joint Surg 68-B:442–446, 1986.
126. Letts, R. M. Degloving injuries in children. J Pediatr Orthop 6:193–197, 1987.
127. Levine, A. M.; Drennan, J. C. Physiological bowing and tibia vara. The metaphyseal-diaphyseal angle in the measurement of bowleg deformities. J Bone Joint Surg 64-A:1158–1163, 1982.
128. Ligier, J. N.; Metaizeau, J. P.; Prévot, J.; Lascombes, P. Elastic stable intramedullary pinning of long bone shaft fractures in children. Z Kinderchir 40:209–212, 1985.
129. Lock, T. R.; Aronson, D. D. Fractures in patients who have myelomeningocele. J Bone Joint Surg 71-A:1153–1157, 1989.
130. Lodge, T. Bone, joint, and soft tissue changes following paraplegia. Acta Radiol 46:435–445, 1956.
131. Mabrey, J. D.; Fitch, R. D. Plastic deformation in pediatric fractures: Mechanism and treatment. J Pediatr Orthop 9:310–314, 1989.
132. MacEwen, G. D.; Zionts, L. E. Proximal tibial fracture in children. In: Uhthoff, H. K.; Wiley, J. J., eds. Behavior of the Growth Plate. New York, Raven Press 1988, pp. 141–152.
133. Mahnken, R. F.; Yngve, D. A. Valgus deformity following fracture of the tibial metaphysis. Orthopaedics 11:1320–1322, 1988.
134. Makin, M. Tibio-fibular relationship in paralysed limbs. J Bone Joint Surg 47-B:500–506, 1965.
135. Matejczyk, M. B.; Rang, M. Fractures in children with neuromuscular disorders. In: Houghton, G. R.; Thompson, G. H., eds. Problematic Musculoskeletal Injuries in Children. London, Butterworths, 1983, pp. 178–192.
136. Matin, P. The appearance of bone scans following fractures, including immediate and long-term studies. J Nucl Med 20:1227–1231, 1979.
137. Matsen, F. A., III. A practical approach to compartmental

syndromes. Part I. Definition, theory, and pathogenesis. Instr Course Lect 32:88–91, 1983.
138. Matsen, F. A., III; Clawson, D. K. The deep posterior compartmental syndrome of the leg. J Bone Joint Surg 57-A:34–39, 1975.
139. Matsen, F. A., III; Staheli, L. T. Neurovascular complications following tibial osteotomy in children. Clin Orthop 110:210–214, 1975.
140. Matsen, F. A., III; Krugmire, R. B., Jr.; King, R. V. Increased tissue pressure and its effects on muscle oxygenation in level and elevated human limbs. Clin Orthop 144:311–320, 1979.
141. Matsen, F. A., III; Winquist, R. A.; Krugmire, R. B. Diagnosis and management of compartmental syndromes. J Bone Joint Surg 62-A:286–291, 1980.
142. Maurer, D. J.; Merkow, R. L.; Gustilo, R. B. Infection after intramedullary nailing of severe open tibial fractures initially treated with external fixation. J Bone Joint Surg 71-A:835–838, 1989.
143. McIvor, W. C.; Samilson, R. L. Fractures in patients with cerebral palsy. J Bone Joint Surg 48-A:858–866, 1966.
144. Meland, N. B.; Fisher, J.; Irons, G. B.; et al. Experience with 80 rectus abdominis free-tissue transfers. Plast Reconstr Surg 83:481–487, 1989.
145. Mellick, L. B.; Reesor, K. Spiral tibial fractures of children: A commonly accidental spiral long bone fracture. Am J Emerg Med 8:234–237, 1990.
146. Mellick, L. B.; Reesor, K.; Demers, D.; Reinker, K. D. Tibial fractures in young children. Pediatr Emerg Care 4:97–101, 1988.
147. Meurman, K. O. A.; Elfving, S. Stress fracture in soldiers: A multifocal bone disorder. Radiology 134:483–487, 1980.
148. Micheli, L. J.; Gerbino, P. G. Etiologic assessment of stress fractures of the lower extremity in young athletes. Orthop Trans 4(1):51, 1980.
149. Morton, K. S.; Starr, D. E. Closure of the anterior portion of the upper tibial epiphysis as a complication of tibial-shaft fracture. J Bone Joint Surg 46-A:570–574, 1964.
150. Mubarak, S. J. A practical approach to compartmental syndromes. Part II. Diagnosis. Instr Course Lect 32:92–102, 1983.
151. Mubarak, S. J.; Carroll, N. C. Volkmann's contracture in children. Aetiology and prevention. J Bone Joint Surg 61-B:285–293, 1979.
152. Mubarak, S. J.; Hargens, A. R. Diagnosis and management of compartmental syndromes. In: American Academy of Orthopaedic Surgeons: Symposium on Trauma to the Leg and its Sequelae. St. Louis, C. V. Mosby, 1981.
153. Mubarak, S. J.; Owens, C. A.; Hargens, A. R.; et al. Acute compartment syndromes: Diagnosis and treatment with the aid of the Wick catheter. J Bone Joint Surg 60-A:1091–1095, 1978.
154. Mueller, M. E.; Allgower, M.; Schneider, R.; Willenegger, H. Manual of Internal Fixation, 2nd ed. New York, Springer Verlag, 1979.
155. Navarre, J. R.; Cardillo, P. J.; Gorman, J. F.; et al. Vascular trauma in children and adolescents. Am J Surg 143:229–231, 1982.
156. Ogden, J. A. Skeletal Injury in the Child. Philadelphia, W. B. Saunders, 1990, pp. 787–863.
157. O'Neill, J. A., Jr.; Meachan, W. F.; Griffin, P. P.; Sawyer, J. C. Patterns of injury in the battered child syndrome. J Trauma 13:332–339, 1973.
158. Oudjhane, K.; Newman, B.; Oh, K. S.; et al. Occult fractures in preschool children. J Trauma 28:858–860, 1988.
159. Paley, D.; Catagni, M. A.; Argnani, F.; et al. Ilizarov treatment of tibial nonunions with bone loss. Clin Orthop 241:146–165, 1989.
160. Pappas, A. M.; Filler, R. M.; Eraklis, A. J.; Bernhard, W. F. Clostridial infections (gas gangrene). Diagnosis and early treatment. Clin Orthop 76:177–184, 1971.
161. Pappas, A. M.; Anas, P.; Toczylowski, H. M., Jr. Asymmetrical arrest of the proximal tibial physis and genu recurvatum deformity. J Bone Joint Surg 66-A:575–581, 1984.
162. Park, H.-M.; Kernek, C. B.; Robb, J. A. Early scintigraphic findings of occult femoral and tibia fractures in infants. Clin Nucl Med 13:271–275, 1988.
163. Parsch, K.; Rossak, K. Die pathologischen Frakturen bei Spina Bifida. Arch Orthop Unfallchir 68:165–178, 1970.
164. Parrini, L.; Paleari, M.; Biggi, F. Growth disturbances following fractures of the femur and tibia in children. Ital J Orthop Traumatol 11:139–145, 1985.
165. Patzakis, M. J.; Wilkins, J. Factors influencing infection rate in open fracture wounds. Clin Orthop 243:36–40, 1989.
166. Pauwels, F. Grundriss einer Biomechanik der Fraktur Heilung. Verh Dtsch Orthop Ges 34:62–108, 1940.
167. Pollen, A. G.: Fractures and Dislocations in Children. Baltimore, Williams & Wilkins, 1973.
168. Potthoff, H. Ein Beitrag zur Behandlung der Proximalen metaphysären Tibiafraktur in Kindesalter. Aktuel Traumatol 12:127–128, 1982.
169. Prather, J. L.; Nusynowitz, M. L.; Snowdy, H. A.; et al. Scintigraphic findings in stress fractures. J Bone Joint Surg 59-A:869–874, 1977.
170. Ralis, Z. A.; Ralis, H. M.; Randall, M.; et al. Changes in shape, ossification, and quality of bone in children with spina bifida. Dev Med Child Neurol 18(Suppl. 37):29–41, 1976.
171. Rang, M. Children's Fractures. Philadelphia, J. B. Lippincott, 1974, pp. 189–197.
172. Reff, R. B. The use of external fixation devices in the management of severe lower extremity and pelvic injuries in children. Clin Orthop 188:21–33, 1984.
173. Reynolds, D. A. Growth changes in fractured long-bones. A study of 126 children. J Bone Joint Surg 63-B:83–88, 1981.
174. Robert, M.; Khouri, N.; Carlioz, H.; Alain, J. L. Fractures of the proximal tibial metaphysis in children: Review of a series of 25 cases. J Pediatr Orthop 7:444–449, 1987.
175. Roberts, S. M.; Vogt, E. C. Pseudofracture of the tibia. J Bone Joint Surg 21:891–901, 1939.
176. Robin, G. Fracture in childhood paraplegia. Paraplegia 3:165–170, 1966.
177. Rooker, G. D.; Coates, R. L. Deformity after greenstick fractures of the upper tibial metaphysis. In: Houghton, G. R.; Thompson, G. H., eds. Problematic Musculoskeletal Injuries in Children. London, Butterworths, 1983, pp. 1–13.
178. Rooker, G.; Salter, R. Prevention of valgus deformity following fracture of the proximal metaphysis of the tibia in children. J Bone Joint Surg 62-B:527, 1980.
179. Rorabeck, C. H. A practical approach to compartmental syndromes. Part III. Treatment. Instr Course Lect 32:102–113, 1983.
180. Rorabeck, C. H. The treatment of compartment syndromes of the leg. J Bone Joint Surg 66-B:93–97, 1984.
181. Rorabeck, C. H.; MacNab, I. Anterior tibial compartment syndrome complicating fractures of the shaft of the tibia. J Bone Joint Surg 58-A:549–550, 1976.

182. Roub, L. W.; Gumerman, L. W.; Hanley, E. N.; et al. Bone stress: A radionuclide imaging perspective. Radiology 132:431–438, 1979.
183. Russell, W. L.; Apyan, P. M.; Burns, R. P. Utilization and wide clinical implementation using the wick catheter for compartment pressure measurement. Surg Gynecol Obstet 160:207–210, 1985.
184. Russo, V. J. Traumatic arterial spasm resulting in gangrene. J Pediatr Orthop 5:486–488, 1985.
185. Salter, R. B.; Best, T. The pathogenesis and prevention of valgus deformity following fractures of the proximal metaphyseal region of the tibia in children. J Bone Joint Surg 55-A:1324, 1973.
186. Sarmiento, A.; Gersten, L. M.; Sobol, P. A.; et al. Tibial shaft fractures treated with functional braces. J Bone Joint Surg 71-B:602–609, 1989.
187. Savoca, C. J. Stress fractures. A classification of the earliest radiographic signs. Radiology 100:519–524, 1971.
188. Sawmiller, S.; Michener, W. M.; Hartman, J. T. Stress fracture in childhood. Cleve Clin Q 32:119–123, 1965.
189. Schrock, R. D. Peroneal nerve palsy following derotation osteotomies for tibial torsion. Clin Orthop 62:172–177, 1969.
190. Shaker, I. J.; White, J. J.; Signer, R. D.; et al. Special problems of vascular injuries in children. J Trauma 16:863–867, 1976.
191. Shannak, A. O. Tibial fractures in children: Follow-up study. J Pediatr Orthop 8:306–310, 1988.
192. Singer, J.; Towbin, R. Occult fractures in the production of gait disturbance in childhood. Pediatrics 64:192–196, 1979.
193. Skak, S. V.; Toftgard, T.; Torben, D. P. Fractures of the proximal metaphysis of the tibia in children. Injury 18:149–156, 1987.
194. Smillie, I. S. Injuries of the Knee Joint, 2nd ed. Baltimore, Williams & Wilkins, 1951.
195. Soutter, F. E. Spina bifida and epiphyseal displacement. J Bone Joint Surg 44-B:106–109, 1962.
196. Spiegal, P. G.; Mast, J. W. Internal and external fixation of fractures in children. Orthop Clin North Am 11:405–421, 1980.
197. Stanford, T. C.; Rodriguez, R. P.; Hayes, J. T. Tibial-shaft fractures in adults and children. JAMA 195:1111–1114, 1966.
198. Steel, H. H.; Sandrow, R. E.; Sullivan, P. D. Complications of tibial osteotomy in children for genu varum or valgum. J Bone Joint Surg 53-A:1629–1635, 1971.
199. Steinert, V. V.; Bennek, J. Unterschenkelfrakturen im Kindesalter. Zentralbl Chir 91:1387–1392, 1966.
200. Stern, M. B.; Grant, S. S.; Isaacson, A. S. Bilateral distal tibial and fibular epiphyseal separation associated with spina bifida. Clin Orthop 50:191–196, 1967.
201. Swaan, J. W.; Oppers, V. M. Crural fractures in children. Arch Chir Neerl 23:259–272, 1971.
202. Tauton, J. E.; Clement, D. B.; Webber, D. Lower extremity stress fractures in athletes. Physician Sports Med 9:77–86, 1981.
203. Taylor, S. L. Tibial overgrowth: A cause of genu valgum. J Bone Joint Surg 45-A:659, 1963.
204. Teitz, C. C.; Carter, D. R.; Frankel, V. H. The problems associated with tibial fractures with intact fibulae. J Bone Joint Surg 62-A:770–776, 1980.
205. Tenenbien, M.; Reed, M. H.; Black, G. B. The toddler's fracture revisited. Am J Emerg Med 8:208–211, 1990.
206. Thompson, G. H.; Wilber, J. H. Fracture management in the multiply injured child. In: Marcus, R. E., ed. Trauma in Children. Rockville, MD, Aspen Publishers, 1986, pp. 99–146.
207. Thompson, G. H.; Wilber, J. H.; Marcus, R. E. Internal fixation of fractures in children and adolescents. A comparative analysis. Clin Orthop 188:10–20, 1984.
208. Tolo, V. T. External skeletal fixation in children's fractures. J Pediatr Orthop 3:435–442, 1983.
209. Townsend, P. F.; Cowell, H. R.; Steg, N. L. Lower extremity fractures in children simulating infection in myelomeningocele. Clin Orthop 144:255–259, 1979.
210. Trotter, M.; Gleser, G. C. Estimation of stature from long bones of American whites and Negroes. Am J Phys Anthropol 10:463–514, 1952.
211. Tscherne, H.; Gotzen, L. Fractures with Soft Tissue Injuries. Berlin, Springer Verlag, 1984.
212. Tscherne, H.; Oestern, H. J. Die Klassifizierung des Weichteilschadens bei offenen und geschlossenen Frakturen. Unfallheilkunde 85:111–115, 1982.
213. Tupman, G. S. A study of bone growth in normal children and its relationship to skeletal maturation. J Bone Joint Surg 44-B:42–67, 1962.
214. Verhelst, M. P.; Spaas, F. M.; Fabry, G. Progressive valgus deformity of the knee after resection of an exostosis at the proximal medial tibial metaphysis. A case report. Acta Orthop Belg 41:689–694, 1975.
215. Verstreken, L.; Delronge, G.; Lamoureux, J. Orthopaedic treatment of paediatric multiple trauma patients. Int Surg 73:177–179, 1988.
216. Vinz, H. Die Behandlung offener Frakturen bei Kindern. Zentralbl Chir 105:1483–1493, 1980.
217. Vinz, H.; Kurz, W. Die offene diaphysäre Unterschenkefraktur im Kindesalter. Zentralbl Chir 105:32–38, 1980.
218. Visser, J. D.; Veldhuizen, A. G. Valgus deformity after fracture of the proximal tibial metaphysis in childhood. Acta Orthop Scand 53:663–667, 1982.
219. Voto, S. J.; Pigott, J.; Riley, P.; Donovan, D. Arterial injuries associated with lower extremity fractures. Orthopaedics 11:357–360, 1988.
220. Wagner, H. Pediatric Orthopaedic International Seminar, 1969.
221. Walton, J. N.; Warrick, C. K. Osseous changes in myopathy. Br J Radiol 27:1–15, 1954.
222. Weber, B. G. Fibrous interposition causing valgus deformity after fracture of the upper tibial metaphysis in children. J Bone Joint Surg 59-B:290–292, 1977.
223. Weber, B. G.; Brunner, C.; Freuler, F., eds. Treatment of Fractures in Children and Adolescents. Berlin, Springer Verlag, 1980.
224. Whitesides, T. E., Jr.; Haney, T. C.; Morimoto, K.; Harada, H. Tissue pressure measurements as a determinant for the need of fasciotomy. Clin Orthop 113:43–51, 1975.
225. Willhoite, D. R.; Moll, J. H. Early recognition and treatment of impending Volkmann's ischemia in the lower extremity. Arch Surg 100:11–16, 1970.
226. Wiltse, L. L. Valgus deformity of the ankle: A sequel to acquired or congenital abnormalities of the fibula. J Bone Joint Surg 54-A:595–606, 1972.
227. Wolma, F. J.; Larrieu, A. J.; Alsop, G. C. Arterial injuries of the legs associated with fractures and dislocations. Am J Surg 140:806–809, 1980.
228. Wood, D.; Hoffer, M. M. Tibial fractures in head-injured children. J Trauma 27:65–68, 1987.
229. Yasko, A.; Wilber, J. H. Open tibial fractures in children. Orthop Trans 13:547–548, 1989.

230. Yasko, A. W.; Thompson, G. H.; Wilber, J. H. Ipsilateral fractures of the femur and tibia in children. Presented at the Combined Meeting of Pediatric Orthopaedic Society of North America and the European Pediatric Orthopaedic Society. Montreal, Sept. 6–8, 1990.
231. Zionts, L. E.; MacEwen, G. D. Spontaneous improvement of post-traumatic tibia valga. J Bone Joint Surg 68-A:680–687, 1986.
232. Zionts, L.; Harcke, T. H.; Brooks, K. M.; MacEwen, G. D. Post-traumatic tibia valga: A case demonstrating asymmetric activity of the proximal growth plate on technetium bone scan. J Pediatr Orthop 7:458–462, 1987.

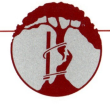

Alvin H. Crawford, M.D., F.A.C.S.

14

Fractures and Dislocations of the Foot and Ankle

*F*ractures and injuries about the foot and ankle in children are important. A pain-free and deformity-free foot and ankle following injury allows the child the freedom to run, play, explore the environment, and satisfy his or her unlimited personal curiosities. If there is a residual deformity following injury, the child limps. This causes agony for the parents, who feel, perhaps, that they did not do enough to prevent their child's angular deformity; the child is teased and taunted by peers or has an arthritic problem that causes pain and leads to unfulfilled wishes—whether it be simply walking across a meadow and smelling the flowers, or being a great athlete like Michael Jordan, "skying" above the towering giants of the National Basketball Association. My collected thoughts and those of my 85 referenced colleagues are intended to guide the reader to a safe resolution of foot and ankle injuries in children.

Relevant Anatomy

The ankle joint is a true mortise joint, or a modified hinge joint, consisting of three bones: the tibia, fibula, and talus. The joint essentially moves in only one plane from plantar flexion to dorsiflexion. The lateral malleolus allows minimal rotation to accommodate the changing width of the talar dome. The talar dome is broader anteriorly than posteriorly and, as a result, allows minimal rotation when the foot is in plantar flexion. The anatomic relationships and limited joint motion render the distal fibular epiphysis particularly vulnerable to crushing and twisting injuries (Fig. 14–1).

The ligaments about the ankle are attached to the epiphyses (Fig. 14–2). The deltoid ligament arises from the tip of the medial malleolus distal to the growth plate; it consists of two sets of fibers—superficial and deep. The superficial fibers are attached to the navicular bone, talus, and sustentaculum tali. The deep portion inserts into the medial surface of the talus. On the lateral side of the ankle, the support is provided by three separate ligaments. Their tension and spatial orientation change according to the position of the ankle joint: plantar flexion, neutral, or dorsiflexion. These ligaments have their origin in the fibula distal to the physis. The anterior talofibular ligament runs anteriorly and medially from the anterior margin of the lateral malleolus to the talus anteriorly. The posterior talofibular ligament runs horizontally from the sulcus on the back of the lateral malleolus to the posterior aspect of the talus. The calcaneofibular ligament extends downward and slightly posterior from the tip of the lateral malleolus to a tubercle on the lateral aspect of the calcaneus; it is in close relationship to the peroneal tendons and their sheath. The growth plate is more likely than the ligaments to fail during the years of skeletal development. The tibiofibular syndesmosis consists of four ligaments—the anterior and posterior inferior tibiofibular ligaments, the interosseous ligament, and the anterior transverse ligament—in addition to the interosseous membrane. The anterior tibiofibular ligament runs downward between the anterior margin of the tibia and

450 14 / Fractures and Dislocations of the Foot and Ankle

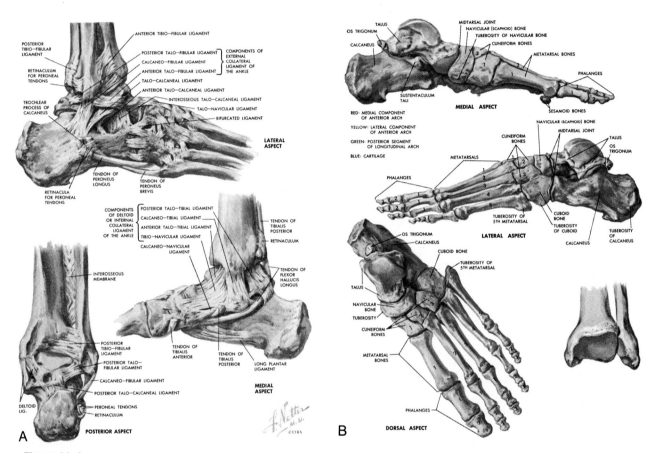

Figure 14–1

A–B, The anatomic bones of the foot and ankle; anteroposterior and lateral views, including ligaments. (From Clin Symp 17:1, 1965. Ciba-Geigy Corporation.)

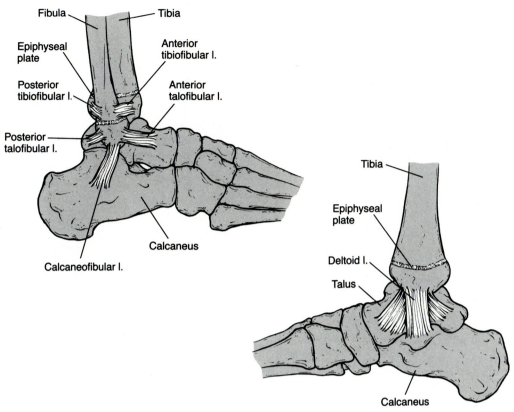

Figure 14-2

The ligaments of the foot. Medial and lateral views of ankle indicating ligamentous anatomy. (From McNealy G. A.; Rogers, L. F.; Hernandez, R.; Pozananski, A. K. Injuries of the distal tibial epiphysis: Systematic radiographic evaluation. AJR 138:683, 1982.)

fibula; its origin in the fibula is also distal to the growth plate.

The distal tibial physis begins its closure about 18 months prior to complete cessation of tibial growth, closing first in its midportion, then medially, and finally laterally. Longitudinal growth of the distal tibial epiphysis ceases at about age 12 years in girls and 13 years in boys.[36] The fusion process does not occur uniformly but rather is asymmetric (Fig. 14-3). Fusion begins in the area of the tibial "hump," which is located centrally, and is seen in the anteroposterior view as a small bump over the area of the medial edge of the talus. As fusion progresses, the medial part of the plate closes, then it progresses posteriorly, and finally, the anterolateral part of the plate fuses. The average period of fusion is 18 months. The fused part of the epiphyseal plate is no longer weak and prone to fracture but becomes an area of relative strength.[36] The irregular fusion pattern and the resulting areas of relative strength and weakness are responsible for the unusual fracture patterns, specifically the juvenile Tillaux and the triplane fracture.

Accessory ossicles of the malleoli are common in skeletally immature individuals. They usually appear between the ages of 7 and 10 years and eventually fuse with the secondary ossification center of the malleolus at skeletal maturity.[54] The lateral ossicle has been termed the os subfibulare. Most of these ossification variations are identified only fortuitously, when radiographs are taken to evaluate injury to the ankle or foot. They may be confused with a sleeve fracture avulsion of the medial or lateral malleolus. If the patient is symptomatic and the lesion is in question, a positive technetium bone scan may support a diagnosis of injury.[13]

Incidence and Mechanism of Injury

Injuries are commonly caused by indirect violence, with the fixed foot being forced into eversion-inversion, plantar flexion, external rotation, or dorsiflexion. Fractures also may be sustained by direct violence, the usual history being an automobile

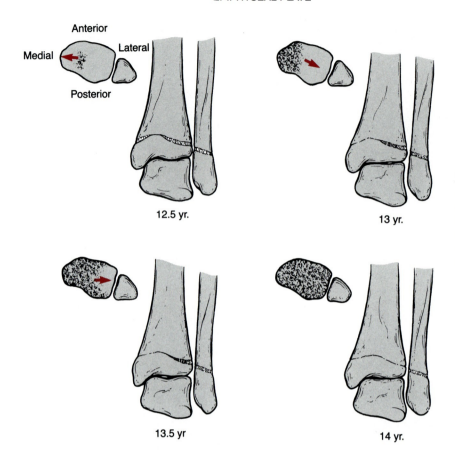

Figure 14–3
Average age of onset and normal fusion pattern in distal tibial epiphysis. (From McNealy, G. A.; Rogers, L. F.; Hernandez, R.; Pozananski, A. K. Injuries of the distal tibial epiphysis; Systematic radiographic evaluation. AJR 138:683, 1982.)

accident, a fall from a height, or participation in contact sports. Injuries to the lower leg and foot are more common in boys and usually occur between the ages of 10 and 15 years.[16, 33, 57, 70] Those about the ankle constitute 10 to 25% of all physeal injuries.[47] The distal tibial and fibular epiphyseal and physeal injuries account for 4% of all ankle injuries. Fractures of the distal tibia often involve the articular surface and the physis (growth plate). If left unreduced, these injuries can predispose to articular and growth deformities and eventually arthritis. The distal tibial epiphysis is the second most common site of epiphyseal fracture in children, after the distal end of the radius.[57] The bone of a child is more capable of elastic and plastic deformation than is adult bone.[62] Ligamentous injuries are rare because the ligaments are stronger than the physes. Adduction injuries are most common (15%) and also account for the highest rate of complications. The patterns of separation of the epiphyseal plate, when it is subjected to indirect trauma, are usually from avulsive or rotational forces applied to the fixed foot and leg, resulting in the transmission of shearing and sliding forces to the epiphyseal plate.

These forces are transmitted to the medial part of the tibia by the ligamentous pull of the deltoid ligaments. Laterally, forces are transmitted by the anterior and posterior tibiofibular ligaments, the anterior and posterior talofibular ligaments, and the calcaneofibular ligaments.[30] There is also a greater tendency for physeal compression during adduction injury. With an adduction injury, the medial migration of the talus is usually blocked by the medial malleolus, causing a fracture through the medial malleolus. Pronation injuries involve eversion and external rotation. Pronation injury results from an abduction force in 40% of the cases.[28] External rotation injuries are seen in 25% of leg and foot injuries.

Consequences of Injury

The prognosis for injuries to the foot and ankle involves several criteria. The skeletal maturity of the patient determines the resulting bone, ligament, or growth plate injury. At different skeletal ages, the same mechanical twisting, torsional force, or related trauma to the foot and leg will cause different injuries. Children are more prone to epiphyseal injuries, which, of course, are subject to more complications than shaft or metaphyseal injuries. The more severe the injury (e.g., compound, grossly contaminated, comminuted with or without soft tissue crushing), the greater the possibility of secondary devitalization with consequent delayed union, nonunion, pseudarthrosis, or osteomyelitis. The adequacy of reduction directly influences the rate of union; the more bony contact, the less healing time is required. All things considered, anatomic reduction is especially important for epiphyseal fractures, in which anatomic alignment will reduce the incidence of angular deformity and shortening secondary to growth arrest as well as degenerative arthritis secondary to persistent joint incongruity and instability. The prognosis following fractures involving the distal end of the tibia in children is dependent on the skeletal maturity of the patient, the severity of the injury, the fracture type, the degrees of comminution and displacement of the fracture, and the adequacy of reduction.[70]

Radiologic Evaluation

Anteroposterior and lateral views should always be taken of the injured area. If there is swelling and no injury can be seen, an oblique view is recommended. One should assess the soft tissue very carefully. The normal fat stripe surrounding a bone may be thickened following a nondisplaced fracture. Also, joint effusion following nondisplaced articular fractures may result in a positive fat pad, or synovial, sign; this is especially true of the anterior ankle over the talar neck or posterior ankle with displacement of the Achilles tendon fat stripe (Fig. 14–4). Computed tomography (CT) is recommended for articular fractures when plain films show displacement of greater than 2 mm. Polycycloidal tomography is still preferred for mapping out a physeal bar following premature growth arrest. Even though the C-arm image intensifier is excellent for achieving reductions in the operating room, I recommend permanent plain x-rays following reductions and prior to awakening the patient.

When following fractures about the ankle in children, it is extremely important to observe the Park-Harris growth arrest lines. The lines represent calcification of physeal cartilage during the injury repair. The lines will be parallel to the physis if growth is occurring normally (Fig. 14–5). If there has been physeal damage, the line may be tented or angular. Special attention to this phenomenon is indicated in the Salter-Harris III and IV injuries to the medial malleolus (Fig. 14–6).

Classification

In 1898, Poland, based on an anatomic study of amputation specimens, showed that pure separation of the epiphysis at the physis was rarer than sepa-

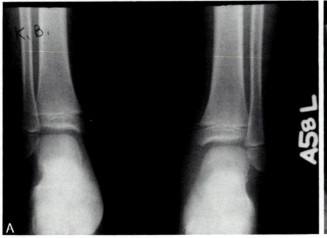
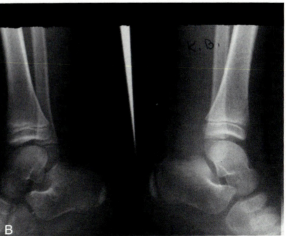

Figure 14–4

Radiographic evaluation of foot with notation to the fat stripe (soft tissue shadows). *A,* The right side is normal. Note the increase in soft tissue density adjacent to and below the medial malleolus on the left side. *B,* The left lateral ankle view (right side) shows an increase in the soft tissue posterior to the ankle joint. The soft tissue density is limited by the fat stripe just anterior to the Achilles tendon shadow.

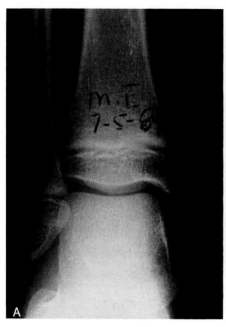
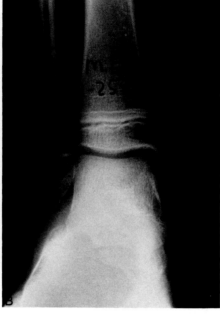

Figure 14–5

"Sprain" injury to ankle with subsequent development of Park-Harris lines. *A*, X-rays taken at the time of injury demonstrate soft tissue swelling below malleoli. *B*, Six months later there is a horizontal Park-Harris line just superior to the physis of both tibia and fibula. This is the Park-Harris growth arrest line. The line should always be horizontal and parallel to the physis when growth is normal.

ration of the epiphysis with a fracture of the metaphysis.[59] Ashhurst and Bromer in 1922 presented a classification of the mechanisms of fractures of the leg bones involving the ankle.[3]

In 1932, Bishop classified the physeal injuries of the ankle based on the Ashhurst-Bromer classification according to the direction of the force that produced the fracture: external rotation, abduction, adduction, axial compression, and direct injury.[5] Each mechanism was subdivided as followed: external rotation, first-, second-, and third-degree; abduction, first-, second-, and third-degree; and adduction, first-, second-, and third-degree. This classification was confusing and often inaccurate, and as a result, it is rarely used today.

Aitken in 1936 classified fractures of the physeal cartilage into three distinct types according to the relationship of the fracture line to the various zones of the physis.[1]

Lauge-Hansen, in 1950, through a series of experimental studies and clinical observations, proposed a new classification for ankle fractures in adults.[37] According to his study, three elements are important in ankle injury: axial load, position of the foot at the moment of trauma, and direction of abnormal forces.

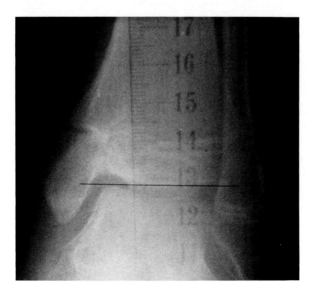

Figure 14–6

Scanogram of left ankle taken 1 year following a Salter-Harris IV fracture of the medial malleolus illustrating a physeal bar. The physis is obliterated just above the medial corner of the mortise, and trabeculae can be seen connecting the epiphysis to the metaphysis. The Park-Harris growth arrest line can be seen lateral to the bony bar and is angulated, indicating an arrest on the medial side.

In 1955, Carothers and Crenshaw added the plantar flexion mechanism to the classification of Bishop.[10] This system describes five mechanisms of injury: plantar flexion, external rotation, abduction, adduction, and direct injury/axial compression. They described six cases in which no fracture of the fibula accompanied the posterior displacement of the entire tibial physis.

Salter and Harris in 1963 classified the physeal injury into five types.[65] Ogden classified physeal injuries into seven types with subgroupings.[53] Although more anatomically inclusive, the Ogden classification has not gained widespread use; the Salter-Harris classification is the most generally accepted and widely used.

In 1978, Dias and Tachdjian introduced a new classification using the Lauge-Hansen concepts for children's fractures.[16] In order to classify the fracture properly, x-rays are necessary; anteroposterior (AP), lateral, and oblique views must be taken, and tomograms may also be necessary. In their classification (Table 14–1), the first term describes the position of the foot at the moment of trauma, and the second term notes the abnormal force applied to the ankle joint: i.e., (1) supination-inversion (SI); (2) pronation–eversion–external rotation (PEER); (3) supination–plantar flexion (SPL); (4) supination–external rotation (SER) (Fig. 14–7).

Spiegel and co-workers (Fig. 14–8) followed 184 of a series of 237 fractures of the distal end of the tibia or fibula, or both, for an average of 28 months after injury.[70] Using the Salter-Harris classification, three groups were identified according to the risk of developing shortening of the leg, angular deformity of the bone, or incongruity of the joint. The low-risk group consisted of 89 patients, 6.7% of whom had complications; this group included all type I and type II fibular fractures, all type I tibial fractures, type III and type IV tibial fractures with less than 2 mm of displacement, and epiphyseal avulsion injuries. The high-risk group consisted of 28 patients, 32% of whom had complications; this group included type III and type IV tibial fractures with 2 mm or more of displacement, juvenile Tillaux fractures, triplane fractures, and comminuted tibial epiphyseal fractures (type V). The unpredictable group was made up of 66 patients, 16.7% of them with complications; only type II tibial fractures were included. The incidence and types of complications were correlated with the type of fracture (Salter-Harris classification), the severity of displacement or comminution, and the adequacy of reduction.[70]

In this chapter the Salter-Harris classification will be used to describe the injuries to the growth plates. X-rays must be studied carefully to determine the type of Salter-Harris physeal injury and the direction of displacement of the epiphyseal-metaphyseal fracture fragments in relation to localized swelling and tenderness. Various published studies noting the importance of the mechanism of injury will be cited. Unfortunately, my clinical experience has been that the child is seldom able to recall the exact position of the foot and leg at the time of injury (Fig. 14–9).

Salter-Harris Fractures of the Distal Tibia

TYPE I FRACTURE

The type I injury is rare and is most often noted in neurologically impaired children or those subjected to child abuse. Most of the type I injuries are diagnosed as an ankle sprain or strain on the initial x-rays because no definite fracture can be identified.

Physical Examination. As the patient presents with pain and swelling around the ankle, there is very little detectable deformity, if any. An adequate range of motion of the ankle is usually possible but may be limited by pain.

Radiographic Examination. The radiographs may show some displacement of the tibial epiphysis on the metaphysis or may show only a mild widening of the tibial physis (Fig. 14–10). No special studies are required for this injury, as the diagnosis appears to be fairly straightforward.

Management. The child often has been treated initially with an Ace bandage for a sprain but returns in 2 or 3 days complaining of continued pain and swelling. X-rays then reveal a widening of the growth plate and an increase in density of the metaphyseal border. The child is treated for 4 weeks with a below-knee walking cast. The patient is relieved of pain, and the growth plate is restored to its normal thickness. The fibula may also be involved. I recommend follow-up in 6 months to rule out growth arrest of the distal tibia.

Three cases of rotational displacement of the lower tibial epiphysis due to trauma have been reported. The injury is a Salter-Harris I fracture to the distal tibia. This is a rare injury to the distal tibial growth plate whereby there is true rotational displacement of the distal tibial epiphysis with posterior displacement of the fibula but without fracture of the fibula.[6, 41, 52] The fibula in these cases appears

Table 14–1
Classification of Physeal Injuries of the Ankle in Children (Modified from Lauge-Hansen)

Type	Grade	Position of Foot	Injuring Force	Pattern of Fracture	Comment
Supination-inversion	1	Supinated	Inversion	Usually Salter-Harris I or II fracture-separation of distal fibular physis Occasionally rupture of lateral ligament or fracture of tip of lateral malleolus	Displacement minimal and almost always medial
	2	Supinated	Inversion	Usually Salter-Harris III or IV of medial part of tibial epiphysis Rarely Salter-Harris I or II with medial displacement of entire tibial epiphysis	Caution! Asymmetric growth arrest causes varus ankle
Supination–plantar flexion	1	Supinated	Plantar flexion	Commonly Salter-Harris II of tibial epiphysis Rarely Salter-Harris I of tibial physis No associated fracture of fibula Metaphyseal fragment and displacement posterior Fracture line best seen in lateral x-ray	Prognosis good Caution! Do not damage growth plate by forced manipulation. Posterior displacement will remodel
Supination–lateral rotation	1	Supinated	Lateral rotation	Salter-Harris II of distal tibial epiphysis with long spiral fracture of distal tibia starting laterally at distal tibial growth plate	Distinguishing feature is direction of fracture line starting laterally and running medially and proximally
	2	Supinated	Lateral rotation	Grade I plus spiral fracture of distal fibular shaft	—
Pronation–eversion–lateral rotation	1	Pronated	Eversion–lateral rotation	Salter-Harris II of distal tibial epiphysis Metaphyseal fragment lateral or posterolateral Displacement lateral or posterolateral Fibular fracture short, oblique, 4 to 7 cm from tip of lateral malleolus	
Miscellaneous					
Adolescent Tillaux	—	? Neutral?	Lateral rotation	Salter-Harris III of lateral part of distal tibial epiphysis Should not be any metaphyseal fragment Displacement anterolateral	Medial part of distal tibial physis closed
Triplane three-fragment	—	?	Lateral rotation	Fracture in three planes—coronal, sagittal, and transverse Combination of Salter-Harris II and III Fracture produces three fragments	Medial part of distal tibial physis open
Triplane two-fragment	—	?	Lateral rotation	Fracture in three planes—coronal, sagittal, and transverse Combination of Salter-Harris II and III Fracture creates two fragments	Medial part of distal tibial physis usually closed
Comminuted fracture of distal end of tibia	—	?	Crushing injuries Direct violence	Comminuted fracture involving distal tibial epiphysis Physis often damaged Fibular fracture at various levels	Poor prognosis

From Tachdjian, M.O. Pediatric Orthopedics, 2nd ed. Philadelphia, W. B. Saunders, 1990.

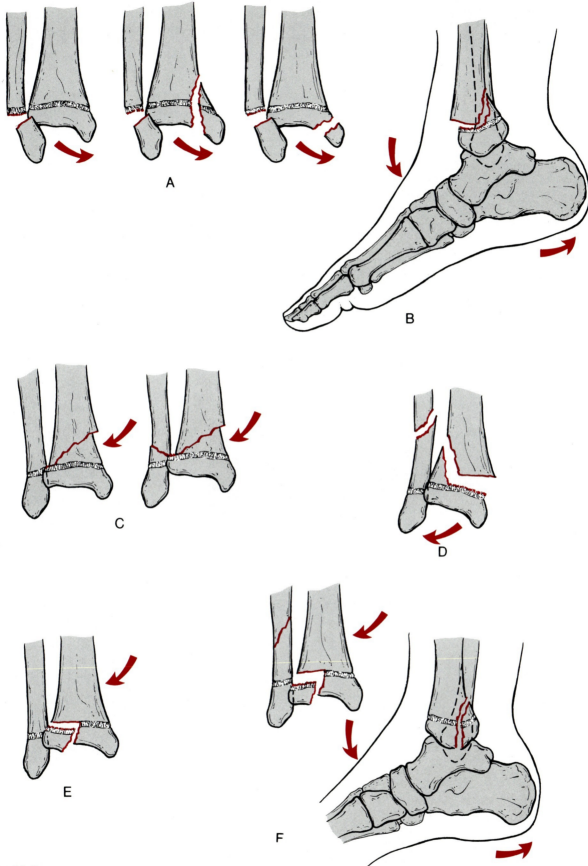

Figure 14–7

A, Supination-inversion. B, Supination–plantar flexion. C, Supination–external rotation. D, Pronation-eversion. E, Salter-Harris III, distal tibial epiphysis. F, Triplane fracture. (From Dias, L. S.; Tachdjian, M. O. Physeal injuries of the ankle in children: Classification. Clin Orthop 136:230, 1978.)

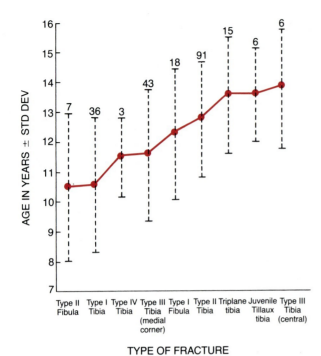

Figure 14–8

Type of fracture based on age (age vs. type of fracture). (From Spiegel, P. G.; Cooperman, D. R.; Laros G. S. Epiphyseal fractures of the distal ends of the tibia and fibula. J Bone Joint Surg 60-A:8, 1978.)

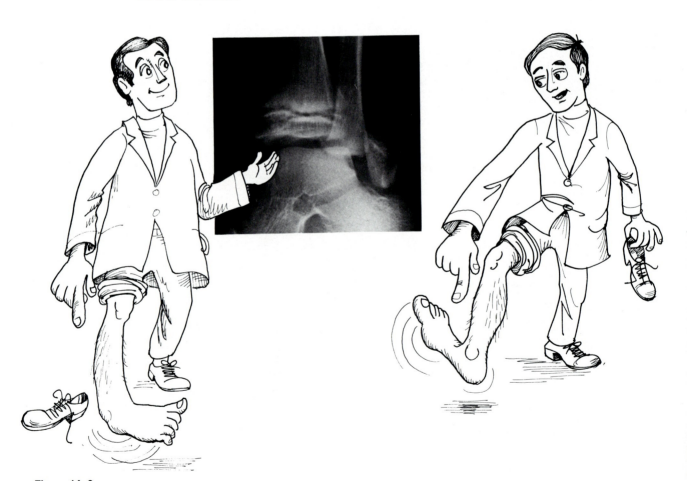

Figure 14–9

One surgeon demonstrating to another the mechanism of an ankle injury. (From Rang, M. Children's Fractures. Philadelphia, J. B. Lippincott, 1974.)

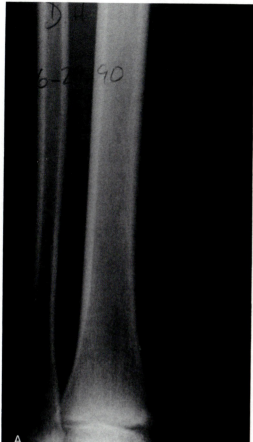
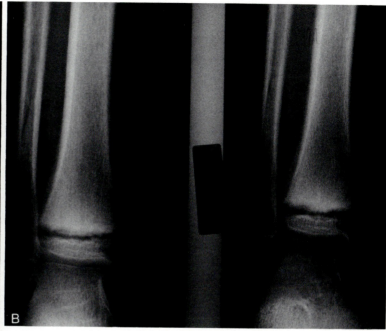

Figure 14–10

Salter-Harris I fracture of the distal tibia and fibula. *A*, The initial x-ray shows only soft tissue injury; there is no evidence of fracture. *B*, Follow-up x-ray 2 months later show widening of the physis as well as some deposition of bone or early callus in the interosseous space. The ankle was asymptomatic.

to be plastic enough to twist without breaking. The reduction is achieved with an audible click, probably caused by the fibula snapping back into the metaphyseal portion of the incisura fibularis, having retained its normal relationship and attachments to the displaced tibial epiphysis. No permanent damage to the growth plate was noted with these injuries.

TYPE II FRACTURE

The type II injury is the most common injury. It is usually caused by a fixed supination and external rotation force. The fibula is often fractured with it. The ankle is swollen and painful, and there is obvious deformity of the ankle. The circulation and motor-sensory nerve function are documented, and x-rays are obtained.

Radiographic Evaluation. The metaphyseal spike Thurston-Holland sign is usually seen on the distal medial tibia; however, the metaphyseal fragment may pull off the lateral side (Fig. 14–11). The fibula may or may not be injured.

Management. A closed reduction is usually easily performed if relaxation is achieved. The majority of these reductions can be achieved under fentanyl analgesia and a muscle relaxant. The distal fragment may be rotated, and the rotatory displacement is not appreciated on x-ray. An oblique x-ray view will usually identify any displacement of the distal fragment. Unlike the shoulder or hip joint, the ankle is a single-action hinge joint. Malalignment in the plane of motion of the ankle joint will correct spontaneously in the young. Most important is the fact that neither rotation nor varus or valgus malalignment will correct spontaneously. Reduction usually can be achieved by closed methods; however, it may be necessary to perform an open reduction in some cases. An above-knee cast with 30 degree knee flexion is indicated for immobilization. The cast is changed at 2 weeks, and a below-knee walking cast is applied. Because malalignment in the plane of motion will correct spontaneously, it is far better to accept a less than perfect reduction than to risk physeal damage by delayed or repeated manipulation.

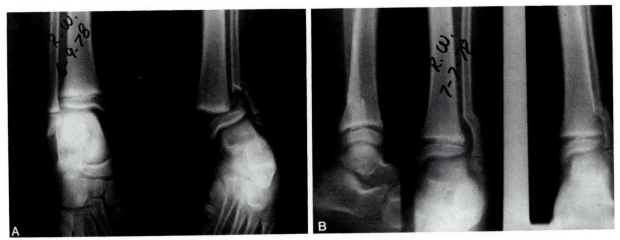

Figure 14–11

Salter-Harris II fracture of the distal tibia with fibular shaft fracture. *A,* This Salter-Harris II fracture is an abduction injury. The Thurston-Holland fragment sign from the distal tibia is on the lateral side. *B,* Following the reduction, the injury healed with no difficulty.

TYPE III FRACTURE

Salter-Harris III and IV injuries of the medial malleolus are somewhat unusual.[17] These injuries are usually the result of a supination-inversion force to the ankle. After separation of the distal fibular epiphysis, the inversion-adduction force of the talus striking the medial malleolus will produce either of these two fracture patterns. The child presents complaining of pain and swelling over the medial aspect of the ankle. The fibula may be involved and may also be painful. The injury occurs most often in children under 10 years of age or before the growth plate begins to close.

Radiographic Evaluation. Type III injuries are less common to the medial malleolus, but do show the fracture to involve less than one-third the medial-lateral distance across the epiphysis. The fracture line extends vertically to the physis and exits medially through the physis (Fig. 14–12).

Management. Closed reduction can usually be achieved under fentanyl anesthesia with good muscle relaxation. Failure to reduce the interfragmentary gap to less than 2 mm has been associated with growth arrest and angular deformity.[33] An anatomic reduction is required, followed by application of an above-knee cast with 30 to 40 degrees of knee flexion. I recommend reduction under general an-

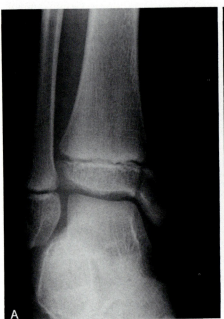
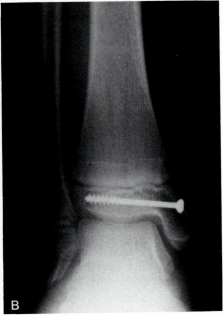

Figure 14–12

Salter-Harris III fracture treated by percutaneous interfragmentary screw. *A,* This was an adduction injury with the fracture occurring just above the superomedial aspect of the talar dome. The fracture line of the epiphysis ends at the physis. *B,* The injury was treated by closed reduction and a percutaneous interfragmentary screw. Note the horizontal Park-Harris line, indicating normal growth following treatment. The screw should never obliquely cross an open growth plate.

esthesia if the displacement of the subchondral surface is greater than 3 mm. The greater muscle relaxation obtained under general anesthesia should enable a more anatomically correct reduction. Determining the precise extent of displacement in these fractures is crucial, for a significant gap may lead to arrest growth. As the fracture unites, the ossification process above and below the physis may span the growth plate, forming a bony bridge anchored in the metaphyseal and epiphyseal calluses. The width and, in turn, the strength of that bridge depend on the size of the residual interfragmentary gap. A thin, weak bridge may have no adverse effect on growth, disruption of which requires substantial force.[17]

Open reduction under general anesthesia is performed if there is greater than 2 mm displacement *following reduction*. Because of the potential instability following reduction, internal fixation is advisable. I recommend a cannulated 3.5-mm interfragmentary screw or percutaneous threaded Steinmann pins.

The interfragmentary screw, which can be inserted quite neatly when cannulated, allows excellent control and can be inserted percutaneously if closed reduction within 2 mm is achieved. The problem with the interfragmentary screw is that often, when one attempts to remove the screw, it has been overgrown with healing callus. I feel that it is quite acceptable to leave the screw in. Percutaneous pinning is less traumatic, operative exposure with potential vascular compromise and infection is avoided, and the reduction is adequately stabilized. Another advantage of the percutaneous Steinmann pin is that it can be removed in 3 to 4 weeks at the time of cast change.

TYPE IV FRACTURE

Using general anesthesia and image-intensification control, an open reduction is carried out in the operating room. One should make an effort to insert the transfixion implant from the epiphysis to the epiphysis or the metaphysis to the metaphysis. Every effort should be made to avoid placing the screw from the epiphysis across the physis into the metaphysis unless the physis is closing. Physeal arrest may occur following oblique cross-physeal pinning, as is performed for adult fractures. An above-knee, non–weight bearing cast is used for 3 weeks, followed by weight bearing for 3 weeks. I recommend removal of the fixation implant at 1 year. If the screw is not removed within 1 to 1 1/2 years, exuberant callus may overgrow it. Removing it would then subject the extremity to more trauma than simply leaving the pin in place.

Following anatomic reduction of type IV injuries (Fig. 14–13), one should place transverse epiphysis-

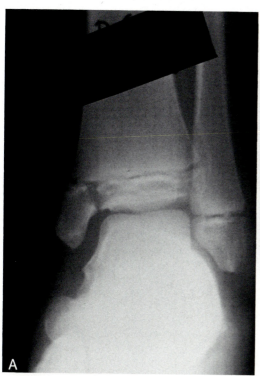
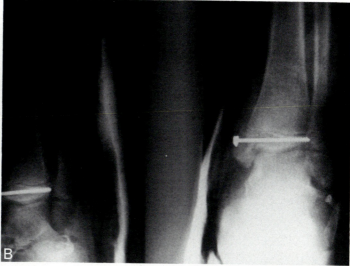

Figure 14–13

Salter-Harris IV fracture treated by open reduction and interfragmentary screw fixation. *A*, Initial x-ray shows the vertical fracture through the epiphysis with a small metaphyseal fragment. There is increased soft tissue density. *B*, X-ray in plaster showing anatomic reduction and screw placement.

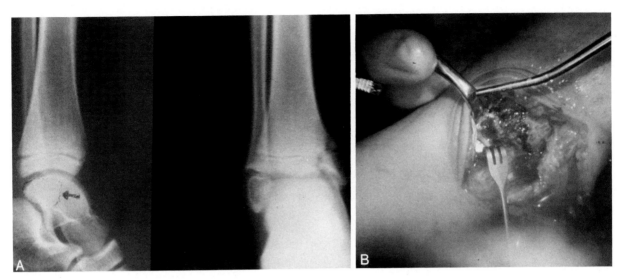

Figure 14–14

This Salter-Harris IV fracture required open reduction and anatomic repair. *A*, This is a Salter-Harris IV fracture of the tibia with the vertical component extending through the epiphysis and obliquely through the metaphysis. There is a Salter-Harris I fracture of the lateral malleolus. *B*, Note the articular surface of the talus, the bony epiphysis, and the physeal line on the operative photograph. The metaphyseal fragment should be discarded if it prevents anatomic reduction.

to-epiphysis or metaphysis-to-metaphysis Steinmann pins or cannulated 3.5 mm or 4 mm screws. Because the metaphyseal fragment is often warped or fragmented, it may be necessary to discard it in order to ensure anatomic reduction of the epiphysis. Removing the fragment also prevents the formation of a bony bridge (Fig. 14–14). Following reduction, an above-knee, nonwalking cast is applied for 3 weeks, followed by an above-knee walking cast for 3 weeks.

If a percutaneous Steinmann pin is used, it should be removed at the changing of the cast. If interfragmentary screw fixation has been used, the screw may be removed at or about 1 year following treatment. I have no experience with the use of bioabsorbable implants for the management of these fractures. Closed reduction of this injury is associated with successful results if anatomic reduction is achieved (Fig. 14–15) and maintained.

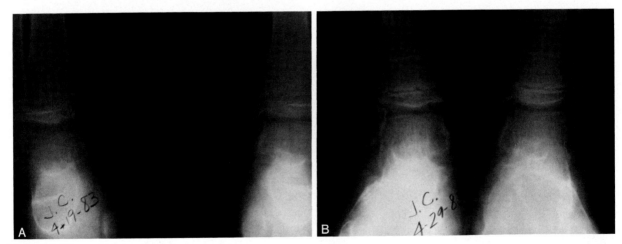

Figure 14–15

Salter-Harris III fracture of the right ankle and Salter-Harris IV fracture of the left ankle treated by closed reduction and followed for 1 year. *A*, Initial x-rays showing less than 2 mm displacement of either fracture. The positions were accepted, and bilateral fiberglass casts were applied. *B*, X-rays 1 year later show both fractures to be healed. The horizontal Park-Harris lines show that no physeal bar developed.

TYPE V FRACTURES

These injuries are extremely rare. They appear to result from axial compression. The Salter-Harris type V injury supposedly causes partial or complete physeal arrest by virtue of a crush injury to the germinal cells of all or a portion of the physis. In such an injury, there is no obvious fracture of the epiphysis or metaphysis, and the initial x-ray may show no evidence of injury. The diagnosis of a type V injury is therefore a retrospective one, made only after premature closure has been established in a growth plate previously considered uninjured. There is believed to be unrecognized damage to physeal cells either directly or secondary to injury to the blood supply of the germinal cell layer of the physis. Controversy surrounds the contribution of premature closure of the growth plate to crush injury of the germinal cell layers alone.

Two cases of tibial fracture have been reported in which both patients had symmetric premature closure of the entire proximal tibial physis, causing a leg length discrepancy without any angular deformity.[56] A compression injury to the entire physis would be unlikely unless a uniform longitudinal force were the mechanism of injury, as in a fall from a height. However, the clinical history and the configuration of the associated fractures were not consistent with a purely longitudinal force in their cases. Peterson and Burkhart considered the assumption that premature closure of the growth plate due to compression at the time of the accident is speculative. Furthermore, the two cases cited by Salter and Harris[65] did not show a normal radiographic appearance at the time of injury and, therefore, could have been another type. They further concluded that all cases of type V injuries reported in the literature involved the knee. Upon review of the literature they concluded that the common factor in all these conditions, including the trauma cases, seemed to be prolonged immobilization. Thus, the intriguing possibility is that posttraumatic physeal fusions are not always due to direct damage to the growth plate at the time of injury, but rather to factors associated with the immobilization.

Peterson and Burkhart considered symmetric premature closure of the physis following trauma and found that, when treated by immobilization, premature closure is more likely to be due to ischemia secondary to immobilization rather than to physeal compression.[56] Furthermore, the type V classification may unwittingly be stifling investigation into equally plausible mechanisms of premature growth arrest. Bone scan at the time of injury has been proposed as an investigative modality to aid and confirm a crush injury.[80] I have not encountered this injury. The most severe compression injury in my experience resulted in an angular deformity (Fig. 14–16).

TYPE VI FRACTURE

Ablation of the perichondrial ring has been categorized as a type VI injury. Avulsion or compression injury to the lateral side of the physis is rarely seen. Lawn mower and degloving injuries, as occurs when the leg is dragged across concrete or pavement, may remove the perichondrial ring. The ensuing callus may cause the development of a bridge between the metaphysis and epiphysis as described by Kessel.[60] I have not encountered this fracture about the ankle.

Juvenile Fracture of Tillaux

The juvenile fracture of Tillaux is an isolated fracture of the lateral portion of the distal tibial epiphysis. It usually occurs early in the second decade, when the medial half of the distal growth plate is closed and the lateral portion remains open. This fracture is usually the result of an external rotation force. When displacement of the fragment is minimal, the vertical and horizontal fracture lines may be difficult to visualize. It is a Salter-Harris type III epiphyseal fracture. The pattern of the injury is thought to result from the closure sequence of the distal tibial physis.[32]

The distal physis of the tibia closes first on its medial half at the age of 13 or 14 years; the lateral part closes at 14 1/2 to 16 years. Closure of the distal tibial physis occurs first in the middle, then the medial, and finally the lateral physis. Because the lateral physis is still open, the fracture crosses through it. The fracture line extends from the articular surface proximally, transversing the epiphysis, and then continuing along the physis laterally; it is equivalent to the Tillaux lesion in the adult. There may be local tenderness and swelling over the anterolateral distal tibial epiphysis.

A variably sized portion of the anterolateral bony epiphysis is pulled off by the anterior tibiofibular ligament when the foot is forcibly externally rotated; it is a variation of a supination–external rotation mechanism. If the fragment is large enough, a residual deformity in the joint surface may lead to an increased risk of osteoarthritis. The importance of preventing this problem in an adolescent cannot be overstated.[12]

Management. The reduction may be performed

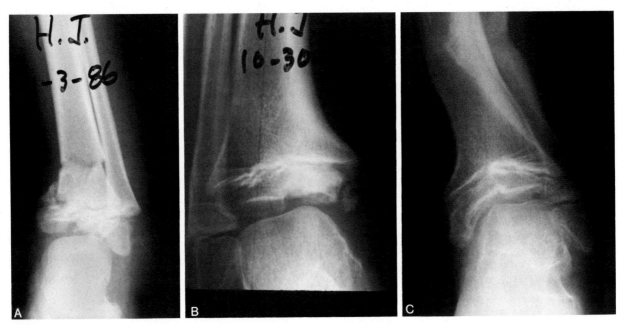

Figure 14–16

Axial compression injury with multiple fractures around the metaphyseal-physeal-epiphyseal juncture that resulted in angular deformity treated by osteotomy. *A,* Initial x-ray shows soft tissue swelling and markedly comminuted tibial epiphyseal fracture. The fibular epiphysis is medially displaced. *B,* Nine months later there is a dense bone scar over the medial physis with angulation of the lateral Park-Harris line; the ankle is in varus. Note the horizontal Park-Harris line of the fibula. *C,* A valgus overcorrection osteotomy was performed and resulted in good clinical alignment. Note the medial bone scar and the multiple Park-Harris lines over the lateral tibial metaphysis. The deformity subsequently recurred.

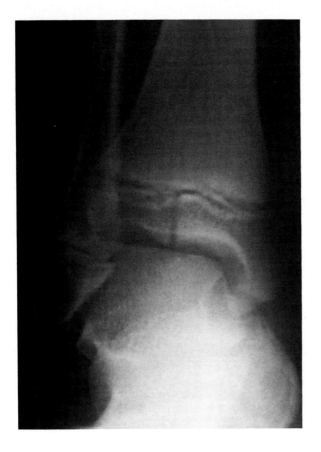

Figure 14–17

This nondisplaced Salter-Harris III fracture was treated by cast immobilization with an uneventful outcome.

under analgesia and muscle relaxant if done within the first 24 hours. The reduction usually is achieved by gentle internal rotation of the foot. An above-knee cast is applied for 3 weeks, followed by a below-knee walking cast for 3 weeks (Fig. 14–17). If the gap following reduction appears to be less than satisfactory (>3 mm), further radiographic studies are indicated (Fig. 14–18). CT scanning provides an accurate assessment of the reduction; three-dimensional re-formation produces a readily interpretable image that does not require a mental reconstruction of two-dimensional films and provides a permanent record of the reduction.[38] If closed reduction is not satisfactory, an open reduction with transfixion may be required. The screw or percutaneous Steinmann pin can cross the physis in this particular situation because the middle and medial sections of the growth plate are usually closed. If the growth plate is not closed or closing, the implant should not cross the physis. Growth discrepancy is an unusual sequela to this injury because most of the physis has closed. The more

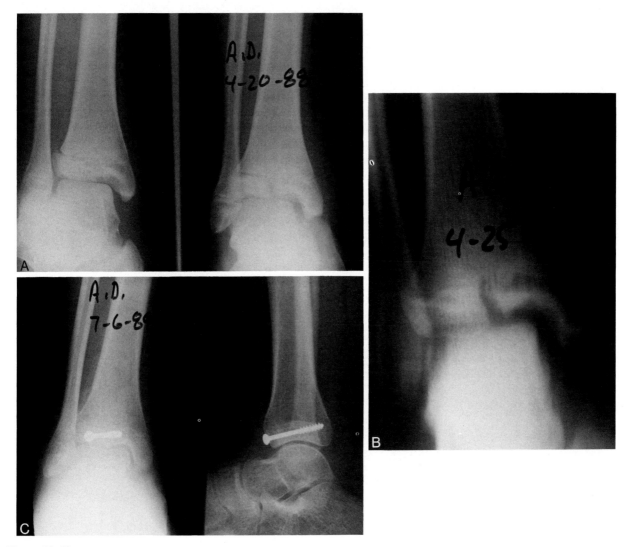

Figure 14–18

This child sustained a Salter-Harris III fracture of the lateral tibial epiphysis that required open reduction and internal fixation. A, A mortise and anteroposterior view of a juvenile Tillaux fracture. B, Polytomogram following closed reduction shows that the fracture-separation at the subchondral surface was greater than 3 mm; therefore, an open reduction was performed. C, Complete closure of the physis occurred within 3 months following the open reduction.

significant complication is arthritis resulting from either a step-off of the articular surface or a residual interfragmentary gap of greater than 3 mm.

Triplane Fractures

The triplane fracture is an injury unique to the closing of the distal tibial growth plate. The fracture line crosses the articular surface through the epiphysis, the physis, and finally the posterior tibial metaphysis in the coronal, sagittal, and transverse planes. The multiplanar Salter-Harris type IV injury created is felt to be caused by external rotation of a supinated foot.

Radiographic Evaluation. Triplane fractures of the distal tibia are sometimes quite difficult to identify on plain radiographs. AP, lateral, and mortise views should be taken. On x-ray, the fracture appears to be a Salter-Harris type III on AP view and a Salter-Harris type II on lateral projection. In the AP projection, the fracture can be seen as a vertical line crossing the central area of the epiphysis with widening of the mortise. The appearance in this projection is remarkably similar to that of the juvenile Tillaux fracture, and care must be taken not to confuse the two. The mortise views may show more displacement than the AP ones.[18] This radiographic fracture pattern in a growing child should always suggest a triplane fracture. CT studies have simplified identification of all facets of this injury. The fracture may consist of two or three fragments, directly as a result of the closure of the distal tibial physis. The fracture usually involves three parts in children less than 10 years old and two parts in children over 10 years.

This unusual fracture was first reported by Marmor, who noted widening of the ankle mortise after closed reduction of what appeared to be a Salter-Harris II fracture.[44] Upon reduction, he observed that the fracture extended in three planes—sagittal, transverse, and coronal—and involved three parts of the distal tibia: the shaft, an anterolateral epiphyseal fragment, and an unattached fragment consisting of the remainder of the epiphysis with a metaphyseal spike.

The triplane fracture was named by Lynn, who reported two fractures with a three-dimensional configuration that required open reduction and internal fixation.[42] Torg and Ruggiero also noted that the fracture was intrinsically unstable and needed internal fixation.[76] Cooperman and colleagues felt that most triplane fractures had no free anterolateral epiphyseal fragment and were, therefore, two-part fractures in three planes (Fig. 14–19).[11] Dias and Giegerich postulated that the same mechanism—external rotation of the foot on the leg—causes both triplane fractures and the juvenile Tillaux fractures and felt that the resulting injury is solely determined by the patient's age.[15] The triplane fracture occurs

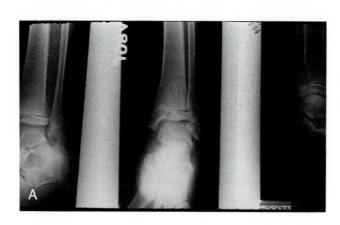
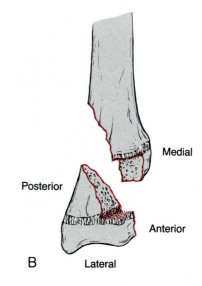

Figure 14–19

Radiograph and artist's drawing of two-part triplane fracture. *A*, On ankle composite view, the mortise view shows little evidence of bony injury. The anteroposterior view reveals the Salter-Harris III fracture of the distal tibial epiphysis and an anterior view of the medial tibial metaphyseal triangular fragment. On the lateral view, the Salter-Harris II fragment of the distal tibia is seen. *B*, Artist's rendition of the two-fragment triplane fracture. (*B* from McNealy, G. A.; Rogers, L. F.; Hernandez, R.; Pozananski, A. K. Injuries of the distal tibial epiphysis: Systematic radiographic evaluation. AJR 138:688, 1982.)

earlier in adolescence than the juvenile Tillaux fracture because the epiphyseal plate is still completely open in early adolescence, thus allowing the horizontal fracture to run through its entire anterior portion. On the other hand, in the older group, the growth plate's medial area has already closed, so the horizontal break extends only through its anterolateral portion and is met by the vertical fracture near the closed medial epiphyseal line.[18] Ertl and co-workers completed a long-term (3 to 13 years) follow-up of this intraarticular fracture and found it to be the predecessor to significant arthritis in adults when less than anatomic reduction was achieved.[18] Although symptoms were absent on early follow-up, about half their patients were symptomatic on long-term evaluation. When the epiphyseal fracture extended into the weight-bearing arch of the ankle, residual displacement of greater than 2 mm was associated with suboptimal results. Anatomic reduction by either closed or open means is mandatory in the treatment of triplane fractures.

The choice between open and closed reduction depends on the amount of residual displacement following reduction. Impending growth arrest is not usually a consideration because the growth plate is approaching closure. Even though this fracture seems to be intrinsically unstable, it is only at the articular surface, where permanent disruption will definitely predispose to degenerative joint disease, that loss of reduction is crucial. Anatomic reduction of the articular surface is mandatory. Ertl and colleagues found that none of their patients with initial displacement of greater than 3 mm on AP or mortise x-rays had successful closed reduction.[18] Interposition of soft tissue at the fracture site was responsible for the failure of closed reduction in six of eight open operations. The soft tissue was identified as periosteum in five patients and was found to be the extensor hallucis longus tendon in one.[18] A diastasis or step-off of more than 3 mm in any plane at the articular surface requires anatomic reduction.

Management. General anesthesia is required for complete relaxation. The knee is flexed to 90 degrees, and the foot is plantar flexed and internally rotated. If anatomic reduction is achieved, I prefer percutaneous threaded Steinmann pin fixation (Fig. 14–20). The extremity is placed into an above-knee, non–weight bearing cast for 4 weeks, at which time the pin is removed, followed by a below-knee cast for 2 to 3 weeks.

If the interfragmentary gap following reduction is greater than 3 mm, an open reduction is necessary. Open reduction is not easy and may require anterolateral and posteromedial approaches to reduce the fractures under direct vision. Only after the posteromedial fragment is reduced can the anterolateral (Tillaux) fragment be reduced. Through an anterolateral approach, the anterolateral fragment is identified and displaced. The posteromedial fragment, if displaced, is first reduced under direct vision by internal rotation and dorsiflexion of the foot. When reduced, the posteromedial fragment is fixed with a percutaneous Steinmann pin or cancellous screw placed in an anteroposterior direction through the anterior tibial metaphysis into the posterior metaphyseal fragment. If the posteromedial fragment cannot be reduced by manipulation, it should be reduced under direct vision through a medial incision. If displaced, the fibular fracture is next reduced. Finally, the displaced anterolateral fragment (Tillaux) is reduced and fixed with a Steinmann pin or screw.[33] A non–weight bearing above-knee cast is applied for 3 weeks, followed by a below-knee walking cast for 4 weeks. If percutaneous Steinmann pins are used, they are removed at the time of cast change.

Distal tibial growth is nearly completed when this injury occurs, so shortening from growth arrest is rarely a problem. Ertl's long-term reevaluation showed marked deterioration with time if there was a failure of reduction of the articular surface. At an average of more than 6 years after injury, the result was that of 15 patients had declined at least one grade.[18] None of these patients improved during follow-up after injury to the articular cartilage. Even in those individuals with anatomic reduction, there were delayed long-term symptoms. Granted, the symptomatic patients followed for 20 years were only in their third decade and could possibly experience continued deterioration. Residual displacement of 2 to 3 mm of the articular cartilage in the weight-bearing area may result in late-onset degenerative arthritis.[18]

Fractures of the Distal Fibula

Isolated distal fibular shaft injuries are somewhat uncommon and are more often associated with tibial fractures. The Salter-Harris type I distal fibular injury is the most common type of ankle fracture in children.[70] If the injury occurs through the physis, diagnosis may be difficult because displacement is usually minimal. There is usually pain and swelling ("goose egg") over the lateral malleolus.

Radiographic Evaluation. Fragment displacement is usually minimal. The soft tissue ("goose egg")

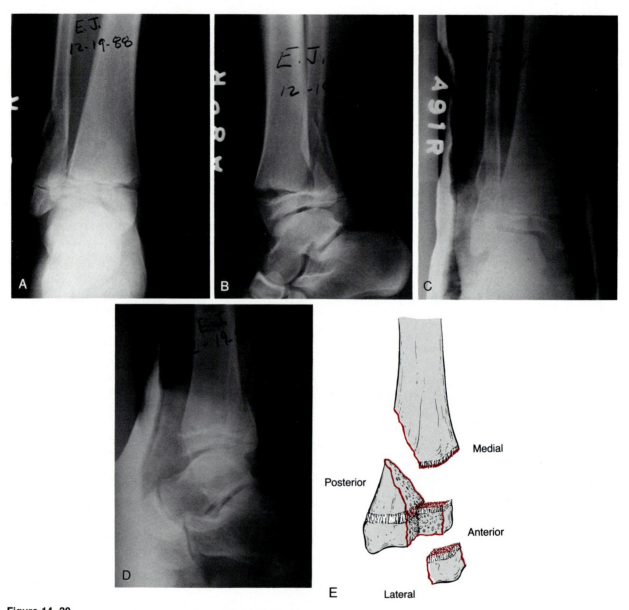

Figure 14–20

Triplane fracture treated by closed reduction and percutaneous Steinmann pinning. A, Anteroposterior x-ray shows Salter-Harris III fracture of the distal tibia and nondisplaced distal fibular fracture. B, Lateral x-ray showing an apparent Salter-Harris II fracture of the distal tibia. C, Anteroposterior x-ray following closed reduction revealing less than anatomic reduction of the Salter-Harris III fracture of the distal tibia. D, Lateral x-ray following closed reduction, with Salter-Harris II component slightly posterior and Salter-Harris III component slightly anterior. This was not considered to be acceptable. E, Artist's rendition of three fracture fragments and three planes of fracture.

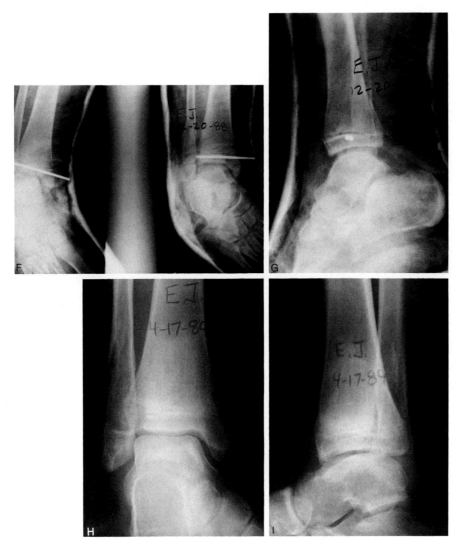

Figure 14–20 *Continued*

F, Anteroposterior and mortise views following closed reduction and percutaneous Steinmann pin fixation. *G,* Lateral view following closed reduction and percutaneous Steinmann pin fixation. Reduction is anatomic. *H,* Anteroposterior x-ray 3 months following pin removal. Subchondral surface is anatomic. *I,* Lateral x-ray 3 months following pin removal. (*E* from McNealy, G. A.; Rogers, L. F.; Hernandez, R.; Pozananski, A. K. Injuries of the distal tibial epiphysis: Systematic radiographic evaluation. AJR 138:689, 1982.)

appearance over the lateral malleolus is usually diagnostic (Fig. 14–21).

Management. A compression dressing of three layers of Webril and an Ace bandage is used for 1 week to diminish swelling. A below-knee walking cast is then applied for 3 weeks. Many of these injuries are misdiagnosed as a sprain or strain and are thus treated initially with a compression bandage. When the patient is reevaluated at 10 days to 2 weeks, there may be ecchymosis extending down the lateral aspect of the lower third of the leg into the foot. These patients usually tend to do well. Fractures that are displaced, unstable, and not treated may undergo a chronic nonunion that gives rise to an epiphysiolysis. This is an extremely rare problem, except for patients with neurologic disorders.

Isolated distal fibular shaft fractures above the tibiofibular syndesmosis are uncommon in children. They are most often associated with injuries to the deltoid ligament (pronation injuries) if no fracture of the tibia is seen. Failure to recognize the medial ligamentous instability associated with distal-third isolated fibular fractures has been responsible for the development of chronic instability and early degenerative joint disease. I recommend open re-

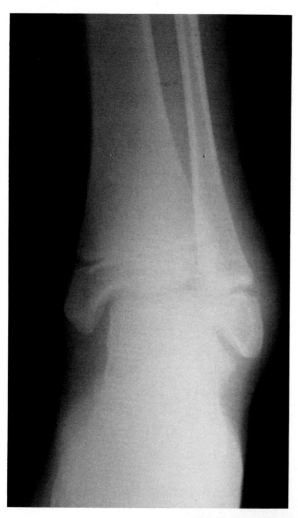

Figure 14–21

An anteroposterior x-ray of ankle with soft tissue swelling "goose egg" over a nondisplaced fibular Salter-Harris I fracture.

Figure 14–22

A, An anteroposterior x-ray of the ankle 2 months following injury shows a delayed union of the distal fibula and horizontal Park-Harris lines of the tibial metaphysis. The ankle was asymptomatic. B, Anteroposterior x-ray of this 14-year-old male's ankle following a sprain. There is soft tissue swelling and an ossicle beneath the fibula. The child is an avid soccer player with a history of repeated sprains. The ossicle is round and smooth, probably representing an old nonunited fracture.

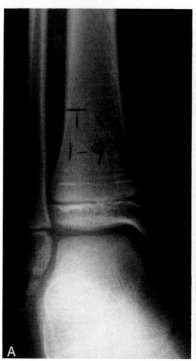

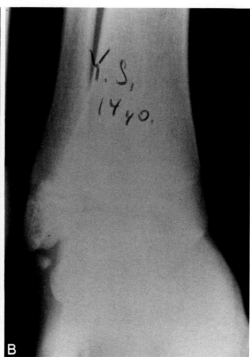

duction and compression plate fixation for these injuries. An above-knee, non–weight bearing cast is applied initially for 3 weeks, followed by a below-knee walking cast; the plate is removed at 1 year.

A small chip fracture of the inferior tip of the epiphysis may occur from an initial ankle injury and not be diagnosed; this is especially true if the fracture occurs through the cartilaginous epiphysis. The history given is that the patient sustained an ankle sprain and, although the x-rays were negative, the patient continues to experience pain and instability. A repeat x-ray shows a small rounded ossicle just inferior to the epiphysis. This ossicle, the os subfibulare, is felt to be a posttraumatic development and not a normal variant. A below-knee walking cast or Aircast may relieve the symptoms, but rarely does the ossicle unite to the fibula. Occasionally the problem progresses to chronic pain and instability. Removal of the ossicle and ligamentous repair followed by a below-knee walking cast for 4 weeks are recommended (Fig. 14–22).

The Foot

ANATOMY

The foot has 26 bones and a variable number of sesamoids and accessory ossicles (Fig. 14–23). All are held together by interconnecting ligaments. The five rays of the foot each contain a metatarsal and its phalanges—two for the first toe and three for the others. The epiphysis of the first metatarsal is located at its proximal end, similar to a phalanx, rather than at the distal end as it is for the other metatarsals.

The first three rays have a cuneiform bone at the base; the fourth and fifth share the cuboid bone at

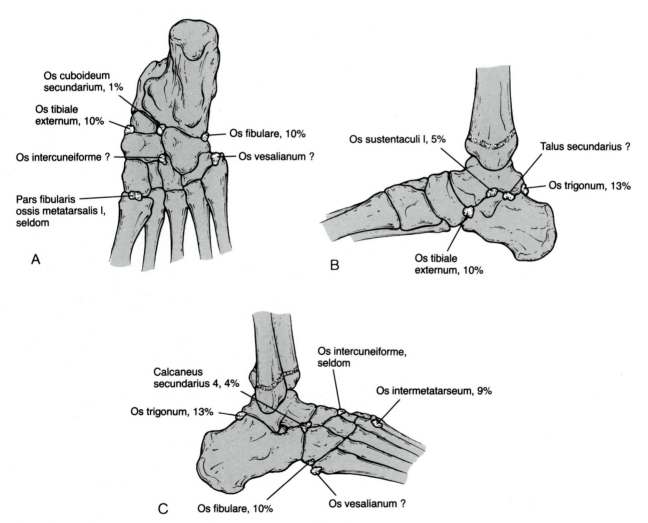

Figure 14–23

Bones of the foot. The normal bones and accessory ossicles. (From Tachdjian, M. O. Pediatric Orthopedics, 2nd ed. Philadelphia, W. B. Saunders, 1990.)

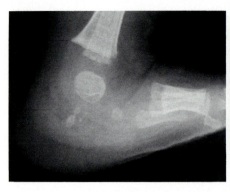
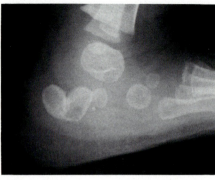

Figure 14–24

The presence of multiple calcaneal centers usually implies a malformation syndrome. This patient with four calcaneal centers, which eventually fused, had Williams' (Beuran's) elfin facies syndrome. (From Oestrich, A. O.; Crawford, A. H. Atlas of Pediatric Orthopaedic Radiology. New York, Thieme, 1985.)

the base. The tarsal navicular is interposed between the head of the talus and the cuneiform, and the talus sits "sidesaddle" on the calcaneus. Thus, the talus lies roughly in the axis of the first ray, and the calcaneus lies in the axis of the fourth ray.

The foot is customarily divided into the forefoot, midfoot, and hindfoot (metatarsus, midtarsus, and tarsus). The forefoot contains the 5 metatarsals and 14 phalanges; it is separated from the midfoot by the tarsometatarsal joint (of Lisfranc). The midfoot contains the three cuneiforms, the navicular, and the cuboid, and it is separated from the hindfoot by the transverse midtarsal joint of Chopart. The hindfoot contains two bones: the talus and the calcaneus. The reader is referred to the comprehensive articles by Mann[43] and Morris[50] for a thorough description and discussion of foot and ankle biomechanics.

The foot presents a myriad of interesting anatomic features. It is not well ossified at birth. Of the tarsal bones present at birth, only the calcaneus and talus are fully ossified; however, the cuboid ossifies shortly after birth. The calcaneus may be bifid in certain syndromes (e.g., Larsen, Williams) (Fig. 14–24), which may be interpreted as a fracture. There is extensive retention of the cartilaginous model.

The reduction of foot deformities following fractures in children is important. Remodeling cannot always be predicted with growth. Fifty percent of mature length has been achieved in 1-year-old girls and 1 1/2-year-old boys. In contrast, the femur and tibia do not reach 50% of their length until 3 years before comparable physeal closure in the long bones.[72] Following foot fractures, not enough time is usually available for severe malalignment to correct spontaneously.

OSTEOCHONDROSES

There are several osteochondroses that may or may not be anatomic variants. *Sever's disease* has been considered to be an epiphyseal ischemic necrosis of the calcaneal apophysis; this area may be the site of trauma as well as developmental problems. The clinical condition usually occurs in very active youngsters and presents as heel pain. Radiographs show fragmentation of the calcaneal apophysis. We have found identical fragmentation in the calcaneal apophysis (Fig. 14–25) of asymptomatic feet in children x-rayed for other reasons; therefore, this finding is not diagnostic. The clinical condition most likely results from an overuse syndrome. Sympto-

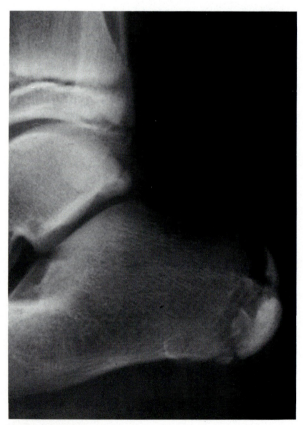

Figure 14–25

Sever's disease. Note the fragmentation of the calcaneal apophysis. The author believes that the condition of heel pain diagnosed as Sever's disease is an overuse syndrome.

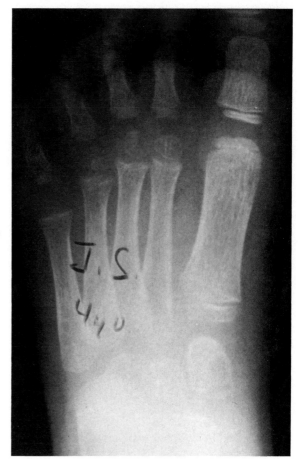

Figure 14–26

A pseudoepiphysis on the distal aspect of the first metatarsal. The normal epiphysis is located at the proximal end of the first metatarsal.

matic treatment and an explanation to the child and parents are usually successful. Treatment ranges from rest to a 1/4-inch heel lift, to a sponge cushion heel insert.

A pseudoepiphysis may occur at the distal end of the first metatarsal and may be interpreted as a fracture. The epiphysis of the first metatarsal is proximal; the other metatarsals (2 through 5) develop secondary ossification centers distally (Fig. 14–26). The base of the fifth metatarsal may have an ossification center just lateral to it, commonly called the os vesalianum, or os peronei; it is quite frequently mistaken for an avulsion fracture (Fig. 14–27). The middle phalanges may occasionally lack secondary ossification centers.

The appearance and variance of ossification of

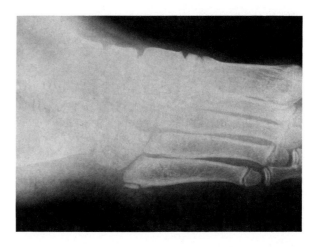

Figure 14–27

The os vesalianum is an oblique bony ossicle found just lateral to the base of the fifth metatarsal ray. It is normal.

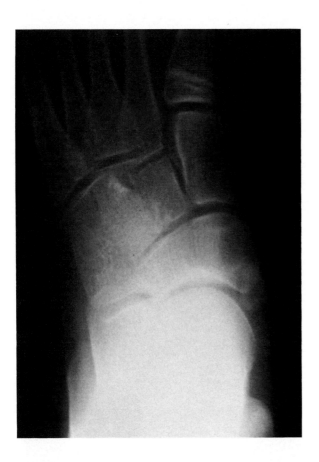

Figure 14–28

An accessory navicular ossicle is seen on the proximal medial aspect of the navicular bone; this one has round, smooth edges. The accessory navicular may be either separate from the bone and found in the posterior tibialis tendon or partially attached to the navicular bone itself. Those that are partially attached are usually thought to have injury to the attachment as a result of overuse and the pull from the posterior tibialis tendon, which causes the patient to be symptomatic.

anatomic structures are commonplace. Ossification of the lateral cuneiforms usually occurs by the end of the first year. The navicular ossification center appears between 3 and 5 years and is the last of the ossification centers of the foot to appear. The secondary ossification centers of the metatarsals and phalanges appear by 5 years of age. The calcaneal apophysis appears by 6 to 10 years of age and tends to unite with the body of the calcaneus at 15 to 18 years of age. An accessory navicular is found on x-ray in 10% of feet[53] and may present clinically because of either trauma or repetitive overuse syndrome (Fig. 14–28). The os trigonum is a posterior lateral process of the talus found at the same level as the groove for the flexor hallucis longus; it may occasionally be separated and interpreted as a fracture on x-ray (Fig. 14–29). Structural variations in ossification patterns are the rule rather than the

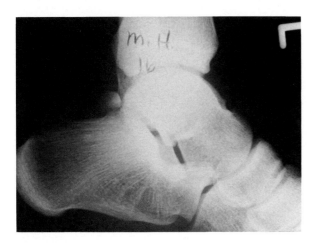

Figure 14–29

Note the round ossicle "os trigonum" just posterior to the talus. The os trigonum is considered to be a normal component of the posterior lateral process of the talus. A bone scan will determine whether there is current injury or fracture.

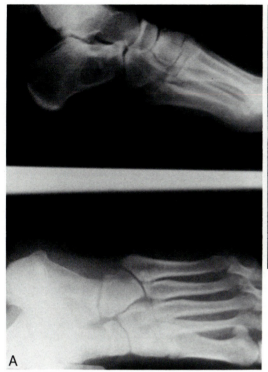
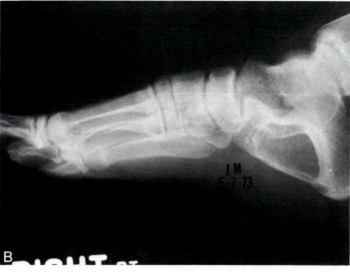

Figure 14–30

Two calcaneal x-rays showing cystic lesions. *A*, The appearance of a simple bone cyst of the calcaneus. The oblique view is not as convincing. This may be a normal finding related to the convergence of the trabecular patterns. *B*, An example of a true unicameral bone cyst of the calcaneus. Note the pathologic fracture on the proximal inferior cortex.

exception and may occur in 22% of children. The orientation of the trabecular patterns in the os calcis may mimic a unicameral bone cyst (Fig. 14–30).

TYPES OF INJURIES

A review of foot injuries managed by the resident service at The Children's Hospital Medical Center, Cincinnati, was undertaken in December 1990[14] (Table 14–2). Two hundred fifteen patients were identified, and their charts and x-rays were pulled; 175 patients with definitive fractures and follow-up to completion of treatment were identified and reviewed by the author. *Metatarsal* fractures accounted for 90% of the fractures, with 60% occurring in the lesser second through fifth metatarsals, 22% in the isolated base of the fifth metatarsal, and 8% at the base of the first metatarsal, with or without other injuries. *Phalangeal* fractures (18%) were the next most common group, including proximal (64%), distal (39%), and middle (7%) phalanges. The *navicular* (5%) was the most common tarsal bone fracture, followed by the *talus* (3%) and *cuboid* (2%). Coexistent unrecognized fractures of the distal tibia and fibula occurred in 8% of all fractures studied. Dislocation of the phalanges occurred in 3%, and conditions initially mistaken as fractures were talofibular ligament tear, tarsal coalition, foreign body, and a sesamoid fracture, each

Table 14–2

**Distribution of 175 Foot Injuries
Cincinnati Children's Hospital
Resident Fracture Service 1990 (14)
Boys 62%   Girls 38%
Left 64%   Right 36%**

Area of Injury	Number		Percentage
Metatarsals			
Lesser (2–4)	104	(49.038)	59.42
Buckle base	14	(13.46)	8
Base of 5th	39	(37.5)	22.2857
Navicular	9		5.14
Talus	4		2.285
Calcaneus	4		2.285
Cuboid	2		1.42
Cuneiform	1		0.571
Phalanges	31		17.71
Proximal	20	64.51	(11.4285)
Distal	9	29.0	(5.14285)
Middle	2	6.45	(1.14285)
Talofibular ligament	1		0.571
Fibula	8		4.57
Sesamoid	1		0.571
Tarsal coalition	1		0.571
Foreign body	1		0.571
Medial malleolus	3		1.71
Distal tibial articular surface	2		1.42
Dislocation (MP/IP)	4		2.285

Crawford, A.H. Fractures about the foot in children. A radiographic analysis. Cincinnati, The Children's Hospital Medical Center, 1991 (unpublished data).

occurring once. There were 62% males and 38% females in this study. The left side was involved in 64% of cases; the right side in 36%.[14] This study will be referred to during the discussion of foot fractures. There are very few firm guidelines for treatment of foot injuries in children. The most common fractures occur to the metatarsals, phalanges, and proximal fifth metatarsal. Injury to the chondro-osseous components of the child's foot is uncommon.

The majority of foot fractures result from direct violence, such as a crush from a falling object, being run over by the wheel of an automobile, a fall, or jumping from a height. The foot is so flexible and resilient that force applied to it is usually transmitted higher up, causing ankle and leg injuries. The soft tissue component of a foot injury is most important, and if the area is swollen and tense, elevation and decompression should be employed very early. Preservation of soft tissues, particularly the ligaments essential to long-term function of the longitudinal and transverse arches, is just as important as actual fracture reduction in restoring complete function to the injured foot. Fractures involving a joint surface carry a worse prognosis than nonarticular fractures, especially when tarsal bones are involved. Articular fractures to mobile joints require anatomic reduction to prevent early degenerative arthritis.

THE TALUS

Fracture of the talus, infrequent in the child, is a potential problem injury because of the precarious blood supply.[51] The posterior tibial artery gives off small branches that enter the region of the posterior tubercle to supply a portion of the body of the talus. The anterior tibial artery creates small branches that enter the superior surface of the head and neck of the talus. The formation of the primary talar ossification center depends on a functioning vascular supply (Fig. 14-31). In the child there appears to be less dominance of a single system with retrograde flow from the neck into the body compared with the adult, and avascular (ischemic) necrosis is a rare complication following talar fracture. Much of its surface is covered by articular cartilage, leaving only the constricted neck to accept the majority of nutrient vessels. Unfortunately, this is the area where most injuries occur. A displaced fracture of the neck of the talus is consistent with impending avascular necrosis.[8] Talar neck fractures can be overlooked in children and may become apparent only after the onset of osteonecrosis (Fig. 14-32). Avascular necrosis may not be appreciated for up to 6 months following injury.

Types of Fractures

Talar Neck Fractures. The most common talar fracture occurs through the neck and is slightly angulated, usually with minimal displacement. There is ankle pain with swelling and decreased joint motion. Weight bearing is not tolerated. X-rays will reveal the injury in most cases (Fig. 14-33). Angulation of up to 30 degrees usually can be accepted. The apex of the angulation is in a plantar direction. Gentle, maximum plantar flexion using image-intensification control under general anesthesia should be carried out if the angulation is greater than 30 degrees. One has to weigh the risk of further displacement and vascular compromise against acceptance of the angulation. Rarely does the angulation inhibit ankle motion. If plantar flexion is required to maintain the reduction, a non–weight bearing above-knee cast is worn for 3 to 4 weeks, followed by an Aircast. Treatment also consists of a below-knee walking cast for 3 to 4 weeks. The x-rays should be monitored for evidence of subchondral osteopenia of the distal fragment. The vascular resorption Hawkins sign is indicative of the blood supply being intact.[24]

Displaced talar neck fractures tend to occur in older children (Fig. 14-34). They require open anatomic reduction. Early reduction by open or closed means will enhance fracture healing but may not influence avascular necrosis. Because the distal tibial growth plates are closing, a medial malleolar osteotomy may be used to allow direct visualization of the fracture. Reduction is stabilized with interfragmentary screws, and the osteotomy is repaired. An above-knee cast is applied with the knee flexed 30 degrees and the ankle plantar flexed 20 degrees for 4 to 6 weeks, followed by a below-knee weight-bearing cast. The parents should be *strongly* advised of the possibility of avascular necrosis. X-rays of the talus should be monitored for evidence of subchondral osteopenia of the distal fragment. If there is no Hawkins sign and the distal fragment becomes sclerotic, I recommend a patellar tendon–bearing brace to prevent talar collapse.

Compression Fracture of the Dome of the Talus. This injury is rare in children. The cartilage-to-bone ratio tends to cushion the impact of the tibial and subtalar joints, and the bone is well protected in the mortise. The compression fracture is most common

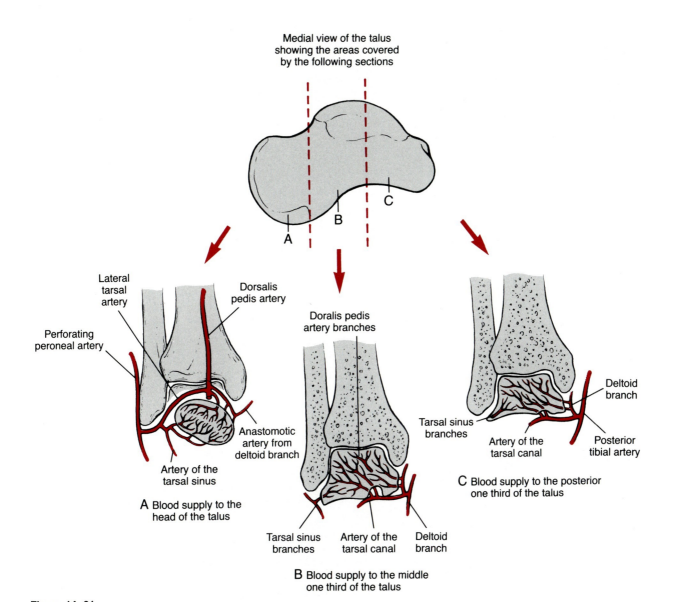

Figure 14–31
Diagram to show the blood supply to the talus in coronal sections. (From Mulfinger, G. L.; Trueta, J. The blood supply of the talus. J Bone Joint Surg 52-B:160–167, 1970.)

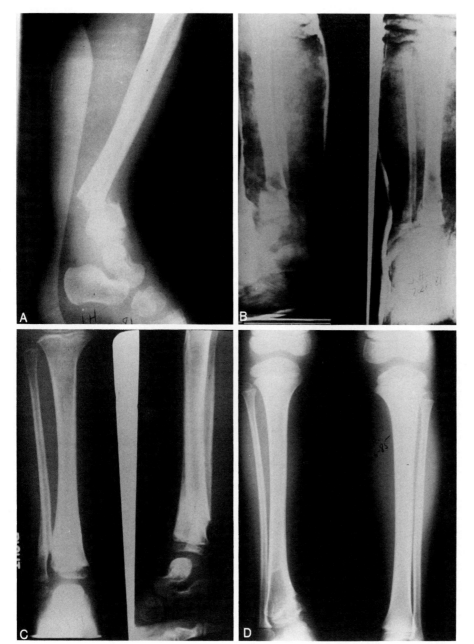

Figure 14–32

An example of unrecognized injury to the talus resulting in osteonecrosis. This child sustained a tibial fracture that was reduced and healed uneventfully. He was subsequently noted to have an avascular necrosis of his talus over the dome of the talus. Another unrecognized injury was a Salter-Harris IV injury to the medial malleolus that resulted in a severe varus deformity, which finally caused his return to the hospital. *A,* Lateral x-ray of leg showing displaced, posteriorly angulated distal tibial fracture. The talar fracture was not recognized. *B,* Anteroposterior and lateral x-ray of the leg showing adequate reduction. *C,* Anteroposterior and lateral leg x-ray 2 months later showing avascular necrosis of the talar dome that had not been recognized. *D,* The patient was seen in consultation 3 1/2 years following the injury because of an ankle varus deformity secondary to a growth arrest of the medial malleolar fracture. The talus was collapsed, and there was very little motion of the ankle or subtalar joint.

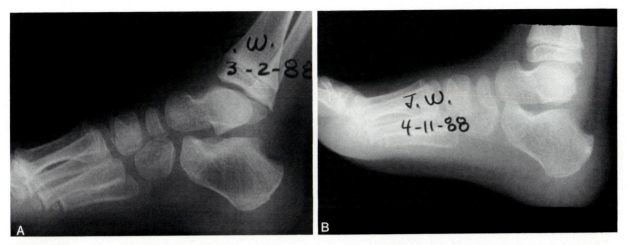

Figure 14–33

Minimally angulated talar neck fracture in a 6-year-old following dorsiflexion injury to his foot. *A,* Lateral x-ray at the time of injury. There is minimal plantar angulation. *B,* Lateral x-ray at the time of healing. The neck remains slightly angulated.

in older adolescents and young adults; thus, it will not be discussed here.

Lateral or Medial Process Fractures. These may occur following a twisting injury to the ankle. The patient complains of pain beneath the malleolus. Rarely does displacement occur, and treatment consists of immobilization and avoidance of weight bearing until the patient is comfortable. The process fragment may not unite, but the patient is usually asymptomatic.

Transcondylar Fractures (Osteochondritis Dissecans). This entity will be discussed separately under Osteochondral Fractures.

Os Trigonum

The lateral tubercle, also called the os trigonum, sometimes separates, usually at the attachment of the talocalcaneal ligament. The os trigonum may be considered a developmental analogue of a secondary ossification center, similar to the posterior calcaneal apophysis.[22] The normal ossification process within the body of the talus is characterized by a progressive posterior extension toward the posterior tubercle. Radiographic studies have suggested that the incidence may be as high as 14 to 25% and that the condition is usually bilateral.[27]

Hindfoot pain may be due to myriad causes and may be acute or chronic; x-rays will show evidence of chondro-osseous separation (see Fig. 14–29). A bone scan can be used to determine whether the lesion should be treated as an undisplaced fracture with probable microscopic delayed union or nonunion. A below-knee weight-bearing cast is indicated for symptomatic treatment; although the x-rays may not change, the patient becomes asymptomatic. On rare occasions excision may be indicated.

Avascular Necrosis

The talus is the anatomic keystone for the ankle joint; it is the linchpin between the anatomic foot and ankle. Collapse of the talar dome may occur following avascular necrosis of the talus, but this condition is extremely rare in children under 10 years of age. The anatomy and function of the talus are usually stable until the collapse occurs. The subsequent alteration of its shape leads to ankle joint incongruity, instability, and subsequent degenerative joint disease. A bone scan is indicated following the treatment of all displaced talar fractures to rule out avascular necrosis. There is a question as to whether the avoidance of weight bearing has an effect on the outcome of talar avascular necrosis. Management is usually similar to that for Legg-Perthes disease with no weight bearing and active motion in a patella tendon–bearing (PTB) articulated ankle brace until there is evidence of revascularization.

Osteochondral Fractures

In 1888, Konig first used the term "osteochondritis dissecans" to describe loose bones in the knee joint.[35] It was not until 1932 that Rendu reported

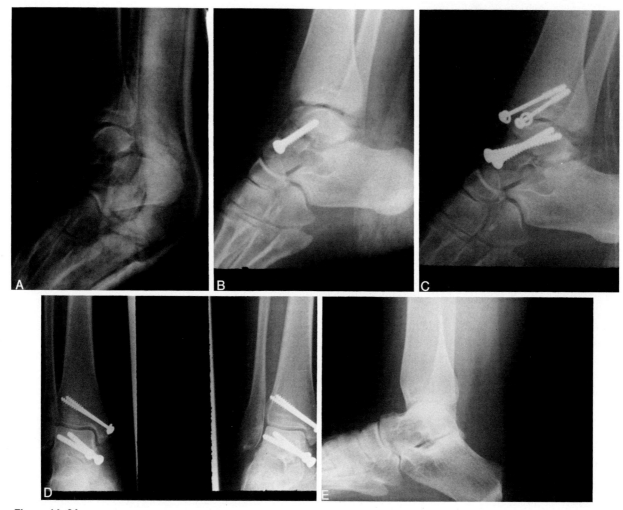

Figure 14–34

This adolescent female was in an automobile accident, sustaining injury to her foot. The talar neck fracture was displaced. As a result, she underwent open reduction and internal fixation. The open reduction was performed through a medial malleolar osteotomy. Because of avascular necrosis, the child was maintained in a brace for 1 1/2 years; she healed uneventfully. *A,* Original lateral x-ray of foot in a posterior plaster splint showing a displaced talar neck fracture. *B,* Intraoperative x-ray showing anatomic reduction of the talar neck fracture with cortical screw fixation. *C,* Final postoperative x-ray showing fixation of the talar neck fracture as well as medial malleolar osteotomy. *D,* Anteroposterior and mortise view x-ray 3 months post injury. Note the absence of subchondral osteopenia (Hawkins sign). The talus had undergone avascular necrosis. *E,* Lateral view of ankle 3 years later. The ankle was protected with a PTB brace for 2 years. There is a loss of ankle joint space.

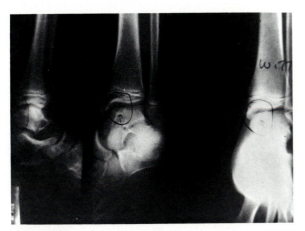

Figure 14-35

These composite x-rays of the ankle show a medial talar osteochondritis dissecans in a 3-year-old child. This child was treated with a below-knee walking cast, and the lesion healed.

an intraarticular fracture of the talus that appeared to be similar in nature to that described by Konig.[61] The condition occurs most frequently in the second decade; however, it has been seen in a 3-year-old (Fig. 14-35). Osteochondral fractures of the talus usually result from eversion-inversion injuries.[4, 7] The presenting complaint is usually ankle pain and an associated limp. The association of trauma is still controversial. The condition has been reported in siblings and has been associated with dwarfism[2, 58, 82, 84] and with endocrine abnormalities.[77] Medial osteochondritis dissecans, which is thought to be benign, is usually a deeper lesion, and the clinician is not always able to elicit a history of injury. Lateral osteochondritis dissecans is usually caused by a more significant injury; however, it is also more shallow. There is also a greater tendency for the lateral fragment to displace into the joint.

Berndt and Harty coined the term "torsional impaction," which is useful in understanding the mechanism of injury in these lesions.[4] They classified the lesion into four stages: (1) a small area of compression of subchondral bone; (2) a partially detached osteochondral fragment; (3) a completely detached osteochondral fragment remaining in the crater; and (4) a displaced osteochondral fragment (Fig. 14-36). They suggested that the lesion may represent nonunion of an osteochondral fracture or separation of articular cartilage and underlying subchondral bone by means of a localized vascular insult. They produced the posteromedial lesion by inversion and plantar flexion of the foot, combined with external rotation of the tibia. Traumatic inversion and ankle dorsiflexion, and compression of the

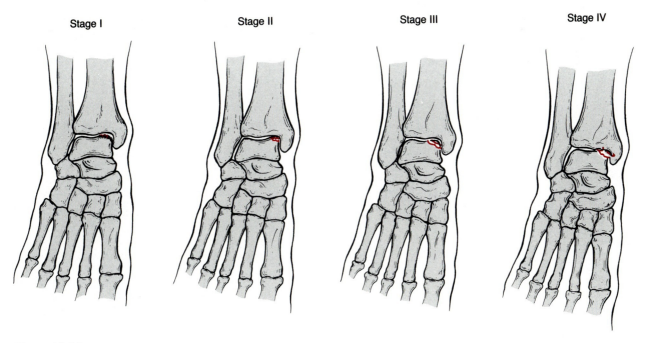

Figure 14-36

The four stages of the osteochondral lesion of the talus according to the classification of Berndt and Harty. Stage I—A small area of subchondral compression; stage II—a partially detached fragment; stage III—a completely detached fragment remaining in the crater; stage IV—a fragment that is loose in the joint. (From Canale, S. T.; Belding, R. M. Osteochondral lesions of the talus. J Bone Joint Surg 62-A:1, 1980.)

talus against the lateral malleolus, produce the anterolateral lesion that may be accompanied by rupture of the fibular collateral ligaments. The posteromedial lesion is slightly more common. The osteochondritic fragment consists of viable hyaline cartilage with underlying necrotic bone. The radiolucent line between the dead bone and the remainder of talus is formed by a dense layer of fibrous connective tissue that acts as a barrier to capillary ingrowth. The primary objective of any treatment is to obtain bony union between the osteochondritic fragment and the remainder of the talus. Magnetic resonance imaging (MRI) is superior to CT arthrography if detachment or displacement of the fragment cannot be identified on plain x-ray (Fig. 14–37).

Canale and Belding recommended that undisplaced lesions be treated conservatively with casts and that displaced lesions be treated with excision and curettage.[7] The literature is pessimistic about the use of a cast and no weight bearing to obtain healing of medial osteochondritis.[4,7] We have been successful in the treatment of nondisplaced lesions in children under 10 years of age with application of an above-knee, non–weight bearing cast for 3

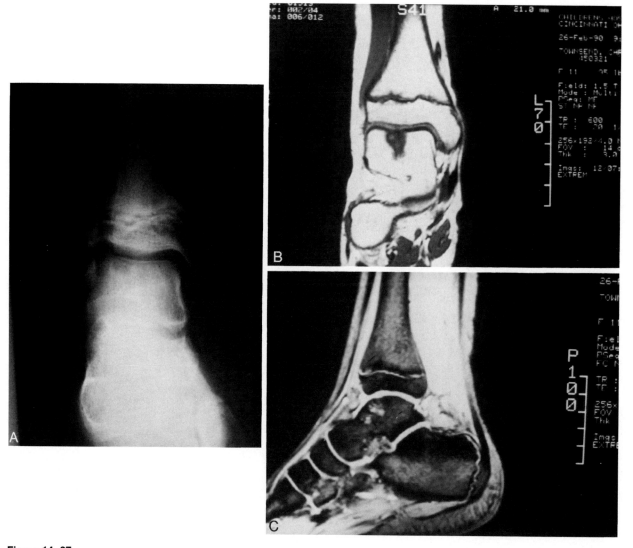

Figure 14–37

An example of a symptomatic osteochondritis dissecans of the talus evaluated by x-ray and MRI. *A*, Anteroposterior x-ray of ankle showing lateral talar osteochondritis dissecans. *B*, T_2 weighted MRI reveals a more extensive lesion than does plain x-ray. *C*, Lateral T_1 weighted image reveals further extensive involvement of osteochondritis dissecans. (Case referred by D. R. Roy, M. D., Cincinnati, OH.)

months. If the lesion does not respond to non-weight bearing and can be approached through arthroscopy, I advocate this method. For larger lesions, surgery is advised. Surgery allows either open curettage of the base and bone grafting via transmalleolar osteotomy or arthroscopic spongialization.[40] If the fragment is completely detached and the bed of the defect is forming granulation tissue, only excision of the fragment may be indicated.

Complications

The complications of talar fractures depend on the location of the fracture line and the amount of displacement. Commonly, following reduction of fractures with significant displacement, the complication is avascular necrosis. Five of the 17 children with nondisplaced fractures of the talus developed avascular necrosis, as reported by Canale and Kelly,[8] and by Letts and Gibeault,[39] leading Gross[23] to suggest that children may be as much at risk as adults for the development of avascular necrosis following nondisplaced fractures. These reports contradict the prevailing philosophy that avascular necrosis is unusual in children because displacement is unusual in children (see Fig. 14-32).

Hawkins, in 1970, detailed his experience with a series of 57 fractures of the talus in adults and outlined a useful classification.[24] Type I fractures were nondisplaced, and in his series avascular necrosis did not appear. Type II fractures were displaced with a subtalar dislocation or subluxation. All united, but the rate of avascular necrosis was 42%. Type III fractures were accompanied by subluxation or dislocation at the subtalar and ankle joints, and a 91% rate of avascular necrosis was found in this group.[24] Following injury and reduction, the Hawkins sign, a radiolucent subchondral line, is usually an indication that the blood supply is intact even though avascular necrosis may have occurred. Since this sign goes together with disuse atrophy, it may be absent in children immobilized for only a brief period. A bone scan will determine whether avascular necrosis has occurred and has been used by Canale and Kelly to determine when weight bearing can be resumed.[8] We have treated talar avascular necrosis by PTB bracing in an effort to prevent collapse. This method has not been completely successful; in one child the talus underwent flattening with stiffness of the ankle and shortening of the extremity. Pain has not been a consistent complaint, but 5 years following the injury the child is only 10 years old.

CALCANEUS

Schofield reviewed 2025 fractures of the calcaneus; his youngest patient was an 18-year-old boy.[67] Essex-LoPresti reported only 12 patients between the ages of 9 and 20 years of 241 fractures of the calcaneus.[19] Thomas, in 1969, reported five boys aged 6 to 12 years who had sustained fractures of the calcaneus.[74] Matteri and Frymoyer reported three fractures of the calcaneus in children.[45] Schmidt and Weiner discovered 59 fractures of the calcaneus in patients less than 20 years old, 46 of which were in skeletally immature children.[66] One third of their patients had associated injuries; three sustained lumbar vertebral fractures. Ten percent of adults with calcaneal fractures will have spinal injuries, whereas only 5% of children will have spinal injuries. This does not mean that the injury should not be looked for in children. Calcaneal fractures were initially unrecognized in 16 of the 59 fractures reviewed. Most of these were minimal, leading to the conclusion that the injury had a very benign prognosis.

Classification

The patterns of fracture modified from Rowe by Ogden (Table 14-3) include type 1, fracture of the tuberosity, sustentaculum tali, or anterior process; type 2, a beak fracture or avulsion fracture of the tendo Achillis insertion; type 3, an oblique fracture in the posterior portion of the bone not involving the subtalar joint, and similar to a metaphyseal fracture of a longitudinal bone; type 4, involvement of the subtalar region with or without actual articular

Table 14-3
Calcaneal Fracture Patterns

Type	Description
Type 1	Fracture of the tuberosity
	Fracture of the sustentaculum tali
	Fracture of the anterior process
Type 2	"Beak" fracture
	Avulsion fracture of the tendo Achillis insertion
Type 3	Oblique fracture in the posterior portion not involving the subtalar joint; corresponds to a metaphyseal fracture of a longitudinal bone
Type 4	Fracture involving the subtalar region with or without actual articular involvement
Type 5	Central depression with varying degrees of comminution
Type 6	Involvement of the secondary ossification center

From Rowe, C.R.; et al. Fracture of the os calcis. JAMA 184:920, 1963.

involvement; type 5, a central depression fracture with varying degrees of comminution; and type 6, involvement of the secondary ossification center.[53]

Consequence of Injury

The calcaneus is largely cartilaginous in children. Fracture of the calcaneus is a common, disabling injury in adults, yet it is rarely reported either in infancy or in early childhood.[45,75] However, it is probably the most frequent tarsal injury seen in children.[66] Fracture of the calcaneus occurred in 4 of 175 patients seen at the residents' fracture clinic at the Children's Hospital Medical Center in Cincinnati.

Stress fractures may occur; beware of the young child who refuses to bear weight or who limps, especially when there is no x-ray evidence of fracture. Depending on the degree of primary ossification, stress fracture is extremely difficult to diagnose early. Later, a sclerotic oblique line may be seen over the trabecular pattern, indicating the reparative process. It is possible that a bone scan would identify the problem early. A below-knee, weight-bearing cast for 3 to 4 weeks is usually sufficient treatment.

Heel pain may be a result of overuse or a symptom of systemic disease such as osteomyelitis or leukemia. The appearance of the secondary ossification center of the calcaneus is often fragmented on x-ray and leads one to assume that there is an injury. This pattern of fragmentation of the apophysis in young children is more the rule than the exception. The clinical condition of pain about the heel with this x-ray finding carries the diagnosis of Sever's disease. The author considers Sever's disease to be an overuse syndrome or the result of repetitive microtrauma (see Fig. 14–25).

Most calcaneal fractures result from a significant fall. X-rays are usually taken in AP, lateral, and axial planes, although internal and external oblique views of the foot as well as a CT scan may be necessary. If there was a significant fall from a height, AP and lateral views of the thoracolumbar spine should be taken to rule out vertebral fracture (Fig. 14–38). Calcaneal injuries may also result from vehicular and lawn mower accidents (Fig. 14–39) or from a heavy object falling onto the foot (Fig. 14–40).

Intraarticular injuries will affect the subtalar joint and are most often caused by the inferior protruding lateral process of the talus (Fig. 14–41). The process jams superiorly into the calcaneus during impact, cracking the calcaneus in a dorsal-plantar direction. The majority of young children with a fracture of the calcaneus will be assumed to have an ankle sprain. The initial x-rays may not show the fracture. In suspected cases a bone scan is indicated. A nondisplaced fracture of the calcaneus is treated by immobilization. This injury in children has produced minimal disability in comparison with fractures of the calcaneus in adults.[46] For the displaced calcaneal fracture, the initial treatment should be directed toward the soft tissue swelling, which may be extensive. One should make every effort to achieve anatomic reduction of all articular surfaces to prevent subsequent degenerative joint disease. Following reduction, the foot and ankle should be immobilized in a well-padded compression dressing and the leg elevated for 2 to 3 days. A cast should not be applied until the bulk of the swelling has subsided. A below-knee walking cast is sufficient for immobilization of most calcaneal fractures not requiring open reduction. Following open reduction, a well-padded above-knee cast is indicated for 3 to 4 weeks, followed by a below-knee walking cast for 3 to 4 weeks.

Complications

Subtalar arthritis may occur with persistent displacement and instability of osteochondral fractures in the subtalar joint. Late surgery to reduce and align the joint surfaces is rarely successful, and subtalar or triple arthrodesis may be required. Injury to the growth plate has been noted following open fracture secondary to lawn mower injury (see Fig. 14–39); otherwise, growth plate injury to the calcaneus is extremely rare.

NAVICULAR BONE

The tarsal navicular bone is injured only occasionally in children, and the fracture is rarely displaced. Nine navicular fractures were seen in 175 fractures reviewed from the Cincinnati Children's Hospital.

Because of the variability in ossification, a fracture may be confused with Köhler's disease. The x-ray presentation of a sclerotic, thin, fragmented tarsal navicular bone, commonly called Köhler's disease, may represent repetitive microtrauma, an abnormal ossification pattern, or an overuse syndrome (Fig. 14–42). In Waugh's study of 52 boys and 52 girls, with x-rays taken at 6-month intervals from 2 to 5 years, 10 boys and 16 girls showed abnormal ossification.[81] X-rays taken of the foot for other reasons often show irregularity of tarsal navicular ossification. There remains a question as to whether Köhler's disease is a normal variant or represents over-

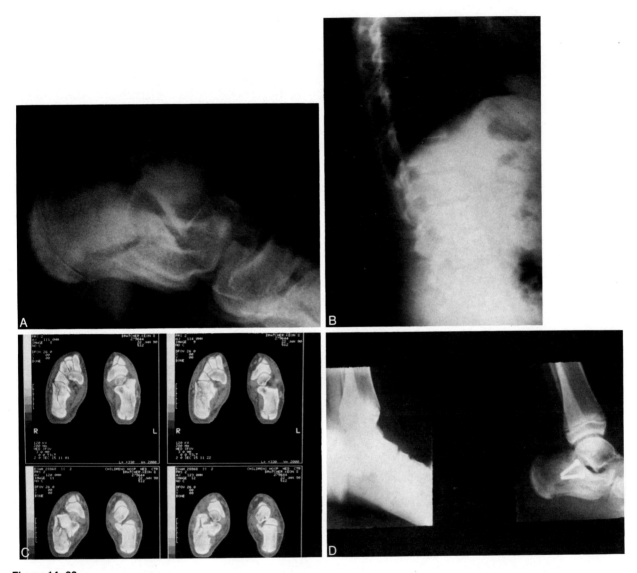

Figure 14–38

A comminuted calcaneal fracture in association with a thoracolumbar spine injury. This child jumped from a height, sustaining a calcaneal fracture; he also had back pain at the time. The lateral thoracolumbar spine film shows a compression injury to the T12–L1 junction. The calcaneal fracture was treated by open reduction and internal fixation. A, Lateral view of foot showing comminuted dorsally displaced calcaneal fracture. B, Lateral thoracolumbar spine x-ray showing mild compression fractures of T12, L1, and L2. C, Multiple coronal view CT scans of both feet revealing comminuted right calcaneal fracture and nondisplaced fractures of the left calcaneus. D, Pre- and postoperative lateral views of the right foot show reduction and fixation with two cortical screws.

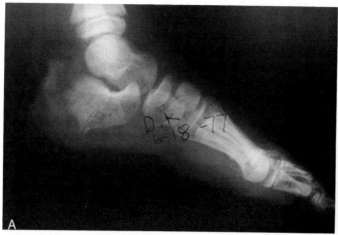
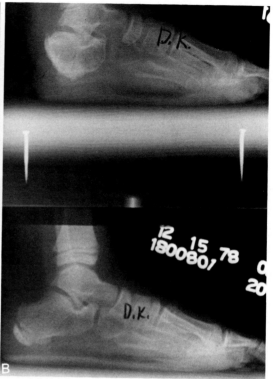

Figure 14–39

This child sustained a lawn mower injury that clipped away the posterior half of the calcaneus. There was minimal posterior growth of the bone after injury. A, Lateral x-ray of foot showing extensive soft tissue and bony injury to the posterior calcaneus. The wound was debrided and the Achilles tendon sutured to bone. Unfortunately, the apophysis was crushed and had to be discarded. B, Comparison lateral views of both feet 1 1/2 years later showing loss of calcaneal apophysis and failure of continued posterior growth of the bone.

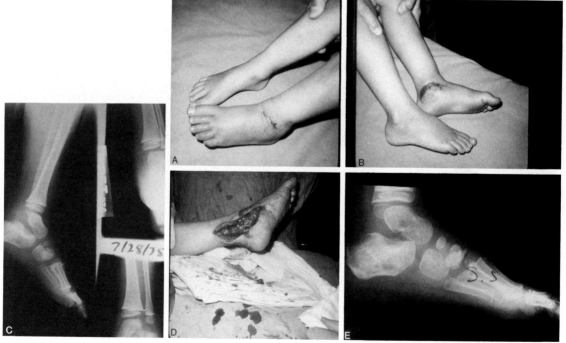

Figure 14–40

This child was watching her father erect a wall of concrete blocks when one of the blocks fell on her left foot. There was tremendous swelling of the foot and toes. Immediate decompression was carried out to save the foot. The fracture healed uneventfully. The swelling and congestion of the foot and toes is a surgical emergency. A, Anterior clinical photograph of both feet showing the tension edema of the foot and toes. B, Side view showing swelling of medial right foot with focal blanching "ischemia" on plantar aspect. C, Anteroposterior, lateral, and mortise views. D, Operative photograph at time of decompression. E, Follow-up lateral x-ray of foot. The calcaneus is healed. The wounds were approximated by delayed primary closure.

Figure 14–41

Fracture through the medial facet of the calcaneus. This fracture is thought to be caused by the lateral process of the talus impacting between the posterior and medial facets. This injury healed uneventfully.

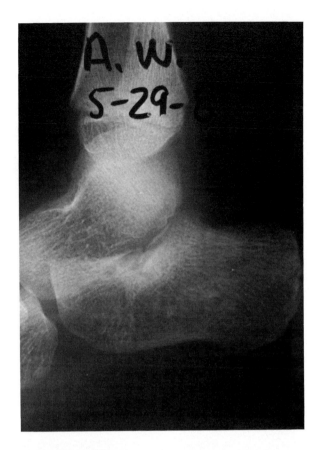

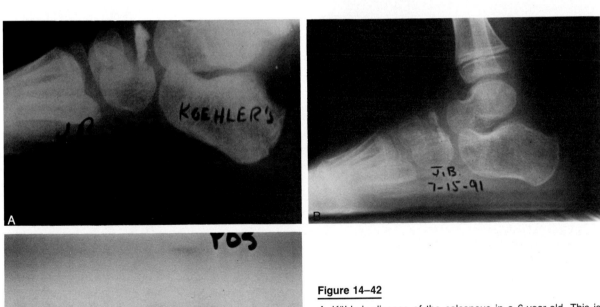

Figure 14–42

A, Köhler's disease of the calcaneus in a 6-year-old. This is believed to be an inflammatory condition; however, there have been asymptomatic feet with similar radiographic findings. B, Lateral x-ray illustrating osteopenia of tarsal navicular. C, Bone scan of patient's foot showing photopenic tarsal navicular. I do not recommend bone scanning to investigate this condition.

use. The treatment of this injury is usually uncomplicated because there is very minimal, if any, displacement of the bone.

The most frequent navicular fracture in children is a dorsal proximal chip fracture seen best on the lateral x-ray of the foot (Fig. 14–43). This injury may represent an avulsion pull-off of an apophyseal fragment from the dorsal tarsal ligament. The treatment of this injury is usually uncomplicated because there is minimal, if any, displacement. A below-knee walking cast is applied for 3 to 4 weeks. Even though the small chip may not unite to the navicular body, the symptoms subside.

Displaced fractures of the tarsal navicular bone in children are usually associated with severe trauma and possibly a dislocation. I recommend anatomic reduction and percutaneous pinning with a threaded Steinmann pin. If closed anatomic reduction cannot be achieved, open reduction and internal fixation are indicated. If there is soft tissue injury, compression and elevation are required until the problem is resolved. A below-knee, non–weight bearing cast is then applied.

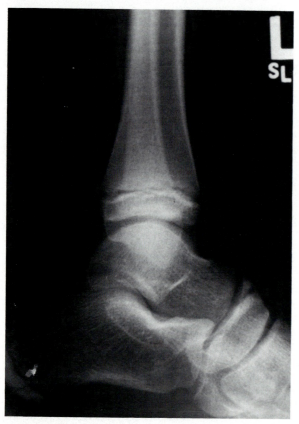

Figure 14–43

This lateral foot x-ray shows a dorsal chip fracture of the navicular. The dorsal chip fracture is the most common of the navicular fractures in children.

TARSOMETATARSAL FRACTURES

These injuries are rare[83] and usually result from (1) indirect injury, such as violent plantar flexion and dorsiflexion found in toe-walking or trying to break speed when sledding or tobogganing; or (2) direct injury, which is more common, secondary to an object falling onto the foot. The unique pattern of tarsometatarsal joint injuries described by numerous authors is related to the anatomic features of this joint complex and the mechanism of injury. The most relevant anatomic features are the fixed, mortised position of the base of the second metatarsal and the ligamentous attachments to its base. A fracture of the base of this metatarsal is a sentinel feature of a tarsometatarsal joint injury.[83] Trillat and associates reviewed 81 fracture-dislocations of the tarsometatarsal joint and concluded that "the lesion is not seen in children."[78] Wiley reported 18 tarsometatarsal injuries in children under 16 years of age.[83]

Mechanism of Injury

Wiley has described three basic mechanisms of injury[83] (Fig. 14–44):

1. *Traumatic impact while in the tiptoe position.* An example of this would be jumping from a height to the ground, and landing on the toes. This usually causes metatarsal joint dislocation plus fracture of the base of the second metatarsal.
2. *Heel-to-toe compression.* In this instance, the victim is in a kneeling position when the impact load strikes the heel. There may be lateral dislocation of the second, third, fourth, and fifth metatarsals, and fracture of the second metatarsal base.
3. *The fixed forefoot.* In this situation, the patient falls backward while the forefoot is fixed to the ground by a heavy weight. The patient's heel resting on the ground becomes the fulcrum for the forefoot injury.

There is no specific injury pattern; the pattern depends upon the character of the impact and the distance. The soft tissue injury is most important.

Lisfranc's joint is rarely injured, but when injury does occur, it usually involves the second metatarsal. There is swelling, and its potential for further damage is most important. Decompression of soft tissue may be necessary. Extensive soft tissue injury, particularly involving disruption of major vessels, may require amputation, although this complication is extremely rare in children.

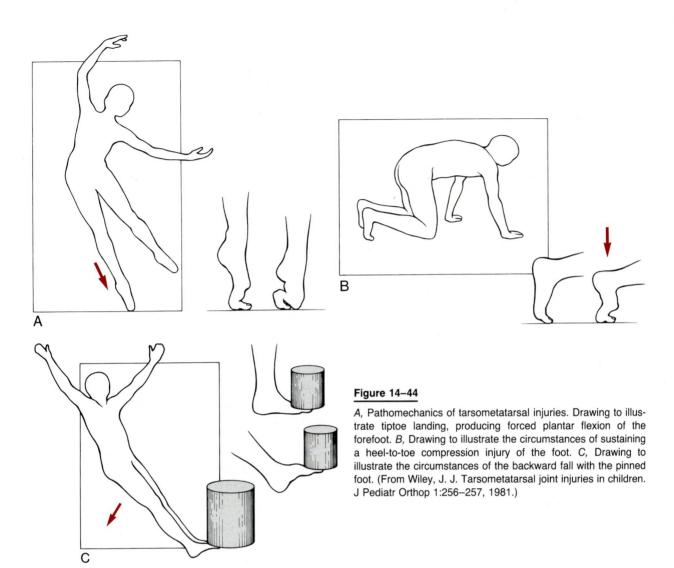

Figure 14-44

A, Pathomechanics of tarsometatarsal injuries. Drawing to illustrate tiptoe landing, producing forced plantar flexion of the forefoot. *B*, Drawing to illustrate the circumstances of sustaining a heel-to-toe compression injury of the foot. *C*, Drawing to illustrate the circumstances of the backward fall with the pinned foot. (From Wiley, J. J. Tarsometatarsal joint injuries in children. J Pediatr Orthop 1:256–257, 1981.)

Management

One should always obtain AP, lateral, and oblique x-rays. A fracture of the base of the second metatarsal fracture implies a more severe injury. The combination of a fracture at the base of the second metatarsal and the cuboid bone usually has resulted from a tarsometatarsal dislocation.

Treatment should consist of not only reduction of the fracture, if it is displaced, but also elevation of the extremity and compression. Then, a below-knee walking cast is applied when the swelling is down and the patient is comfortable. A closed reduction should be performed for displacement. The key to reduction involves aligning the base of the second metatarsal anatomically. Percutaneous pinning may be used to obtain stability of the reduction, especially when there is swelling. A compression dressing is applied until the swelling subsides, followed by a short leg walking cast.

METATARSAL FRACTURES

Metatarsal fractures accounted for 90% of the fractures of the foot seen in the pediatric foot fracture study from the Cincinnati Children's Hospital.[14] The injury usually occurs as a result of direct trauma from a falling object. Indirect trauma following torsional stresses may result in oblique fractures. Avulsion fracture of the base of the fifth metatarsal is the most common isolated metatarsal injury in children. Stress fractures do occur in the foot subjected to repetitive trauma, such as jogging and track-and-field activities. The injury occurs most commonly to the second metatarsal, although other metatarsals may be involved.

The necks of the metatarsals are rarely injured. The fracture pattern may be oblique, transverse, or linear. If the articular surface or condylar epiphysis is not injured, the injury usually resolves readily.

Treatment consists of a below-knee walking cast for 3 weeks.

Metatarsal shaft fractures usually occur from a direct crushing blow. Solitary fractures are usually undisplaced. Reduction of shaft injuries requires particular attention. Lateral displacement of metatarsal fractures is acceptable, but dorsal and plantar angulation is not. Residual dorsal angulation or plantar angulation may give rise to subsequent problems because of abnormal weight distribution. Malunion as well as nonunion is rare but may occur.

The base of the metatarsal usually is injured only when there are other associated injuries, except for the bases of the first and fifth metatarsals. The isolated fracture of the first metatarsal base is not uncommon, but this injury may predispose to growth plate injury. The child's symptoms are usually swelling, pain, or ecchymosis across the forefoot. There may or may not be evidence of fracture on initial x-rays. Fractures of the base of the fifth metatarsal are more common in adolescent athletes involved in jumping sports.

Displaced fractures of the base of the metatarsals are usually caused by a strong, avulsive force. It is important to appreciate the fibrous compartment of the interossei and short plantar muscles with foot injuries, especially when there is significant swelling. One should consider early fasciotomies similar to those performed in the hand when there is marked swelling with the skin stretched and taut or when there is significant venous congestion of the toes. One should be especially wary if there are multiple fractures and should not hesitate to perform fasciotomies.

Growth plate injuries to the metatarsals are rare but do occur under certain conditions: (1) The chondroepiphysis may be avulsed; (2) there may be a fracture into the epiphysis; and (3) the secondary ossification center condylar surface may be avulsed. The treatment for these injuries, more often than not, is a below-knee walking cast for 3 to 4 weeks. Growth inhibition is unusual; overgrowth is more common. Condylar fractures rarely require open reduction. The growth rates may be affected differently according to the type of injuries.

Treatment

Significant displacement is rare. If swelling is present, one should refrain from the immediate use of a circular cast around the ankle, which would lead to dorsal pressure and a tourniquet effect. One should consider a *bulky dressing only* very early in all cases, even those with minimal displacement. Following reduction of swelling, a below-knee cast is applied. Skeletal traction can be used for the severely swollen foot with multiple displaced fractures to achieve alignment and decrease swelling (Fig. 14–45). Open reduction and internal fixation must be avoided at all costs.

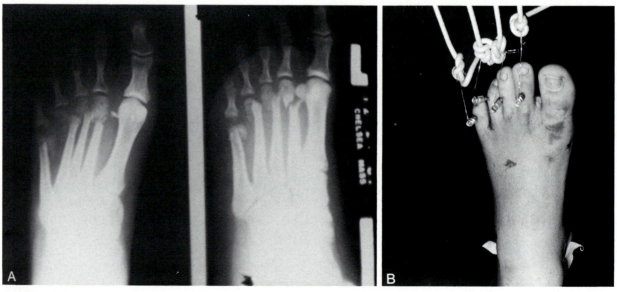

Figure 14–45

Skeletal traction for the management of severe injuries to the foot. This child presented with a tremendously swollen foot and multiple metatarsal neck fractures. Pins were placed through the distal phalanges, and the foot was hung in traction. The swelling receded, and adequate alignment was obtained. *A*, Anteroposterior x-ray of the foot showing multiple metatarsal neck fractures. *B*, Clinical photograph of the foot in traction; 18-gauge needles were placed through phalanges and 22-gauge wires attached to traction.

Severe soft tissue injury may occur with injury to the interossei and short plantar flexor muscles contained in the tightly closed fascial compartments of the foot. Fasciotomy is indicated if swelling is severe. Similar to injuries to the hand, the clinical indications for fasciotomy are marked swelling, taut skin, and decreased sensation. I have no experience with the measurement of compartment pressures in the foot. The incisions should be generous and should extend down to the bone. A medial and lateral longitudinal incision is made over the second and fourth metatarsals; they are packed open and the foot is elevated. C-wire fixation can be used to stabilize the bones but is rarely necessary. A delayed primary closure is carried out in 5 to 7 days.

Management of Specific Injuries

First Metatarsal

The first metatarsal is often fractured. The injury occurs most frequently in the first decade, and as a result the mechanism of injury is elusive. The child presents with a limp, and the parents may simply state that he "fell on the foot." The x-ray shows a buckle at the base of the metatarsal just distal to the physis, which I have termed "buckle base" (Fig. 14–46), similar to the "torus" radius forearm fracture. One should look carefully at the physis for evidence of injury. As opposed to the other metatarsals, the physis occurs on the proximal end of the first metatarsal. A pseudoepiphysis may occur at the distal end. If the physis is injured, shortening may result causing a deficiency on the longitudinal arch with further growth of the other bones. The "buckle base" injury may appear to be isolated on initial x-ray; however, on follow-up, callus may be noted over other metatarsals, indicating healing of nondisplaced fractures. A below-knee walking cast is all that is needed once the swelling is down.

Osteochondritis of the first metatarsal has been reported but is extremely rare.[20] Four cases of painful osteochondritis of the basal epiphysis of the first metatarsal have been reported; the children are usually active in running sports. Radiographic findings are usually noted at the time of presentation, and bone scan, if necessary, confirms the diagnosis. Treatment is symptomatic with immobilization in plaster, with arch supports providing adequate management. Subtle x-ray changes of slight irregularity of the subchondral surface of the first metatarsal in a child with transitory foot pain should be investigated for this condition. The technetium 99m bone scan is diagnostic.

Second Metatarsal

Isolated fractures of the second metatarsal are rare. Fracture of this bone was associated with fractures of other metatarsals in 30 of 51 fractures of the lesser second through fifth metatarsals in a recent review.[14] The most common mechanism of injury

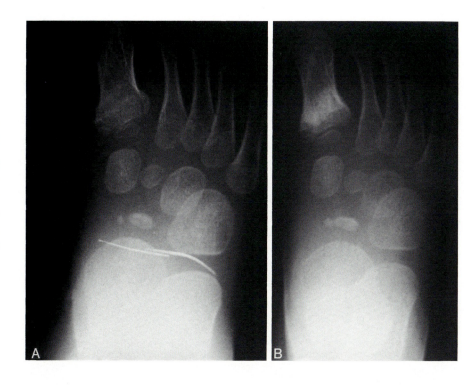

Figure 14–46

Fractures of the base of the first metatarsal tend to buckle and have been termed the buckle base injury; these injuries heal uneventfully. *A,* Initial anteroposterior x-ray showing buckle fracture to base of first metatarsal. *B,* Follow-up anteroposterior x-ray 3 weeks later; the fracture has healed, and remodeling is taking place.

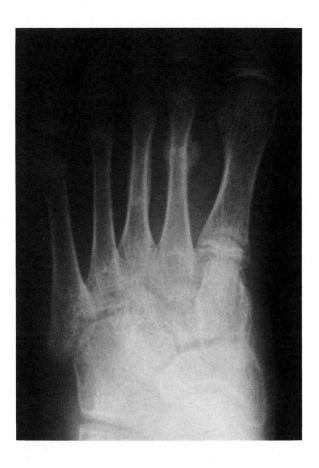

Figure 14–47

Evidence of stress fracture. This child had an excision of a calcaneonavicular bar and was required to be immobile for 6 weeks and not participate in sports. She was an avid soccer player and upon return to soccer noted foot pain and swelling. The anteroposterior x-ray of the foot shows a stress fracture with exuberant callus of the second metacarpal and healing callus over the shaft of the third metatarsal.

was indirect, such as jumping from a height of less than 5 feet. Other direct mechanisms included objects falling on the foot, such as a rock, table, or chair. The fractures were rarely displaced except with severe trauma, e.g., foot run over by car or lawn mower. Most of these fractures could be treated with a below-knee walking cast once the swelling was down.

The second metatarsal is more often subject to a stress fracture. The injury occurs early in the second

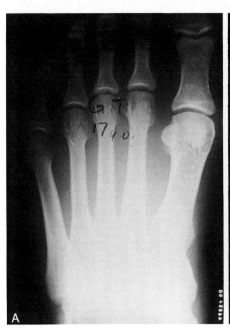 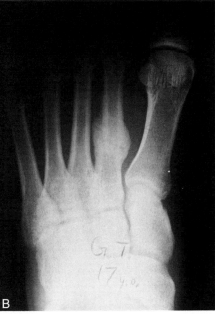

Figure 14–48

Stress fracture of the second metatarsal. *A,* Initial x-ray reveals nondisplaced proximal second metatarsal fracture. *B,* On follow-up, bulbous callus is noted around fracture line at the base of the second metatarsal.

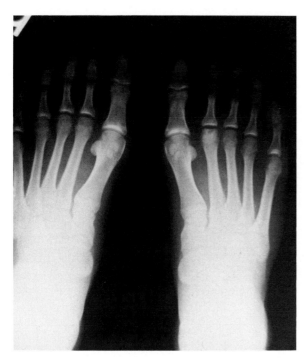

Figure 14–49

This example of Freiberg's disease was noted in an avid soccer player; the head of the second metatarsal of the left foot is flattened. The patient was treated by a hard toeplate in the soccer shoe and continued playing with minimal difficulty.

This can be achieved only if the debridement is done very early; otherwise, if there are multiple fragments in various stages of union, open debridement is not indicated. I recommend rest as the early treatment if there is an acute injury, but following that a hard toeplate should be inserted in the shoe to allow the child to participate in sports activities if desired. I have had no experience with shortening of the metatarsal for this condition.

Fractures of the chondroepiphysis of the second metatarsal occur most frequently as Salter-Harris II fractures of the neck. The injury is rarely displaced. Even those fractures with plantar flexion tend to remodel. The condylar fractures are usually oblique Salter-Harris IV fractures and rarely result in growth injuries (Fig. 14–50). All these injuries have been treated by a below-knee cast with good results.

Third and Fourth Metatarsals

The third and fourth metatarsals are injured not infrequently, usually as the result of indirect trauma; these injuries may occur anywhere along the shaft.

decade. The stress fracture, commonly called a march fracture, usually occurs in runners. We have seen the injury in sedentary children who suddenly increase their walking or running activity (Fig. 14–47). The child complains of persistent pain under the metatarsal arch. The initial x-rays may be negative, but a bone scan is positive. Periosteal cortical hypertrophy or new bone is usually present within 2 weeks following complaints of pain (Fig. 14–48). Treatment most often consists of wearing a hard-soled shoe; rarely is a cast indicated. There is hardly ever a displacement of the fragments.

Freiberg's disease, an osteochondrosis of the second metatarsal head, may be confused with a fracture.[21] The second metatarsal is the longest and most rigidly fixed metatarsal (Fig. 14–49). Repetitive trauma to the articular surface of the distal second metatarsal may cause this injury. The injury usually occurs following intensive training for running sports and has been seen in avid young soccer players. Conservative treatment by rest or wearing a below-knee walking cast is recommended. Small osteochondral fragments may be left in the second metatarsophalangeal joint. Open debridement may be necessary to prevent degenerative joint disease.

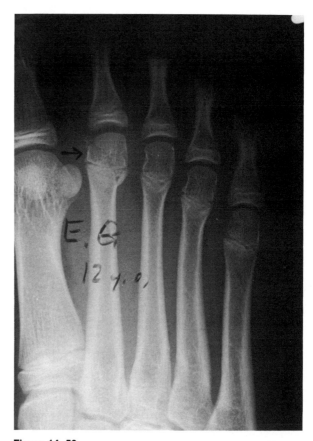

Figure 14–50

A condylar fracture of the metatarsal head; this is a Salter-Harris IV fracture. It healed uneventfully.

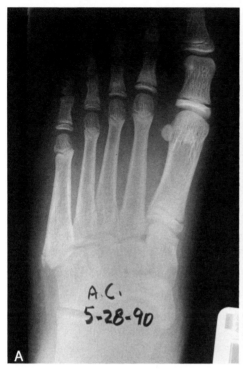
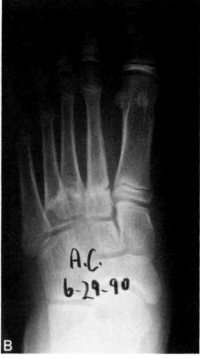

Figure 14–51

Nondisplaced fractures of the base of the metatarsals. The child presented with pain across the base of the forefoot; however, no fractures were noted. The child was placed in a below-knee walking cast and upon return 3 weeks later was noted to have fracture healing lines of the second, third, and fourth metatarsals. *A*, Anteroposterior x-ray of foot showing soft tissue swelling but little evidence of fracture. *B*, Anteroposterior x-ray 1 month later showing healing bone scars at base of inner metatarsals.

More often than not, these fractures are nondisplaced and may not even be seen on initial x-rays (Fig. 14–51). Exceptions are those cases following severe trauma such as vehicular or lawn mower accidents. Persistence of plantar displacement or angulation following reduction is to be avoided because of the prominence over the weight-bearing surface with development of painful callosities. Nonunion of these metatarsals has been noted following severely displaced fractures, but tends to be asymptomatic (Fig. 14–52).

Fifth Metatarsal

The fifth metatarsal is a relatively common area of fracture. This bone was injured in 39 of 104 children and adolescents with metatarsal fractures; the average age was 12 years. The most common mechanism of injury was jumping during an athletic activity, such as basketball or volleyball.[14] The patient may complain acutely of pain over the base of the lateral aspect of the foot and ceases the activity immediately, or the child may present with a painful limp several days later. The initial x-rays may be negative and show only soft tissue swelling over the lateral aspect of the foot. The presence of the os vesalianum in this age group may cause it to be confused with a fracture. The os vesalianum has an oblique distribution or a sagittal line between it and the metatarsal (Fig. 14–53). The true fracture through the metatarsal usually has a transverse orientation (Fig. 14–54). There is a question of avulsion of the base of the fifth metatarsal by the action of the peroneus brevis at its insertion, but this usually applies to the Jones fracture, which is a proximal diaphyseal fracture that occurs in 15- to 20-year-olds; it is not an avulsion fracture.

Kavanaugh and colleagues have emphasized that the Jones fracture is a fracture of the proximal part of the diaphysis of the fifth metatarsal and not an avulsive fracture of the base (despite the incorrect common use of the term).[29] The Jones fracture appears to result from a combination of a vertical loading and medial lateral forces, with the patient weight bearing on the metatarsal heads, concentrating the forces at the proximal fifth metatarsal (Fig. 14–55).

There is a possibility that the avulsion fracture that occurs in the child is the result of the tendinous portion of the abductor digiti minimi and the tough lateral cord of the plantar aponeurosis inserting into the base. The majority of these fractures can be treated by a below-knee walking cast. Nonunion is rare, although it occasionally takes longer than 4 to 6 weeks for radiographic bony union (Fig. 14–56). Those patients not showing union are immobilized only until they are pain-free and then are allowed to return to their athletic activity.

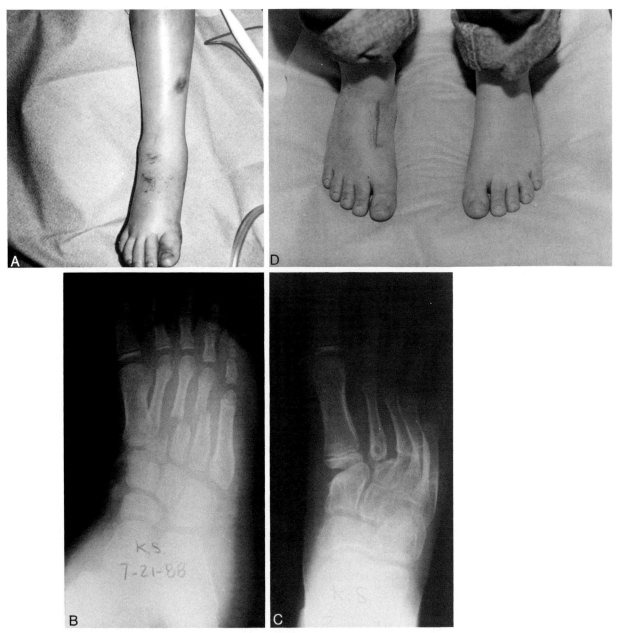

Figure 14–52

This child's foot was run over by a car. She presented with severe swelling and multiple fractures. Immediate decompression was achieved with two longitudinal incisions over the lateral aspect of the first ray and the medial aspect of the fifth ray. The patient did quite well; the wounds were closed with delayed primary closures. She has some tendency to varus positioning of her metatarsals and a nonunion of the base of the second metatarsal; however, she is asymptomatic. *A,* Clinical photograph at time of injury. Forefoot was tense. *B,* Initial x-rays showing soft tissue swelling and displaced metatarsal fractures. *C,* X-rays 18 months later showing union of third and fourth metatarsals and tenuous union of second metatarsal. *D,* Clinical photograph at last follow-up; patient was asymptomatic.

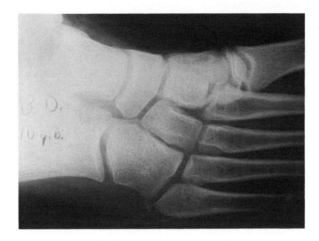

Figure 14-53

Fracture of the os vesalianum. This is an unusual fracture through the accessory apophysis.

Figure 14-54

Fracture to the base of the fifth metatarsal. The oblique x-ray shows anatomic alignment. The anteroposterior view shows minimal displacement.

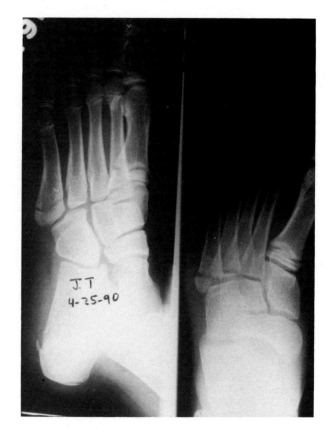

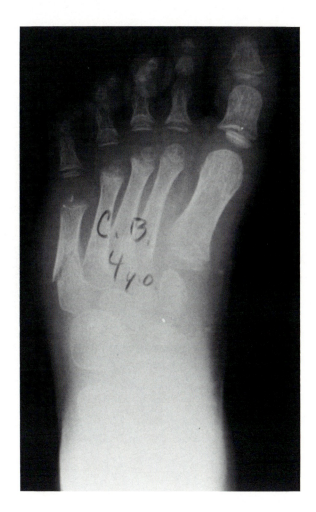

Figure 14–55

Jones fracture through the proximal portion of the fifth metatarsal. The true Jones fracture is quite rare in children, who most often sustain a fifth metatarsal base avulsion fracture.

PHALANGEAL FRACTURES

Phalangeal fractures occurred in 31 of 175 children with fractures about the foot. Twenty fractures (64%) occurred to the proximal phalanges, nine (29%) in the middle, and two (6.4%) to the distal. Indirect trauma, such as stubbing a toe, or direct trauma from a falling object was the usual mechanism of injury. Rarely is operative reduction of a phalangeal fracture necessary; usually traction, manipulative reduction, and taping are all that is needed (Fig. 14–57). If the swelling will allow, wearing a hard-soled shoe is all that is necessary; if not, a below-knee walking cast will suffice.

Fracture of the growth plate of the great toe proximal phalanx may involve the articular surface (Fig. 14–58). The percentage of articular surface involved and its displacement determine the need for anatomic reduction. Open reduction and internal fixation of the fragment is indicated when greater

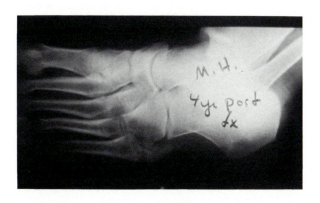

Figure 14–56

An avulsion fracture of the base of the fifth metatarsal. Example of a nonunion of the base of the fifth metatarsal. These injuries are treated only until they are asymptomatic. This child was asymptomatic when seen for another problem approximately 4 years after his initial treatment.

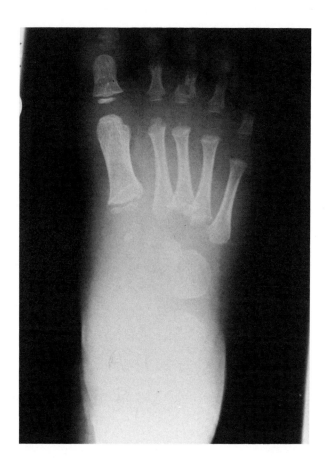

Figure 14–57

A 3-year-old child with a third-ray proximal phalangeal fracture. These injuries may be buddy-taped and tend to do well.

Figure 14–58

A Salter-Harris III fracture through the articular surface of the proximal phalanx. Reduction and fixation are indicated if the fracture involves greater than one third of the articular surface and shows more than 2 mm of separation following reduction.

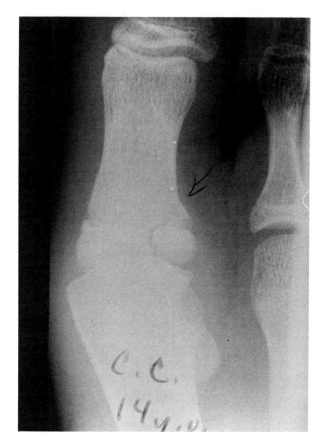

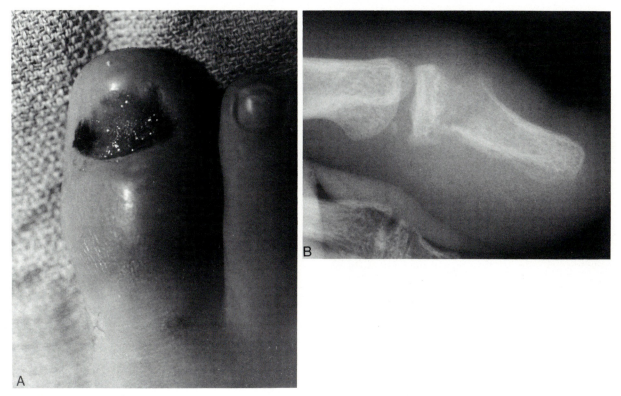

Figure 14–59

"Stubbed-toe" osteomyelitis should be assumed when there is a great toe distal phalangeal injury that extends through the nail matrix. Prophylactic antibiotics are indicated. This child was thought to have an ingrown toenail and the toenail was removed, at which time the treating foot health care professional noted pus draining from the base and referred the child to Children's Hospital. *A,* Clinical photograph of great toe following removal of nail. *B,* Lateral x-ray of great toe showing changes consistent with osteomyelitis at the fracture site.

than 30% of the articular surface is involved or displacement is greater than 3 mm. Following anatomic reduction, the fragment should be pinned to prevent displacement. If this is not done, instability may occur, causing a step-off of the fragments. Degenerative arthritis and hallux rigidus may occur. Rarely does incomplete reduction result in bony bridge formation.

The distal phalangeal epiphyseal fracture of the great toe may be open because of its proximity to the nail matrix (Fig. 14–59). The crushing nature of the injury leaves cracks or breaks in the skin that allow bacterial contamination. The possibility of osteomyelitis should be recognized. Prophylactic antibiotics are recommended for 10 days following this injury. Other management may include (1) irrigation and debridement; (2) reduction, which is rarely necessary if the fracture is not particularly displaced; (3) buddy-taping; (4) a hard-soled shoe; or (5) a below-knee walking cast.

Fractures of the proximal phalanges of the lateral four toes rarely require more than symptomatic treatment. They are rarely displaced enough to require operative treatment. Buddy-taping tends to work well for these fractures. They occasionally will become malaligned, and the angulation does not always correct. Fortunately, these disturbances rarely cause clinical problems.

Open fractures of the phalanges will require debridement and irrigation. The patient should be given parenteral broad-spectrum antibiotics, a tetanus booster, adequate aggressive thorough debridement, and wound dressing changes. It is better to return to the operating room for delayed primary closure than to perform immediate closure of these injuries. Internal fixation is indicated only if the neurovascular bundles are torqued or under tension and do not adequately perfuse at the time of surgery. It is better to have a malunion or growth plate injury in these patients than osteomyelitis.

DISLOCATIONS

Dislocations of the joints of the foot are extremely rare. Only four patients with dislocation of the bones

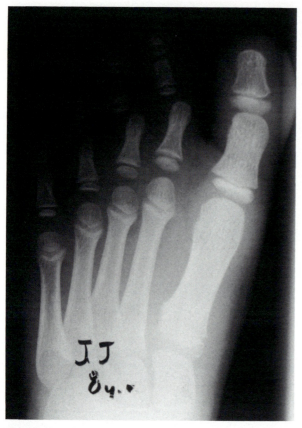

Figure 14–60

Interphalangeal joint dislocations of the second and third toes. Reduction was easily accomplished by longitudinal traction and maintained by buddy-taping.

crunching sound in the rotor blades. The force of injury causes soft tissue contamination by grass, shoe leather, socks, and various other debris. One should never make an early decision concerning the sterility or the ultimate viability of the tissue. The force may cross the physis at multiple levels, possibly even excising the growth center. The injury may include a loss of the articular surfaces and the collateral ligaments. Vigorous debridement and irrigation are carried out immediately. Avulsed tissue is usually less vital than it appears when first seen. This severe trauma may involve degloving of the bone and detachment of the perichondrial rings, permitting a callus bridge to form between the epiphysis and metaphysis, resulting in bar formation across the physes.[60] A vigorous debridement, delayed primary closure, and split-thickness or skin graft (initially with mesh), followed by a cast, brace, or splint, are indicated (Fig. 14–62). I urge resistance against early aggressive closure (e.g., crossleg pedicle) until the issue of wound viability and sterility is resolved.

of the foot were seen in 175 children diagnosed with fractures and other injuries about the foot[14]; three of the four were over 10 years old. All except one sustained proximal interphalangeal joint dislocations of the second and third digits (Fig. 14–60). One child dislocated the metatarsophalangeal joint of the fifth ray (Fig. 14–61). Reductions of all were uneventful; treatment consisted of a buddy-taping and a hard-soled shoe.

LAWN MOWER INJURIES

Lawn mower and threshing machine injuries are quite common in children in rural communities. Considerable judgment is required when managing these injuries. Most often the child is riding on the mower with one of the parents rather than with a sibling. The usual history is that the child will leave to take a break, such as to go to the bathroom. Because of the noise from the mower, the parent is not aware when the child returns, until hearing a

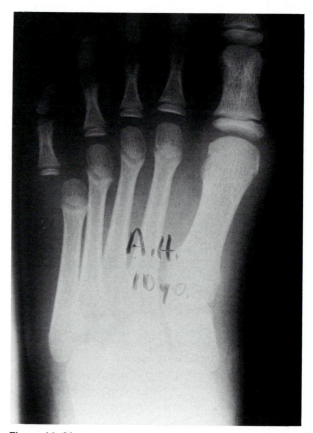

Figure 14–61

A metatarsophalangeal dislocation of the fifth toe. Reduction was achieved by traction and was stable.

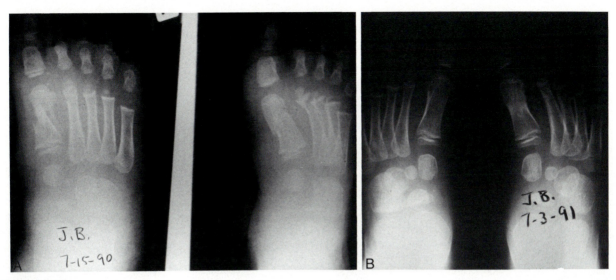

Figure 14–62
This child's foot was run over by a lawn mower. Treatment consisted of irrigation and debridement followed by delayed primary closure. *A*, Initial anteroposterior and oblique x-rays showing markedly comminuted fracture of the first metatarsal and Salter-Harris II fractures of the third and fourth metatarsal necks with marked soft tissue swelling. A pseudoepiphysis occurs at the distal first metatarsal. *B*, Anteroposterior x-ray 1 year later showing healing of all fractures.

LACERATION INJURIES TO THE FOOT

Laceration of soft tissue structures may occur in association with open fractures to the foot. One should carefully examine the limb for injury to nerves, vessels, or tendons. Laceration injuries to the foot may result in deformity, especially if the heel cord, the anterior tibialis tendon, or the posterior tibialis tendon is involved. These are the only tendons requiring immediate or delayed repair. There is little indication for direct repair of the extensor hallucis longus, the long-toe flexor, or the long-toe extensors, because little disability occurs.

PUNCTURE WOUNDS

Puncture wounds require adequate debridement, tetanus toxoid, and a broad-spectrum antibiotic. A small puncture wound may be all that is evident on clinical inspection (Fig. 14–63). If there is a history of stepping on a nail, the diagnosis is clear; if not, an x-ray to rule out a radiopaque foreign body is indicated. Careful exploration of the wound, open Wick catheter drainage, and antibiotics usually resolve the problem. If there is persistent pain and swelling, there is a possibility of osteomyelitis (Fig. 14–63*B* and *C*). If there is a question of osteomyelitis, one should perform a bone scan with either technetium or gallium. *Pseudomonas* is the most common organism cultured from children who have stepped on a nail.[48] The age-old question of tennis sneaker glue harboring *Pseudomonas* has not been answered. With osteomyelitis, there is usually local pain and swelling for 2 or 3 days following the puncture and about 5 to 10 days before local reaction becomes more apparent. One should perform a surgical incision and drainage with aggressive debridement to remove any contaminated tissue. Carbenicillin and gentamicin are the antibiotics of choice. The wound should be left open with a drain inserted. One should be aware of the possibility of premature physeal arrest or avascular necrosis at the epiphysis. If the metacarpophalangeal joint is involved, early chondrolysis of the articular surfaces with fibrosis and subsequent arthritis may occur. The family should be informed of the possibility of growth plate involvement and advised to continue follow-up examination. Several times each year a child presents with a short third or fourth toe with a vague history of stepping on a nail, or with an occult foot injury incurred at an earlier age. It appears in retrospect that osteomyelitis, avascular necrosis, and growth arrest occurred (Fig. 14–64).

FOREIGN BODY

If the child complains of pain and has a persistent limp with no clear history of injury, one has to consider the possibility of a retained foreign body. The object may or may not be visible on x-ray. Although CT scan and MRI have been used in the

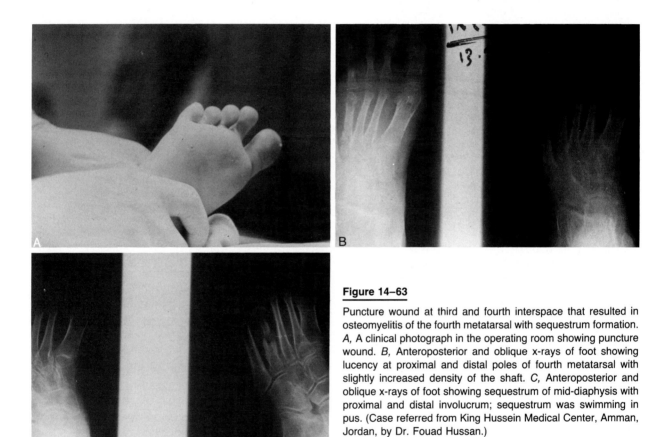

Figure 14–63

Puncture wound at third and fourth interspace that resulted in osteomyelitis of the fourth metatarsal with sequestrum formation. *A,* A clinical photograph in the operating room showing puncture wound. *B,* Anteroposterior and oblique x-rays of foot showing lucency at proximal and distal poles of fourth metatarsal with slightly increased density of the shaft. *C,* Anteroposterior and oblique x-rays of foot showing sequestrum of mid-diaphysis with proximal and distal involucrum; sequestrum was swimming in pus. (Case referred from King Hussein Medical Center, Amman, Jordan, by Dr. Fouad Hussan.)

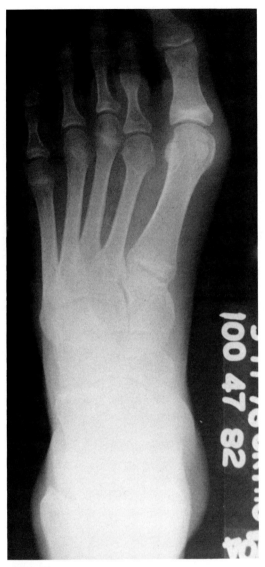

Figure 14–64
This child was seen because the foot was developing a shorter second toe. The history revealed that a nail had penetrated the child's foot when he was younger and the toe became infected. I believe the retrospective history to be that of an osteomyelitis involving the physis with subsequent growth arrest of the metatarsal.

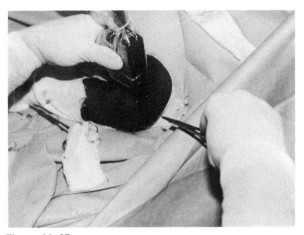

Figure 14–65
The use of ultrasound to remove foreign bodies has allowed us to visualize nonradiopaque as well as radiopaque objects. I strongly recommend its use to prevent the extensive dissection occasionally required to remove nonopaque foreign bodies.

past to localize the object, we now use ultrasound. Ultrasound will pick up both radiodense and radiolucent lesions. The object may be localized and removed under ultrasonic control (Fig. 14–65). Occasionally, a foreign body, such as a needle, is seen in the foot of an asymptomatic patient who receives an x-ray for other reasons (Fig. 14–66). I do not recommend removal of these asymptomatic objects.

Shells from gunshot wounds are a notorious type of foreign body (Fig. 14–67). Most often the wound is accidental, self-inflicted, and located in the forefoot. Depending upon the size and caliber of the bullet, there may be a large amount of soft tissue injury as well as debris, such as shoe leather and socks. There also may be segmental loss of bone. The wound should be vigorously irrigated and debrided but not closed. Multiple dressing changes are carried out, followed by mesh skin graft coverage. Reconstructive procedures should be considered only after all wounds are cleaned and closed, which might take 6 to 8 months.[71]

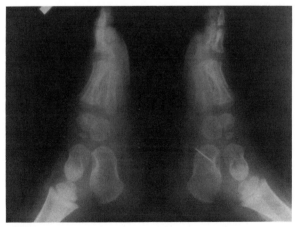

Figure 14–66
A needle in the foot. This child was seen for another problem; the needle had apparently lodged in the foot several years earlier. Removal of an incidentally seen asymptomatic foreign body is contraindicated and is to be condemned.

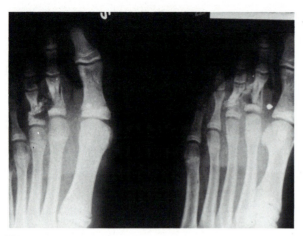

Figure 14–67

A gunshot wound to the forefoot. Note the significant soft tissue swelling, phalangeal fractures, and metallic fragments. Most such injuries are self-inflicted through accident. They require extensive debridement with the possibility of later skin grafting. Amputation is indicated for vascular compromise distal to the metatarsophalangeal joint.

MISCELLANEOUS CAUSES OF FOOT PAIN

Foot pain with reluctance to bear weight with no direct history of trauma should lead one to consider other conditions, including tarsal coalitions, stress fractures, tumors, and early inflammatory arthritis. The cause of pain is usually age-related. If plain x-rays are normal, a bone scan is indicated. The pediatric orthopaedist is often faced with vague nondescript pain, known by the six P's: puzzling and perplexing pain problems in pediatric patients. The bone scan has been of tremendous benefit in these situations.

Tarsal Coalition

This condition is usually heralded by the complaint of repeated ankle sprains and strains in the 8- to 12-year-old child; it is more common in boys than in girls. Because girls have become more active in sports, we now see coalitions in young females. Most often the children are involved in running sports. The most common coalitions are the calcaneonavicular and talocalcaneal. The child may present with lateral foot pain and a flatfoot, the so-called peroneal spastic flatfoot. The pain may be localized to the area of the coalition or may be more diffuse over the midfoot and hindfoot. The pain is activity-related and responds poorly to antiinflammatory drugs. The differential diagnosis must include juvenile rheumatoid arthritis, osteoid osteoma, trauma, infection, neoplasm, and idiopathic peroneal spastic flatfoot. The calcaneonavicular bar is found in younger children, the talocalcaneal in older ones.

The physical examination will show a limitation of subtalar motion. Plain x-rays may show talar beaking on the lateral film for either condition, or there may be an "anteater nose" sign present on the lateral view in the calcaneonavicular coalition (Fig. 14–68). The specific views on plain films that best illustrate the lesions are the Slomann lateral oblique view (Fig. 14–69) for the calcaneonavicular coalition and the axial Harris view (Fig. 14–70) for the talocalcaneal coalition. The CT scan identifies both lesions easily but is most often indicated for the talocalcaneal coalition (Fig. 14–71).

The initial treatment for these lesions consists of immobilization by cast, brace, or shoe inserts. If the pain is not resolved, excision of the bar is indicated. The calcaneonavicular coalition responds best to excision. I recommend excision of the talocalcaneal bar in young adolescents,[49] although better results are reported following triple arthrodesis. If excision does not result in resolution of the symptoms, triple arthrodesis is recommended. Fracture of a tarsal coalition has been reported but is quite rare.[64]

Stress Fractures

Stress fractures usually occur after a sudden increase in activity in a skeletally maturing adolescent who is starting to participate in intensive or repetitive sports training. The condition may be seen as early as 8 to 12 years of age. The most frequent sites are

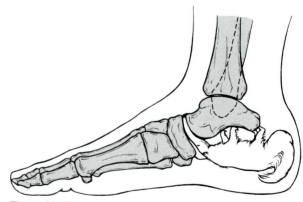

Figure 14–68

The "anteater nose" on plain films illustrating the calcaneonavicular coalition. (From Oestrich, A. E. How to Measure Angles from Foot Radiographs: A Primer. New York: Springer-Verlag, 1990.)

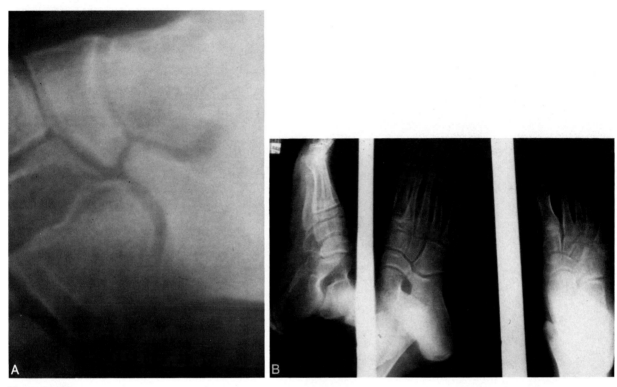

Figure 14–69

A, The Slomann view, an oblique view, which shows an extension of the anterior calcaneal process ("anteater nose") toward the navicular consistent with a calcaneonavicular bar. B, Frame 1—Lateral view showing anterior prolongation of the calcaneal process, "anteater nose." Frame 2—Slomann view showing extension of posterolateral process of the navicular and anterolateral calcaneus. Frame 3—Anteroposterior view showing false articulation between the calcaneus and navicular.

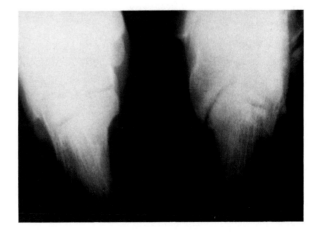

Figure 14–70

The Harris view, an axial view of the subtalar joints illustrating the obliquity of the middle facet on one side in a child with a unilateral talocalcaneal coalition. The image on the left shows the normal middle and posterior facets.

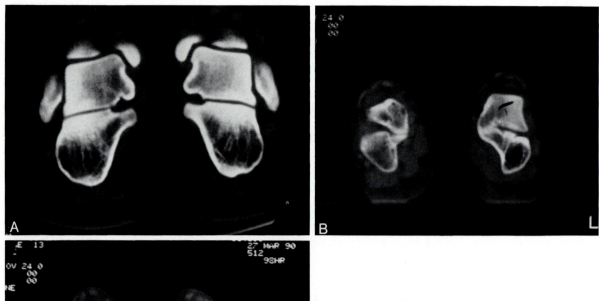

Figure 14–71

A coronal CT scan illustrating the talocalcaneal coalition and its subsequent excision. *A*, Coronal cut through normal subtalar joints. *B*, CT scan showing complete talocalcaneal coalition on the right and partial on the left. The cuts on the right and left are at different levels. *C*, CT scan following excision of talocalcaneal coalition on the left.

the proximal tibia in the 10- to 15-year-old, the distal fibula in the 2- to 5-year-old, and the second metatarsal in older adolescents (see Figs. 14–47 and 14–48).

Pathologic Fractures

Metabolic disease such as end-stage renal osteodystrophy may cause weakening of the bone at the metaphyseal-epiphyseal junction with subsequent fracture following trivial trauma. These same patients may also develop brown tumors following secondary hyperparathyroidism with consequent bone weakening. The bone may also be undermined by constitutional disorders such as idiopathic juvenile osteoporosis, osteogenesis imperfecta, and congenital insensitivity to pain (Fig. 14–72), and therapeutic modalities such as chemotherapy for leukemia or anticonvulsant medication such as phenytoin (Dilantin) for seizure disorders (Fig. 14–73).

Tumors

Tumors rarely present in the lower leg and foot, possibly because they occur most often in the areas of the most active growth plates. There is less activity of the growth plates in the lower leg and foot. The lesions most frequently seen are osteochondromas, nonossifying fibromas, and rarely a

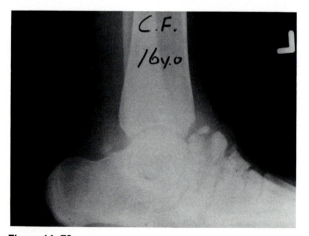

Figure 14–72

This child has familial dysautonomia (congenital insensitivity to pain). This lateral x-ray of the foot and ankle shows Charcot-like joints at the talonavicular cuneiform joints.

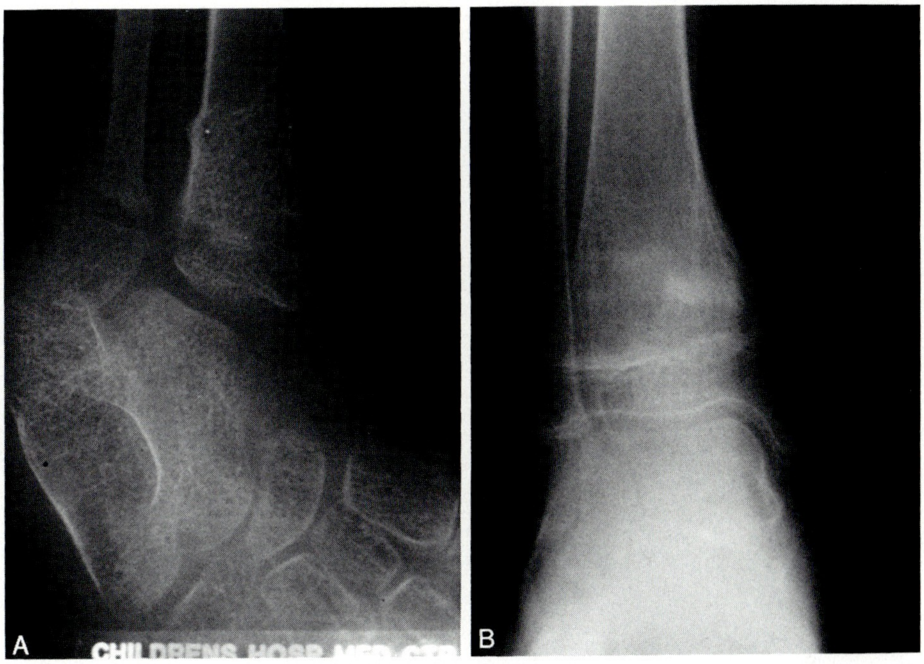

Figure 14–73

Pathologic fractures through osteopenic bone. *A*, A pathologic fracture in a child with Dilantin rickets and abnormal bone. Note the widened fibular and tibial physis. *B*, This anteroposterior x-ray shows horizontal trabecular densities and osteopenia in a young girl diagnosed as having juvenile osteoporosis.

malignancy. Except for the osteochondroma, most lesions will present as pathologic fractures. Several children have presented with what appeared to be recurrent ingrown toenails of the great toe, which have subsequently been diagnosed as subungual exostoses (Fig. 14–74). Osteochondromas are benign bone tumors found in growing children. They may be sessile (broad, flat base) or pedunculated (narrow base with mushroom head) and may be solitary or multiple. Multiple osteochondroma is usually an autosomal dominant hereditary condition, hence, the term multiple hereditary osteochondroma. The occurrence of these lesions around the ankle frequently gives rise to a valgus deformity. The deformity is supramalleolar and usually causes little pain; there is only deformity and decrease in joint motion (Fig. 14–75). Night pain in the foot relieved by aspirin is an unusual clinical presentation. A suspicious bone scan in one patient led to an excisional biopsy, which revealed an osteoid osteoma (Fig. 14–76). The occasional rare malignancy in the ankle and foot is preferably treated by amputation rather than limb salvage procedures (Fig. 14–77).

Bicycle Spoke Injuries

These injuries occur in early walkers, usually between 2 and 8 years of age. A fracture, if present, is not often as important as the soft tissue injury. Initially, the foot may appear to be normal with no significant injury because none of the bones is broken.[26] The foot subsequently tends to swell and exhibit soft tissue problems. This pathobiologic picture is similar to that seen in the crush injury due to a washing machine wringer. I recommend that soft tissue decompression be done early, if necessary, followed by delayed primary closure or skin graft. It is more important to resolve the issue of crush injury to the tissue than to manage the fracture in this situation.

Child Abuse

Child abuse injuries are not uncommon in our society today. In 1860, Tardieu published the first article that clearly identified features associated with the battered child syndrome.[73] Silverman clearly defined the traumatic nature of the lesions.[69] King and co-workers reviewed 429 fractures in 189 battered children and found that 50% of patients had a single fracture.[31] The battered child syndrome is very difficult to diagnose in a child with a single, acute fracture. The orthopaedic surgeon should not discount the possibility of child abuse when there is only a single, fresh diaphyseal fracture.[31] Child battering should be suspected when there is significant swelling in and about the foot and ankle, especially in a child who has not started walking. X-rays reveal evidence of metaphyseal corner fractures, which represent periosteal new bone formation. These metaphyseal corner fractures, "Silverman's rings," are usually indicative, if not diagnostic, of child

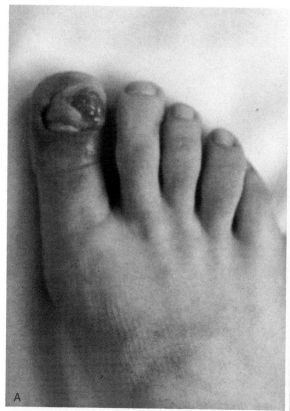 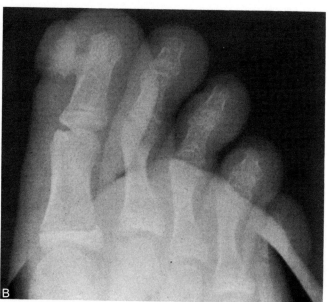

Figure 14-74

An example of subungual exostosis of the great toe. Several children who presented with this lesion were subsequently diagnosed with multiple hereditary exostosis. *A*, The child complained of an ingrown toenail that had recurred three times. *B*, An oblique x-ray of the toe. Excision of the exostosis resulted in complete relief. (From Crawford, A. H. Pediatric Orthopaedic Surgery, 2nd ed. Burbank, CA, Science Communications, 1988.)

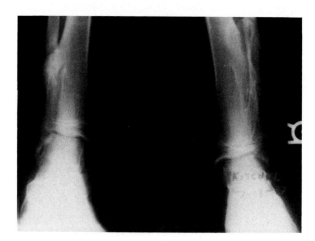

Figure 14-75

Multiple hereditary osteochondroma causing ankle valgus. Painless foot and ankle valgus deformity is a common finding in multiple hereditary osteochondroma. The more affected limb is often shorter.

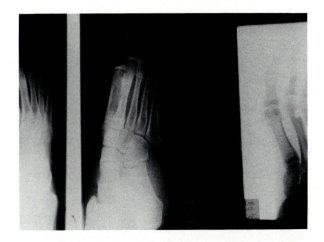

Figure 14–76

Although the foot is an unusual location for an osteoid osteoma, this child presented with foot pain at night that was relieved by aspirin. *Frame 1*—Anteroposterior x-ray showing increased density of distal second metatarsal with small lucent nidus. *Frame 2*—Oblique view shows a circumscribed density of the second metatarsal. *Frame 3*—Postexcision x-ray. The pathologic diagnosis was osteoid osteoma.

abuse (Fig. 14–78). The injury usually can be treated by immobilization; however, it is most important to separate the child from his or her environment. The potential for reinjury and possible death makes separation mandatory.

Complications of Injuries to the Distal Tibial and Fibular Growth Plates

1. *Angular deformity secondary to asymmetric arrest of the distal tibial growth plate.* The deformity is usually varus and is most frequently seen with the Salter-Harris III and IV medial malleolar injuries. The adduction injury most commonly results in a varus deformity. Following an adduction injury, a direct compressive force is applied to the epiphyseal plate by the talus, resulting in premature closure of that part of the plate, leading to angular deformity (Fig. 14–79). Anatomic reduction by open or closed means is necessary when the fracture involves the medial malleolus (Salter-Harris III or IV) because incomplete anatomic reduction will result in subsequent deformity.[34] Anatomic reduction and fixation will usually prevent this problem. Creative

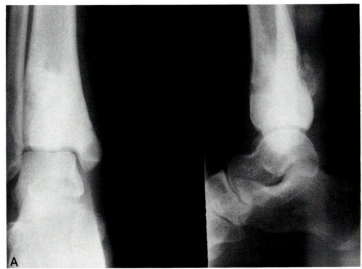
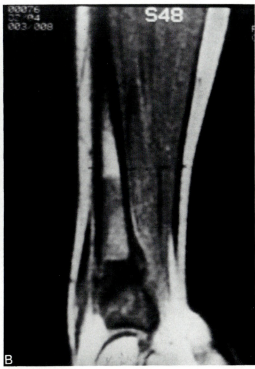

Figure 14–77

Osteogenic sarcoma of the distal tibia. *A,* Lateral x-ray of foot and ankle; note sunburst lesion with breakthrough of posterior cortex. *B,* MRI shows canal involvement of neoplasm. I recommend against limb salvage for these tumors because the BK prosthesis is much more functional.

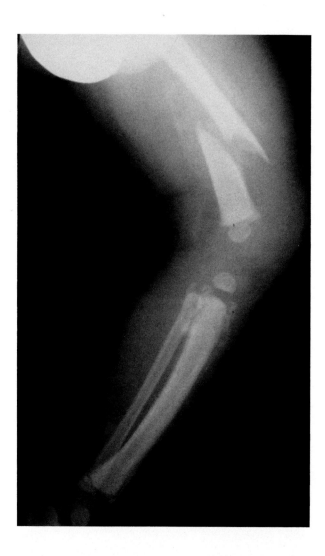

Figure 14-78

This lateral x-ray of the leg and foot of a battered child shows an obvious displaced femoral fracture; there are other characteristic, if not diagnostic, signs. The calcific densities at the proximal and distal tibial epiphyses represent the periosteal new bone response to torsional twisting injuries. The periosteal new bone that surrounds the epiphysis is called Silverman's rings, considered to be diagnostic of battered child syndrome.

opening or closing wedge osteotomies have been used successfully to lessen the leg length discrepancy caused by partial growth arrest when there is minimal discrepancy. An epiphysiodesis of the distal tibia and fibula may be performed to prevent an angular deformity if the child has less than 2 years of growth remaining. Correction by epiphysiolysis may be successful if less than 50% of the cross-sectional area of the physis is involved.[55] Epiphysiolysis is an adequate, if not excellent, procedure to perform when there has been a partial growth arrest of the distal tibia. The child should have more than 3 years of growth remaining. The amount of involvement of the growth plate can be well documented graphically by the use of anterior and lateral polycycloidal tomography to map out the physeal bar. When performing epiphysiolysis, one has to remember that the fibula is more often than not abnormally remodeled, and osteotomy may be necessary. If the angulation of the distal tibia is greater than 20 degrees varus, one should consider a supramalleolar tibial and fibular osteotomy in addition to the epiphysiolysis.

2. *Angular deformity secondary to malunion.* This unusual complication is seen more frequently in the older adolescent. Angulation of less than 20 degrees can be expected to remodel in children under 10 years of age. We tend to give injuries with less than 20 degrees of angulation approximately 2 years to remodel to within 10 degrees, or to within limits acceptable to the parents, prior to considering an osteotomy. Angulation of less than 15 degrees rarely causes functional disability. Residual valgus deformities are usually more acceptable than varus. Angular deformities in the plane of motion tend to remodel more readily. Supramalleolar osteotomy is usually considered when the child is too old for epiphysiolysis and also as a complement to bar excision in the older child, or when residual varus/valgus angulation is greater than 20 degrees.

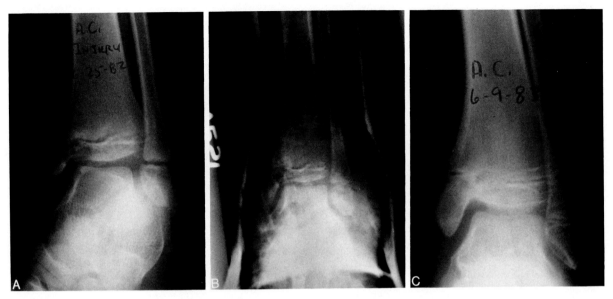

Figure 14–79

This child sustained a Salter-Harris IV medial malleolar fracture of the distal tibia that resulted in a growth plate injury. The growth plate injury in turn resulted in a physeal bar, causing a varus deformity. The bar was removed, fat was interposed, and growth was reestablished. *A*, Initial x-ray of ankle showing minimal displacement. *B*, X-ray through plaster cast consistent with anatomic reduction. *C*, X-ray 1 year later showing bony bar. Note the Park-Harris line angulated from the bar.

3. *Leg length discrepancy.* Direct bone lengthening is another option for the management of growth problems following fractures. From 10 to 30% of lengthening procedures to the lower extremity are carried out for correction of discrepancies following injury to the growth plates. One-stage, step-cut procedures or opening or closing wedge osteotomies may be performed for correction of discrepancies within 1 inch. Greater discrepancy may be addressed by contralateral open or closed epiphysiodesis or ipsilateral leg lengthening. The most frequently used lengthening procedures include the Wagner gradual distraction followed by osteosynthesis,[79] and callotasis techniques of de Bastiani[63] or Ilizarov.[25] The axial distraction osteogenesis or callotasis methods used to lengthen with periosteally stimulated regenerate bone are the most popular at the time of this writing. All have been found to be quite satisfactory in the management of limb length inequality. The most popular techniques utilize the monaxial fixator or the circular frame. The monaxial fixator frame is less bulky than the circular frame lengthener. It is an excellent method to use for the femur. The monaxial fixator may cause the tibia to go into valgus unless it is applied in an anteroposterior direction instead of lateral. The circular frame is preferred when angular and rotational deformity is associated with tibial shortening and length discrepancy.

4. *Osteoarthritis* may occur secondary to persistent residual joint incongruity. The condition usually follows failure to achieve anatomic reduction of interfragmentary gaps greater than 3 mm. The use of current radiographic imaging technology may increase our awareness of this problem and prevent its occurrence. Prevention may be achieved by open or closed anatomic reduction and stabilization.

Another reason for osteoarthritis may be unappreciated damage to the articular cartilage. The impact of the trauma may damage the subchondral plate. Irreversible damage to these cartilage cells causes localized failure of the articular weight-bearing surface, leading to shearing down to subchondral bone and chondrolysis. There may be consequent damage to the articular component of an adjacent structure, e.g., tibia to talar dome.

5. *Rotational deformities.* This complication is unusual and, if significant, can be easily corrected by supramalleolar osteotomy. Both bones should be osteotomized; however, it may not be necessary to transfix the fibula.

6. *Nonunion or delayed union.* These complications

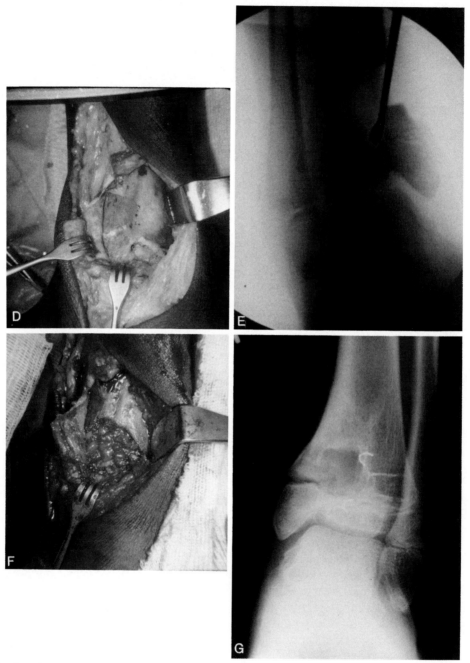

Figure 14–79 Continued

D, Intraoperative photograph showing bone bridge across growth plate. *E*, Intraoperative Polaroid x-ray showing curette across resected physeal bar. *F*, Operative photograph showing fat through bone window. *G*, Anteroposterior x-ray following excision of bar and resumption of growth. The metallic clips are used as markers to monitor future growth.

are extremely rare but may occur. Operative management of nonunion or delayed union rarely has been required for fractures below the distal third of the tibia. Nonunion of the metacarpals may be asymptomatic and thus not require treatment. We have treated segmental loss of a metatarsal following a lawn mower injury by autologous fibular interposition grafting with good results.

7. *Avascular necrosis of the distal tibial physis.* This is an extremely rare condition and has been reported only once in the English language literature.[68]

Aphorisms for Ankle and Foot Injuries

Parents should be made aware of the *possibility of a growth injury any time an epiphysis is fractured.* If the child is seen in the emergency room, the attending physician should impress upon the parents how serious this issue is. The parents must be informed and aware of the injury's potential growth-related problems. The worst development is when growth arrest occurs and the parent has not even been made aware of the possibility.

Closed reduction is usually possible for most injuries around the foot and ankle. If the patient is under general anesthesia and anatomic reduction is accomplished, I very strongly recommend percutaneous Steinmann pinning or percutaneous use of an interfragmentary screw. The new cannulated cancellous screws are optimal for this technique. The need for open reduction is minimal if the injuries are treated within 48 hours.

Soft tissue "goose egg" swelling over the distal fibula usually represents a Salter-Harris type I growth plate injury. The fibular physeal fracture may or may not accompany a distal tibial physeal injury. After several weeks of treating an ankle sprain, the appearance of calcification around the distal fibular metaphysis or in the interosseous ligament is indicative of a previously unrecognized fracture.

Epiphyseal injuries should be reduced within the first 24 to 48 hours; repeat manipulation after 5 or 6 days may be difficult and can cause epiphyseal damage. I would rather accept the malreduction after 1 week than to risk injury to the growth plate.

The distal tibia and fibula ossification centers may vary, and sometimes this causes the diagnosis of fracture to be difficult. In most of these instances, the fracture is very minor with minimal displacement and is adequately treated with simple immobilization. A bone scan will differentiate an anomalous ossification pattern from a fracture.

Close attention must be paid to the direction of growth plate injury displacement, especially the metaphyseal fragment. The direction of displacement of the metaphyseal fragment determines the mechanism of injury in most circumstances.

Epiphyseal articular fragment displacement of greater than 2 mm requires reduction. CT scan can be used not only for the diagnosis of these injuries but also in some cases for assessment of the reduction. It is more important that the reduction of the articular cartilage be anatomic than that of the metaphyseal-epiphyseal junction, which tends to remodel unless angulation is excessive or there is a growth plate arrest. If the metaphyseal fragment of the medial malleolar Salter-Harris IV fracture cannot be reduced, it can usually be discarded so long as the epiphyseal fracture is anatomically reduced.

An eccentric bony bridge is more likely to cause angular deformity than to significantly slow growth in a distal tibial injury because the central growth plate is too strong.

Following injury, one should look closely at the growth arrest lines (Park-Harris) for evidence of bony bridging. These lines should be horizontal, and any tendency toward angulation into the fracture site indicates bony bridge formation.

A residual deformity of greater than 2 mm displacement of the weight-bearing articular surface following reduction has not been consistent with a good result. A greater than 3 mm interfragmentary gap on initial x-ray has not been consistent with successful closed reduction. Open reduction should be considered if manipulation under general anesthesia does not enable better fragment apposition. After having achieved anatomic reduction, one should be alert to possible instability; bearing this in mind, I very strongly recommend a percutaneous pin or percutaneous interfragmentary screw to maintain stability.

Unrecognized damage to the articular cartilage at the time of injury may lead to chondrolysis and long-term symptoms in spite of adequate reduction and normal-appearing x-rays. The articular cartilage has poor remodeling potential, and injury tends to lead to arthritic changes.

Growth arrest is rare in the triplane fracture. The child is usually an adolescent without much longitudinal growth remaining. The major residual problem is joint incongruity or an interfragmentary gap greater than 3 mm, resulting in degenerative arthritis. All x-rays of the ankle should be made in no fewer than three planes; if necessary, a polytomogram or a limited CT scan can be used to determine the direction and reduction of the fracture fragments.

Mandatory follow-up of growth plate injuries in children under 12 years of age for 1 year is necessary. Managed health care plans are becoming more prevalent, with patients constantly switching physicians as the plan dictates. This movement makes it extremely difficult to follow patients who may or may not have a current problem but have suffered a growth plate injury with predictable future disability. One must be aware of "disappearing patients."

Angular deformity and shortening are usually asymptomatic. The patient returns because of deformity and not pain. Joint incongruity and articular cartilage injury leading to degenerative joint disease are more significant long-term problems that do cause pain.

The compartments of the foot are tight. Decompression is indicated for any persistent swelling, venous congestion, or taut skin or when multiple bones are involved.

Displacement of metatarsal fractures is rare, but nonunion is not uncommon. Lateral displacement of the middle metatarsal (second through fourth) fracture fragments with varus or valgus is acceptable, tends to remodel, and does not cause problems. Dorsal or plantar displacement is not acceptable because the resulting angular deformity will alter the weight-bearing pattern, leading to painful callosities.

One should avoid a primary circular cast for most ankle injuries; this may cause a tourniquet effect. I recommend the use of a bulky dressing for initial management of these injuries. After several days, when the swelling is decreased, a well-molded cast is satisfactory.

Open reduction and internal fixation of foot fractures are rarely indicated and should be avoided, if possible. Growth inhibition in and around the foot is unusual; overgrowth is more common. Usually the only indications for open reduction of foot fractures are open injuries and significant soft tissue injury.

Acknowledgment

Kind appreciation is extended to Ms. Beverly DeFiglia for her indefatigable support with preparation of this manuscript.

REFERENCES

1. Aitken, A. P. Fractures of the epiphyses. Clin Orthop 41:19–23, 1965.
2. Anderson, D. V.; Lyne, E. D. Osteochondritis dissecans of the talus: Case report on two family members. J Pediatr Orthop 4:356–357, 1984.
3. Ashhurst, A. P.; Bromer, R. S. Classification and mechanism of fractures of the leg bones involving the ankle. Arch Surg 4:51, 1922.
4. Berndt, A. L.; Harty, M. Transchondral fractures (osteochondritis dissecans). J Bone Joint Surg 41-A:988–1020, 1959.
5. Bishop, P. A. Fractures and epiphyseal separation fractures of the ankle: Classification of 332 cases according to mechanism of their production. Am J Roentgenol 28:49–67, 1932.
6. Broock, G. J.; Greer, R. B. Traumatic rotational displacements of the distal tibial growth plate. J Bone Joint Surg 52-A:1666–1668, 1970.
7. Canale, S. T.; Belding, R. H. Osteochondral lesions of the talus. J Bone Joint Surg 62-A:97–102, 1980.
8. Canale, S. T.; Kelly, F. B., Jr. Fractures of the neck of the talus. Long-term evaluation of 71 cases. J Bone Joint Surg 60-A:143–156, 1978.
9. Carlson, W. O.; Wenger, D. R. A mapping method to prepare for surgical excision of a partial arrest. J Pediatr Orthop 4:232, 1984.
10. Carothers, C. O.; Crenshaw, A. H. Clinical significance of a classification of epiphyseal injuries at the ankle. Am J Surg 89:879–887, 1955.
11. Cooperman, D. R.; Spiegel, P. G.; Laros, G. S. Tibial fractures involving the ankle in children: The so-called triplane epiphyseal fracture. J Bone Joint Surg 60-A:1040–1046, 1978.
12. Crawford, A. H.: Triplane fracture. Orthop Consult 68:12, 1983.
13. Crawford, A. H. Pediatric Orthopaedic Surgery. Burbank, Science Image Communications, 1988.
14. Crawford, A. H. Fractures about the foot in children: A radiographic analysis. Cincinnati, The Children's Hospital Medical Center, 1991 (unpublished data).
15. Dias, L. S.; Giegerich, C. R. Fractures of the distal tibial epiphysis in adolescence. J Bone Joint Surg 65-A:438–444, 1983.
16. Dias, L. S.; Tachdjian, M. O. Physeal injuries of the ankle in children: Classification. Clin Orthop 136:230–233, 1978.
17. Erlich, M. G. The problem: Distal tibial fracture in a child. Orthop Consult 7:1–10, 1986.
18. Ertl, J. P.; Barrack, R. L.; Alexander, A. H.; Van Buecken, K. Triplane fracture of the distal tibial epiphysis: Long-term follow-up. J Bone Joint Surg 70-A:967–976, 1988.
19. Essex-LoPresti, P. The mechanism, reduction technique, and results in fractures of the os calcis. Br J Surg 39:395–419, 1952.
20. Falkenberg, M. P.; Dickens, D. R.; Menelaus, M. B. Osteochondritis of the first metatarsal epiphysis. J Pediatr Orthop 10:797–799, 1990.
21. Freiberg, A. Infraction of the second metatarsal bone, a typical injury. Surg Gynecol Obstet 19:191–193, 1914.
22. Grogan, D. P.; Walling, A. K.; Ogden, J. A. Anatomy of the os trigonum. J Pediatr Orthop 10:618–622, 1990.
23. Gross, R.: Fractures and dislocations of the foot. In: Rockwood, C. A.; Green, D. P., eds. Fractures. Philadelphia, J. B. Lippincott, 1975.

24. Hawkins, L. G. Fractures of the neck of the talus. J Bone Joint Surg 52-A:991–1002, 1970.
25. Ilizarov, G. A.; Devitav, A. A. Operative elongation of the leg with simultaneous correction of deformities. Ortop Travmatol Protez 30:32, 1969.
26. Izant, R. J., Jr.; Rothmann, B. F.; Frankel, V. H. Bicycle spoke injuries of the foot and ankle in children: An underestimated "minor" injury. J Pediatr Surg 4:654–656, 1969.
27. Johnson, R. P.; Collier, B. D.; Carrera, G. F. Os trigonum syndrome: Use of bone scan in the diagnosis. J Trauma 24:761–764, 1984.
28. Karrholm, J.; Hansson, L. I.; Laurin, S. Pronation injuries of the ankle in children: Retrospective study of radiographical classification and treatment. Acta Orthop Scand 54:1–17, 1983.
29. Kavanaugh, J. H.; Brower, T. D.; Mann, R. V. The Jones fracture revisited. J Bone Joint Surg 60-A:776–782, 1978.
30. Kaye, J. J.; Bohne, W. H. A radiographic study of the ligamentous anatomy of the ankle. Radiology 125:659–667, 1977.
31. King, J., Diefendorf, D., Apthorp, J., et al. Analysis of 429 fractures in 189 battered children. J Pediatr Orthop 8:585–589, 1988.
32. Kleiger, B.; Mankin, H. J. Fracture of the lateral portion of the distal tibial epiphysis. J Bone Joint Surg 46-A:25–32, 1964.
33. Kling, T. F., Jr.: Operative treatment of ankle fractures in children. Orthop Clin North Am 21:381–392, April 1990.
34. Kling, T. F., Jr.; Bright, R. W.; Hensinger, R. N. Distal tibial physeal fractures in children that may require open reduction. J Bone Joint Surg 66-A:647–657, 1984.
35. Konig F. Ueber freie Korper in den Gelenken. Dtsch Z Chir 27:90–109, 1888.
36. Kump, W. L. Vertical fractures of the distal tibial epiphysis. Clin Orthop 73:132–135, 1970.
37. Lauge-Hansen, N. Fractures of the ankle. Combined experimental-surgical and experimental-roentgenological investigations. Arch Surg 60:957–985, 1950.
38. Leitch, J. M.; Cundy, P. J.; Paterson, D. C. Case report: Three-dimensional imaging of a juvenile Tillaux fracture. J Pediatr Orthop 9:602–603, 1989.
39. Letts, R. M.; Gibeault, D. Fractures of the neck of the talus in children. Foot Ankle 1:74–77, 1980.
40. Letts, R. M.; Greenspoon, J.; Rosman, M. Medial osteochondritis of the talus in children: Review and new surgical management. J Pediatr Orthop 7:705–708, 1987.
41. Lovell, E. S. An unusual rotatory injury to the ankle. J Bone Joint Surg 50-A:163–165, 1968.
42. Lynn, M. D. The triplane distal tibial epiphyseal fracture. Clin Orthop 86:187–190, 1972.
43. Mann, R. A. Biomechanics of the foot. In: American Academy of Orthopedic Surgeons: Atlas of Orthotics. Biomechanical Principles and Applications. St. Louis, C. V. Mosby, 1975, pp. 257–266.
44. Marmor, L. An unusual fracture of the tibial epiphysis. Clin Orthop 73:132–135, 1970.
45. Matteri, R. E.; Frymoyer, J. W. Fracture of the calcaneus in young children: Report of 3 cases. J Bone Joint Surg 55-A:1091–1094, 1973.
46. McFarland, B. Industrial aspect of fractures of os calcis. Br Med J 1:607–610, 1937.
47. McNealy, G. A.; Rogers, L. F.; Hernandez, R.; Pozananski, A. K. Injuries of the distal tibial epiphysis: Systematic radiographic evaluation. AJR 138:683, 1982.
48. Miller, E. H.; Semian, D. W. Gram-negative osteomyelitis following puncture wounds of the foot. J Bone Joint Surg 57-A:535–537, 1975.
49. Morgan, R. C., Jr.; Crawford, A. H. Surgical management of tarsal coalition in adolescent athletes. Foot Ankle 7:183–193, 1986.
50. Morris, J. M. Biomechanics of the foot and ankle. Clin Orthop 122:10, 1977.
51. Mulfinger, G. L.; Trueta, J. The blood supply of the talus. J Bone Joint Surg 52-B:160–167, 1970.
52. Nevelos, A. B.; Colton, C. L. Rotational displacement of the lower tibial epiphysis due to trauma. J Bone Joint Surg 59-B:331–332, 1977.
53. Ogden, J. A. Skeletal Injury in the Child. Philadelphia, Lea & Febiger, 1982, pp. 621–641.
54. Ogden, J. A.; Lee, J. Accessory ossification patterns and injuries of the malleoli. J Pediatr Orthop 10:306–316, 1990.
55. Peterson, H. A. Partial growth plate arrest. In: Morrissy, R.T., ed. Lovell and Winter's Pediatric Orthopaedics, 3rd ed, Vol. 1. Philadelphia, J.B. Lippincott, 1990.
56. Peterson, H. A.; Burkhart, S. S. Compression injury of the epiphyseal growth plate: Fact or fiction? J Pediatr Orthop 1:377–384, 1981.
57. Peterson, C. A.; Peterson, H. A. Analysis of the incidence of injuries to the epiphyseal growth plate. J Trauma 12:275–281, 1972.
58. Pick, M. P. Familial osteochondritis dissecans. J Bone Joint Surg 37-B:142–145, 1955.
59. Poland, J. Traumatic separation of the epiphysis. London, Smith, Elder and Company, 1898.
60. Rang, M. Children's Fractures. Philadelphia, J. B. Lippincott, 1974.
61. Rendu A. Fracture intra-articulaire parcellaire de la poulie astragalienne. Lyon Med 150:220–222, 1932.
62. Renner, R. R.; Mauler, G. G.; Ambrose, J. L. The radiologist, the orthopedist, the lawyer, and the fracture. Semin Roentgenol 13:7–18, 1978.
63. Renzi-Brivio, L.; Lavini, F.; de Bastiani, G. Lengthening in the congenital short femur. Clin Orthop 250:112–116, 1990.
64. Richards, R. R.; Evans, J. G.; McGoey, P. F. Fracture of a calcaneonavicular bar: A complication of tarsal coalition. A case report. Clin Orthop 185:220–221, 1984.
65. Salter, R. B.; Harris, W. R. Injuries involving the epiphyseal plate. J Bone Joint Surg 45-A:587–622, 1963.
66. Schmidt, T. L.; Weiner, D. S. Calcaneal fractures in children: An evaluation of the nature of the injury in 56 children. Clin Orthop 171:150–155, 1982.
67. Schofield, R. O. Fractures of os calcis. J Bone Joint Surg 18-B:566–580, 1936.
68. Siffert, R. S.; Arkin, A. M. Post-traumatic aseptic necrosis of the distal tibial epiphysis. J Bone Joint Surg 32-A:691–694, 1950.
69. Silverman, F. N. Unrecognized trauma in infants, the battered child syndrome, and the syndrome of Ambrose Tardieu. Radiology 104:337–353, 1972.
70. Spiegel, P. G.; Cooperman, D. R.; Laros, G. S. Epiphyseal fractures of the distal ends of the tibia and fibula. A retrospective study of 237 cases in children. J Bone Joint Surg 60-A:1046–1050, 1978.
71. Stucky, W.; Loder, R. T. Extremity gunshot wounds in children. J Pediatr Orthop 11:67–71, 1991.
72. Tachdjian, M. O. Pediatric Orthopedics, 2nd ed. Philadelphia, W. B. Saunders, 1990.
73. Tardieu, A. Etude medico-legale sur les services et mauvais traitments exercés sur des enfants. Ann Hyg Publ Med Leg 13:361–398, 1860.

74. Thomas, H. M. Calcaneal fracture in childhood. Br J Surg 56:664–666, 1969.
75. Tomaschewski, H. K. Ergebnisse der Behandlung des posttraumatischen Fehlwuchses des Fusses bei Kindern und Jugendlichen. Beitr Orthop Traumatol 22:90, 1975.
76. Torg, J. S.; Ruggiero, R. A. Comminuted epiphyseal fracture of the distal tibia. A case report and review of the literature. Clin Orthop 110:215–217, 1975.
77. Trias, A.; Ray, R. D. Juvenile osteochondritis of the radial head. Report of a bilateral case. J Bone Joint Surg 45-A:576–582, 1963.
78. Trillat, A.; Lerat, J. L.; LeClerc, P.; Schuster, P. Tarsometatarsal fracture-dislocations. Rev Chir Orthop 62:685–702, 1976.
79. Wagner, H. Operative lengthening of the femur. Clin Orthop 136:125, 1978.
80. Walter, E.; Feine, U.; Anger, K.; et al. Szintigraphische diagnostik und verlaufskontrolle bei epiphysenfugen verletzunger. Fortschr Geb Rontgenstr Nuklearmed Erganzungsband 132:309–315, 1980.
81. Waugh, W. The ossification and vascularisation of the tarsal navicular and their relation to Köhler's disease. J Bone Joint Surg 40-B:765–777, 1958.
82. White, J. Osteochondritis dissecans in association with dwarfism. J Bone Joint Surg 39B:261–267, 1957.
83. Wiley, J. J. Tarsometatarsal joint injuries in children. J Pediatr Orthop 1:255–260, 1981.
84. Zellweger, V. H.; Ebnother, M. Uber eine familiare Skelettstorung mit multilocularen, aseptischem Knochennekrosen, insbesondere mit Osteochondritis dissecans. Helv Paediatr Acta 6:95–111, 1951.

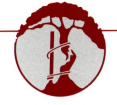

Neil E. Green, M.D.

15

Child Abuse

Child abuse is a serious problem that touches the lives of many people yearly. Although the actual incidence of child abuse is not known with certainty, it is suspected that for every reported case of child abuse, many others go unreported. It is estimated that every year more than 1 million children in the United States are seriously abused by their parents, guardians, or others and that between 2000 and 5000 children die annually as a result of injuries sustained from abuse.[23] The National Committee for Prevention of Child Abuse reported that the number of confirmed deaths from child abuse increased from 1253 in 1990 to 1383 in 1991.[13] For the purposes of this chapter we will deal only with physical abuse, which is estimated to occur more than 125,000 times each year. Other types of abuse are also recognized, and the orthopaedic surgeon should be familiar with them, because recognition of signs of neglect, sexual abuse, or emotional maltreatment may direct attention to the possibility that the trauma being treated may not be the result of accidental injury.

Recognition of abuse is extremely important in order to protect the involved child as well as any siblings. It has been stated that 10% of emergency room trauma in children under 3 years of age is nonaccidental, as are 30% of head and limb injuries and fractures in this age group.[27] Between 30 and 50% of physically abused children are seen by orthopaedic surgeons.[41] Abused children are likely to be the victims of repeated abuse, and the second incident may be fatal for as many as 10% of them.

History

Although the radiographic findings of child abuse have been known for more than a century, it was not until 1946 that Caffey studied six children with chronic subdural hematomas and fractures of long bones with no history of injury.[7] He stated that they did not have a systemic disease that could explain the radiographic findings and felt that injury to the children was responsible for the findings. He further suggested that children with unexplained long bone fractures should be investigated for chronic subdural hematoma, and vice versa.

In 1953 Silverman described periosteal new bone formation associated with irregular fragmentation of the metaphyses in children and believed that this was part of the syndrome that Caffey originally described.[46] In 1960, Altman and Smith reported cases of unrecognized trauma in children, and in 1972 Kempe and Helfer coined the term "battered child syndrome."[4,28] Since that time the definition has been expanded to include forms of abuse other than physical.

Legal Aspects

Physicians and other health care professionals are required by law to report suspected incidents of child abuse. The law affords them immunity from litigation stemming from the act of reporting; however, maliciously reporting abuse when it is not the cause of injury may expose an individual to the risk of litigation. In addition, civil suits have been filed against physicians for failure to report acts of child abuse.[23] The law is therefore clear: One must report suspected child abuse. Thus, the examining physician must be aware of the syndrome in order to recognize it.

Identification of At-Risk Individuals

Although child abuse is pervasive, affecting all strata of society, certain individuals are at greater risk. Low-income families are perceived to be more vulnerable; however, this may be due to underreporting in middle- and upper-income families. Socially isolated families with no external support system tend to be more abusive. Abuse also is more common in families in which the parents are involved in a violent interpersonal relationship. Adults who were childhood victims of abuse are more likely to become abusive parents as are those with unrealistic expectations (i.e., expectations inconsistent with the child's developmental or intellectual abilities) for their children. Families with increased stress are vulnerable. For example, drug or alcohol abuse by the parents enhances the likelihood of child abuse, as does mental illness in the parents.

Children who were born prematurely are at increased risk of abuse, as are those born to adolescent parents. Infants who suffer from colic, which makes them irritable, likewise are at higher risk. The presence of any condition that interferes with the normal parent-child bonding, such as congenital deformities or abnormalities or hospitalization of the neonate with lack of normal parental contact, will also increase the risk of child abuse.

Risk increases as the age of the child decreases. Drvaric and associates found that 65% of the children in their series who were abused were 18 months of age or younger.[15] In the most recent report of the National Committee for Prevention of Child Abuse, 79% of deaths due to abuse occurred in children under the age of 5 years; 54% of them were age 1 year or younger.[13] Therefore, fractures in children younger than 18 months, and certainly in children younger than 1 year, should be carefully evaluated for the possibility of abuse.

Signs of Child Abuse

Signs of Physical Abuse. Physical abuse is defined as the nonaccidental injury of a child. This ranges from minor bruises and lacerations to severe bone and neurologic trauma and death. It is the most easily recognizable form of child abuse and the type most commonly seen by physicians. Characteristically, the injuries sustained are more severe than would normally be expected with the given history.[11,18] Because it is likely that orthopaedic surgeons will be confronted with children who have sustained musculoskeletal injuries as a result of abuse, it is imperative that they be aware of the syndrome of child abuse so that the family and the circumstances surrounding the injury can be investigated appropriately.

The physical signs of abuse include bruises and welts over any part of the body. Areas particularly subject to trauma are the face, head, and neck, including the lips, mouth, ears, and eyes. Bruises about the trunk, back, buttocks, and thighs are also common. Bruises may be seen on multiple body surfaces and may form regular patterns resembling the shape of the object that was used to inflict the injury, such as a hand, fist, belt or belt buckle, or electrical cord.

Burns are also commonly seen and may be noted in conjunction with bone injuries. Cigarette burns may be present, especially on the palms, soles, back, or buttocks. Immersion burns form a regular pattern. If the child is pushed into a tub or sink of very hot water, the burns will occur around the buttocks and genitalia. However, if one of the extremities is dipped in hot water, a stocking-glove distribution of the burn will be seen. Pattern burns may result if the child is burned with an instrument such as an iron, grill, or some other hot object with a recognizable shape.

Lacerations may occur anywhere on the body, but some common types are rope burns on the wrists, ankles, neck, or torso. Lacerations about the head and face are frequently seen and may even be inside the mouth or ears. One must also look for injuries to the genitalia and other body surfaces.

Injuries to the abdomen and to the components of the abdominal cavity may result from child abuse. Bruises of the abdominal wall and bleeding within the wall of the small intestine may be seen. Rupture of an abdominal viscus has been reported, including intestine, spleen, liver, pancreas, and blood vessels. The kidneys and bladder may also be injured.

Trauma to the central nervous system is common and may be severe. Subdural hematoma may result from either blunt trauma or violent shaking of the infant. However, a subarachnoid hemorrhage is more commonly the result of the so-called shaken baby. An ophthalmologic examination may demonstrate the presence of retinal hemorrhage.

The orthopaedic manifestations of abuse may include any bone injury; however, so-called corner fractures of the metaphyseal and physeal areas are typical of abuse. In addition, multiple fractures in different stages of healing are considered to be characteristic of child abuse. A third typical injury is the fracture of ribs posteriorly in the infant.

Behavioral Changes. The abused child is likely to demonstrate behavioral problems that may be the result of physical or emotional abuse.[12] Abused children are said to be less compliant, more negative, and more unhappy than the average child. They tend to be angry, feel isolated, and show destructive behavior. They are abusive toward others and have difficulty developing normal relationships. Parental separation is frequently difficult, but occasionally the abused child will be indifferent to separation from the parents. These children may constantly seek attention and may show developmental delays as well.[12]

Physical Neglect. Physical neglect may be even more common than physical abuse. Child neglect may be defined as the failure of a parent or other legal guardian to provide for the child's basic needs and to provide an adequate level of care.[12] Neglect tends to be chronic, leading to an inadequate level of love, food, clothing, shelter, medical care, safety, and education.

Physical signs of physical neglect include malnutrition, pica, constant fatigue and listlessness, poor hygiene, and inadequate clothing for the circumstances.[12] Behavioral signs of physical neglect include lack of appropriate adult supervision and even "role reversal," in which the child becomes the parental caretaker. Other signs include drug or alcohol abuse, poor school attendance, and exploitation by the parents, such as being forced to beg or steal.[12]

Sexual Abuse. Child sexual abuse is the sexual exploitation of a child for the gratification or profit of an adult. Sexual exploitation is usually perpetrated by someone known to the child and frequently continues over a prolonged period. It is very prevalent and is estimated to have an incidence of 100,000 to 250,000 cases per year; however, this type of abuse is difficult to detect and confirm.[12] A description of the physical signs of sexual abuse is beyond the scope of this text; however, the behavioral signs should be recognized because their presence may alert the physician that the child is a victim of sexual abuse.

The child who is a victim of sexual abuse may become withdrawn and have poor peer relationships. These children may demonstrate low self-esteem and seem frightened, especially of adults. They may have feelings of shame or guilt, and their academic performance may deteriorate. They may also show pseudomature personality development. Regressive behavior and even attempted suicide may be the result of child sexual abuse. These children may also become sexually promiscuous and may sexually abuse a sibling.

Management

Evaluation of suspected child abuse is best handled by a multidisciplinary team of health care professionals. The team may include a pediatrician, a social worker, a psychiatrist, a nurse, an attorney, and a pediatric orthopaedic surgeon. Consultants may include a pediatric radiologist and a gynecologist. One individual, such as the social worker, should be designated as the contact person for the child abuse team. This will facilitate reporting of suspected abuse in that all initial contacts are made through the same person or office.

The physician who suspects child abuse must first be aware of the signs of abuse so that identification is possible. Treatment of the initiating medical problem is necessary. If the child presents because of fracture of one or more of the long bones, the orthopaedic surgeon must suspect abuse. Next, a skeletal survey of all the long bones, the spine, the ribs, and the skull should be performed to identify any other fractures. Accurate documentation of the injuries is necessary for future legal proceedings.

Throughout the examination, the physician should remain nonjudgmental and, if possible, should attempt to establish a normal relationship with the family. If a child presents with a suspicious fracture, the physician should explain to the family that this type of fracture is one that may be seen in children who have been abused. One should never accuse the family but rather explain in a matter-of-fact way the legal need for investigation of the injury. Most of the time, if the injury is truly accidental, the family will be understanding. If the family becomes argumentative, one's suspicion of abuse increases.

The child should be hospitalized, if possible, if there is a strong suspicion of abuse, even though the injury may not require it. If necessary, the child may be placed in emergency foster care. Abuse of siblings must also be considered, and care must be provided for them, if necessary. Although the orthopaedic surgeon usually will not assume the primary responsibility for the complete evaluation and reporting of suspected child abuse, he or she should be aware of the process so that appropriate steps will be taken to assure the future safety of the abused child.

It is legally mandated that suspected child abuse be reported to the designated community agency. Although the exact reading of the law in various communities may differ, all statutes require prompt identification of the child suspected of having been abused. Physicians are granted immunity from civil and criminal liability if a report is made in good faith. Most laws impose a criminal penalty for failure to report suspected child abuse.

Injuries From Physical Abuse

Fractures of almost any bone may occur; however, fractures of long bones, ribs, and skull are most frequently seen. In one series, fractures of the long bones accounted for 68% of all fractures in patients who were the victims of child abuse.[10] Physical abuse occurs in younger children and infants much more frequently than in older children. Most of the children who are abused are less than 2 years of age, and approximately one third are less than 1 year old. Bone injuries are the most common type of abuse seen in infants. Skeletal injuries resulting from abuse occur in infants under 1 year of age more than 50% of the time. Conversely, less than 10% are over 5 years of age.[35]

Fractures of the long bones of the arms and legs are the most common type of skeletal injury, fractures of the ribs and the skull being the next most frequent type. In one review, the femur, tibia, fibula, skull, and humerus were the most commonly fractured bones. The authors also found that long bone fractures accounted for 68% of all fractures.[10] The long bone injuries may involve the epiphyseal and metaphyseal areas of the bone, or the diaphysis may be the site of trauma.

EPIPHYSEAL-METAPHYSEAL FRACTURES

Epiphyseal-metaphyseal fractures may be almost diagnostic of child abuse. True physeal injuries, however, are uncommon in the abused child except in the distal humerus, proximal humerus, and proximal femur. Salter-Harris type I fractures of the distal humerus may occur in the newborn as a result of a traumatic delivery. After this age this injury has been considered to be most often the result of abuse.

Type I Fractures of the Distal Humerus

Incidence. The exact incidence of this type of fracture is not known because it is underdiagnosed.[14] In 1979 Macafee reported three cases of infantile supracondylar fractures that were actually fracture-separations of the distal humeral physis.[14] At one time this injury was thought to be very rare; however, it is now recognized more frequently.

Mechanisms of Injury. Two clear mechanisms of injury seem to be the cause of this fracture: birth trauma and abuse. Child abuse is the likely cause after the neonatal period. Holda and colleagues reported that a fall from a height was the cause of the fractures in their series.[26] However, three of their seven patients were under the age of 1 1/2 years, making child abuse more likely. DeLee and co-workers reported that child abuse was proved or suspected in 6 of their 16 patients.[14] One must therefore strongly suspect the possibility of child abuse when one sees this fracture in a young child.[36]

Diagnosis. These children present with marked swelling about the elbow, and the physical appearance of the elbow resembles a dislocation. Gentle manipulation of the elbow will reveal a muffled crepitus, which is the result of two cartilaginous surfaces rubbing against one another. It must be distinguished from bony crepitus.

On the anteroposterior (AP) radiograph the radius and ulna are displaced in relation to the humerus. However, the radius and ulna are in their normal relationship to each other (Fig. 15–1). This injury must be distinguished radiographically from an elbow dislocation, a displaced fracture of the lateral condyle of the distal humerus, and a supracondylar fracture of the distal humerus.

Treatment. Unlike the supracondylar fracture, this fracture is usually stable because it occurs through the thicker distal end of the humerus below the thin supracondylar region. Therefore, cubitus varus deformity is less likely to occur than it is after a supracondylar fracture.[14] Holda and co-workers, on the other hand, found that five of their seven patients developed a cubitus varus deformity.

DeLee and associates recommend closed reduction if the fracture is fresh; however, if the fracture is old, they recommend splinting the arm until the

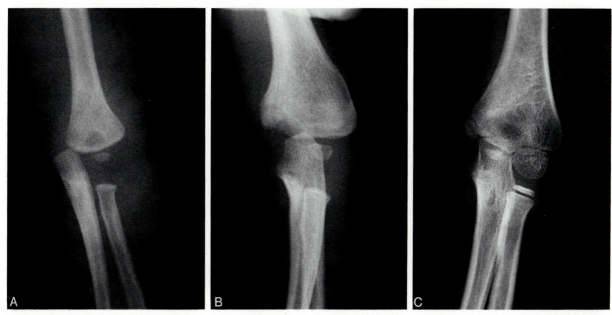

Figure 15–1

Displaced fracture of the distal humeral physis. *A*, Anteroposterior radiograph of the distal humerus at the time of injury demonstrating the medial displacement of the capitellum. Note that the longitudinal axis of the radius intersects the capitellum. *B*, Anteroposterior radiograph of the elbow 3 months after injury. The displacement was not corrected at the time of immobilization. *C*, Follow-up radiograph 5 years post injury demonstrating remodeling of the distal humerus. The patient clinically had full mobility in the elbow.

fracture is solid, without attempts at reduction.[14] The results presented by Holda and colleagues tend to corroborate this because their results with more aggressive treatment were poor.[26] Mizuno and coworkers obtained good results with open reduction through a posterior approach.[36]

Our preference is to investigate for the possibility of child abuse first. The child may be admitted to the hospital to facilitate this investigation, if necessary. Admission may also be warranted to observe for circulatory change. If reduction is required, closed reduction is performed by placing gentle traction on the forearm. The medial displacement of the distal fragment is then corrected. Any malrotation is corrected, and the elbow is flexed to 90 degrees with the forearm pronated, because the medial displacement recurs if the forearm is supinated.[14] The arm is splinted for 3 weeks, after which unrestricted motion is allowed.

Type I Fractures of the Proximal Femur

Type I fractures of the proximal femur are very rare and are usually the result of significant trauma, such as a motor vehicle accident or a fall from a great height. These displaced type I fractures are frequently associated with dislocation of the femoral head. The prognosis is generally poor because of the extremely high incidence of avascular necrosis.

If a type I fracture of the proximal femur is seen and the history of injury does not include violent trauma, the orthopaedic surgeon should be suspicious of child abuse, especially in the child under the age of 5 years. Obviously, acute slipped capital femoral epiphysis may occur without a violent injury and is not the result of intentional trauma; however, this entity generally occurs in an older age group.

Minimally displaced type I fractures of the proximal femoral physis in young children and infants without a substantiated history of violent trauma should be thoroughly investigated for the possibility of child abuse. Although the prognosis for the markedly displaced type I fracture is poor, that for the minimally displaced fracture of the proximal femoral physis has been good, in our experience. A recent report by Forlin and colleagues documents the incidence of child abuse in type I fractures of the proximal femur in young children.[19] These investigators also found that avascular necrosis of the femoral head is not as common as once feared if the femoral head is not dislocated. They are in accord with treatment of these fractures in spica casts until union is complete. Because of the wide range of motion of the hip joint, remodeling of the

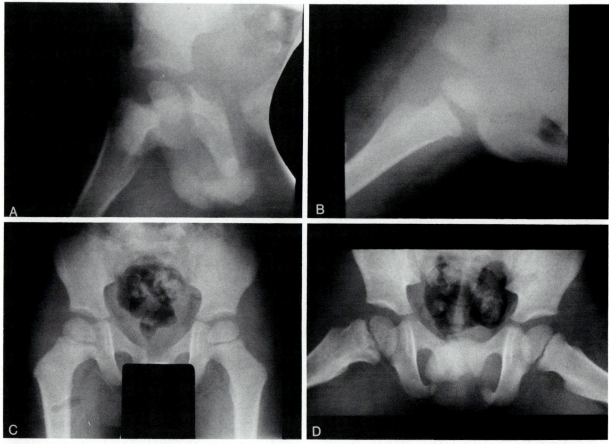

Figure 15–2

A 3-year-old child sustained a type I physeal injury of the proximal femur as the result of child abuse. *A,* Anteroposterior radiograph demonstrates the angulation of the fracture but without complete displacement. *B,* Lateral radiograph of the hip and proximal femur also shows the displacement of the fracture. *C,* Anteroposterior radiograph of both hips shows nearly complete remodeling of the fracture 1 1/2 years after the injury. The fracture was not reduced, but the child was placed in a hip spica cast for 6 weeks. There is no evidence of avascular necrosis of the femoral head. *D,* Lateral radiograph of both hips demonstrates the near-complete remodeling of the fracture.

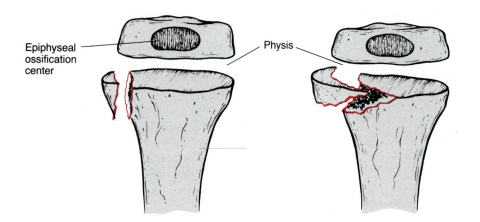

Figure 15–3

The metaphyseal avulsion fractures occurring at the junction of the metaphysis and the physis that are seen in child abuse. The injuries are caused by sudden twisting of the limb. The fracture may be a simple corner fracture *(A)* or a so-called bucket-handle fracture *(B)*.

fracture should be extensive; therefore, reduction is not generally required (Fig. 15-2).

Other Salter-Harris injuries of the physis are commonly seen in children as a result of accidental trauma but are only rarely seen in victims of child abuse.

The epiphyseal-metaphyseal fractures that are common in childhood victims of physical abuse are the so-called corner and bucket-handle fractures. These injuries result from a combination of traction and torsion directed to the metaphysis and physis of a long bone. Because this force is not generated through accidental trauma, these fractures are considered typical of child abuse (Fig. 15-3). It is felt that because of the loose attachment of the periosteum to the diaphysis, it is easily stripped; however, the periosteum becomes tightly attached to the metaphysis of the bone. Torsional and traction force is therefore transmitted to the metaphysis, resulting in the corner fracture (Fig. 15-4).

DIAPHYSEAL FRACTURES

Although not seen exclusively in the victims of child abuse, diaphyseal fractures of long bones are much more common than the more typical corner fractures

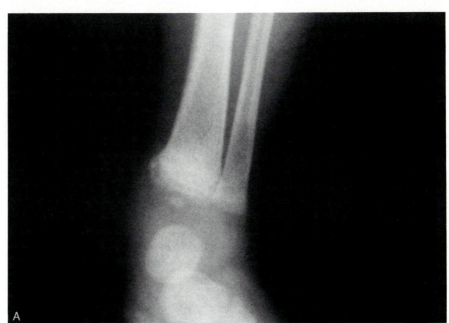
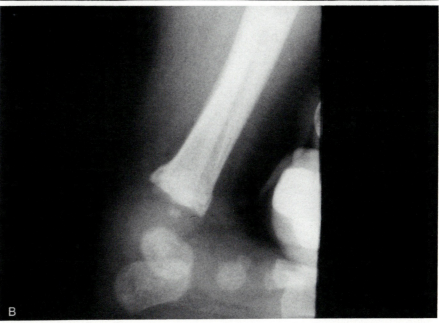

Figure 15-4

Corner fractures of the distal tibia in an infant who was abused. *A,* Anteroposterior radiographs that show the corner fractures of both sides of the metaphysis at the level of the physis. There is evidence of new bone formation, which indicates that the fracture is more than a week old. *B,* Lateral radiograph of the same ankle that also shows the corner fractures.

of the metaphyseal-epiphyseal area. Spiral, oblique, and transverse fractures of the shaft of a long bone may result from accidental or nonaccidental trauma. Children under the age of 1 year with a diaphyseal fracture should be thoroughly investigated for the possibility of abuse, because accidental injuries of this type are very uncommon before the age of ambulation. These fractures may take any form. Although they typically have been characterized as long spiral fractures, almost any pattern may be seen as the result of either accidental or nonaccidental trauma (Fig. 15–5). Therefore, the type of diaphyseal fracture of the femur does not necessarily suggest the cause of the injury (Fig. 15–6). Other factors, such as associated injuries, age of the patient, circumstances surrounding the injury, and history of the injury, must be used for making the diagnosis of child abuse. Long spiral fractures of the femur are common in the toddler as the result of accidental trauma and should not be considered solely as the result of abuse (Fig. 15–7).

The so-called toddler's fracture of the tibia typically occurs in the second and third years of life and is the result of accidental trauma. Unfortunately, the history of trauma is not always clear when these children are seen, and one should not be too quick to diagnose child abuse. Not infrequently, the parents are unaware of the trauma because it occurred out of their sight. Frequently we are confronted with a child who has been picked up from daycare, carried into the car, and then taken into the house. The child may eat and then go to bed without walking, but in the morning the parents are aware that the child will not walk, and at that time they seek medical attention. Normally the delayed diagnosis and lack of a clear history of trauma alert the physician to possible child abuse; however, this is usually not the case in this injury. As a matter of fact, it may be difficult to identify the fracture on a plain radiograph because it is nondisplaced. Sometimes oblique radiographs will help demonstrate the oblique fracture of the mid- and distal tibia. In some instances, even this view fails to show the fracture, and empirical treatment for a suspected toddler's fracture is necessary. Repeat radiographs 2 to 3 weeks later will show the periosteal healing about the fracture (Fig. 15–8).

Fracture of the diaphysis of a long bone in a nonambulatory child suggests child abuse until proved otherwise. Abuse should be suspected if there is either an unreasonable history of cause of the fracture, such as fracture with diaper change, or no true history of trauma. Abuse should also be suspected if there is an inappropriate delay in seek-

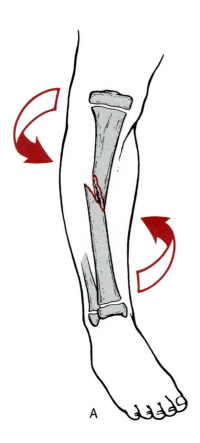
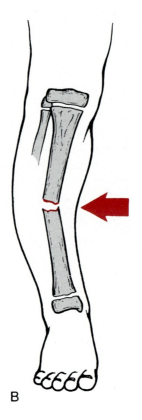

Figure 15–5

The mechanism of injury that will produce either a spiral fracture, which is the result of a twisting injury (A), or a transverse fracture, which is the result of a direct blow to a long bone (B).

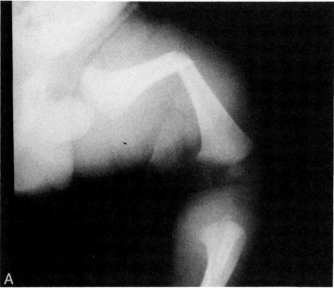
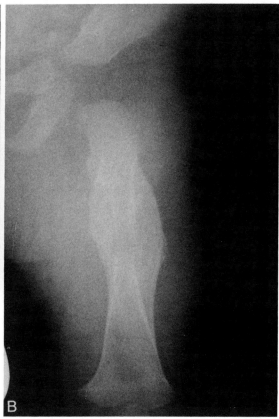

Figure 15-6

Fracture of the midshaft of the femur in an infant that was caused by nonaccidental trauma. *A*, Radiograph of the femur demonstrates the midshaft fracture of the femur with marked angulation of the fracture. Fractured femurs in infants that result from child abuse may be spiral fractures but also may be simple transverse diaphyseal fractures such as seen here. This fracture undoubtedly was the result of significant force. *B*, Healing of the fracture is demonstrated after the fracture had been reduced and the limb immobilized in a hip spica cast.

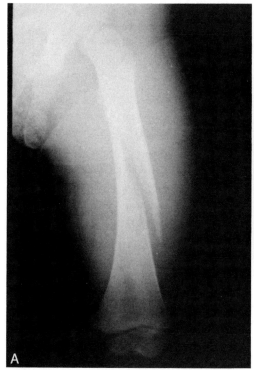
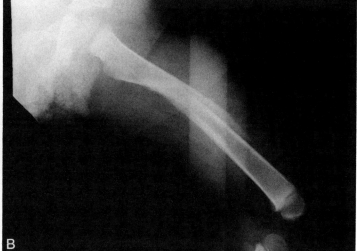

Figure 15-7

Fracture of the femur in a toddler that occurred as the result of accidental trauma. *A*, Anteroposterior radiograph of the femur of a 2-year-old child who tripped while running. This fracture pattern is quite typical of fractures in the toddler age group. The investigation of the family showed no evidence for suspicion, and the child had no other injuries or warning signs of abuse. *B*, Lateral radiograph that demonstrates the long spiral fracture of the femur.

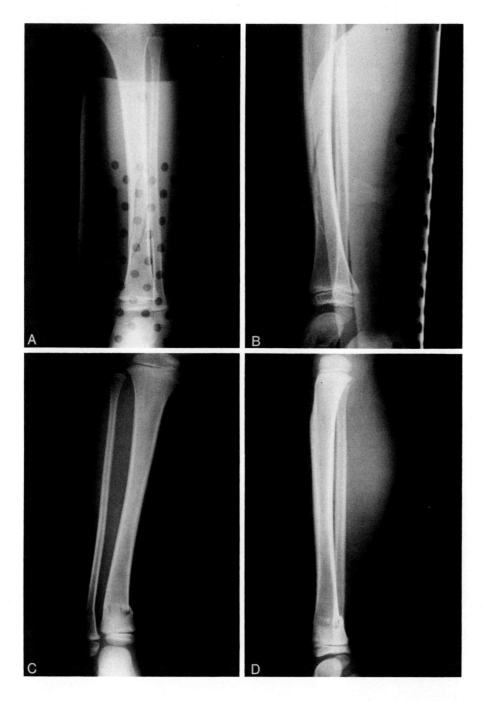

Figure 15–8

Fractures of the tibia are commonly seen as the result of accidental trauma in young children. *A–B,* Anteroposterior and lateral radiographs of the tibia of a 2-year-old child who sustained this spiral fracture of the tibia when she fell while running. This typical so-called toddler fracture is well seen on these radiographs, but the fracture may be much more subtle and very difficult to see except on oblique radiographs. Sometimes the fracture may not be seen on any initial radiograph, but in follow-up, periosteal healing of the fracture may be demonstrated. *C–D,* Anteroposterior and lateral radiographs of the tibia of a child who sustained a fracture of the distal tibia in a fall. This fracture, while less common than the spiral fracture, is also the result of accidental trauma. The child and family were investigated, and no suspicion of child abuse was found. The fracture was treated with simple immobilization.

ing medical care of if there is physical evidence of other trauma. Diagnosis of abuse should be made if there is, in addition to a diaphyseal fracture, radiologic evidence of fractures in varying stages of healing or multiple acute fractures without evidence of accidental trauma or bone disease.

Fracture of the diaphysis of the femur in children under the age of 1 year has been considered typical of child abuse. In a series reported by Gross and Stranger, 17 of 26 fractures of the femur in children less than 1 year old were the result of child abuse.[24]

Fractures of the shaft of the humerus are so uncommon as the result of accidental trauma in this age group that they are considered to be distinctly characteristic of child abuse.[49] Worlock and colleagues found that no child under the age of 5 years sustained an accidental humeral shaft fracture, all such injuries seen in this age group being due to abuse. In contrast, all the supracondylar and condylar fractures of the distal humerus in their series were the result of accidental trauma.[53]

Treatment. Diaphyseal fractures of the long bones

are usually treated with immobilization. Fractures of the shaft of the femur are best treated with application of an immediate spica cast. Some fractures of the shaft of the femur may be very unstable if the trauma has been significant enough to disrupt the periosteum. Therefore, close observation with repeat radiographs is necessary until union of the fracture is complete, usually within 6 weeks. Hospitalization is frequently necessary for completion of a social service investigation of the family and the circumstances of the injury.

Humeral shaft fractures should also be treated with closed immobilization. This is best accomplished with the application of a Velpeau bandage. This fracture also will heal very quickly in the infant (Fig. 15–9).

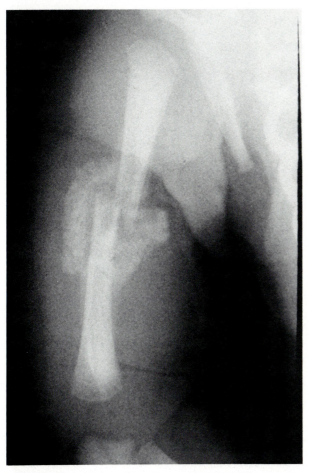

Figure 15–9

Fracture of the humerus in an infant. The anteroposterior radiograph of the humerus demonstrates a transverse, mid-diaphyseal fracture of the humerus that was the result of nonaccidental trauma. When the child was seen, the fracture was already healing, as demonstrated by the radiograph. The child was found to have other skeletal and soft tissue injuries.

CLAVICLE AND RIB FRACTURES

Fractures of the clavicle are rarely seen in the victims of child abuse; however, fractures of the shaft of the clavicle have been seen in such children. These fractures must be differentiated from those associated with trauma sustained during delivery of the infant. Fractures of the distal end of the clavicle are said to be more characteristic of child abuse.[32] These avulsion fractures are thought to be due to sudden and forceful traction on the upper extremity and are associated with injury to the proximal humerus.[32]

The ribs are the third most common site for skeletal injury in children who are abused.[34, 35] Accidental fractures of the ribs in young children are rare.[10, 52, 53] The relatively pliant rib cage of the infant and toddler affords protection against fracture of the ribs from falls and other accidental trauma. Worlock and associates found that none of the rib fractures in the infants and toddlers in their series was the result of accidental trauma.[53] In addition, they found that all the children and infants who had sustained one or more rib fractures had also sustained another skeletal injury and that most of the rib fractures were identified incidentally on skeletal surveys.

Rib fractures are frequently multiple in battered children and most frequently occur posteriorly adjacent to the costovertebral junction. Because of this location these fractures are difficult to identify radiographically, and this led to the early impression that rib fractures were not common in child abuse. These fractures are seen best after fracture callus is evident, making identification easier (Fig. 15–10). Rib fractures occur as a result of sudden, violent compression of the chest laterally (Fig. 15–11). Lateral rib fractures are much less commonly seen in child abuse than are posterior rib fractures and are felt to be caused by anterior compression of the chest.

SKULL FRACTURES

Skull fractures are common in children who have been physically abused. These fractures are second in frequency only to fractures of the long bones.[23, 24] Skull fractures are far more often a result of abuse than of accidental trauma.[26, 32] They occur most commonly in the first year of life and are rare after age 2.[32, 35] Characteristic skull injuries include multiple fractures, complex fractures, depressed fractures, and wide fractures.[17]

Cerebral damage associated with the skull injury is of greatest concern. Although one most commonly

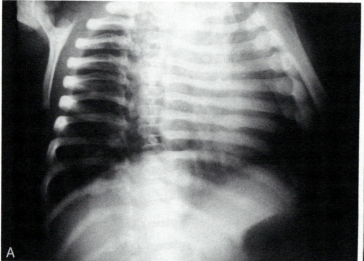
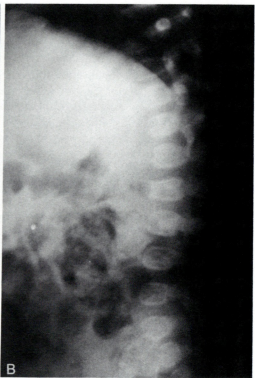

Figure 15–10

This infant sustained multiple fractures, including multiple rib fractures and a compression fracture of the lumbar spine. A, Multiple posterior fractures of ribs on both sides of the chest in this infant were seen on the radiograph of the ribs taken on the day of admission to the hospital. These fractures were all healed, evidence that these injuries had occurred prior to admission. B, Lateral radiograph of the spine demonstrates a compression fracture of the second lumbar vertebra. Both these injuries were thought to be the result of intentional trauma.

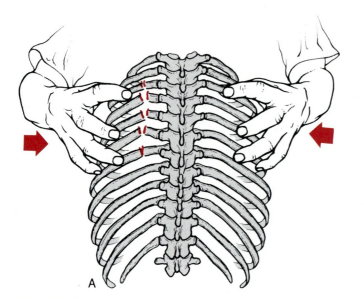
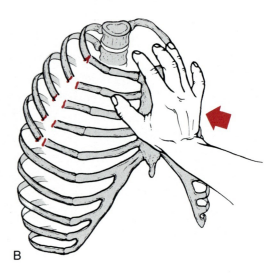

Figure 15–11

Mechanism of injury that produces rib fractures. Anteroposterior compression of the chest will most commonly result in fractures of the ribs laterally (A). Compression of the ribs from the side, however, will produce posterior rib fractures (B). This mechanism of injury is most commonly seen in children who have been abused, because of the side-to-side compression of the infant by the adult's hands.

associates cerebral injury with trauma to the skull, in 1974 Caffey coined the term "whiplash shaken infant syndrome."[9] The most widely used term today is "shaken baby syndrome." This entity refers to cerebral and retinal bleeding in an infant caused by vigorous shaking. These children do not have external signs of head trauma, but computed tomography (CT) scans show sustained subarachnoid and subdural hematomas, especially in the posterior hemispheric fissure.[16]

Crying is the most commonly cited provocation for the injury.[17] The infant is most commonly held by the thorax and shaken, resulting in cerebral and retinal bleeding in addition to fractures of the posterior ribs.[17] If the child is held by the extremities when shaken, the result will be metaphyseal avulsions and subperiosteal hemorrhage caused by the traction and shearing forces.[17] If the shaking is violent enough, injury to the spine and spinal cord is possible.[17]

DIFFERENTIAL DIAGNOSIS

Obstetric trauma may possibly be mistaken for child abuse; however, multiple fractures are not common in birth trauma. Usually, the obstetrician is aware of the injury. In addition, the neonate will not use the injured extremity immediately after birth, allowing detection in the nursery.

Accidental trauma sustained by toddlers initially may produce confusion. However, the type of fractures sustained by these children through accidental trauma differs from the injuries that result from child abuse. Children who are not yet walking rarely sustain accidental trauma. The toddler, on the other hand, frequently fractures the tibia or femur as the result of a fall. The tibia fracture, as previously mentioned, is almost always nondisplaced and may be very difficult to see radiographically. Tibia fractures that result from abuse are usually readily seen on radiographs. Fractures of the femur, also common in toddlers, are usually long spiral fractures. Although femoral fractures that are nonaccidental may also be spiral, other signs may be present. Multiple fractures, especially if they are in different stages of healing, make differentiation easier. Fractures of the posterior ribs or skull also provide strong clues to the actual cause of the injuries.

Congenital syphilis may be mistaken for child abuse, because of the periosteal new bone formation and the corner metaphyseal erosions that may be mistaken for corner fractures (Fig. 15-12). The bone lesions of congenital syphilis are usually symmetric, and a positive serologic test result will confirm the presence of the disease.

Other conditions may theoretically mimic child abuse; however, the differentiation should not be difficult. Scurvy will be manifested radiographically

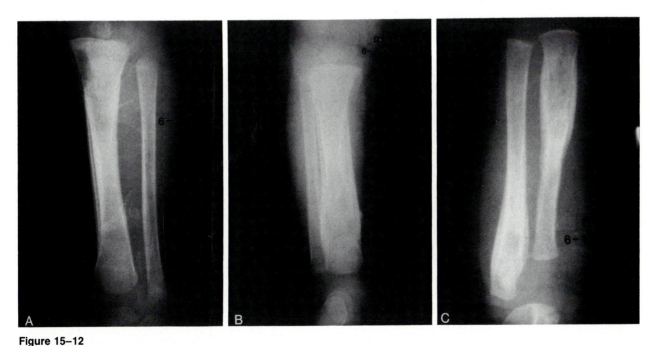

Figure 15-12

Radiographs of multiple bones of an infant with congenital syphillis. *A–B*, The radiographs show periosteal new bone in both tibias. *C*, Periosteal new bone formation in the radius and ulna.

with subperiosteal new bone formation because of the periosteal elevation that results from the subperiosteal bleeding. Hypervitaminosis A may produce periosteal elevation and should be ruled out by history taking. Another relatively rare cause of periosteal new bone is Caffey's disease (infantile cortical hyperostosis), in which there is extensive new bone formation in the diaphyses of long bones but with metaphyseal sparing (Fig. 15–13). The mandible is involved in 95% of cases. Because of associated evidence of inflammation, Caffey's disease is more commonly confused with osteomyelitis.

Osteogenesis imperfecta (OI) is the disease that may most closely mimic child abuse. It is divided into four main types that can be subclassified further.[14, 29–32] Type I is most common, accounting for 80% of all cases.[33] It is inherited as an autosomal dominant disorder.[14] The scleras are blue in this type. It is a milder form of the disease, with fewer fractures and less bone deformity than are seen in other types.

Type II is also inherited as an autosomal dominant disorder. It is a very severe form of the disease that leads to intrauterine or early infant death. Type III is similar to type II but milder; however, both types are characterized by extreme bone fragility, with fractures at birth and obvious bony deformity. Therefore, neither of these two types is likely to be mistaken for child abuse.

Type IV is more like type I in that there is less bone fragility than in types II and III. The scleras are normal or faintly blue in infancy, although they become more blue in adulthood. Types I and IV are most likely to be mistaken for child abuse.[14, 29–32] One should look for telltale signs of OI, such as wormian bones and osteopenia. Occasionally both are absent, making diagnosis difficult. Gahagan and Rimsza have reported that metaphyseal corner-type fractures may occur in children with OI.[21] If, in addition, the child is a member of an at-risk family, one may be quick to diagnose child abuse.

A history that is incompatible with the injury is one of the hallmarks of child abuse; however, that is also the case in patients with OI. Fractures in these children may be sustained with minimal, even trivial, trauma. A careful family history is important. However, because of the occurrence of new mutations, a negative history does not exclude the diagnosis of OI. Therefore, accurate diagnosis may require biochemical analysis of skin fibroblast collagen to identify the abnormalities of type I collagen seen in children with OI.

REFERENCES

1. Akbarnia, B. A.; Akbarnia, N. O. The role of the orthopedist in child abuse and neglect. Orthop Clin North Am 7:733–742, 1976.
2. Akbarnia, B.; Torg, J. S.; Kirkpatrick, J.; Sussman, S. Manifestations of the battered-child syndrome. J Bone Joint Surg 56-A:1159–1166, 1984.
3. Alffram, P. A.; Bauer, G. C. H. Epidemiology of fractures of the forearm: A biomechanical investigation of bone strength. J Bone Joint Surg 44-A:105–114, 1962.
4. Altman, D. H.; Smith, R. L. Unrecognized trauma in infants and children. J Bone Joint Surg 42-A:407–413, 1960.
5. Anderson, W. A. The significance of femoral fractures in children. Ann Emerg Med 11:174–177, 1982.
6. Beals, R. K.; Tufts, E. Fractured femur in infancy: The role of child abuse. J Pediatr Orthop 3:583–586, 1983.
7. Caffey, J. Multiple fractures in the long bones of infants suffering from chronic subdural hematoma. Am J Roentgenol 56:163–173, 1946.
8. Caffey, J. On the theory and practice of shaking infants. Am J Dis Child 124:161–169, 1972.
9. Caffey, J. The whiplash shaken infant syndrome: Manual shaking by the extremities with whiplash-induced intracranial and intraocular bleedings, linked with residual permanent brain damage and mental retardation. Pediatrics 54:396–403, 1974.
10. Cameron, J. M.; Rae, L. J. An Atlas of the Battered Child Syndrome. Edinburgh, Churchill Livingstone, 1975.
11. Child Abuse. Guidelines for Intervention by Physicians and Other Health Care Providers. Seattle, Washington State Medical Association, 1990.
12. Council on Scientific Affairs. AMA diagnostic and treatment guidelines concerning child abuse and neglect. JAMA 254(6):796–800, 1985.
13. The National Center on Child Abuse Prevention Research. Current Trends in Child Abuse Reporting and Fatalities:

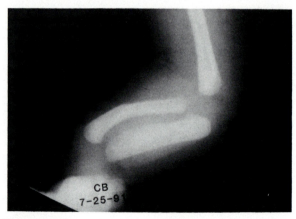

Figure 15–13
Caffey's disease is a rare cause of periosteal new bone formation. The radiograph of the forearm in this infant shows periosteal new bone formation in both the radius and, especially, the ulna. Frequently the children may have fever and evidence of local inflammation, which makes the differential diagnosis of osteomyelitis more common than child abuse.

The Results of the 1991 Annual Fifty State Survey. A Program of the National Committee for Prevention of Child Abuse. Working Paper No. 808:1–24, 1992.
14. DeLee, J. C.; Wilkins, K. E.; Rogers, L. F.; Rockwood, C. A. Fracture-separation of the distal humerus epiphysis. J Bone Joint Surg 62-A:46–51, 1980.
15. Drvaric, D. M.; Morrell, S. M.; Wyly, J. B.; et al. Fracture patterns in the battered child syndrome. J South Orthop Assoc 1(1):20–25, 1992.
16. Duhaime, A. C.; Gennarelli, T. A.; Thibault, L. E.; et al. The shaken baby syndrome: A clinical, pathological, and biomechanical study. J Neurosurg 66:409–415, 1987.
17. Dykes, L. J. The whiplash shaken infant syndrome: What has been learned? Child Abuse Negl 10:211–221, 1986.
18. Everything You Always Wanted to Know about Child Abuse and Neglect. Washington, D. C., National Center on Child Abuse and Neglect, 1991.
19. Forlin, E.; Guille, J.; Kumar, S.; Rhee, K. Transepiphyseal fractures of the neck of the femur in very young children. J Pediatr Orthop 12:164–168, 1992.
20. Franken, E. A.; Smith, J. A. Roentgenographic evaluation of infant and childhood trauma. Pediatr Clin North Am 22:301–315, 1975.
21. Gahagan, S.; Rimsza, M. E. Child abuse or osteogenesis imperfecta: How can we tell? Pediatrics 88(5):987–992, 1991.
22. Galleno, H.; Oppenheim, W. L. The battered child syndrome revisited. Clin Orthop 162:11–19, 1982.
23. Green, F. C. Child abuse and neglect, a priority problem for the private physician. Pediatr Clin North Am 22:329–339, 1975.
24. Gross, R. H.; Stranger, M. Causative factors responsible for femoral fractures in infants and young children. J Pediatr Orthop 3:341–343, 1983.
25. Habibian, A.; Sartoris, D. J.; Resnick, D. The radiologic findings in battered child syndrome. J Musculoskeletal Med 4:16–33, 1988.
26. Holda, M. E.; Manolia, A.; LaMont, R. L. Epiphyseal separation of the distal end of the humerus with medial displacement. J Bone Joint Surg 62-A:52–57, 1980.
27. Holter, J. C.; Friedman, S. B. Child abuse. Early case finding in the emergency department. Pediatrics 42:128, 1968.
28. Kempe, C. H.; Helfer, R. E. Helping the Battered Child and His Family. Philadelphia, J. B. Lippincott, 1972.
29. King, J.; Diefendorf, D.; Apthorp, J., et al. Analysis of 429 fractures in 189 battered children. J Pediatr Orthop 8:585–589, 1988.
30. Kogutt, M. S.; Swischuk, L. E.; Fagan, C. J. Patterns of injury and significance of uncommon fractures in the battered child syndrome. AJR 121:143–149, 1974.
31. Landin, L. A. Fracture patterns in children: Analysis of 8,682 fractures with special reference to incidence, etiology and secular changes in a Swedish urban population 1950–1979. Acta Orthop Scand (Suppl) 202:1–109, 1983.
32. Leonidas, J. Skeletal trauma in the child abuse syndrome. Pediatr Ann 12:875–881, 1983.
33. McClellan, C. Q.; Kingsbury, G. H. Fractures in the first year of life: A diagnostic dilemma? Am J Dis Child 136:26–29, 1982.
34. Merten, D. F.; Kirks, D. R.; Ruderman, R. J. Occult humeral epiphyseal fracture in battered infants. Pediatr Radiol 10:151–154, 1981.
35. Merten, D. F.; Radkowski, M. A.; Leonidas, J. C. The abused child: A radiological reappraisal. Radiology 146:377–381, 1983.
36. Mizuno, K.; Hirohata, K.; Kashiwagi, D. Fracture-separation of the distal humeral epiphysis in young children. J Bone Joint Surg 61-A:570–573, 1979.
37. O'Neill, J. A., Jr.; Meacham, W. F.; Griffin, J. P.; et al. Patterns of injury in the battered child syndrome. J Trauma 13:332–339, 1973.
38. Paterson, C. R.; McAllion, S. J. Osteogenesis imperfecta in the differential diagnosis of child abuse. Br Med J 299:1451–1454, 1989.
39. Radkowski, M. A.; Merten, D. F.; Leonidas, J. C. Abused child: Criteria for the radiologic diagnosis. Radiographics 3:262–297, 1983.
40. Rosenberg, N.; Bottenfield, G. Fractures in infants: A sign of child abuse. Ann Emerg Med 11:178–180, 1982.
41. Sheinkop, M. B.; Gardner, H. R. Child abuse as seen by the orthopaedic surgeon. Paper presented before the 41st Annual Meeting of the American Academy of Orthopaedic Surgeons, Dallas, 1974.
42. Sillence, D. O. Abnormalities of density of modelling in the skeleton. In: Behrman, R. E., Vaughan, V. C., eds. Nelson's Textbook of Pediatrics. Philadelphia, W. B. Saunders, 1983, pp. 1645–1647.
43. Sillence, D. O. Osteogenesis imperfecta: An expanding panorama of variants. Clin Orthop 159:11–25, 1983.
44. Sillence, D. O.; Barlow, K. K.; Cole, W. G.; et al. Osteogenesis imperfecta type III. Delineation of the phenotype with reference to genetic heterogeneity. Am J Med Genet 23:821–832, 1986.
45. Sillence, D. O.; Senn, A. S.; Danks, D. M. Genetic heterogeneity in osteogenesis imperfecta. J Med Genet 16:101–116, 1979.
46. Silverman, F. N. The roentgen manifestations of unrecognized skeletal trauma in infants. Am J Roentgenol 69:413–427, 1953.
47. Smith, R. Osteogenesis imperfecta. Br Med J 289:394–395, 1984.
48. Swischuk, L. E. Spine and spinal cord trauma in the battered child syndrome. Radiology 92:733–738, 1969.
49. Thomas, S. A.; Rosenfield, N. S.; Leventhal, J. M.; Markowitz, R. I. Long-bone fractures in young children: Distinguishing accidental injuries from child abuse. Pediatrics 88(3):471–476, 1991.
50. Thompson, G. H.; Gesler, J. W. Proximal tibial epiphyseal fracture in an infant. J Pediatr Orthop 4:114–117, 1984.
51. Wilkinson, W. S.; Han, D. P.; Rappley, M. D.; Owings, C. L. Retinal hemorrhage predicts neurologic injury in the shaken baby syndrome. Arch Ophthalmol 107:1472, 1989.
52. Worlock, P.; Stower, M. Fracture patterns in Nottingham children. J Pediatr Orthop 6:656–660, 1986.
53. Worlock, P.; Stower, M.; Barbor, P. Patterns of fractures in accidental and nonaccidental injury in children: A comparative study. Br Med J 293:100–102, 1986.

Index

Note: Page numbers in *italics* refer to illustrations; page numbers followed by t refer to tables.

A

AARF (atlantoaxial rotatory fixation), 294–296, *295*
Abdomen, hemorrhage in, 80–82, 81t
  multiple injury and, 71t, 80–82, 81t
Accidents, 68–70
  bicycle, 68t, 70, 411–413, *413*, 507
  falling, 68t, 70
  femoral fracture and, 346–347, 524–526, *525*
  gunshot injury and, 503, *503*, *504*
  incidence of, 346
  lawn mower, 500, *501*
  motor vehicle, 68t, 68–70, 300, 301–304, *302*, *303*
  motorcycle, 68t
  multiple injury and, 68t, 68–70
  pedestrian, *66*, 68t, 70
  spinal injury due to, 300, 301–304, *302*, *303*
  train, 68t
Acetabulum, *308*, *312*. See also *Pelvis*.
  anatomy of, *308*
  fracture of, 307–326
    classification of, *312*, 313t
    complications of, 326
    incidence of, 307
    management of, 315–317, 319t, 324
    mechanism of, 307–309
    multiple injury and, 307–310
    pathophysiology of, 307
    radiology in, 314–315, *316*
  shallow, 112, 309, *309*
Achilles tendon, 453, *453*
Acid-base balance, bicarbonate therapy and, 78
Acromioclavicular joint, 262–263
  injury to, 262–263, *263*
    type I, 262, *263*
    type II, 262, *263*

Acromioclavicular joint *(Continued)*
    type III, 262–263, *263*
Acromion, *262*, 262–263, *263*
  anatomy of, *263*, 263–264
  fracture of, 265
  fusion failure of, 263, *264*, 265
Acute lymphocytic leukemia, spinal fracture and, 300, *301*
Age, anatomic proportion and, 65–67, *67*, *75*, 77t
  blood volume and, 77t
  injury mechanism and, 70
  vital signs and, 77t
Airway, multiple trauma and, 71t, 72t, 74–76
Allman's classification, 262–263, *263*
Amputation, vascular injury and, 99–101
Anesthesia, hand injury and, 199
Angle(s), Baumann's, 214, *214*, 223
  elbow, *214*, 214–216, 233
  humeral fracture and, 233
  patella and, 391, *391*
  Q, 391, *391*
  trochlear groove and, 233
Ankle, 449–514. See also *Foot*; specific bones.
  anatomy of, 449–451, *450*, *451*
  fracture of, 449–467
    approach in, 513–514
    osteochondral, 479–483, *481*, *482*
    physeal injury due to, 453–471, 456t, *457–462*, *464–466*
  ligaments of, 449, *450*, *451*
  movement of, 449
  tumor affecting, 506–507, *508*, *509*
  valgus deformity of, 436–437, 507, *508*
  varus deformity of, 476, *478*, 509–511, *511*
Ankylosis, elbow and, 104, *104*
"Anteater nose" appearance, 504, *504*, *505*

Antibiotics, open fracture and, 89–90, 425, 430
Apophysis, 16
  athletic injury to, 48–51, *49*, *50*
  calcaneal, 48
  humeral epicondylar, *50*, 51
  iliac, 48–49, *49*
  injury to, 48–51
  ischial, 48–49, *49*
  muscle attachment to, 48
  patellar, 48
  pelvic, 49, *49*, 308
  tendon attachment to, 48–51
  tibial tuberosity, 48, *371*, *391*, 391–393, *393*
  vertebral ring, 49–50, *50*
Apophysitis, 48–51. See also *Growth disturbance*.
  calcaneal, 48–49, 472, *472–473*
  femoral, 49, *49*
  foot affected by, 48–49, 472–475, *472–475*
  humeral, 48, *50*, 51
  iliac, 49, *49*
  ischial, 49, *49*
  patellar, 48
  tibial, 48
  traction, 48
  vertebral, 49–50, *50*
Arm. See also specific bones and structures.
  compartment syndrome of, 83, *83*, *101*, 101–102, 149–150, *150*
Arteriography, popliteal, 388, *388*
Artery(ies), 99–101
  brachial, 99, *100*, 214, *214*
  Doppler pressure index for, 82
  elbow and, 214, *214*
  femoral, 99
  fracture complication and, 82–83, 99–101, *100*, 387–388, *388*

533

Artery(ies) *(Continued)*
　injury to, 82–83, 99–101, *100*, 387–388, *388*
　interosseous, elbow and, 214, *214*
　　forearm and, *131*, 214, *214*
　knee and, *387*, 387–388, *388*
　mesenteric, cast syndrome role of, 104, *105*
　　duodenum compressed by, 104, *104*
　peroneal, 387, 397
　popliteal, 387–388, 397
　　femoral fracture and, 99–101, *100*
　　knee and, 82, 99, *100*, 369, *387*, 387–388
　　tibial fracture and, 99, *387*, 387–388, *388*, 397
　radial, 214, *214*
　tibial, 387, 397
　ulnar, 214, *214*
Athletics, apophyseal injury in, 48–51, *49*, *50*
　metatarsal injury and, 489–494, *489–494*
　physeal injury in, 16, 48–51
Atlantoaxial joint, 283–286
　dislocation of, 284–285, 293–294
　rotatory fixation of, 294–296, *295*
Atlanto-occipital joint, 283–286, *289*, 293, *293*
Atlas, 283–285
　anatomy of, 283–285, *284*, *289*
　development of, 283, *284*
　fracture of, 296, *297*
　rotatory fixation affecting, 294–296, *295*
Atrophy, Sudeck, 121
Autonomic nervous system, forearm fracture and, 150–151
　reflex dystrophy and, 121–122, 150–151
Axis, 283–285
　anatomy of, 283–285, *284*, *289*
　development of, 283, *284*, 285
　fracture of, 296–298, *298*
　rotatory fixation affecting, 294–296, *295*

B

Backboard, child patient and, *75*, 75–76
　occiput space in, *75*, 75–76
Bacteria, open fracture and, 428–430
　tetanus caused by, 429, 429t
　wound infection and, 428–430
Bado's classification, 175–177
Bands, Mach, spinal fracture vs., 287, *287*
Bankart lesion, 268
Basion, 287–289, *289*
　odontoid relation to, 286–287, *289*
Battered child syndrome. See *Child abuse*.

Baumann's angle, 214, *214*, 223
Bayonet apposition, femur and, 6, *7*
　fracture healing and, 6, *7*
Beck's triad, 76
Bell-Tawse procedure, 186–188, *187*
Berndt-Harty classification, 481, *481*
Bicarbonate, acid-base balance and, 78
Bicycle spoke injury, 414–415, *415*, 507
Birth, infant spine injury during, 289–290, *290*
　newborn clavicle fracture and, 258–260, *260*
Bleeding, abdominal, 80–82, 81t
　evaluation of, 77, 80–82, 81t
　multiple injury and, 77, 80–82, 81t
Blood pressure, 77t
　arterial injury and, 82
　Doppler index using, 82
　multiple injury and, 76–77, 77t
　shock and, 76
　spinal cord injury and, 80
　trauma evaluation and, 72t, 82
Blood volume, age vs., 77t
Body proportion, age vs., 65–67, *67*, 75, 77t
　trauma injury and, 65–67, *67*, 75, 77t
Body weight, 77t
　acid-base balance and, 78
　age vs., 77t
Bone(s), 1–9. See also *Joint(s)*; *Ossification*; *Physis*; specific bones and joints.
　accessory ossicular, 471–475, *471–475*
　acromion, 262, 262–263, *263*
　　anatomy of, *263*, 263–264
　　fracture of, 265
　　fusion failure of, 263, *264*, 265
　calcaneus. See *Calcaneus*.
　carpal, 130, *130*
　　anatomy of, 130, *130*, *160*, 161
　　dislocation of, 196, *197*, 199
　　fracture of, 196, *197*, *198*, 199
　　radioulnar joint and, 130, *130*, *160*, 161
　cartilage model for, 4–5
　clavicle. See *Clavicle*.
　coalition of, calcaneonavicular, 504, *504*, *505*
　　talocalcaneal, 504, *505*, *506*
　costal, 67
　　first, 69, 259
　　fracture of, 69, *259*, 527, *528*
　　　child abuse and, 527, *528*
　　　multiple injury and, 69
　cranial, fracture of, 527–529
　　spine junction with, 283–286, *289*
　cuboid, 450, *471*, 471–472
　cuneiform, *450*
　dysplasia of, 57, *58*
　ectopic, 103–104, *104*
　embryonic, 3–6
　enchondral, 4–6
　femur. See *Femur*.
　fibula. See *Fibula*.

Bone(s) *(Continued)*
　growth of, 1–6, 15–18, *16*
　healing of, 1, *2*, *3*, 4–8
　hip. See *Hip*; *Pelvis*.
　humerus. See *Humerus*.
　ilium, 307, *308*
　　apophysitis affecting, 49, *49*
　　fracture of. See *Pelvis, fracture of*.
　ischium, 307, *308*
　　apophysitis affecting, 49, *49*
　　fracture of. See *Pelvis, fracture of*.
　membranous, 3
　metacarpal, 203–205, *208*
　metatarsal. See *Metatarsals*.
　navicular, *450*
　　accessory ossicle of, 474, *474*
　　coalition affecting, 504, *504*, *505*
　　fracture of, 475, 475t, 484–488, *487*, *488*
　patella. See *Patella*.
　pathologic conditions and, 57–64, 418–421, 529–530
　pelvic. See *Pelvis*.
　periosteum formation of, *3*, 3–6
　　disorders inducing, *529*, 529–530, *530*
　phalanx. See *Phalanges*.
　physiology of, 1–2, 15–16, *16*
　pubic, 307, *308*
　　fracture of, *311*, 323, *323*
　radius. See *Radius*.
　remodeling of, 4–8, *7*, 30–31, 135
　scaphoid, 196–198, *197*, *198*
　scapula. See *Scapula*.
　sesamoid, *450*
　spinal. See *Spine*; *Vertebra*.
　spongy, 15–16, *16*
　talus. See *Talus*.
　tarsal, *450*, 471, *472*
　tibia. See *Tibia*.
　ulna. See *Ulna*.
　vertebral. See *Spine*; *Vertebra*.
Brachial artery, 99, *100*
Bright classification, 44–45, *45*
Bruises, child abuse and, 518
Burns, child abuse and, 518

C

Caffey's disease, 530, *530*
Calcaneus, *450*, *451*
　anatomy of, *450*, *451*
　apophysitis affecting, 48–49, *472*, 472–473
　coalition affecting, 504–506, *504–506*
　fracture of, 475, 475t, 483t, 483–484, *485–487*
　multiple centers of, 472, *472*
　ossification of, 472, *472*, 474, *474*
　secundarius, 471
Calcium, immobilization affecting, 103
Cancer, fracture with, 57–64, 62t, *63*

Capitellum, *233*
 child abuse injury of, 520–521, *521*
 elbow fracture and, *230*, *231*, *233*–236
 formation of, 213, *213*
 lines and angles using, *214*, 214–216, *215*, *233*
 sulcus of, *233*
Carpometacarpal joint, 205, *206*
Carpus, *130*
 anatomy of, 130, *130*, *157*, *160*, 161
 dislocation of, 196, *197*, 199
 fracture of, 196, *197*, *198*, 199
 radioulnar joint and, 130, *130*, *157*, *160*, 161
Cartilage, 4–6. See also *Physis*.
 bone formation and, 4–6, 15–16, *16*
 physeal, 3–6, 15–16, *16*
 triangular, 130, *130*
 triradiate, *308*, *312*. See also *Acetabulum*.
  anatomy of, *308*, *312*
  arrest of, *309*
  fracture of, 27, *28*, 109–112, 307–326, *312*
Cast syndrome, 104
 mesenteric artery in, 104, *105*
 pathophysiology of, 104, *105*
 treatment of, 104
Casts. See also *Fixation*.
 duodenal obstruction due to, 104
 femur fracture and, 350–352, *351*, 370–372, 375–378
 forearm fracture and, 143, *143*, *144*, 161, *161*
 humerus fracture and, 222–223
 tibia fracture and, 430
Cavity, glenoid, 263–264
  anatomy of, 263–264
  fracture of, 265, *266*
  humerus and, 265–270
Chance fracture, 69, 303
Chest, child abuse injury to, 527, *528*
 child body proportion and, 65–67, *67*, 77t
 multiple injury and, 69, 71t, 80
Child abuse, 517–530
 clinical signs of, 518–519
 diagnosis of, 414, *529*, 529–530, *530*
 fracture due to, 520–529
  clavicular, 527, *528*
  differential diagnosis in, *529*, 529–530, *530*
  femoral, distal, 370
    proximal, 521–523, *522*
    shaft, 346–347, *510*, 523–529, *525*
  foot injury and, 507–509
  humeral, 520–521, *521*, 527, *527*
  pelvic, *29*, 522
  physeal injury in, *29*, 520–523, *521*–523
  rib, 527, *528*
  skull, 527–529
  spinal, 300, *301*, *528*
  tibial, *29*, 413–414, *510*

Child abuse *(Continued)*
  shaft, *510*, 523–529, *524*, *525*
  toddler's vs., 414, 524, *525*, *526*
 history in, 346–347, 414, 524–529
 legal aspects of, 517–520
 management of, 519–520
 risk factors for, 518
 sexual, 519–520
 Silverman's rings in, 507–509, *510*
Chondroclasts, 4
Chondrocytes, *16*, 17
Chopart's joint, 472
Clavicle, 257–263
 anatomy of, 257, *263*
 fracture of, 257–262
  birth-related, 258–260, *260*
  child abuse and, 527, *528*
  classification of, *262*, 262–263, *263*
  diagnosis of, 257–260
  distal, 261–262, *262*, *263*
  fixation of, 260–261, *261*
  mechanism of, 257, 258, 260, 261
  medial, 257–261, *259*–*261*
  physeal injury due to, 257, *259*
  pseudoparalysis with, 258, *260*
  "serendipity" view of, 258, *259*, 260
  treatment of, 258, 260–262
 ligaments of, 257
 muscles of, 257
Clostridial infection, 429, 429t
Coalition, calcaneonavicular, 504, *504*, *505*
 foot pain and, 504, *504*–506
 talocalcaneal, 504, *505*, *506*
Coma, fixation indicated by, 106
 Glasgow scale for, 71, 72t
Compartment syndrome, *101*, 101–102
 causes of, 101–102
 duration of, 101–102
 femoral shaft fracture and, 366
 forearm fracture and, 149–150, *150*
 lower extremity, 83, *84*, 101–102, 366, 440–443
 multiple trauma and, 83, *83*, *84*
 tibial shaft fracture and, 440–443
 upper extremity, 83, *83*, *101*, 101–102, 149–150, *150*
Computed tomography (CT), abdominal trauma and, 81t, 81–82
Contracture, ischemia and, *101*, 101–102
 Volkmann's, *101*, 101–102
Coracoid process, anatomy of, 263–264
 fracture of, 265, *267*
Coronoid fossa, *215*, *233*
Coronoid process, *131*
Crepitation, open fracture and, 429–430
Cricothyrotomy, multiple trauma and, 75
 needle, 75
Cross union, correction of, 109, *110*
 radioulnar, 109, *110*, 171
Cubitus, valgus deformity of, *19*, 237–239, *238*

Cubitus *(Continued)*
 varus deformity of, 109, 219, *219*, 226–227, *228*
Cuboid bone, *450*, *471*, 471–472
Cuneiform bone, *450*, *471*, 471–472
Cyst, calcaneal, 475, *475*
 fracture caused by, 62t
 humeral, 274, *276*
 spinal, 300, *301*
 tibial, 421

D

Debridement, soft tissue injury and, 90–91, 425–430, *426*, *427*
 tibial fracture and, 425–430, *426*, *427*
Deformity, genu recurvatum, 48, 437–438
 gunstock, 227
 Madelung, 156
 overgrowth and, 151, 365, 438
 pseudo-Madelung, 156
 shortening, femoral fracture and, 352, *353*
  tibial fracture and, 438, 511
  toe and, 501, *503*
 valgus, ankle with, 436–437, 507, *508*
  elbow with, *19*, 237–239, *238*
  knee with, 109, *111*, 400–405, *406*, 436–437
 varus, ankle with, 436–437, 476, *478*, 509–511, *511*
  elbow with, 109, 219, *219*, 226–227, *228*
  metatarsal fracture and, *495*
Delbet classification, 327, *328*
Dens. See *Odontoid process*.
Diaphysis, 8
Dias-Tachdjian classification, 455, 456t, *457*
Diphtheria toxoid, 429, 429t
Disk disease, apophysitis and, 49–50, *50*
Dislocation, atlantoaxial, 284–285, 293–294
 carpal, 196, *197*, 199
 carpometacarpal, 199
 cervical spine, 284–285, 293–294, 298–300, *299*, *300*
 elbow, *39*, 248–254
  classification of, 249–250, *250*
  complications of, *242*, 250–251
  radial head in, 251–254, *252*, *253*
  treatment of, *242*, 250
 fingers affected by, 205–208, *207*, *208*
 foot affected by, 475t, 475–476, 499–500, *500*
 glenohumeral, 265–270, *268*, *269*
 hand affected by, 205–208, *207*, *208*
 knee affected by, 393–394
 metacarpophalangeal, 205–208, *207*, *208*
 metatarsal, 500, *500*

Dislocation *(Continued)*
  metatarsophalangeal, 499–500, *500*
  patellar, 391–393, *393*
  radial head, 251–254, *252*, *253*
  radioulnar, 184–188, 194–196, *196*
  shoulder affected by, 265–270, *268*, *269*
  toes affected by, 499–500, *500*
  vertebral, *293*, 293–294, *300–303*, 300–305
Distraction, bone lengthening by, 42–43
Doppler arterial pressure index, 82
Down syndrome, spinal anomalies in, *286*, 294
Dressing, Robert Jones, 430
  tibial fracture and, 430
Drill, saline-cooled, 356
Dysautonomia, foot and, *506*, 506
Dystrophy, reflex sympathetic, 121–122
  diagnosis of, 121
  forearm affected by, 150–151
  treatment of, 122

E

Ectopia, bone and, 103–104, *104*
Elbow, 213–254
  anatomy of, 213–216, *213–216*, *233*
  angle of, *215*, 215–216
  ankylosis of, 104, *104*
  arteries and, 214, *214*
  carrying angle of, 215–216
  dislocation of, *39*, 248–254
    classification of, 249–250, *250*
    complications of, 250–251
    congenital, 251–253, *253*
    divergent, 251, *252*
    mechanism of, 249, *250*
    radial head in, 251–254, *252*, *253*
    recurrent, 251
    treatment of, *242*, 250
  ectopic bone formation in, *104*
  fat pads of, 214
  floating, 171, *173*, *174*
  fracture of, 36–42, *39–42*, 213–248
    condylar, *230*, 230–243, *233–238*, *240*
    epicondylar, 239–243, 241t, *242*, *243*
    nerve injury in, 119–121
    olecranon, 248, 248t, *249*
    radial, *244*, 244–245, 245t, *246–248*
    supracondylar, 216–227, *220*, *225*, *228*
  lines and angles of, *214*, 214–216, *215*, *220*, *230*
  Little Leaguer's, 48, *50*, *51*
  "nursemaid's," 253–254
  radiographic lines of, *214*, 214–216, *215*, *220*
  valgus deformity of, *19*, 237–239, *238*

Elbow *(Continued)*
  varus deformity of, 109, 219, *219*, 226–227, *228*
Embolism, fat, 102–103
  fracture and, 102–103
  symptoms in, 103
  treatment of, 103
Epicondyle, humeral, 42, *50*, *51*, *151*
  lateral, *151*
    fracture of, 42
  medial, *50*, *51*
    apophysitis affecting, *50*, 51
    avulsion of, *50*, 51
Epiphyseodesis, 42–43
Epiphyseolysis, 44, *46*
Epiphysis, 15–17, *16*
  blood supply of, 16, *16*
  injury to. See *Physis, injury to.*
Essex-Lopresti fracture, forearm and, 188, *193*
Exostosis, toe affected by, 507, *508*
Extremities, 67. See also specific bones and joints.
  lower, 67
    compartment syndrome of, 83, *84*, 101–102, 366, 440–443
    length inequality in, 352, *353*, 438, 511
    multiple injury and, 71t, 82–83
  upper, 67
    compartment syndrome of, 83, *83*, *101*, 101–102, 149–150, *150*
Eye, opening of, coma and, 72t

F

Face, multiple injury and, 71t, 79
Falls, accidental, 68, 68t
Fasciotomy, arm decompression and, 149–150, *151*
  Henry approach in, 83, *83*
  leg decompression and, 83, *84*
Fat, Achilles tendon and, 453, *453*
  bony bar inhibited by, 45–46
  cast syndrome treatment and, 104
  embolism due to, 102–103
  globules, 380, *380*
  knee fracture and, 380, *380*
  retroperitoneal, 104
  stripe, 453, *453*
  synostosis correction and, 109, *110*
Femoral artery, 99
Femur, 326–337, 345–366
  anatomy of, 326–327, 345–346, 369
  angle of, neck-shaft, 346
  anteversion of, 346
  apophysitis affecting, 49, *49*
  development of, 345–346
  fracture of, 326–337, 345–366
    child abuse and, 346–347, 370, 521–527, *522*, *525*
    distal, 369–382

Femur *(Continued)*
  condylar, 380, *380*, *381*
  diagnosis of, 370
  fixation in, cast and, 370–372, 375–378
    cast-brace and, 371–372
    external, 372–373, *373*
    internal, 375–380, *376–378*
    traction and, 370–371, *371*, *373*
  management of, 370–380, *371*, *373*, *376–378*
  mechanism of, 370
  osteochondral, 380, *380*
  physeal injury due to, 369, 374–380, *376–381*
  pathologic, 57–64, *59*, *60*, *62*
  proximal, *29*, *316*, 326–337, 521–523
    aftercare in, 334–336, 336t
    classification of, 327, *328*
    complications of, *34*, 112, 336–337
    management of, 329–334, 330t, *332*, *333*, *335*, *340*
    physeal injury due to, *29*, *34*, 521–523, *522*
    type I, 329–330, 330t
    type II, 329–331, 330t
    type III, 329, 330t, 331–333, *332*, *333*
    type IV, 329, 330t, 333–334, *335*
  shaft, 345–366, 523–527
    classification of, 348–349
    diagnosis of, 346–348, 523–527
    fixation in, external, 354–355, *355–357*
      flexible rod and, 360–361, *362*
      medullary nailing and, 355–361, *358–362*
      plate and, 361–363, *364–365*
      spica casting and, 350–352, *351*
      traction and, 350, 352–354, *353*
    history in, 346–347, 523–527
    malunion of, 106, *108*
    management of, 349–363
    mechanism of, 346, 523–527, *524*, *525*
    multiple injury with, 363, 365–366
    overgrowth in, 365
    physical examination in, 347
    radiology in, 348, 524–526, *525*
    shortening due to, 352, *353*
    tibial fracture with, 417–418, *418–419*, 436
  toddler's, 524–526, *525*
  vascular damage in, 99–101, *100*
Fibrous ring of Lacroix, 4
Fibula, 397–443
  blood supply to, 397
  bone graft from, *118*, 119
  collateral ligament of, 25
  fracture of, 397–443
    diagnosis of, 399–400

Fibula *(Continued)*
    distal, 456t, *457*, *459*, 467–471, *470*, 509–513
    incidence of, 398
    management of, 400–434
    mechanism of, 398
    open, 422–434, *426*, *427*, *434–436*
        fixation in, *427*, 430–433, *434–436*
        treatment of, 424–434
        type I, 422, 424t
        type II, 422–423, 424t
        type III, 422–423, 424t
    pathologic, 57–64, *61*
    physical examination in, 399–400
    shaft, 415–416
        isolated, *421*, 421
        management of, 405–410, 407t
    soft tissue injury in, 424, 425t
    stress, 415–416
Fingers, contracture of, *101*, 101–102
    dislocation of, 205–208, *207*, *208*
    fracture of, 199–203, *202–204*
    index, 205–208, *208*
    interosseous nerve palsy and, 119–121, *121*
    mallet deformity of, 201
    traction traps for, *197*
Fixation. See also *Plate(s)*; *Traction*.
    acetabular fracture and, 324
    atlantoaxial joint and, 294–296, *295*
    clavicular fracture and, 260–261, *261*
    comatose patient and, 106
    distraction using, 42–43
    femoral fracture and, 354–363, 370–380, 417–418
    fibular fracture and, *427*, 430–433, *434–436*
    floating knee and, 417–418, *418*, *419*
    forearm fracture and, *133*, 164–171, *166–170*
    hand injury and, 200
    humeral fracture and, 36–42, 223–226, 271–278
    multiple injury fracture and, 85t, 87–88, 91
    olecranon fracture and, 248, *249*
    pelvic fracture and, *320*, 321–324, *323*
    radial fracture and, 165, *166–170*, 168–169
    refracture and, 88, 91
    three-point, *133*, 133
    tibial fracture and, 35–36, 421–422, 430–432
    ulnar fracture and, 165, *166–170*, 168–169
Fluids, multiple injury and, 77t, 77–78
Foot, 449–514
    anatomy of, 449–451, *450*, *451*, *471*, *471–472*
    bicycle spoke injury to, 507
    coalition affecting, 504, *504–506*
    dislocation of, 475t, 475–476, 499–500, *500*

Foot *(Continued)*
    forefoot segment of, 472
    fracture of, 475–499
        approach in, 513–514
        calcaneal, 475, 475t, 483t, 483–484, 485–487
        child abuse causing, 507–509, *510*
        incidence of, 475t, 475–476
        metatarsal, 475, 475t, 489–494, *490–497*
        navicular, 475, 475t, 484–488, *487*, *488*
        osteochondral, 479–483, *481*, *482*
        pathologic, 506, *506*, *507*
        phalangeal, 475, 475t, 497–499, *498*, *499*
        physeal injury due to, 453–471, 456t, *457–462*, *464–466*
        sites of, 475t, 475–476
        stress, 492, 492–494, 504–506
        talar, 475t, 475–483, *478–482*
        tarsometatarsal joint, 475, 475t, 488–489, *489*
        traction in, 490, *490*
    hindfoot segment of, 472
    lawn mower injury to, 500, *501*
    ligaments of, 449, *450*, *451*
    midfoot segment of, 472
    movement of, 449
    ossicles of, 471–475, *471–475*
    osteochondroses of, 472–475, *472–475*
    puncture wound of, 501, *502–504*
    swelling of, *486*, *490*, *495*
    tumor affecting, 506–507, *508*, *509*
Forearm, 127–194
    anatomy of, 127–133, *128–131*
    compartment syndrome of, 83, *83*, *101*, 101–102, 149–150, *150*
    contracture affecting, *101*, 101–102
    fracture of, 127–194
        buckle, 135, *139*
        casting principles in, 143, *143*, 144, 161, *161*
        complete, 135, *136*, 142, *143*, *144*
        complications of, 83, 101–102, 106, 144–151, 155–156, 170–171
        deforming forces in, 133–134, *134*, *160*, *162*
        diagnosis of, 135–141
        distal, 151–162, *154*, *155*, *160–162*
        Essex-Lopresti, 188, *193*
        fixation in, *133*, 164–171, *166–170*
        Galeazzi, 188–194, *191*
        Galeazzi-equivalent, 188–194, *191–193*
        greenstick, 135, *140*, *141*, 142, *158*, *159*
        humeral fracture with, 171, *173*, *174*
        management principles for, *133*, 141–144, *142–144*
        mechanism of, *134*, 134–135
        midshaft, 162–170, *163–170*
        Monteggia, 171–188

Forearm *(Continued)*
        complications of, 186–188, *187*
        management of, 178–186, *181–183*, *185*
        type I, *175*, 175–180, *179*, *181*, *182*
        type II, *175*, 175–177, 180
        type III, *175*, 175–178, 180
        type IV, 175, *175*, 178, 180
        Monteggia-equivalent, 175–177, *176*, 180–186, *183*, *185*
        overgrowth following, 151
        physeal injury in, 106, 151–156, *154–156*
        plastic deformation in, 135, *139*, 141–142, *142*
        proximal, 171–194
        reduction principles for, *129*, 132–133, *133*, 142–144, *143*
        remodeling potential in, 135, *136–138*, 148
        torus, 135, *139*
    function in, *129*, 131–132, *132*
    interosseous membrane of, 131, *131*
    muscles of, 133, *134*, *160*, 161, *162*
    pronation of, *129*, *130*, 131–132, *132*
    supination of, *129*, *130*, 131–132, *132*
Foreign bodies, asymptomatic, *503*
    foot and, 501–503, *503*, *504*
Fossa, coronoid, 215, *216*, 233
    olecranon, *216*
    piriformis, *358*
Foucher classification, 20
Fractures. See also under specific bones and joints.
    biomechanics of, 8–13, *9–12*
    "blow-out," 71t
    "bucket-handle," 370, *522*
    buckle, 9, *10*, 135, *139*
    Chance, 69, 303
    child abuse causing, 520–529, *521–528*
    complete, 10–13
    complications of, 99–122
        cast syndrome and, 104, *105*
        compartment syndrome and. See *Compartment syndrome*.
        deformity and. See *Deformity*.
        ectopic bone formation and, 103–104, *104*
        fat embolism and, 102–103
        growth disturbance and. See *Growth disturbance*.
        hypercalcemia and, 103
        hypertension and, 104–105
        late angulation and, 109, *111*
        ligament injury in, 119, *120*
        malunion and. See *Malunion*.
        nerve injury and. See *Nerve injury*.
        nonunion and. See *Nonunion*.
        refracture and, 119
        soft tissue injury and. See *Soft tissue injury*.
        vascular. See *Vascular injury*.
    compression, 17–18, *20*, *22*, 463, *464*

Fractures *(Continued)*
    "corner," 370, *523*
    Galeazzi, 188–194, *191*
    Galeazzi-equivalent, 188–194, *191–193*
    greenstick, 9–10, 135, *140*, *141*, 142, *158*, *159*
    hangman's, 296–298, *298*
    healing of, 1, *2*, *3*, 4–8
    Jefferson, *297*
    Jones, 494, *497*
    "march," 57, *492*, *493*
    Monteggia, 178–188, *181–183*, *185*, *187*
    Monteggia-equivalent, 175–177, *176*, 180–186, *183*, *185*
    multiple. See *Multiple injury.*
    oblique, 10
    open, 88–91, 390–391, 422–432
        antibiotic therapy in, 89–90, 425
        bone graft in, 91
        classification of, 88–89, 89t, 422–424
        debridement and irrigation in, 90–91, 425–430, *426*, *427*
        fixation in, 91, 361–363, *364*, *365*, 430–432
        gas gangrene in, 429–430
        tetanus and, 89, 90t, 429, 429t
        type I, 88, 89t
        type II, 88, 89t
        type III, 89, 89t
    open-book, *311*, 313t, 319t, 323, *323*
    orbital, 71t
    osteochondral, 380, *380*, 479–483, *481*, *482*
    pathologic, 57–64
        clinical presentation in, 57
        differential diagnosis in, 58–61, *58–61*
        femur and, 57–64, *59*, *60*, *62*
        fibula and, 57–64, *61*
        foot and, 506, *506*, *507*
        humerus and, 57–64, *63*, 274, *276*
        management of, 61–64, *62*, 62t, *63*
        mechanism in, 57–58, 274, 300–301, 418–421, 506
        prevention of, 64
        spine and, 300–301, *301*
        tibia and, 57–64, *58*, *60*, 418–421
    physeal injury due to. See *Physis, injury to.*
    plastic deformation in, 9, *9*, *11*
    "shepherd's crook," 57–58
    "sleeve," 381–382, *382*
    spiral, 10
    stress, 6, *6*, 415–416, *492*, 492–494, 504–506
    Tillaux, 463–466, *465*
    toddler's, 411–413, *413*, 524, *525*, *526*
    torus, 9, *10*, 135, *139*
    transverse, *10*, 10–11, *11*
Freiberg's disease, metatarsal, 493, *493*

G

Galeazzi fracture, 188–194, *191*
Galeazzi-equivalent fracture, 188–194, *191–193*
Gangrene, 429–430
    gas, 429–430
Genu recurvatum, 48, 437–438
Glasgow Coma Scale, 71, 72t
Glenohumeral joint, *264*
    anatomy of, 265–266
    dislocation of, 268–270
        diagnosis of, 268–269
        etiology of, 268, *268*
        incidence of, 267–268
        mechanism of, 268
        recurrence of, 269–270
        treatment of, 269–270
            hippocratic, 269, *269*
            Stimson, 269, *269*
Glenoid cavity, 263–264
    anatomy of, 263–264
    fracture of, 265, *266*
    humerus and, 265–270
"Goose-egg," fibular injury and, 467–471, *470*
Grafts, 92–93, 117–119, 432
    bone, nonunion treated with, 117–119, *118*
        open fracture and, 92, 432, *434–436*
        radius angle and, 156, *157*
    skin, 92–93, 432, *434–436*
    tibial fracture and, 432, *434–436*
Granuloma, eosinophilic, 61–62, *63*
Growth disturbance, 18–20, 42–48, 112–117. See also *Apophysitis; Deformity.*
    leg length inequality and, 352, *353*, 438, 511
    overgrowth and, 151, 365, 438
    periosteal bone and, *529*, 529–530, *530*
    physeal, 18–20, 42–48, 112–117
        central, 44–45, *45*, *114*, 116, *116*, *117*
        classification of, 44–45, *45*, *46*
        Bright, 44–45, *45*
        combined, 44–45, *46*
        distraction in, 42–43
        Harris lines in, 5, 5–6, 43, *43*
        mapping of, *44*, *115*
        peripheral, 44–45, *45*, 116, *116*
        treatment of, 42–48, *46*, *47*, 115–117, *116*, *117*
Growth plate. See *Physis.*
Gunshot wound, foot and, 503, *504*
    knee and, 390–391

H

Hand, 199–208
    anesthesia in, 199

Hand *(Continued)*
    dislocation in, 205–208, *207*, *208*
    fracture of, 199–205, *202–204*, *206*
        physeal injury due to, 200–205, *204*, *206*
Harris lines, growth disturbance and, 5, 5–6, 43, *43*
    physiology of, 5, 5–6
Harris view, 504, *505*
Head injury, child abuse and, 69–70, 527–529
    multiple injury and, 69–70, 71t, 72t, 79
Heel. See also *Calcaneus.*
    apophysitis affecting, 48–49
    pain in, 484
Hemarthrosis, 380, *380*
Hematoma, 4–5
Hemorrhage, abdominal, 80–82, 81t
    evaluation of, 77, 80–82, 81t
    multiple injury and, 77, 80–82, 81t
Henry approach, fasciotomy and, 83, *83*
Heterotopia, osseous, 103–104, *104*
Hip, 307–326, 337–341
    dislocation of, 337–341
        classification of, 337
        complications of, 341
        diagnosis of, 337–338
        management of, 338–341, *340*
        mechanism of, 337
        physical examination in, 338
        radiology of, 338
        recurrence of, 341
    fracture of. See *Pelvis, fracture of.*
Hobb's view, 258
Hormones, bone growth and, 1
Humerus, 213–243
    anatomy of, *213*, 213–216, *215*, *216*, *233*
    apophysitis affecting, 48, *50*, *51*
    fracture of, 213–254
        child abuse and, 520–521, *521*, 527, *527*
        condylar, 230–239
            classification of, 232–236, *233–236*, *239*
            complications of, 237–239, *238*
            diagnosis of, 236–237
            lateral, 230–239
            mechanism of, 230–232, *233*
            medial, 239, *240*
            nonunion in, 237–239, *238*
            treatment of, 237, *238*
            valgus deformity and, 237–239, *238*
        epicondylar, 239–243
            diagnosis of, 241
            fasciotomy and, *151*
            lateral, *151*, 243, *243*
            medial, 239–243, *240*, 241t, *242*
            treatment of, 241–243, *241–243*
        floating elbow and, 171, *173*, *174*
        malunion of, *105*, 105–106
        pathologic, 57–64, *63*

Humerus *(Continued)*
  physeal injury due to, 36–42, 229–230, 270–272, 520–521
  proximal, *270,* 270–278
    classification of, 271, 271t
    deforming force in, *276*
    diagnosis of, 271
    incidence of, 271
    mechanism of, 271
    treatment of, 271–272, *273–275*
  shaft, 272–278, *276, 277, 527*
    bone cyst causing, 274, *276*
    deforming muscle force in, *276*
    fixation in, 274–278, *276, 277*
    treatment of, 274–278, *276, 277*
  supracondylar, 216–227
    anatomy and, 216, *216*
    casting in, 222–223
    classification of, 217–218
    extension position and, 217–226, *225*
    fixation in, 223–226, *225*
    flexion position and, 227, *228*
    management of, *219,* 219–226, *220, 225*
    mechanism of, 216–217
    nerve injury with, 217, 226
    physical examination in, 218
    traction in, 220–222
    varus deformity and, *219,* 226–227
    vascular injury with, 217, 226
    vascular damage in, 99–101, *100*
  lines and angles of, *214,* 214–216, *215, 220, 230*
Hypercalcemia, immobilization and, 103
Hyperemia, fracture site and, 4–5
Hyperesthesia, forearm, 150
Hyperostosis, 530, *530*
Hypertension, traction-induced, 104–105
Hypothermia, management of, 78
  multiple injury and, 78

I

Ilium, 307, *308*
  apophysitis affecting, 49, *49*
  fracture of. See *Pelvis, fracture of.*
Immobilization, hypercalcemia due to, 103
Immunization, tetanus, 89, 90t, 429, 429t
Infection, foot puncture wound and, 501, *502, 503*
  forearm fracture and, 150
  open fracture and, 425, 428–430
  organisms causing, 428–430
  tibial fracture and, 425, 428–430
Inflammation, apophyseal. See *Apophysitis.*
  atlantoaxial, 294–296, *295*

Inflammation *(Continued)*
  fracture site and, 4–5
Interphalangeal joint, 199–208, 499–500
  dislocation of, 205–208, *207, 208,* 499–500, *500*
  foot and, 499–500, *500*
  hand and, 199–208, *207, 208*
Intervertebral joint, 283–286, *285, 289*
  injury to, 284–285, 293–294, 303–304
  C1–C2, 284–285, 293–294
  occiput-C1, 293, *293*
  thoracolumbar, 300–305, *301, 303, 304*
Intubation, multiple trauma and, 74–76
Irrigation, soft tissue injury and, 90–91, 425–430, *427*
Ischemia, compartment syndrome and, *101,* 101–102
  contracture due to, *101,* 101–102
  elbow fracture and, 217, 226
  tibial fracture and, 428
  vascular injury and, 99–101, *100*
Ischium, 307, *308*
  apophysitis affecting, 49, *49*
  fracture of. See *Pelvis, fracture of.*

J

Joint(s), acromioclavicular, 262–263, *263*
  atlantoaxial, 283–286
    dislocation of, 284–285, 293–294
    rotatory fixation of, 294–296, *295*
  atlanto-occipital, 283–286, *289,* 293, *293*
  carpometacarpal, 205, *206*
  ectopic bone formation in, 104, *104*
  elbow. See *Elbow.*
  foot and, *471,* 471–472, 499–500, *500*
  glenohumeral, *264*
    anatomy of, 265–267
    dislocation of, 265–270
      etiology of, 268, *268*
      treatment of, *269,* 269–270
  hip. See *Hip.*
  interphalangeal, 199–208, 499–500
    dislocation of, 205–208, *207, 208,* 499–500, *500*
    foot and, 499–500, *500*
    hand and, 199–208, *207, 208*
  intervertebral, 283–286, *285, 289*
    injury to, 284–285, 293–294, *300–304,* 303–304
    C1–C2, 284–285, 293–294
    occiput-C1, 293, *293*
    thoracolumbar, 300–305, *301, 303, 304*
  knee. See *Knee.*
  metacarpophalangeal, 205–208, *206–208*
  metatarsophalangeal, 500, *500*
  of Chopart, 472

Joint(s) *(Continued)*
  of Lisfranc, 472
    injury to, 488
  radiocarpal, 130, *130, 160,* 161
    angulation in, 156, *157*
    bone graft in, 156, *157*
  radioulnar, 128–132
    articulation of, 128–132, *129–132*
    dislocation of, 184–188, 194–196, *196*
    distal, 130, *130–132, 160,* 194–196, *196*
    ligaments of, 128–130, *130, 131*
    proximal, 128–132, *129–132,* 186–188, *187*
    reconstruction of, 186–188, *187*
  sacroiliac, *308*
    fracture of, 310, *311,* 317–319
  shoulder, 257–278
    anatomy of, 257, *262, 263,* 263–267, *270*
    dislocation of, 265–270, *268, 269*
    fracture of, 257–278
      clavicular, 257–262, *259–263*
      humeral, *270,* 270–278, 271t, *273–277*
      scapular, 263–265, *264–267*
    muscles of, *276*
  tarsometatarsal, 472
    anatomy of, 472
    fracture of, 475, 475t, 488–489, *489*
    management of, 489
    mechanism of, 488, *489*
  wrist, 194–199
    anatomy of, 130, *130, 160,* 161
    dislocation and, 194–196, *196,* 199
    fracture of, 196–198, *197, 198*
    radioulnar joint and, 130, *130, 160,* 161
Jones fracture, fifth metatarsal and, 494, *497*
Jones view, *40*
Judet view, *316*

K

Klippel-Feil syndrome, 286
Knee, 369–394
  anatomy of, 369, *387,* 387–388
  apophysitis affecting, 48
  arteries and, *387,* 387–388, *388*
  dislocation of, 393–394
    diagnosis of, 393
    mechanism of, 393
    patellar, 391–393, *392, 393*
    treatment of, 393–394
  floating, 417–418, *418, 419*
  fracture of, 369–391, 417–418
    femur and, 369–380, *376–381,* 417–418, *418, 419*
    open, 390–391
    patella and, 380, *380–382*

Knee *(Continued)*
   stress, 6, *6*
   tibia and, 382–390, *383*, *384*, *386–388*, 417–418, *418*, *419*
   genu recurvatum and, 48, 437–438
   "jumper's," 48
   ligaments of, 119, *120*, 369
   valgus deformity of, 109, *111*, 400–405, *406*, 436–437
Köhler's disease, calcaneal, 487
   navicular, 484–488, *487*

L

Labor, infant spinal injury in, 289–290, *290*
   newborn clavicular fracture and, 258–260, *260*
Lacroix ring, 4
Ladd procedure, 104
Lauge-Hansen classification, 454, 456t
Lavage, peritoneal, 81t, 81–82
Lawn mower injury, foot affected by, 500, *501*
Leg. See also specific bones and joints.
   compartment syndrome of, 83, *84*, 101–102, 366, 440–443
   length inequality of, femur and, 352, *353*
      tibia and, 438, 511
Letournel classification, 310, *312*
Leukemia, spinal fracture and, 300, *301*
Ligament(s), ankle and, 449, *450*, *451*
   atlantoaxial joint and, 285
   bifurcated, *450*
   calcaneofibular, 449, *450*, *451*
   calcaneonavicular, *450*
   clavicle and, 257
   coracoclavicular, *262*, 262–263, *263*
   cruciate, 369
   deltoid, 449, *450*, *451*
   femur and, 369
   fibular collateral, 25
   foot and, 449, *450*, *451*
   injury to, fracture complication with, 119, *120*
   knee and, 369
   odontoid process and, 285
   patellar, *391*, 391–393, *393*
   planar, *450*
   quadrate, 128–130, *130*, *131*
   radiocarpal collateral, *160*
   radioulnar annular, 128–130, *130*, *131*
      reconstruction of, 186–188, *187*
   talocalcaneal, *450*
   talofibular, 449, *450*, *451*
   talonavicular, *450*
   talotibial, *450*
   tibial, distal, 449, *450*, *451*
      proximal, 119, *120*
   tibiofibular, 449, *450*, *451*
   ulnar collateral, 130, *131*, 241, *241*

Ligament(s) *(Continued)*
   ulnocarpal, 128–130, *130*, *131*
Line(s), anterior coronoid, 215, *215*
   anterior humeral, 215, *215*
   elbow and, *214*, 214–216, *215*, *220*
   Harris, 5–6
      growth disturbance and, *5*, 5–6, 43, *43*
      physiology of, *5*, 5–6
   Park, 5
   Swischuk's, 288, *289*
      spinal pseudosubluxation and, 288, *288*
Lisfranc's joint, 472
   injury to, 488
Little Leaguer's elbow, 48, *50*, *51*
Lloyd-Roberts procedure, 186–188, *187*
Lordosis, cervical, 300, *300*
   loss of, 300, *300*, *302*, 303
   lumbar, *302*, 303
   trauma injury and, 300, *300*, *302*, 303
Lower extremity. See also specific bones and joints.
   compartment syndrome of, 83, *84*, 101–102, 366, 440–443
   length inequality in, 352, *353*, 438, 511

M

Mach bands, spinal fracture vs., 287, *287*
Madelung's deformity, radial epiphyseal injury vs., 156
Malformation syndrome, calcaneus and, 472, *472*
Malleolus, medial, fracture of, 475t
   osteotomy and, *480*
Malrotation, radial fracture and, 106, 145, *146*
   tibial fracture and, 437
Malunion, 105–109, 145, 434–437. See also *Nonunion*.
   femoral, *108*, 109
   forearm fracture and, 106, *107*, 145, *146*, *147*
   humeral, *105*, 105–109
   tibial, 434–437
Membranes, interosseus, 131, *131*, 449
   radioulnar, 131, *131*
   tibiofibular, 387, 397, 449
Meniscus, knee joint, 382–385, *384*
Mesenteric artery, cast syndrome role of, 104, *105*
   duodenum compressed by, 104, *104*
Metabolic rate, 67
Metacarpals, 203–205, *208*
   fracture of, 203–205
Metacarpophalangeal joint, 205–208, *206–208*
Metaphysis, 15–17, *16*
   injury to. See *Physis, injury to*.

Metatarsals. See also *Toes*.
   anatomy of, *450*
   dislocation and, 499–500, *500*
   fifth, 494, *496*, *497*
   first, 491, *491*
   fourth, 493–494, *494*
   fracture of, 475, 475t, 489–494, *490–497*
      "buckle base," 491, *491*
      Jones, 494, *497*
      "march," 57, *492*, 493
      mechanism of, 488, *489*, 491–494, *492*, *495*
      stress, *492*, 492–493
      traction in, 490, *490*
      treatment of, 490–494, *490–497*
      varus deformity with, *495*
   ossicles and, *471*
   pseudoepiphysis of, 473, *473*
   second, 491–493, *492–495*
   third, 493–494, *494*
Metatarsophalangeal joint, 499–500, *500*
Meyers-McKeever classification, 382, *383*
Modified Injury Severity Scale (MISS), 70–71, 71t
Monteggia fracture, 178–188, *181–183*, *185*, *187*
Monteggia-equivalent fracture, 175–177, *176*, 180–186, *183*, *185*
Morel-Lavalée lesion, 310
   pelvic injury and, 310
Motor response, coma and, 72t
Multiple injury, 65–94, *78–79*
   abdomen and, 71t, 80–82, 81t
   airway and, 71t, 72t, 74–76
   anatomic proportions and, 65–67, *67*, *75*, 77t
   chest and, 69, 71t, 80
   classification in, 70–72, 71t, 72t
   coma scale in, 71, 71t, 72t
   extremities in, 71t, 82–83
   face and, 71t, 79
   field management of, 73–78, 74t, *75*
   fracture in, 83–92
      antibiotic therapy and, 89–90
      fixation of, 87–88, 91
      open, 88–92
      physeal plate and, 85–86, *86*
      surgical approach to, 83–92, 85t, 89t
   head and, 69–70, 71t, 79
   incidence of, 67–68
   mechanisms of, 68t, 68–70
   mortality and morbidity in, 72–73
   neurological evaluation in, 71, 71t, 72t, 80
   pelvis and, 71t
   psychological factors and, 93, 93t
   radiography in, 78–79
   rehabilitation following, 92–94
   severity scale in, 70–72, 71t, 72t
   spine and, 69, 71t, 79–80, 290–293, *300*, 300–305, *303*

Muscle(s), biceps, *276*
  brachioradialis, 133, *134, 160,* 161, *162*
  clavicle and, 257
  coracobrachialis, *276*
  deltoid, *276*
  forearm fracture affected by, 133, *134, 160,* 161, *162*
  humeral fracture affected by, *276*
  pectoralis major, *276*
  pronator quadratius, 133, *134, 160,* 161
  pronator teres, 133, *134*
  quadriceps, Q angle and, 391, *391*
  radial, *276*
  shoulder and, *276*
  supinator, 133, *134*
  supraspinatus, *276*
  triceps, *276*
Myelomeningocele, fracture and, 420

N

Nailing. See also *Fixation.*
  medullary, femoral, 355–361, *358–362*
Navicular, *450,* 472
  accessory ossicle of, 474, *474*
  coalition affecting, 504, *504, 505*
  fracture of, 475, 475t, 484–488, *487, 488*
Necrosis, avascular, *34, 35,* 341, *478, 479, 480*
  femur affected by, *34, 35*
  hip and, *34, 35,* 341
  physeal injury and, *34, 35*
  talus affected by, *478, 479, 480*
Neer/Horowitz classification, 271, *271*
Neglect, child, 519. See also *Child abuse.*
Neoplasia, foot affected by, 506–507, *508, 509*
  fracture associated with, 57–64, 62t, *63*
Nerve, interosseous, 119–121, *121,* 188, *189, 190,* 226
  median, 119–121, *121,* 217, 226, 251
  ulnar, 119–121, 188, *189, 190,* 251
Nerve injury, 119–121, *121*
  elbow dislocation and, 119–121, *121,* 217, 226, 251
  forearm fracture and, 119–121, *121,* 188, *189, 190*
  humeral fracture and, 217, 226
  Monteggia fracture and, 188, *189, 190*
  secondary, 121
  spinal cord trauma and, 79–80
  tibial fracture and, 440
Nervous system, reflex dystrophy and, 121–122, 150–151
  sympathetic, 121–122, 150–151
Neuromuscular disease, bone effects of, 418–421

Neurotoxin, tetanus and, 429
Nonunion, 117–119, *118.* See also *Malunion.*
  bone graft in, 117–119, *118*
  forearm fracture and, 149
  humeral fracture and, 117–119, *118,* 237–239, *238*
  tibial fracture and, 117–119, *118,* 434–436
"Nursemaid's" elbow, 253–254

O

Occipitoatlantal joint, 284–285, *289*
Occiput, backboard hollow for, *75,* 75–76
  vertebral joint with, 283–286, *289, 293, 293*
Odontoid process, *289*
  anatomy of, 283–287, *284, 285, 289*
  anomalies of, 285–287, *286*
  basion relation to, 286–287, *289*
  ligaments and, 285
  spinal injury and, 285, 287
Ogden classification, 20–27, *20–27*
Olecranon, apophysitis affecting, 51
  delayed fusion in, 42, *42, 42*
  fossa of, *216*
  fracture of, 42, 248
    classification of, 248, 248t
    elbow and, 248, 248t, *249*
    mechanism of, 248
Open-book fracture, *311,* 313t, 319t, *323, 323*
Os acromiale, 263, *264,* 265
Os calcis. See *Calcaneus.*
Os cuboideum secundarium, *471*
Os fibulare, *471*
Os intercuneiforme, *471*
Os intermetatarseum, *471*
Os odontoideum, 285–287
  axial fracture and, 296–297, *299*
Os subfibulare, 451, *471*
Os sustentaculi, *471*
Os tibiale externum, *471*
Os trigonum, *450, 471, 474, 474,* 479
Os vesalianum, *471,* 473, *473*
  fracture of, *496*
Osgood-Schlatter disease, 48
  tibial fracture vs., 385
Ossicles, foot and, 471–475, *471–475*
Ossification. See also *Physis.*
  calcaneal, 472, *472,* 474, *474*
  clavicular, 257, *259,* 261
  enchondral, 4–6
  femoral, 345–346
  foot and, 472–475, *473–475*
  humeral, *213,* 213–214
  membranous, 4–6
  patellar, 381
  radial, 128, *128*
  scapular, 263, *264*

Ossification *(Continued)*
  spinal, 283–284, *284*
  ulnar, 128, *128*
  vertebral, 283–284, *284*
Osteoarthritis, 341
Osteoblasts, 4
Osteochondritis dissecans, 479–483, *481, 482*
Osteochondroma, ankle affected by, 507, *508*
Osteochondrosis. See *Apophysitis.*
Osteoclasis, forearm, 145, *146*
Osteogenesis imperfecta, 58, *59,* 530
  child abuse vs., 530
Osteoma, foot and, 507, *509*
  osteoid, 507, *509*
Osteomyelitis, foot and, 501, *502, 503*
  fracture due to, 58, *60*
  puncture wound and, 501, *502, 503*
  "stubbed-toe," 499, *499*
Osteonecrosis. See *Necrosis.*
Osteopetrosis, 57, *59,* 61, *62*
Osteoporosis, foot affected by, 506, *507*
Osteosynthesis. See *Fixation; Plate(s).*
Osteotomy, cubitus varus and, 226–227, *228*
  medial malleolar, *480*
  physeal bar resection and, 44–45, *46, 116,* 116–117, *117*
  radial fracture and, 145, *147*
Overgrowth, femoral fracture and, 365
  forearm fracture and, 151
  shortening and, 438
  tibial, 438
Overuse syndrome, calcaneal, 472, *472*
Oxygen therapy, 103

P

Pain, insensitivity to, 506, *506*
Palsy, elbow fracture and, 119–121
  forearm fracture and, 188, *189, 190*
  interosseous nerve and, 119–121, *121,* 188, *189, 190*
  thumb affected by, 119–121, *121*
Paresthesia, compartment syndrome and, 102
  nerve injury and, 119–121, *121*
Park lines, 5. See also *Harris lines.*
Patella, 380–382, 391–398
  anatomy of, *382, 391,* 391–392, *392*
  apophysitis affecting, 48
  bipartite, 381, *381*
  dislocation of, 391–393, *392*
    mechanism of, 391–393
    Q angle in, 391, *391*
    recurrent, 392–393, *393*
    surgical approach in, 392–393, *393*
  fracture of, *27, 380,* 380–382, *382*
    "sleeve," 381–382, *382*
  ligaments of, 392–393, *393*

Pediatric Trauma Score (PTS), 71–72, 72t
Pelvis, 307–326
  anatomy of, 307, *308*
  apophyses of, 49, *49*, *308*
  femoral fracture and, 326–337, *328*, *332*, *333*, *335*
  fracture of, 307–326, *311*, *312*
    A, *311*, 313t
    acetabular, 307–326, *312*, *316*, 319t
    aftercare in, 324–326
    avulsion, 49, *49*
    B, *311*, 313t
    C, *311*, 313t
    child abuse and, 29, 522
    classification of, 310, *311*, *312*, 313t
      Letournel, 310, *312*
      Pennal-Tile, 310, *311*, 313t
      Torode-Zieg, 310
      Trunkey, 310
      Watts, 310
    complications of, 326
    effects of, 308–309, *309*, 326
    fixation in, *320*, 321–324, *323*
    history in, 310
    incidence of, 307
    management of, *314*, 315–326, *317*–*320*, 319t, *323*
      options in, 320–324
    mechanism of, 307–309
    mortality and morbidity in, 325–326
    multiple injury and, 69, *70*, 71t, 307–310, *308*
    open-book, *311*, 313t, 319t, *323*, 323
    physeal injury due to, 28, 29, 307–309, *309*, *312*
    physical examination in, 310–314, *313*
    radiology in, *314*, 314–315, *316*
    traction in, 320–321, 324
Pennal-Tile classification, 310, *311*, 313t
Pericardium, tamponade and, 76–77
Perichondrium, 4–5
Periosteum, *3*, 3–6
  bone growth due to, *3*, 3–6, 8, *529*, 529–530, *530*
  Caffey's disease and, 530, *530*
  formation of, 4–5
  fracture reduction and, 132–133, *133*
  physis union with, 4–5, 15–17
  syphilis affecting, 529, *529*
Peritoneal lavage, 81t, 81–82
Peroneal artery, *387*, *397*
Pertussis toxoid, 429, 429t
Phalanges, 199–208, 497–499
  manual, 199–208
    dislocation of, 205–208, *207*, *208*
    fracture of, 199–203, *202*–*204*
  pedal, *450*, 497–499
    dislocation of, 499–500, *500*
    epiphyseal fissure of, *30*
    fracture of, 475, 475t, 497–499, *498*, *499*

Phenytoin, rickets due to, 506, *507*
Physical therapy, 92–93
Physis. See also *Ossification*.
  anatomy of, 15–16, *16*, *24*
  blood supply to, 16, *16*
  bony bar in, 18–20, *19*, 43–45, *44*–*46*, 113–117, *113*–*117*
  fibular, distal, 456t, *457*, *459*, 509–513
  formation of, 3–4
  growth disturbance and. See *Growth disturbance*.
  injury to, 11–13, 15–51, 112–117
    ankle fracture and, 453–471, 456t, *457*–*462*, *464*–*466*
    biomechanics of, 11–13, 17–18, *23*
    child abuse and, 520–523, *521*–*523*
    classification of, 20–27
      Foucher, 20
      Jakob, 232–236, *236*
      Milch, 232–236, *233*–*235*
      Ogden, 20–27, *20*–*27*
      Poland, 20–21, *22*
      Rang, 21, *22*, *25*
      Salter-Harris, 11–13, *12*, *20*–*24*, *20*–*27*
      Scuderi-Bronson, 25–27, *28*
      Weber, 21, *22*
    compression fracture and, 17–18, *20*, *22*, 463, *464*
    diagnosis of, 27–30, *30*
    femoral fracture and, 35, 114–115, 369, 374–380, 521–523
    fixation in, 31–34, *32*–*34*, 36–42, *38*, *40*–*42*
    foot fracture and, 453–471, 456t, *457*–*462*, *464*–*466*
    forearm fracture and, 151–156, *154*–*157*
    hand fracture and, 200–203, *203*, *204*
    humeral fracture and, 36–42, 229–236, 520–521
    incidence of, 16–17
    management principles for, 30–35, *32*–*34*
    metacarpal fracture and, 203–204, *206*
    phalangeal fracture and, 200–203, *203*, *204*, 497–499, *498*, *501*
    plane of cleavage in, 11, 17–18, *23*
    remodeling and, 30–31
    tibial fracture and, 35–36, 387–389, 437–438, 451–467
    type I, *20*, 21, *22*
    type II, *20*–*22*, 21–25, *23*
    type III, *20*, *22*, *24*, 25, *26*
    type IV, *20*, *22*, *24*, 25
    type V, *20*, *22*, *24*, 25
    type VI, *22*, 25, *25*
    type VII, *22*, 25, *26*
    type VIII, 25
    type IX, 25
    vertebral fracture and, 304, *304*
  periosteal sleeve and, 4, 15–17

Physis *(Continued)*
  pressure-responsive, 15
  traction-responsive, 15
  transplantation of, 46–47
Pins. See *Rods*.
Piriformis fossa, *358*
Plastic deformation fracture, 9, *9*, *11*
  forearm and, 135, *139*, 141–142, *142*
Plate(s). See also *Fixation*.
  clavicle fracture and, 261, *261*
  femoral fracture and, 361–363, *364*–*365*, *418*, *419*
  floating knee and, 417–418, *418*, *419*
  forearm fracture and, 164–171, *168*, *172*
  humeral fracture and, 277
  pelvic fracture and, *323*, 323–324
Pneumothorax, multiple trauma and, 76
  tension, 76
  ventilation and, 76
Poland classification, 20–21, *22*
Polyactide-glycolide copolymer, 33–34
Popliteal artery, 387–388, *397*
  femoral fracture and, 99–101, *100*
  knee and, 82, 99, *100*, 369, *387*, 387–388
  tibial fracture and, 99, *387*, 387–388, *388*, *397*
Process. See also *Tubercle*; *Tuberosity*.
  coracoid, anatomy of, 263–264
    fracture of, 265, *267*
  coronoid, *131*
  odontoid, anatomy of, 283–287, *284*, *285*, *289*
    anomalies of, 285–287, *286*
    basion relation to, 286–287
    ligaments and, 285
    spinal injury and, 285, 287
  styloid, radial, *131*, *132*
    ulnar, *131*, *132*
Pseudoepiphysis, metatarsal, 473, *473*, *501*
Pseudo-Madelung deformity, 156
Pseudoparalysis, arm affected by, 258, *260*
  clavicle fracture and, 258, *260*
  differential diagnosis in, 258, *260*
Pseudosubluxation, spinal, 287–289, *288*, *289*
Psychological factors, multiple injury and, 93, 93t
  reflex sympathetic dystrophy and, 121–122
Pubis, 307, *308*
  fracture of, *311*, *323*, 323
Pulled elbow syndrome, 177, *177*
Pulse rate, 77t
Puncture wounds, foot and, 501, *502*, *503*
  osteomyelitis and, 501, *502*, *503*

Q

Q angle, 391, *391*
Quadriceps tendon, *391*

Quadriceps tendon *(Continued)*
 sleeve fracture and, 382, *382*
 tibia and, *391*, 391–393, *393*

R

Radial artery, 214, *214*
Radiocarpal joint, 130, *130*, *160*, 161
 angulation in, 156, *157*
 bone graft and, 156, *157*
Radiology, acetabular fracture and, *314*, 314–315, *316*
 femoral shaft fracture and, 348, 524–526, *525*
 hip dislocation and, 338
 multiple injury and, 78–79
 pelvic fracture and, *314*, 314–315, *316*
 spine and, 286–288, *287–289*, *528*
 tibial fracture and, 453, *453*, *454*
Radioulnar joint, 128–132
 articulation of, 128–132, *129–132*
 dislocation of, 184–188, 194–196, *196*
 distal, 130, *130–132*, *160*, 194–196, *196*
 ligaments of, 128–130, *130*, *131*
 proximal, 128–132, *129–132*, 186–188, *187*
 reconstruction of, 186–188, *187*
Radius, 127–196. See also *Forearm*.
 anatomy of, 128–132, *128–132*
 development of, 128, *128*
 fracture of, 133–196
  distal, 133–171
  elbow and, *244*, 244–245, 245t, *246–248*
  proximal, 171–194, 244–245
 functioning of, 128–132, *129–132*
 interosseous membrane and, 131, *131*
 ligaments and, 130–131, *130–131*
 muscles and, 133–134, *134*, *160*, 161
 physeal injury in, 151–156, *154–156*
 rotation of, 131–132, *132*
 styloid process of, *131*, *132*, 151
 tuberosity of, 131, *131*, *132*
Rang classification, 21, *22*, *25*
Ranvier's zone, 4, 15–16, *16*
Red blood cells, resuscitation with, 77–78
Reflex sympathetic dystrophy, 121–122
 autonomic nervous system and, 121–122
 diagnosis of, 121
 forearm affected by, 150–151
 psychological factors in, 121–122
 symptoms of, 121
 treatment of, 122
Refracture, 119
Remodeling, bone physiology and, 4–8, *7*
 forearm fracture and, 135, *136–138*, *148*
 fracture healing and, 4–8

Remodeling *(Continued)*
 physeal injury and, 30–31
Respiration rate, 77t
Respiratory distress, fat embolism and, 102–103
Resuscitation, fluid, 77t, 77–78
 multiple trauma and, 74–78, 77t
Ribs, child abuse and, 527, *528*
 first, 69, *259*
 fracture of, 69, *259*, 527, *528*
 multiple injury and, 69
Rickets, phenytoin and, 506, *507*
Ring(s), Lacroix, 4
 pelvic, *308*, *310*, *311*, *314*, *317*, *323*
 Silverman, 507–509, *510*
 vertebral, 49–50, *50*
Robert Jones dressing, 430
Rockwood view, 258, *259*, *260*
Rods, 165. See also *Fixation*.
 biodegradable, 33–34
 flexible, 360–361, *362*
 nailing with, 87, 360–361, *362*
 polyactide-glycolide copolymer, 33–34
 steel, 165
 titanium, 165
 track infection and, 366
Rotation, radioulnar, 128–132, *129–132*
 tibiofibular, 436–437
Roux-Goldthwait procedure, 392–393, *393*

S

Sacroiliac joint, *308*
 fracture of, *310*, *311*, 317–319
Sacrum, *308*, *311*, *314*. See also *Pelvis*.
 fracture of, 307–309, *311*, 319, *320*
Salter-Harris classification, 11–13, *12*, 20–24, 20–27
Sarcoma, tibial, 507, *509*
Scaphoid, 196–198
 fracture of, 196–198, *197*, *198*
Scapula, 263–270
 anatomy of, 263–264
 fracture of, 263–265
  acromial, *264*, 265
  coracoid, 265, *267*
  glenoid, 265, *266*
  thoracic dissociation in, 264–265, *265*
Scheuermann's disease, athletics and, 49–50, *50*
 thoracolumbar spine and, 49–50, *50*
SCIWORA syndrome, 290–291, *291*
Screws. See also *Fixation*; *Plate(s)*.
 epiphyseal placement of, *32*, 36
 metaphyseal placement of, 36
Scuderi-Bronson classification, 25–27, *28*
Seat belt syndrome, 69
 spinal injury and, 301–304, *302*, *303*
"Serendipity" view, 258, *259*

Sesamoid, *450*
Sever's disease, 48–49
 foot affected by, *472*, 472–473, 484
Shaken baby syndrome, 529. See also *Child abuse*.
Shock, multiple injury and, 76
 spinal, 80
 symptoms of, 76
Shortening deformity, femoral fracture and, 352, *353*
 leg length and, 352, *353*, 438, 511
 overgrowth and, 438
 tibial fracture and, 438, 511
 toe and, 501, *503*
Shoulder, 257–278
 anatomy of, 257, *262*, *263*, 263–267, *270*
 dislocation of, 265–270, *268*, *269*
 fracture of, 257–278
  clavicular, 257–262, *259–263*
  humeral, *270*, 270–278, 271t, *273–277*
  scapular, 263–265, *264–267*
 muscles of, *276*
Silverman's rings, 507–509, *510*
Sinding-Larsen-Johansson syndrome, 48
Skeleton, body proportion and, 65–67, *67*, *75*, 77t
 child's, 65–67, *67*, *75*, 77t
Skull, child abuse injury to, 527–529
 fracture of, 527–529
 spine junction with, 283–286, *289*
Sloman view, foot and, 504, *505*
Sodium bicarbonate, acid-base balance and, 78
Soft tissue injury, 425–430. See also *Compartment syndrome*.
 bicycle spoke injury and, 414–415, *415*
 classification of, 425t
 debridement and irrigation in, 90–91, 425–430, *426*, *427*
 fibular fracture with, 424, 425t
 tibial fracture with, 425–430, *426*, *427*
  antibiotics in, 425, 430
  closed, 424, 425t
  distal, 453, *453*, *454*
  open, 422–424, 424t, 425t
Space. See also *Cavity*; *Fossa*; *Sulcus*.
 interosseous, cross union and, 109, *110*, 171
 radioulnar, *131*, 131–132, *132*, 171
 retropharyngeal, 287, *288*
Spinal cord, 285, *286*
 injury to, 79–80, 290–293
  etiology of, 292, 300
  SCIWORA syndrome and, 290–291, *291*
  without radiologic abnormality, 290–291, *291*
 space available to, 285, *286*
Spine, 283–305. See also *Vertebra*.
 anatomy of, 283–286
 anomalies of, 285

544 Index

Spine *(Continued)*
  apophysitis affecting, 49–50, *50*
  development of, 283–286
  injury to, 288–305
    birth-related, 289–290, *290*
    cervical, *293*, 293–300, *295, 297–300*
    child abuse and, 300, *301*, 528, *529*
    incidence of, 288–289
    ligamental, 119, 285
    management of, 290–293
    pathologic fracture in, 300–301, *301*
    patient transport and, 292
    physeal, 304, *304*
    seat belt and, 301–304, *302, 303*
    thoracolumbar, 300–305, *301–304*
  multiple trauma and, 69, 71t, 79–80
  pseudosubluxation of, 287–289, *288, 289*
  radiology of, 286–288, *287–289*, 528
Spleen, trauma injury to, 71–82
Spongiosa, primary, 15–16, *16*
  secondary, 15–16, *16*
Staphylococcal infections, 429, 429t
Stewart-Milford classification, 337
Stimson method, *269*, 269
Stomach, distention of, 76
Styloid process, radial, *131, 132*
  ulnar, *131, 132*
"Sucked candy" appearance, *260*
Sudeck atrophy, 121
Sulcus, capitellotrochlear, *233*
Sustentaculum tali, *450*
Swelling, fibular fracture and, 467–471, *470*
  foot injury and, *486, 490, 495*
  "goose-egg," 467–471, *470*
Swischuk's line, 288, *288, 289*
Sympathetic nervous system, dystrophy and, 121–122, 150–151
Symphysis, pubic, 308
  fracture of, 310, *311,* 323
Synostosis, correction of, 109, *110*
  fat interposition in, 109, *110*
  interosseous space and, 171
  radioulnar, 109, *110,* 171
Syphilis, bone erosion due to, 529, *529*
  child abuse injury vs., 529, *529*

T

Talus, *450, 471*
  avascular necrosis and, *478, 479, 480*
  blood supply to, *476, 477*
  coalition affecting, 504, *505, 506*
  fracture of, 475t, 475–483, *478–482*
    complications of, 483
    compression, 476–479
    neck, 476, *479, 480*
    osteochondral, 479–483, *481, 482*
    types of, 476–479, *479, 480*
    unrecognized, *478*

Talus *(Continued)*
    secundarius, *471*
Tamponade, cardiac, 76–77
Tarsometatarsal joint, 472
  anatomy of, 472
  fracture of, 475t, 475t, 488–489, *489*
    management of, 489
    mechanism of, 488, *489*
Tarsus, *450, 471,* 472
  coalition affecting, 504, *504–506*
Temperature, multiple injury and, 78
Tendon(s), 48–51
  Achilles, 453, *453*
  ankle and, *450*
  bicipital, *130*
  fat stripe of, 453, *453*
  flexor hallucis longus, *450*
  foot and, *450*
    laceration of, 501
  insertion of. See *Apophysis.*
  peroneal, *450*
  quadriceps, *391*
    patellar sleeve fracture and, 382, *382*
    Q angle and, 391, *391*
    tibia and, *391,* 391–393, *393*
  semitendinosus, 392–393, *393*
  tenodesis of, 392–393, *393*
  tibialis, *450*
Tenodesis, 392–393, *393*
Tetanus, bacteria causing, 429
  immunization for, 89, 90t, 429, 429t
  open fracture and, 429, 429t
  symptoms of, 429
Thrombosis, fracture and, 105
Thumb, dislocation of, 208
  forearm fracture and, *160,* 161–162
  fracture of, *204,* 205, *206*
  interosseous nerve palsy of, 119–121, *121*
Thurston-Holland sign, 21, *24*
Tibia, 397–443
  apophysitis affecting, 48
  blood supply to, 397
  fracture of, 397–443
    bone grafting in, 432, *434–436*
    child abuse causing, *523,* 523–525, *524, 526*
    compartment syndrome in, 440–443
    diagnosis of, 399–400, 523–526, *524, 526*
    distal, 421–422, 449–467, 509–513, 523–529
      classification of, 451–467, 456t, *457*
        Dias-Tachdjian, 455, 456t, *457*
        Lauge-Hansen, 454, 456t
        Salter-Harris, *12, 20,* 20–27, 455–463, 456t, *457*
      complications of, 509–513, *511, 512*
      compression and, 456t, *457,* 463, *464*
      fixation in, *423, 436*

Tibia *(Continued)*
      juvenile Tillaux, 463–466, *465*
      mechanism of, 451–452, 456t, *458*
      radiology in, 453, *453, 454*
      triplane, 466, *466–467, 468, 469*
      type of, 455–459
        I, 455–459, 456t, *457, 459*
        II, 456t, *457, 459, 460*
        III, 456t, *457, 460,* 460–461, *462, 464, 465*
        IV, 456t, *457, 461,* 461–462, *462*
        V, 456t, *457, 463, 464*
    femoral fracture with, 417–418, *418, 419, 436*
    incidence of, 398
    management of, 400–434
    mechanism of, 398, 451–452, 456t, *458,* 523–526
    nonunion of, 117–119, *118,* 434–436
    open, 422–434
      classification of, 422–423, 424t
      grafting and, 432, *434–436*
      treatment of, 424–434, *426, 427, 434–436*
    pathologic, 57–64, *58, 60,* 418–421
    physeal injury due to, 11–13, 20–27, 387–389, 451–467
      distal, 11–13, 35–36, 451–467, 523–527
      late angulation and, 109, *111*
      premature closure and, 437–438
      proximal, 20–27, 35, 387–389, 437–438
    physical examination in, 399–400
    proximal, 23–25, 382–390
      arterial damage in, *387,* 387–388, *388*
      intercondylar eminence in, 382–385, *383, 384*
      management of, 400–405, *406*
      tuberosity in, 385–387, *386*
    shaft, 405–443, 523–527
      bicycle spoke injury and, 411–413, *413*
      complications of, 434–443
      femoral fracture with, 417–418, *418, 436*
      fixation in, *419, 427,* 430–433, *434–436*
      isolated, 410–411, *412*
      management of, 405–410, 407t, 424–433, *426, 427, 434–436*
      neuromuscular disorder with, 418–421
      soft tissue injury in, 422–424, 424t, 425t, 453, *453, 454*
      stress, 415–416
      toddler's, 411–413, *413,* 524, *526*
    vascular injury due to, 439–440
  interosseus membrane and, 387, 397, 449

Tibia *(Continued)*
  ligaments of, distal, 449, *450, 451*
    proximal, 119, *120, 391,* 391–393, *393*
  sarcoma of, 507, *509*
Tibial artery, 387, 397
Tillaux fracture, 463–466, *465*
Toddler's fracture, 411–413
  femoral, 524–526, *525*
  tibial, 411–413, *413,* 524, *525, 526*
Toes, *450,* 488–499. See also *Metatarsals.*
  dislocation of, 499–500, *500*
  epiphyseal fissure and, *30*
  exostosis of, 507, *508*
  fracture of, 475, 475t, 488–499, *489–498*
  neoplasia affecting, 507, *508*
  osteomyelitis of, 499, *499*
  shortening deformity of, 501, *503*
  "stubbed," 499, *499*
Torode-Zieg classification, 310
Toxoid, diphtheria, 429, 429t
  pertussis, 429, 429t
  tetanus, 429, 429t
Traction, Dunlop's, 221
  femoral fracture and, distal, 370–371, *371, 373*
    shaft, 350, 352–354, *353*
  finger traps for, *197*
  foot injury and, 490, *490*
  humeral fracture and, 220–222
  hypertension due to, 104–105
  malunion due to, 106–109, *108*
  metatarsal fracture and, 490, *490*
  pelvic fracture and, 320–321, 324
  wrist fracture and, *197*
Transfusion, resuscitation role of, 77–78
Transplantation, physeal, 46–47
Transverse lines of Park, 5. See also *Harris lines.*
Trauma, 65–94. See also *Multiple injury.*
  body proportion in, 65–67, *67, 75,* 77t
  field management of, 73–78, 74t, *75*
  referral to center for, 74t
  severity classification and, 70–72, 71t, 72t
Triangular fibrocartilage complex, 130, *130*
Triplane fracture, *466,* 466–467, *468, 469*
Trochlear groove, *233*
  elbow fracture and, 239, *240*
  formation of, 213, *213*
  humeral, *233*
Trunkey classification, 310
Tubercle, talar, *474, 479.* See also *Os trigonum.*
  ulnar, 131, *131*
Tuberosity, bicipital, 128, 131, *131, 132*
  calcaneal, *450*
  fifth metatarsal, *450*

Tuberosity *(Continued)*
  ischial, apophysitis affecting, 49, *49*
    fracture of, *26,* 307
  navicular, *450*
  radial, 128, 131, *131, 132*
  scaphoid, 198, *198*
  tibial, 48, *391*
    fracture of, 385–387, *386*

U

Ulna, 127–196. See also *Forearm.*
  anatomy of, 128–132, *128–132*
  development of, 128, *128*
  elbow traction using, 221–222
  fracture of, 133–196
    distal, 133–171
    proximal, 171–196
  functioning of, 128–132, *129–132*
  interosseous membrane and, 131, *131*
  ligaments and, 130–131, *130–131*
  muscles and, 133–134, *134, 160,* 161
  physeal injury in, 151–156, *154–156*
  styloid process of, *131, 132*
  tubercle of, *131*
Ulnar artery, 214, *214*
Upper extremity. See also specific bones and joints.
  compartment syndrome of, 83, *83, 101,* 101–102, 149–150, *150*

V

Valgus deformity, ankle with, 436–437, 507, *508*
  elbow with, *19,* 237–239, *238*
  knee with, 109, *111,* 400–405, *406,* 436–437
  osteochondroma and, 507, *508*
  tibial fracture and, 109, *111,* 400–405, *406,* 436–437, 509–511, *511*
Varus deformity, ankle with, 436–437, 476, *478,* 509–510, *511*
  elbow with, 109, 219, *219,* 226–227, *228*
  metatarsal fracture and, *495*
  talus fracture and, 476, *478*
  tibial fracture and, 436–437, *478,* 509–511, *511, 512*
Vascular injury, 99–101
  arterial, 82–83, 99–101, *100,* 387, 387–388, *388*
  elbow dislocation causing, 250–251
  femoral fracture and, *100*
  humeral fracture and, *100,* 217, 226
  ischemia due to, 99–101, *100*
  knee fracture and, 387, 387–388, *388*
  multiple trauma and, 82–83
  thrombosis and, 105

Vascular injury *(Continued)*
  tibial fracture and, 387, 387–388, *388,* 439–440
Ventilation, evaluation of, 76
  gastric distention and, 76
  multiple trauma and, 76
  pneumothorax and, 76
Verbal response, coma evaluation and, 72t
Vertebra, 283–305. See also *Spine.*
  anatomy of, 283–286, *284*
  apophysitis affecting, 49–50, *50*
  atlas, 283–285
    anatomy of, 283–285, *284, 289*
    development of, 283, *284*
    fracture of, 296, *297*
    rotary fixation affecting, 294–296, *295*
  axis, 283–285
    anatomy of, 283–285, *284, 289*
    development of, 283, *284, 285*
    fracture of, 296–298, *298*
    rotary fixation affecting, 294–296, *295*
  development of, 283–286, *284–286*
  dislocation of, 293–294, 300–305
    atlanto-occipital, *293,* 293–294
    thoracolumbar, *300–303,* 300–305
  fracture of, 293–305
    C1–C2, 296–298, *297–298*
    C3–C7, 298–300, *300*
    physeal damage due to, 304, *304*
    thoracolumbar, 300–305, *301, 303, 304*
Vital signs, 77t
Volkmann's contracture, *101,* 101–102

W

Waddell's triad, 65–66, *66*
Watson-Jones approach, femoral neck fracture and, 339–340, *340*
Watts classification, 310
Weber classification, 21, *22*
Williams syndrome, calcaneal centers and, *472, 472*
Wounds, contaminated, 425, 428–430
  gunshot, foot and, 503, *504*
    knee and, 390–391
  open fracture and, 90–92, 425–430, *426, 427*
Wrist, 194–199
  anatomy of, 130, *130, 160,* 161
  dislocation in, 194–196, *196,* 199
  fracture of, 196–198, *197, 198*
  radioulnar joint and, 130, *130, 160,* 161

Z

Zone of Ranvier, 4, 15–16, *16*